Vijay K. Maker

Edgar D. Guzman-Arrieta
Co-Author

Cognitive Pearls in General Surgery

Springer

Vijay K. Maker, MD, FACS, FRCSC
Chairman, Department of Surgery
Advocate Illinois Masonic Medical Center
Executive Program Director
University of Illinois Metropolitan Group Hospitals
Residency in General Surgery
Chicago, IL
USA

Professor of Surgery
University of Illinois at Chicago
Chicago, IL
USA

Co-Author
Edgar D. Guzman-Arrieta, MD, MS, FACS
Vascular Specialists – Hattiesburg Clinic
Hattiesburg, MS
USA

ISBN 978-1-4939-1849-2 ISBN 978-1-4939-1850-8 (eBook)
DOI 10.1007/978-1-4939-1850-8
Springer New York Heidelberg Dordrecht London

Library of Congress Control Number: 2014957721

Printed on acid-free paper

Springer is part of Springer Science+Business Media (www.springer.com)

Foreword

But wisdom is a pearl with most success

Sought in still water, and beneath clear skies

The Task, William Cowper (1781)

For centuries, pearls have been metaphorically linked with wisdom. Both are precious, and both are rare. The pearl is a gemstone formed over many years through the concentric layering of calcium carbonate. Pearls of wisdom, in a sense, represent gems of knowledge shaped over decades by the layers of experience that bring good judgment.

In *Cognitive Pearls in General Surgery,* Dr. Vijay Maker draws on his experience over a professional lifetime as an expert general surgeon and surgical oncologist and as program director of a university-affiliated general surgery residency. Together with his vascular surgeon coauthor Dr. Edgar Guzman, Dr. Maker shares his many surgical insights in a streamlined and highly engaging format.

The practice of surgery cannot be captured as an explicit collection of facts, and surgery cannot be learned merely by memorizing details of anatomy, biological pathways, disease states, and technical particulars. The surgeon must also acquire tacit knowledge—the knowledge that cannot be found in books—those elements of surgical practice that can only be learned in a local context, at the bedside and at the operating table, as an apprentice under the guidance of wise surgical mentors.

Dr. Maker's volume effectively bridges the gap between the explicit and tacit curriculum of surgery. Multiple-choice questions are used to test the reader's current knowledge of embryology, anatomy, and pathophysiology. Following a detailed explanation of the correct answers as well as the incorrect distracters, Dr. Maker illustrates how a deep understanding of these factual details can be applied to clinical decision-making in specific surgical situations. Organized by body region, these cognitive pearls complement standard surgical textbooks and should be of great interest to surgical trainees and established practitioners.

Chicago, IL, USA — Jeffrey B. Matthews, MD, FACS
Norfolk, VA, USA — L.D. Britt, MD, MPH, FACS, FCCM

Preface

The science of surgery involves a thorough understanding of the embryology, anatomy, histology, and pathophysiology of a disease process. In order to make the correct diagnoses and treatment plan, the surgeon must comprehend how these four processes are inter-related. Starting at a cellular level, function defines form, and I have endeavored to demonstrate this through specific examples throughout the body. The increased use of cross-sectional imaging to pinpoint anatomical pathology and evidence-based treatment algorithms to guide surgical therapy has improved our diagnostics and outcomes, but may have removed us from the cognitive elements that define surgical diseases. As a result, I have found that it is now more than ever critical to have a reference to highlight the applicable embryology, anatomy, histology, and pathophysiology of surgical diseases and how these relate to critical tissue planes, surgical pitfalls, and technical pearls.

The present atlas encapsulates my 40 years of continuous general surgery and surgical oncology experience for the perennial student of surgery. Unlike books of similar format, our goal was not to illustrate only the gross anatomy or to describe a specific surgical technique, but rather to demonstrate the underlying cognitive aspects of both in a way that is easy to understand, remember, and apply.

The content is organized by organ system, and the illustrations highlight surgical pearls born of experience and polished by the study of pertinent references. I have hand-drawn and illustrated almost all of the figures to show exact anatomical relationships as we see them in vivo. A question/answer format was chosen to augment the images to allow the reader to actively reflect on the topic and to appraise his/her knowledge in that area. The discussion sections strive to explain not only what the correct answer is but also why the distracters are wrong, in order to motivate discussion and self-reflection. This atlas is the culmination of my surgical experience that has been dedicated to understanding the basis of disease and would have been incomplete without extensive help from Dr. Edgar Guzman, one of my best trainees and now an accomplished vascular surgeon whom I have the privilege of having as my coauthor.

Throughout the book, an effort has been made to make explicit the thought processes and associations that underlie the understanding of the topics at hand, with the intent of enhancing the fun and enjoyment that only an informed and well-grounded practice of surgery can provide.

Chicago, IL, USA Vijay K. Maker, MD, FACS, FRCSC

Acknowledgments

My sincere thanks to my wife and children for letting me borrow enormous amounts of family time to finish this atlas and my son Dr. Ajay Maker for his critical review, expert help, and counseling.

Contents

The Neck

1

1. All of the following are correct *except*:
   (a) The pharyngeal arches are of mesodermal origin.
   (b) The pharyngeal pouches are of endodermal origin.
   (c) The foramen cecum and middle part of the thyroid are of mesodermal origin.
   (d) The branchial membranes bridge the spaces between the pharyngeal arches.
   (e) The superior parathyroids and thyroid share a common origin.

Comments The human branchial apparatus is analogous to the gills found in fish. As mammals developed lungs for breathing, gills lost their respiratory function. However, the branchial apparatus continued to contribute to the formation of head and neck structures. Congenital anomalies of these areas in humans give rise to branchial sinuses, cysts, and other defects (Fig. 1.1). By the fifth week of gestation, only 4 branchial clefts are visible in the human embryos.

The isthmus of the thyroid along with the pyramidal lobe and the anteromedial thyroid lobes is formed by an endodermal extension of the foramen cecum of the tongue, which descends through the hyoid bone. The lateral and posterior aspects of the thyroid lobes develop along with the superior parathyroids from the fourth branchial pouch. Hence, when a superior parathyroid cannot be found, an intrathyroidal location must be confirmed and at times requires ipsilateral thyroid lobectomy. In similar fashion, when an inferior parathyroid cannot be located, an intrathymic location should be suspected, considering the common origin of these two structures in the third pharyngeal pouch.

V.K. Maker, E.D. Guzman-Arrieta, *Cognitive Pearls in General Surgery*,
DOI 10.1007/978-1-4939-1850-8_1, © Springer Science+Business Media New York 2015

Development of the Branchial (Gill) Apparatus in Humans

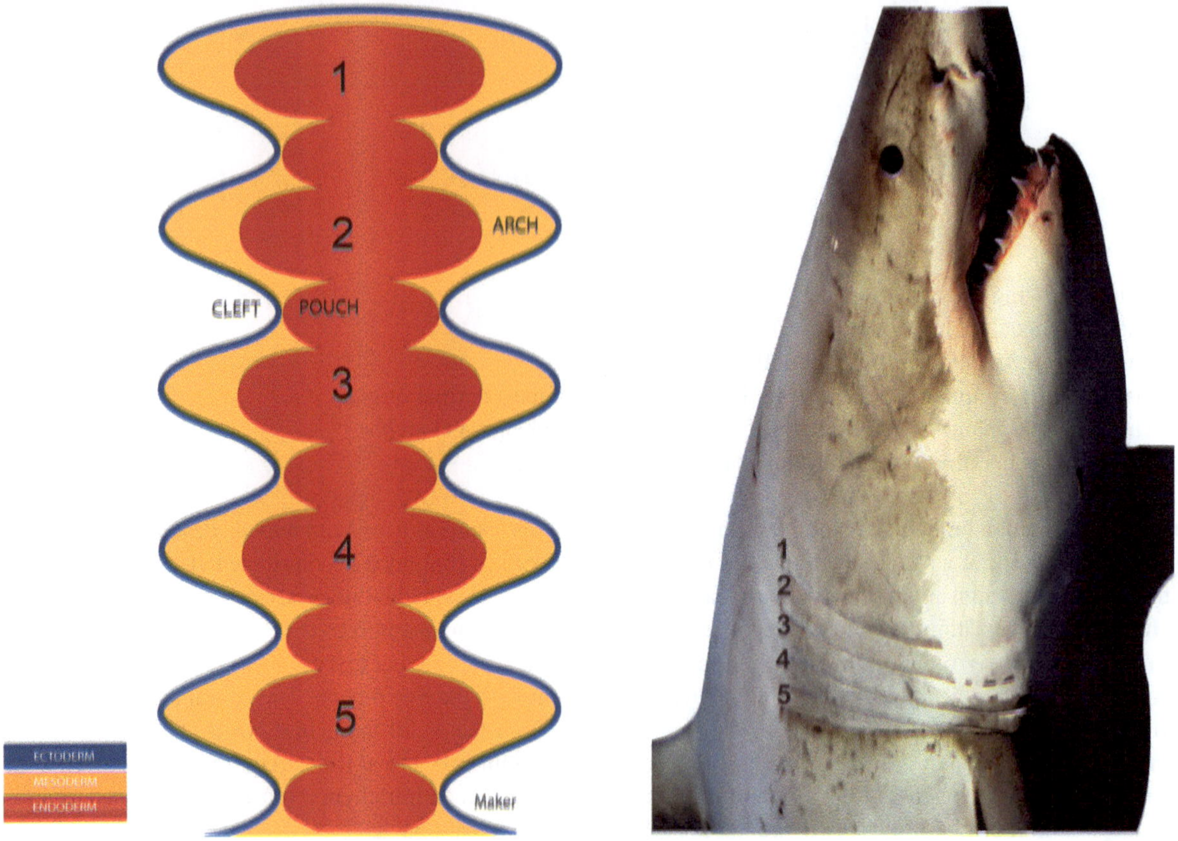

Fig. 1.1 The human embryonic pharynx consists of six paired branchial arches lined by ectodermal clefts and endodermal pouches around an unpaired endodermal ventral floor. Each of these structures forms parts of the face and neck. As these structures develop, overhang, and fuse; the adult components of the face and neck are formed. Embryologic developmental errors in this process present as sinuses, fistulae, cysts, aberrant locations and/or the absence of organs in the face and neck. Many of the anomalies covered in this chapter present a unique set of anatomical relationships which become clinically relevant for their diagnosis and treatment. The very thin membrane that exists between clefts and pouches, phylogenetically representing the gills, has no function in humans

Answer

c

2. All of the following are correct *except*
   (a) The first pharyngeal arch, responsible for the embryogenesis of the muscles of mastication, is innervated by the mandibular branch of the trigeminal nerve and its blood supply is from the facial artery.
   (b) The second pharyngeal arch, responsible for the embryogenesis of the muscles of facial expression, is innervated by the facial nerve and its artery is the external carotid.
   (c) The second pharyngeal pouch gives rise to the tonsils. The second pharyngeal pouch sinuses open into the tonsillar fossa.
   (d) The third pharyngeal pouch is responsible for the formation of the upper parathyroids.
   (e) The fourth pharyngeal arch is responsible for the embryogenesis of the cricothyroid muscle and its nerve supply is through the superior laryngeal branch of the vagus nerve.

Comments The pharyngeal arches are responsible for the mesodermal derivatives of the lower face and neck. Pharyngeal pouches give rise to endodermal elements. Pharyngeal clefts are ectodermal. Only the first cleft persists into adulthood, forming the external auditory canal. In correspondence, the first pharyngeal pouch forms the middle ear. The first pharyngeal cleft may give rise to a persistent preauricular sinus or cyst which courses anterior to the facial nerve towards the external auditory canal.

Most branchial fistulae and cysts originate from the second pharyngeal pouch and cleft. Classically, these fistulae open at the lower third of the medial border of the sternocleidomastoid muscle. These sinus or fistulae typically travel from the tonsillar fossa coursing in between the internal and external carotid arteries to reach the skin (Fig. 1.2).

The third pharyngeal pouch is responsible for the genesis of the inferior parathyroids and thymus. It is interesting to note that the upper parathyroids and thyroid develop from the fourth pharyngeal pouch, while the lower parathyroid and thymus develop from the higher third pharyngeal pouch and migrate caudally [1].

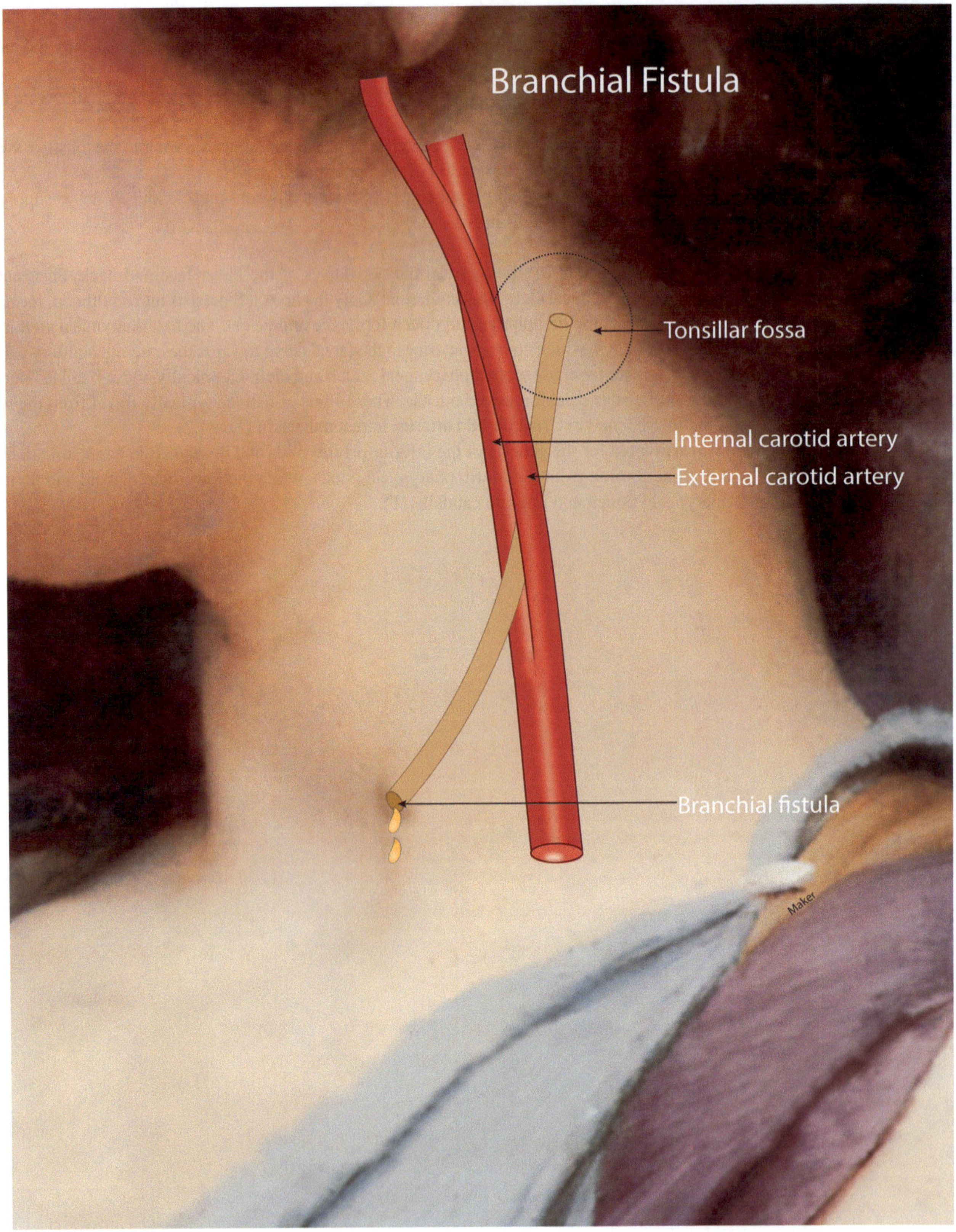

Fig. 1.2 A second branchial fistula typically extends from an external opening in the lower third of the neck, anterior to the sternocleidomastoid muscle. The fistula extends through the bifurcation of the carotid to an internal opening in the tonsillar fossa. Multiple variations exist when the fistula is not complete

Answer
d

3. Select the *incorrect* statement regarding the embryology of the thyroid.
   (a) The median thyroid anlage is derived from the pharyngeal floor and is of endodermal origin. It forms the follicular component of the thyroid.
   (b) The lingual thyroid does *not* have C cells.
   (c) The thyroglossal duct is posterior to the hyoid bone and does not involve it.
   (d) The C cells of the thyroid come from the ultimobranchial bodies.
   (e) The neural crest origin of the C cells of the thyroid explains the association of medullary cancer with other neuroendocrine malignancies.

Comments As discussed in question 1, the follicular elements of the thyroid are of endodermal origin. The middle thyroid anlage descends from the base of the tongue following a trajectory anterior to or through the hyoid bone. The lateral thyroid anlagen are derived from the fourth branchial pouches. The C cells of the thyroid gland are derived from the ultimobranchial body, which is a part of the fourth branchial pouch that is colonized by neuroectodermal cells. They are confined to the lateral aspects of the thyroid.

C cells may give rise to medullary thyroid carcinoma. Reflecting the function of the parent cells, medullary carcinomas may produce calcitonin. This hormone is a useful tumor marker (Fig. 1.3).

Medullary carcinoma of the thyroid may be an isolated familial disease or a component of type 2 multiple endocrine neoplasia (MEN-2) syndromes, together with pheochromocytomas and parathyroid hyperplasia (MEN-2a) or neuromas and marfanoid body habitus (MEN-2b). The underlying theme in these neoplasias is their neuroectodermal origin. This is further substantiated by the pervasive involvement of the RET proto-oncogene.

The RET proto-oncogene is a receptor linked to a tyrosine kinase, normally present in neuroectodermal-derived cells. Mutations leading to its pathologic activation lead to sustained growth signals and tumor development. Interestingly, loss of function mutations of the RET proto-oncogene has been associated with Hirschsprung's disease. In this instance, there is failure of development of the Auerbach's plexus, also derived from the neuroectoderm [2].

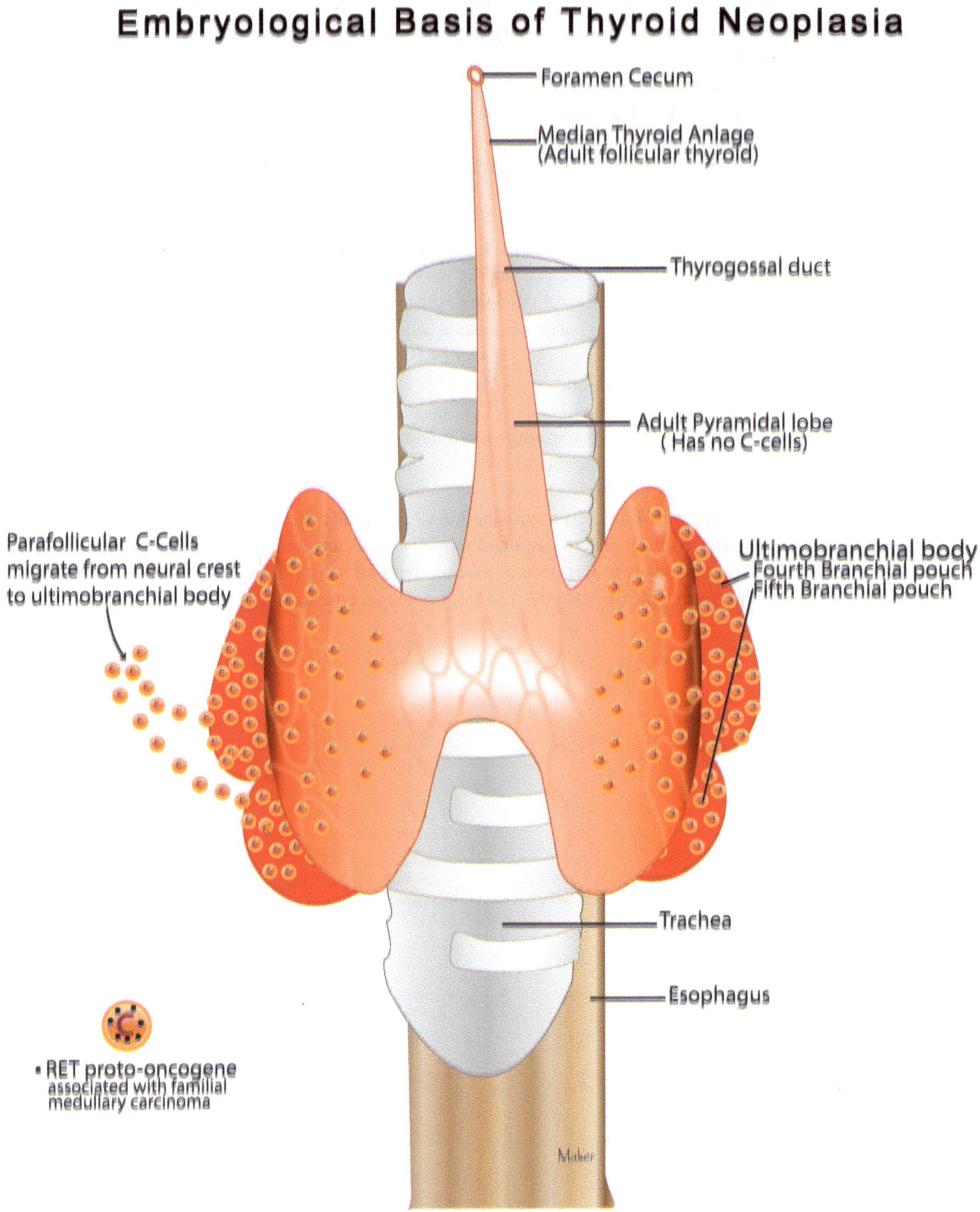

Fig. 1.3 The median thyroid anlage forms all of the follicular thyroid. All differentiated thyroid neoplasms arise from this embryonic origin of the thyroid. The paired lateral anlage arise from the fourth and fifth branchial pouches and fuse with the median anlage. Calcitonin-secreting parafollicular cells, also called C cells, migrate into the lateral anlage from neuroectoderm. C cells disperse in the superior and lateral part of the thyroid and are the parent cells for medullary carcinoma of the thyroid. Thyroid neoplasms maintain many of the characteristics of their embryological cell of origin. For example, papillary carcinoma traps radioactive iodine, and medullary carcinoma over-expresses the RET protein which is derived from embryonic nervous tissue

Answer

c

4. Select the *correct* statement regarding neck surgery.
   (a) The strap muscles are best divided below their upper third to prevent undue denervation.
   (b) A vertical incision in the anterior triangle can be safely extended to the angle of the mandible.
   (c) Vertical incisions provide better cosmetic results.
   (d) Flap creation should be carried along a plane superficial to the platysma muscle.
   (e) The section of the anterior cervical branch of the facial nerve causes permanent drooling.

Comments The innervation of the strap muscles (sternohyoid and sternothyroid) is provided by the ansa cervicalis. The branches of the ansa cervicalis approach these muscles from below; hence, section of the muscle in its lower aspect interrupts the innervation to the majority of the muscle, whereas a cephalad division preserves it. The ansa cervicalis has a unique looping pattern, uniting C1 with C2 and C3 root elements. It may be traced back to the hypoglossal nerve and as such can be a useful anatomical landmark in carotid surgery. On occasion, its presence may impede access to the carotid artery. In this instance, it may be divided without significant consequence (Fig. 1.4).

The mandibular branch of the facial nerve and the anterior ramus of the cervical branch of the facial nerve follow a hammock-like course bellow the angle of the mandible. This exposes them to injury when incisions are made within a 3 cm radius of this landmark (Fig. 1.5).

Injury to the mandibular branch of the facial nerve results in paralysis of the orbicularis oris, producing permanent drooping of the corner of the mouth and drooling. Injury to the anterior cervical branch of the facial nerve produces transient drooling.

Vertical incisions are to be avoided in the neck for cosmetic reasons. Preferably horizontally oriented curvilinear incisions along Langer's lines should be used. All flaps in the neck should be made in the avascular plane deep to the platysma, as the platysma is actually attached to the skin of the neck. The platysma is a remnant of the subcutaneous muscle seen in the animals which can move their skin to ward off insects and birds.

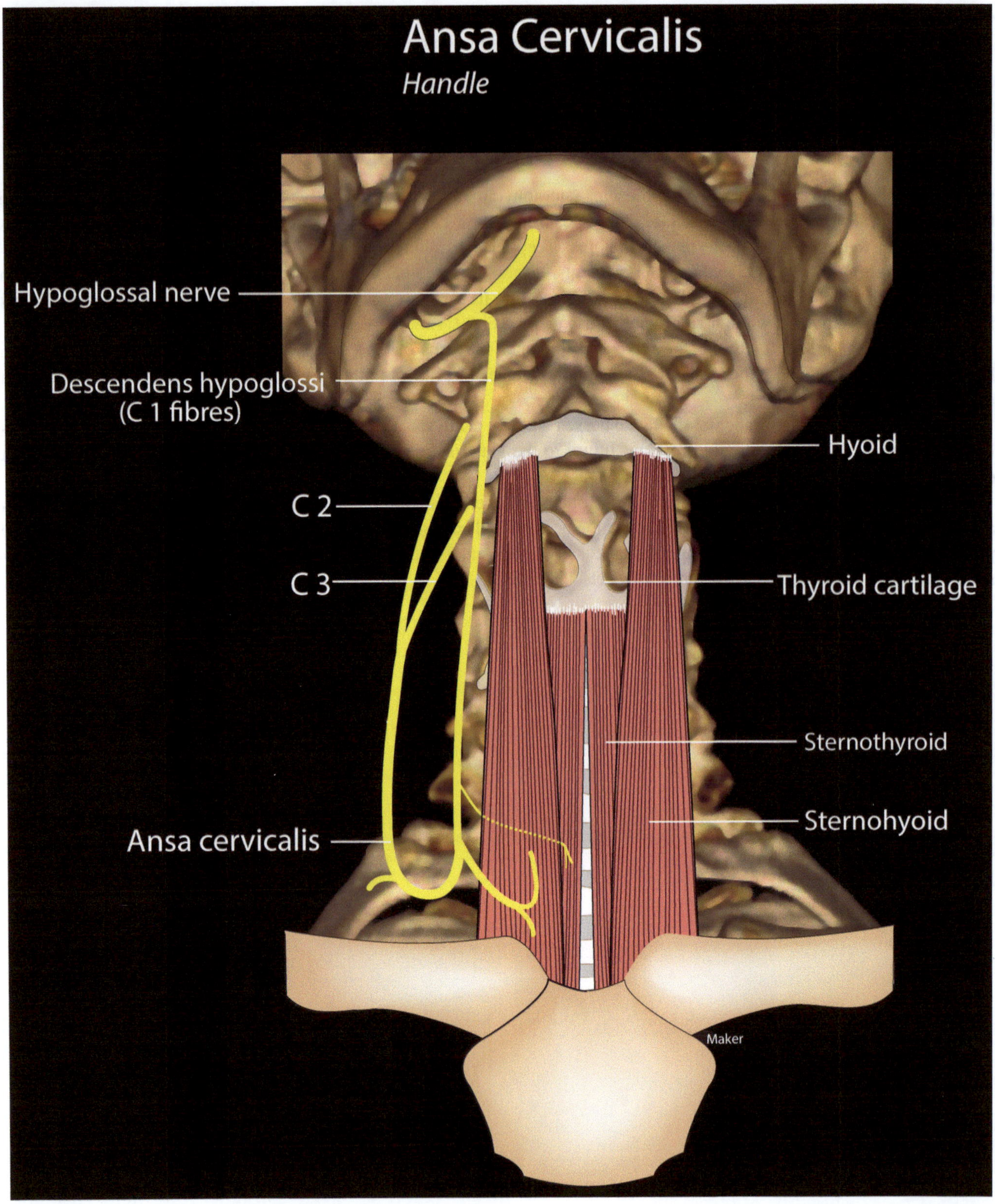

Fig. 1.4 The ansa cervicalis is the handle, or loop, of a nerve connecting C1 fibers from the descendens hypoglossi nerve to the contributions from the C2 and C3 spinal nerves. This loop provides nerve supply to the sternohyoid and sternothyroid muscles, and contributes to the omohyoid

Marginal Mandibular and Cervical Branches (3cm Rule)

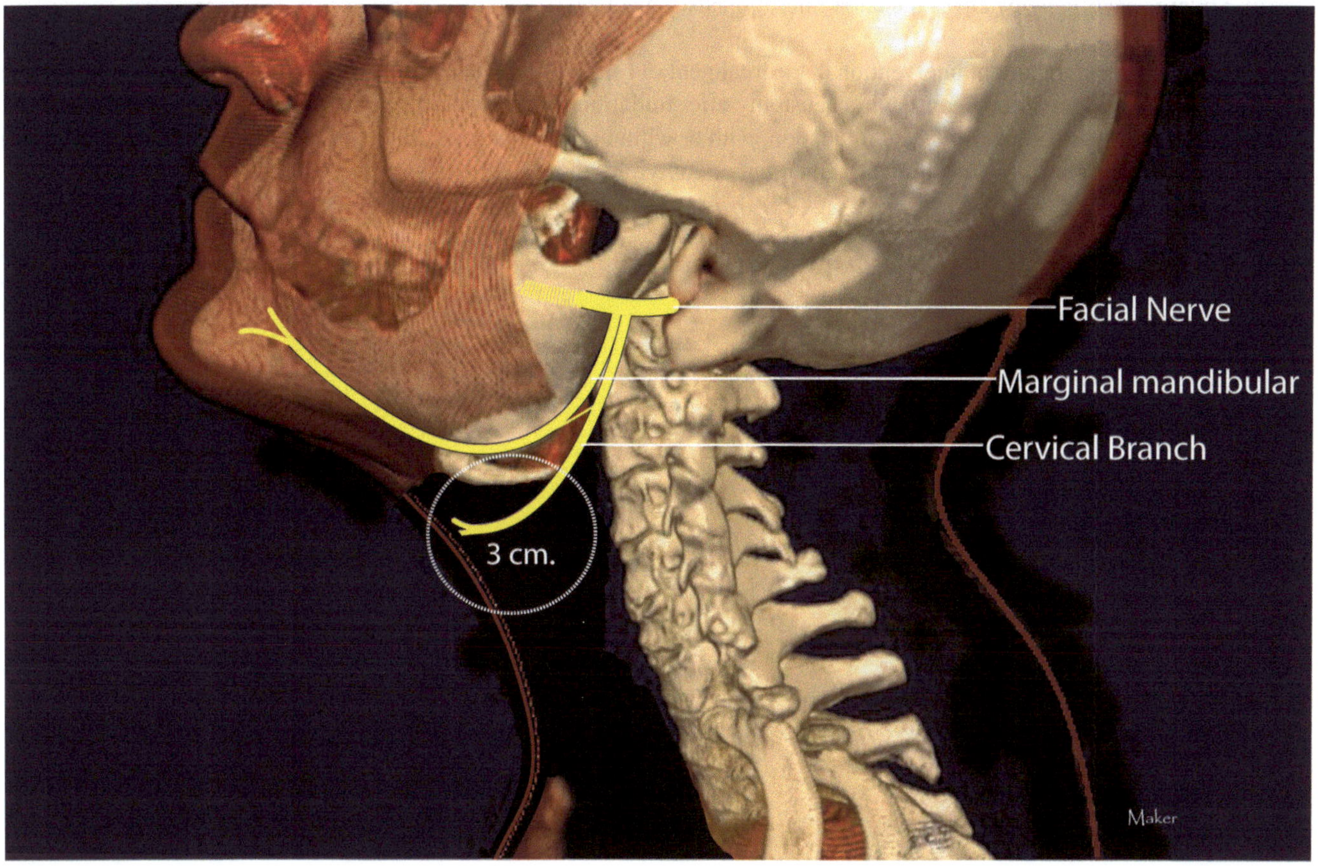

Fig. 1.5 The marginal mandibular branch of the facial nerve is an important nerve for smiling and other facial expressions with the lips. It has multiple variations in branching. To avoid injury to this nerve, a skin incision 3 cm. below the angle of mandible followed by careful dissection of the subplatysmal skin flaps is necessary

Answer

a

5. Select the *incorrect* statement regarding Ludwig's angina causing respiratory distress.
   (a) Incision and drainage is the first therapeutic maneuver.
   (b) The sublingual and submaxillary spaces communicate posteriorly around the mylohyoid muscle.
   (c) Infection can extend to the pharyngomaxillary and retropharyngeal spaces requiring urgent awake tracheostomy.
   (d) The main sources of infection in Ludwig's angina are the lower molars.
   (e) *Streptococcus hemolyticus* is the chief microorganism involved.

Comments The most important intervention in the treatment of Ludwig's angina causing respiratory distress is to secure the airway. This is best done through awake tracheostomy after initiation of gastric acid suppression and cholinergic blockade. Attempts at nasotracheal and orotracheal intubation, with or without bronchoscopic guidance, are likely to fail due to severe anatomic distortion. This same factor makes emergent cricothyroidotomy likely to be unsuccessful [3, 4].

Answer

a

6. Select the *incorrect* statement regarding the carotid sinus and body.
   (a) The carotid sinus is innervated by the glossopharyngeal nerve.
   (b) Carotid sinus distention triggers an elevation of the heart rate and blood pressure.
   (c) The carotid body is located at the carotid bifurcation.
   (d) The carotid body triggers hyperventilation when exposed to high hydrogen ion concentrations.
   (e) Tumors of the carotid body (chemodectomas) are highly vascular.

Comments The carotid sinus and body are often confused as one structure. They are distinct and fulfill separate functions important in regulating nutrient delivery to the brain.

The carotid sinus is a baroreceptor located in the dilated origin of the internal carotid artery. It controls blood flow by decreasing cardiac output when its walls are stretched. This is accomplished by the generation of a vagal reflex (baroreceptor reflex), which can also be triggered by manipulation of this structure in the course of carotid surgery or stenting. The baroreceptor reflex is not to be confused with the Bainbridge reflex, which is triggered by atrial distention, inducing an increase in heart rate.

The carotid body is a chemoreceptor sensitive to low pH and oxygen tension as well as increased carbon dioxide concentration. When stimulated it induces an increase in ventilation to return these parameters to normal levels.

The carotid body originates from the third branchial arch mesoderm and cells of neural crest origin. It is located within the adventitia of the carotid bifurcation. It is innervated by the glossopharyngeal nerve and closely related to the superior laryngeal nerve as well as the hypoglossal nerve. Tumors originating from this structure are very vascular, contraindicating needle biopsies [5].

Answer
b

7. Select the *correct* statement regarding the thoracic outlet.
   (a) The subclavian artery and the brachial plexus course between the posterior and middle scalene.
   (b) Accessory cervical ribs (C7) are a common cause of compression of the subclavian vein.
   (c) Paget–Schroetter syndrome consists of the effort-related thrombosis of the subclavian artery.
   (d) Poststenotic dilatations of the subclavian artery are associated with thrombi formation.
   (e) Anterior scalenectomy has no role in the treatment of thoracic outlet syndrome.

Comments Nomenclature pertaining the thoracic outlet and inlet can be confusing. From a strictly anatomical perspective, the thoracic outlet is the lower border of the rib cage, covered by the diaphragm. In turn, the thoracic inlet is defined as the opening bound by the manubrium, the upper border of T1 and the first rib.

From a clinical perspective, the term thoracic outlet is defined by the passage of the neurovascular elements to the upper extremity. Instead of consisting of a bidimensional ringlike plane, the clinical thoracic outlet is a wedge-shaped volume, occupying the space between the first rib and the clavicle [6] (Fig. 1.6).

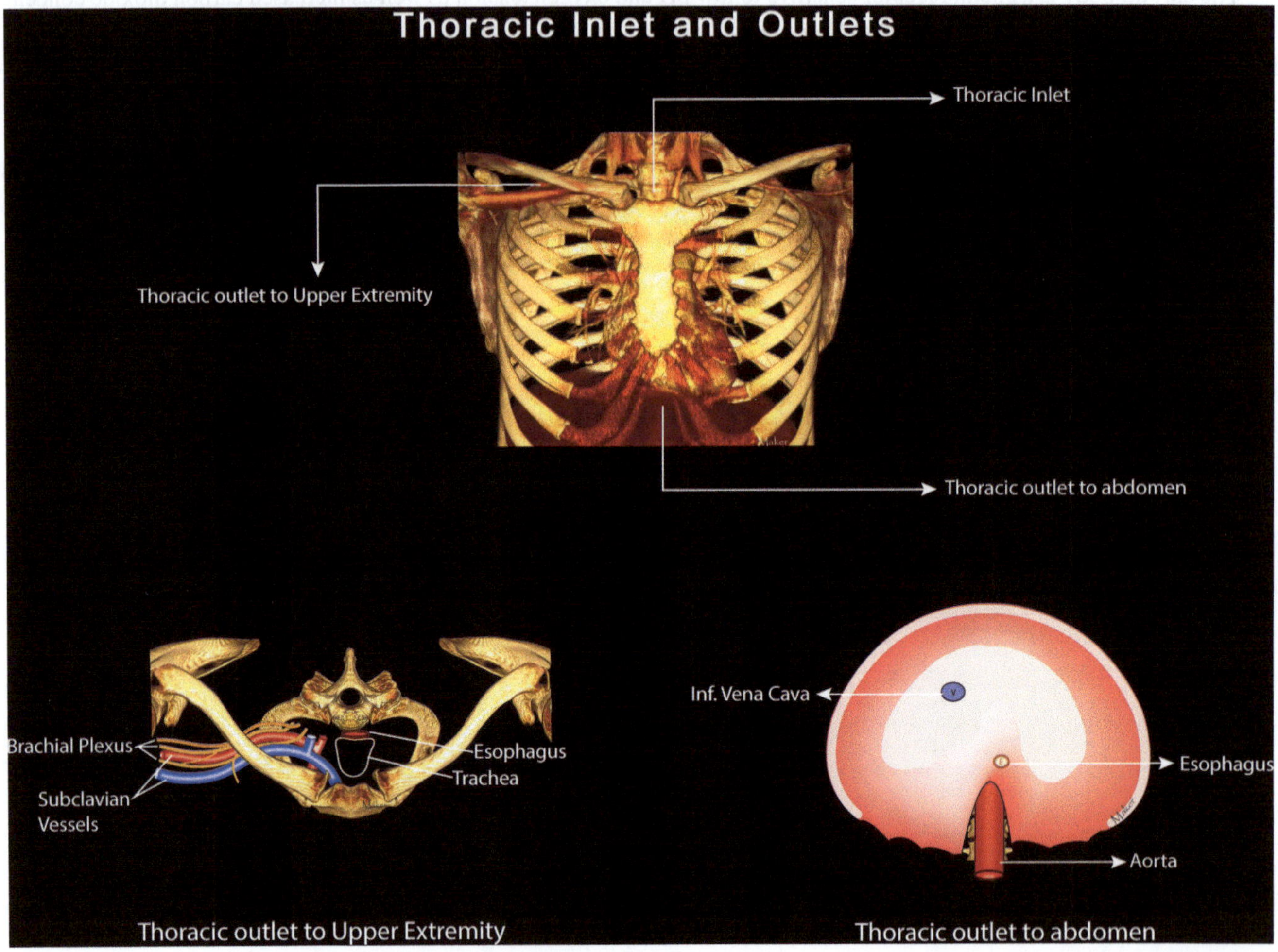

Fig. 1.6 Terminology of the thoracic inlet and outlet is often confusing. We recommend describing the anatomy as follows: the thorax has a single bony inlet bounded by the manubrium anteriorly, the first rib laterally, and the C7–T1 vertebrae posteriorly. The thorax has two outlets, an inferior outlet bounded by the diaphragm, leading to the abdomen, and a superior outlet to the upper extremity bounded by the clavicle and the first rib

The thoracic outlet has three areas of potential compression:

1. The costoclavicular space, between the first rib and the clavicle (partially covered by the subclavius muscle).
2. The interscalene triangle, bound by the first rib inferiorly, the anterior scalene anteriorly, and the middle scalene posteriorly. It contains the subclavian artery and brachial plexus.
3. The subcoracoid space, underneath the pectoralis minor tendon. This muscle marks the transition into the axillary space.

Both the subclavian vein and artery cross over the first rib as they exit the thorax. The subclavian vein courses anterior to the anterior scalene muscle. The subclavian artery crosses behind this muscle, but anterior to the middle scalene muscle, in the space previously defined as the interscalene triangle. Here, it is joined by the elements of the brachial plexus that course in a more superior and slightly more posterior path (Fig. 1.7).

The subclavian vein may be compressed between the first rib, clavicle, and anterior scalene muscle. More laterally, the subclavius muscle may also cause compression against the chest wall. Paget–Schroetter syndrome is effort-related subclavian vein thrombosis caused by repeated strenuous overhead activity, classically, of the dominant arm (Fig. 1.8).

The subclavian artery and brachial plexus can be compressed within the interscalene triangle, bringing about the vascular and neurological manifestations of the thoracic outlet syndrome. This is more likely in the presence of anomalous bands of muscle and tendon or an accessory cervical rib (Fig. 1.9).

Cervical ribs arise from the transverse process of C7 and follow a course that parallels that of the first rib. Cervical ribs may reach the sternum, but more frequently terminate in a ligamentous structure that attaches to the upper margin of the first rib. This ligament may exert compression over the elements of the brachial plexus [7] (Fig. 1.10).

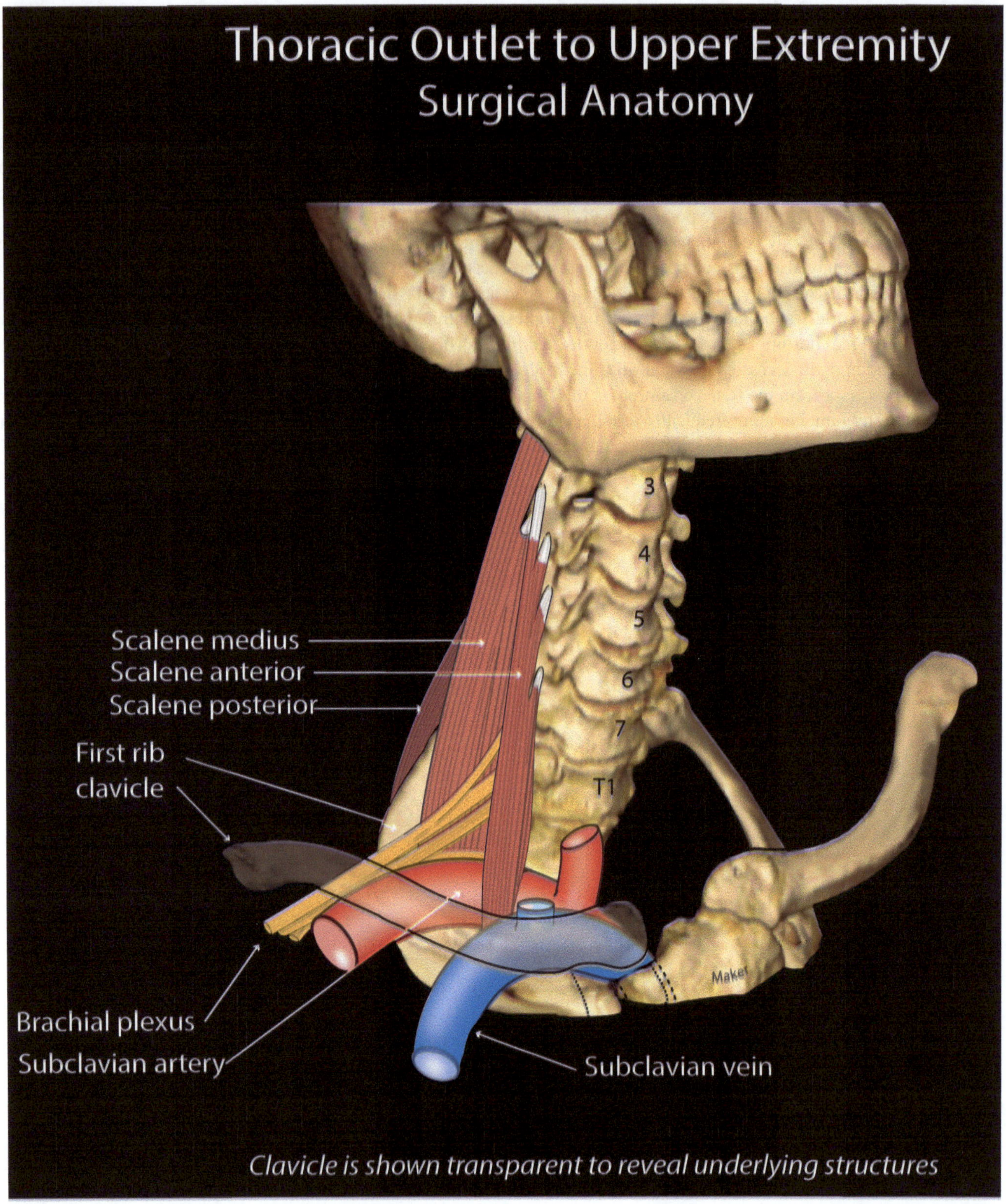

Fig. 1.7 The thoracic outlet is the tight space between the clavicle and the first rib traversed by scalene muscles. The subclavian artery and the brachial plexus are between the scalenus anterior and medius muscles, while the subclavian vein is anterior to the scalenus anterior in the tightest space

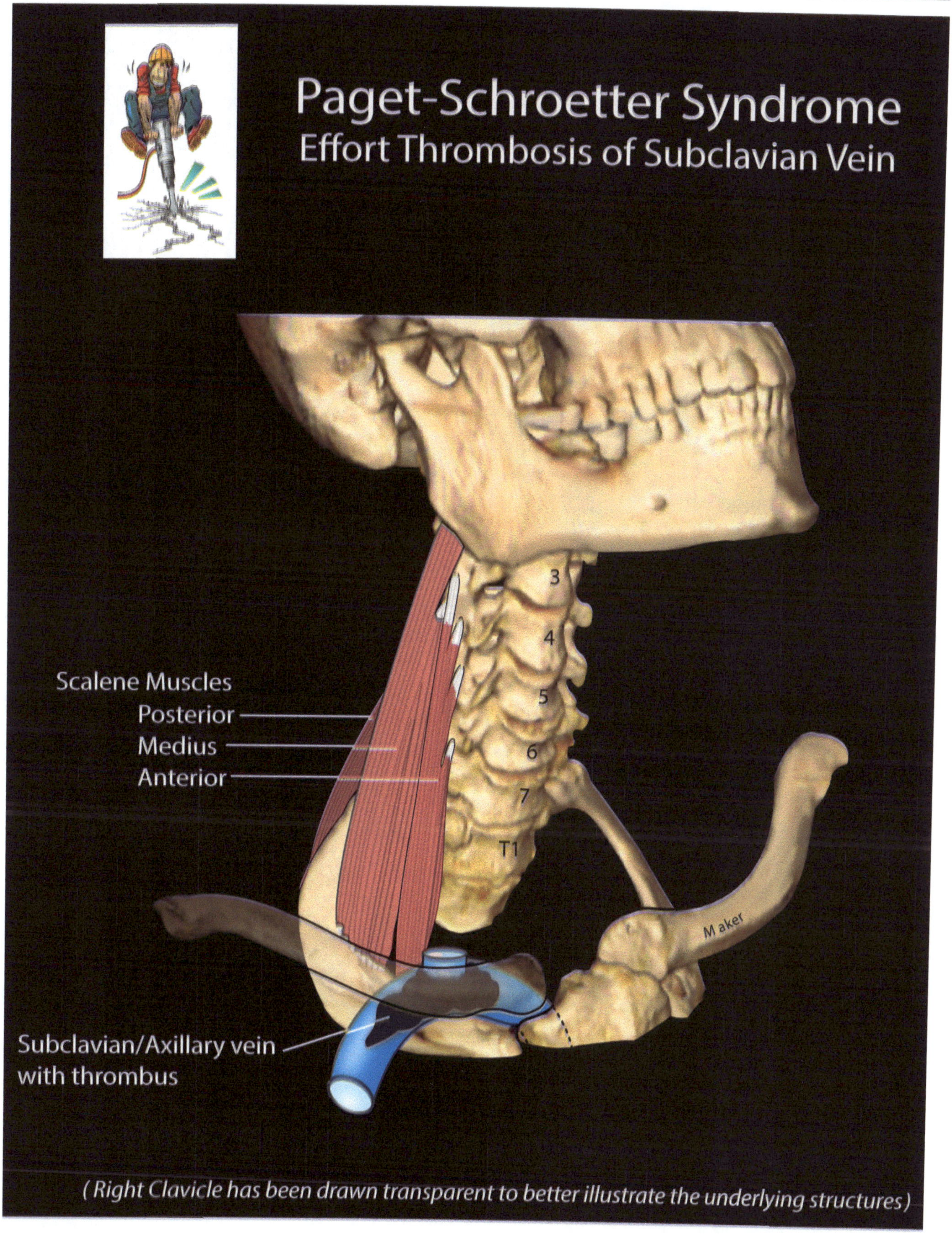

Fig. 1.8 Repetitive strenuous trauma in the tight space between the clavicle and the first rib is the key factor in subclavian–axillary vein thrombosis, also referred to as effort thrombosis or Paget–Schroetter syndrome. Baseball pitchers, manual "jackhammer" operators, swimmers, and other professionals with activities producing this repetitive microtrauma to the subclavian vein endothelium are at higher risk

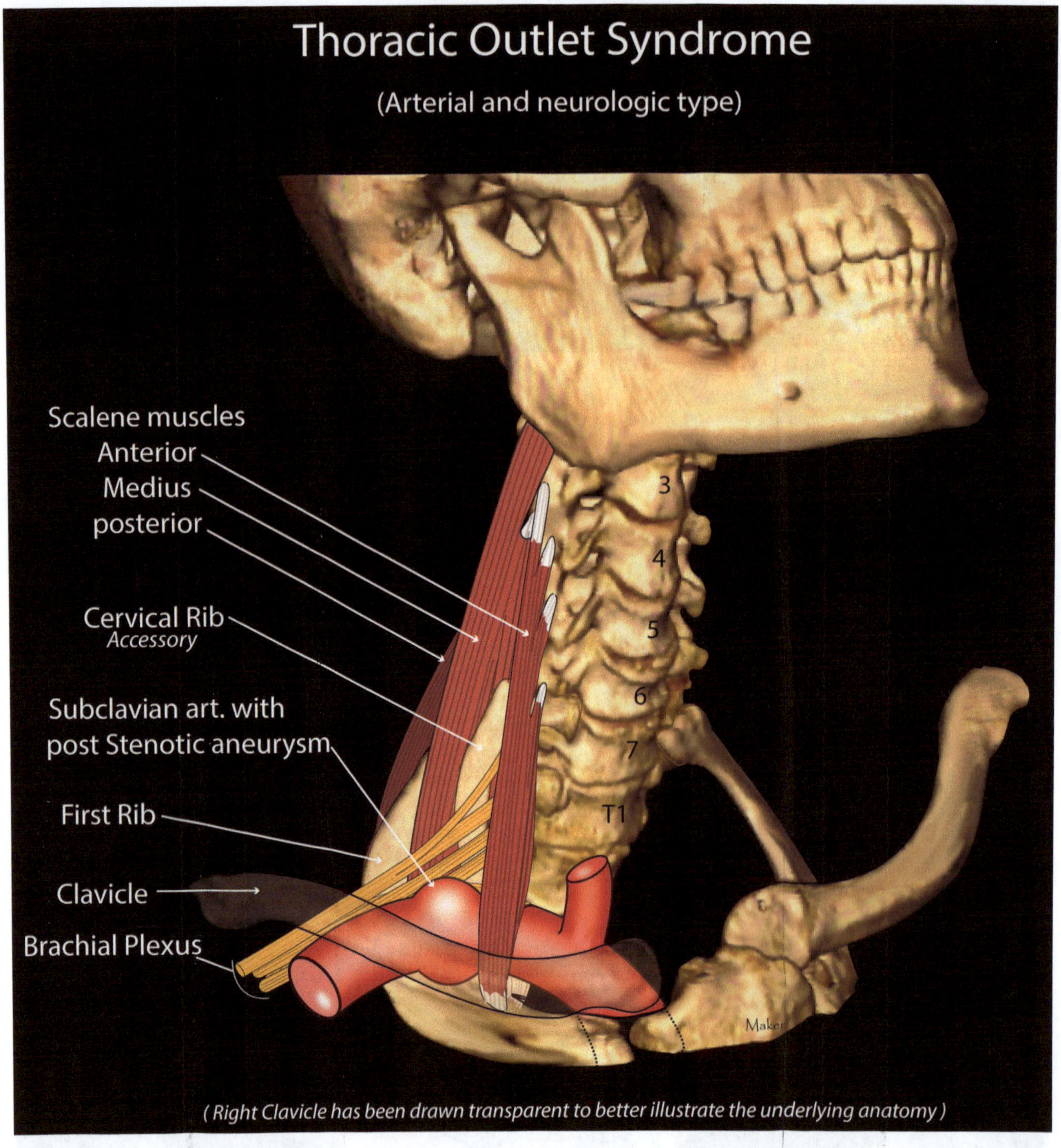

Fig. 1.9 Presence of an accessory cervical rib, as shown above, may significantly narrow the thoracic outlet causing narrowing of the subclavian artery. Resultant poststenotic dilatation can add to the problem with embolic disease. Common associated neurologic problems are compression of C8 and T1

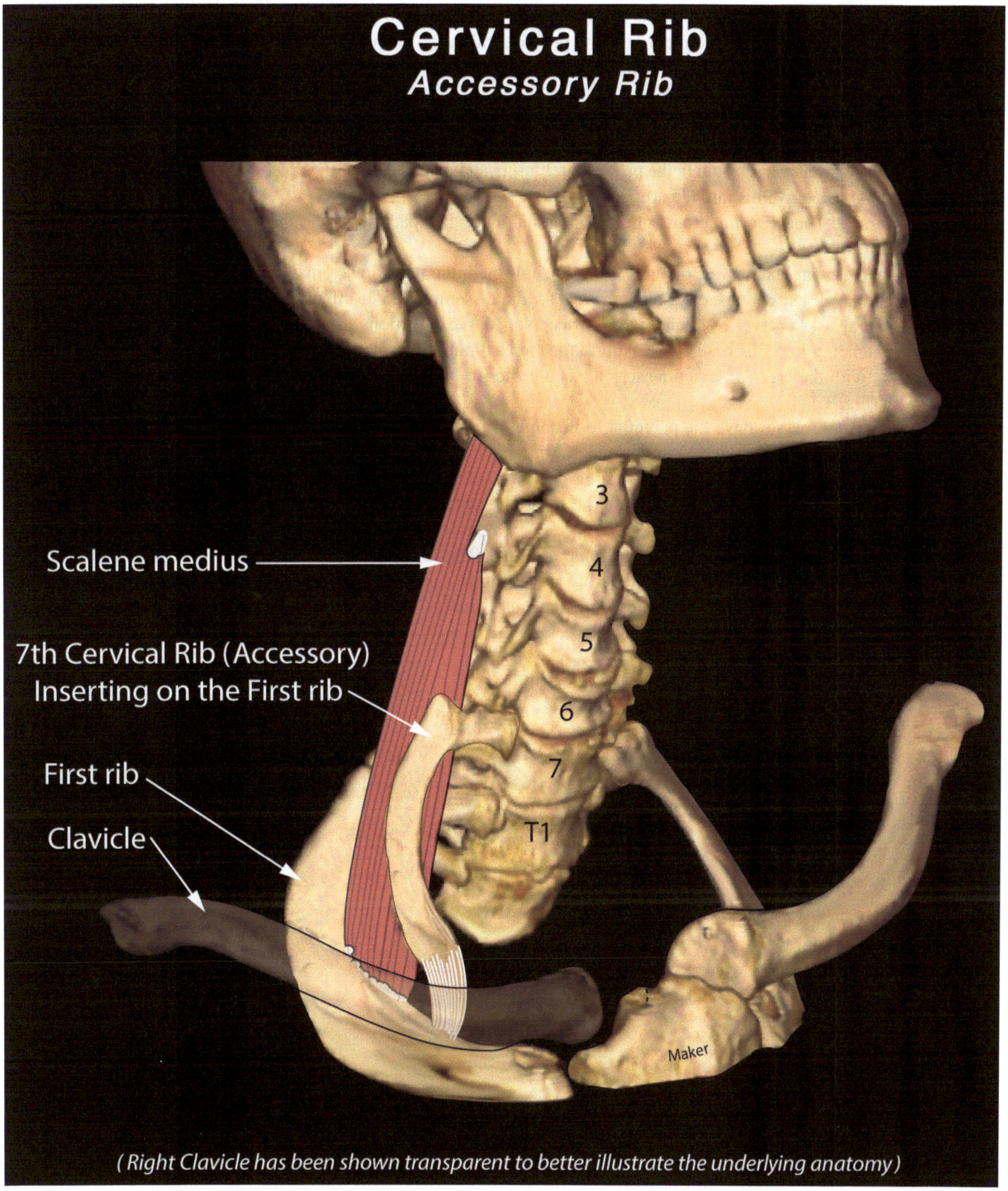

Fig. 1.10 The cervical ribs are seen in about 1 % of the population, are often bilateral, are more common on the left and have three times higher incidence in women. Their extent can be anywhere from a long transverse process of the C7 vertebra to a complete rib inserting on the manubrium. The vast majority are asymptomatic, but the accessory ribs are one of the established causes of the thoracic outlet syndrome causing compression of the lower cord of the brachial plexus and subclavian artery

Answer

d

8. Mark the *incorrect* statement regarding the spaces of the neck and their pathology.
   (a) Retropharyngeal abscesses occur between the prevertebral fascia and the posterolateral wall of the pharynx.
   (b) The retropharyngeal abscesses are acute in nature, secondary to regional infections, esophageal perforations, and pathology of the deep cervical nodes.
   (c) Abscesses between the vertebral bodies and the prevertebral fascia are of chronic nature, secondary to vertebral osteomyelitis.
   (d) The axillary fascia takes origin in the prevertebral fascia and extends along the brachial artery, allowing the extension of vertebral osteomyelitis into the arm.
   (e) The pretracheal space is *not* a route of dissemination of cervical pathology into the mediastinum.

Comments The vascular and nerve structures that course through the neck do so enveloped in sheaths that extend into the head, thorax, and upper extremities, creating pathways for the dissemination of infections.

The prevertebral fascia serves as a landmark for deep soft tissue infections in the neck. The retropharyngeal space lies anterior to it, extending from the base of the skull to the mediastinum. In turn, the prevertebral space is posterior to the prevertebral fascia, with the cervical vertebrae serving as a posterior border. This space extends into the upper arm along the axillary sheath (Fig. 1.11).

Retropharyngeal abscesses have the potential to become life threatening due to airway obstruction, involvement of the carotid sheath, spread into the mediastinum, and septic shock. Mortality rate for this pathology is as high as 50 %. Contamination of this space usually arises from the pharynx, secondary to trauma, foreign bodies, and upper respiratory infections. Children less than 5 years of age are the most affected, but currently, there is an increasing incidence among immunocompromised adults [8, 9].

Prevertebral abscesses are more commonly chronic in nature. The vertebrae themselves are most often the source of contamination, although this space may be seeded during spinal surgery as well [10].

The pretracheal space extends into the middle mediastinum, ending at the pericardium. This space is developed during mediastinoscopy, a procedure that does not confer access to the anterior or posterior mediastinum.

Retropharyngeal and Prevertebral space

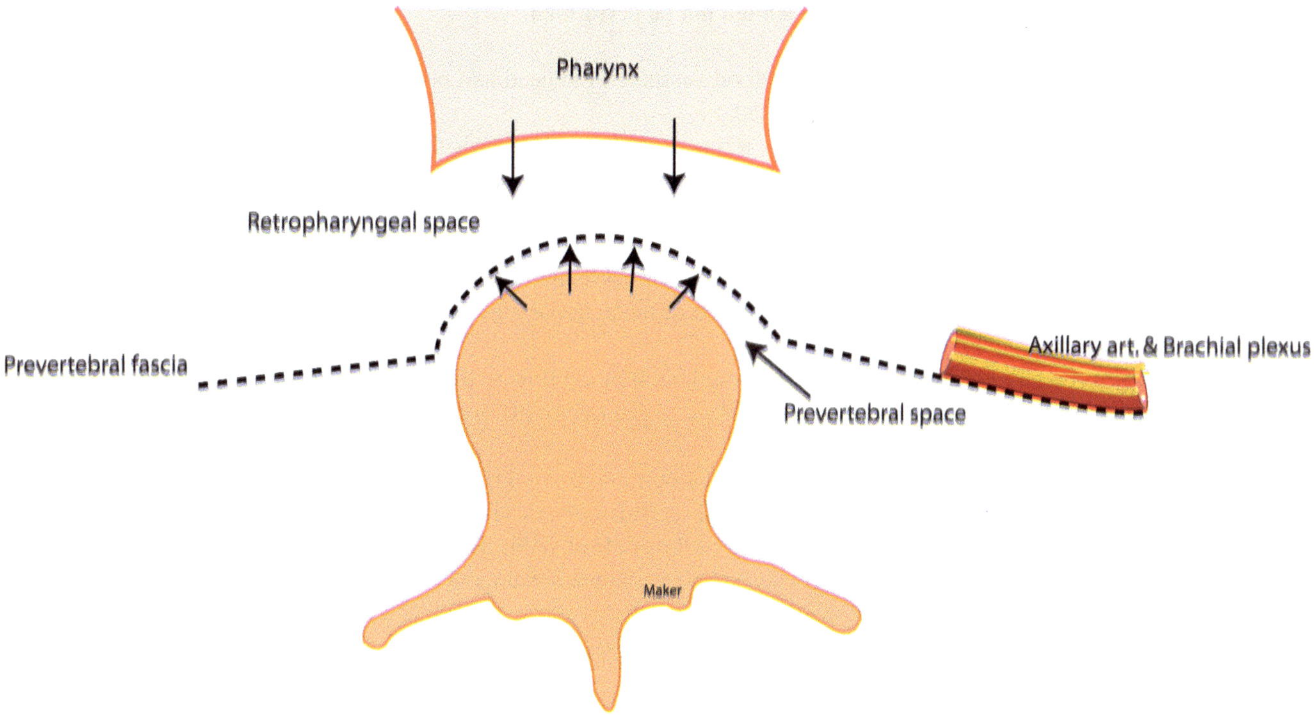

Fig. 1.11 The prevertebral space continues into the arm with the axillary vessels and brachial plexus. The retropharyngeal space may continue into the mediastinum or carotid sheath

Answer
e

9. Regarding the surgical management of vascular injuries in the neck, all of the following are correct *except*:
   (a) The external jugular vein can be ligated if the internal jugulars are intact.
   (b) The internal jugular vein may be ligated unilaterally.
   (c) The external carotid artery can be safely ligated.
   (d) Unilateral ligation of the internal carotid may be safely performed.
   (e) Unilateral ligation of the common carotid should not be performed.

Comments The rich anastomotic networks of the blood vessels in the head and neck allow the preservation of blood flow even when some of the blood vessels are compromised.

When an external jugular vein is ligated, venous return is redirected towards the contralateral vessel, as well as to the ipsilateral internal jugular. Ligation of the external carotid artery is compensated through multiple collaterals to the contralateral external carotid, as well as with the internal carotid artery, through the angular artery.

The internal jugular vein may be ligated unilaterally without a negative impact on intracranial pressure. However, acute simultaneous bilateral ligation results in engorgement of the intracranial venous system, compromising cerebral blood flow. It has been shown in experimental models that preservation of the external jugular veins ameliorates the increase in intracranial pressures [11, 12].

The internal carotid artery behaves as an end artery, although blood flow to the ipsilateral brain can be partially restored through the circle of Willis. Its ligation is associated with a stroke rate of 20 % and a mortality rate as high as 25 %, which makes this maneuver extremely risky.

Although it would seem that ligation of the common carotid artery would result in reconstitution of flow to the internal carotid through the contralateral anastomoses of the external carotid artery, this is unfortunately not the case. What occurs is that flow to the internal carotid on the ligated side is restituted by the circle of Willis. Blood is then diverted from the internal carotid to the external carotid, further compromising brain perfusion in a manner analogous to the subclavian steal syndrome [13].

Answer
d

10. Mark the *incorrect* statement regarding masses in the neck.
    (a) Eighty percent of neck masses are primary tumors.
    (b) Acute (days) neck masses tend to be inflammatory in nature.
    (c) Subacute (months) neck masses are suggestive of neoplasm.
    (d) Chronic (years) neck masses are likely congenital defects.
    (e) Eighty percent of metastatic masses in the upper two thirds of the neck come from supraclavicular sites.

Comments The rich lymphatic network of the neck is fertile soil for metastatic seeding. Up to 80 % of all persistent neck masses are secondary to a primary tumor located in the head or neck. Left supraclavicular masses should raise the suspicion of a primary tumor below the diaphragm.

Fine-needle aspiration is the first diagnostic procedure that should be undertaken to establish the etiology of a persistent neck mass. This modality offers a 95 % accuracy for benign masses and 87 % for malignant masses [14].

Answer
a

11. Regarding the congenital anomalies of the thyroid, all of the following are correct *except*:
    (a) A lingual thyroid lies beneath the epithelium of the tongue, has higher risk of malignancy, and is supplied by lingual arteries.
    (b) Thyroglossal duct cysts are the most common midline congenital masses of the neck.
    (c) It is embryologically unlikely for ectopic thyroid tissue along the thyroglossal tract to contain C cells.
    (d) Aspiration is the treatment of choice for thyroglossal duct cysts.
    (e) Lateral aberrant nodules containing thyroid tissue should be considered metastatic unless proven otherwise.

Comments The most common defect in thyroid development is the persistence of thyroglossal elements forming clusters of ectopic thyroid tissue as well as cystic dilatations.

Thyroglossal duct cysts move with swallowing as well as when the tongue protrudes outside the mouth. Thyroglossal duct cysts typically contain cholesterol crystals like most embryologic tissues. Thyroid tissue derived from the medial thyroid anlage is usually free of C cells [15] (Fig. 1.12).

Adequate treatment of thyroglossal cysts involves complete resection, including the middle portion of the hyoid bone (Sistrunk procedure). Aspiration is fraught with unacceptable rates of cyst recurrence.

It is important to note that ectopic thyroid tissue may be the only functioning thyroid tissue in the patient. Hence, before its removal, a thyroid scan must be undertaken.

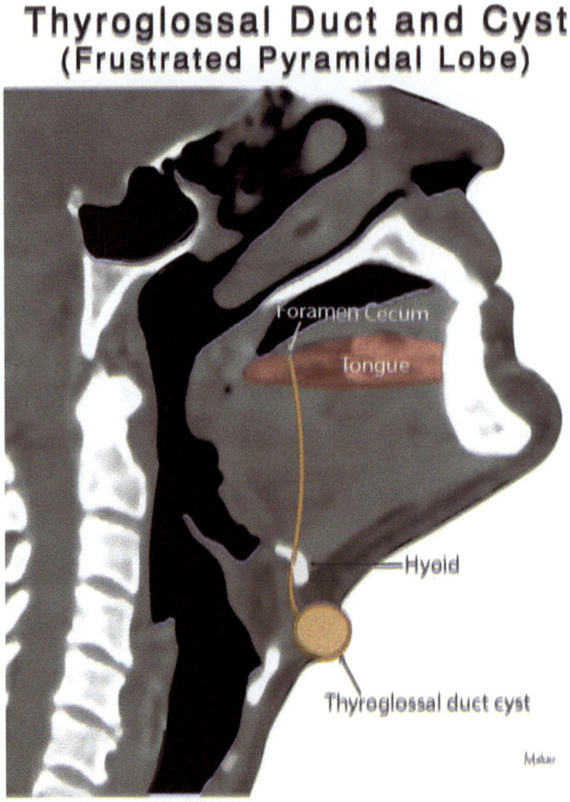

Fig. 1.12 The foramen cecum near the base of the tongue and the pyramidal lobe of the thyroid are the only remnants of the thyroglossal duct in the adult. Protruding the tongue and swallowing move a thyroglossal duct cyst. Thyroid carcinoma can develop in the thyroglossal duct as well as the pyramidal lobes. The thyroglossal duct normally goes through the hyoid bone, and hence, the central part of the hyoid is resected as part of the Sistrunk procedure to decrease recurrence

Answer
d

12. Select the *false* statement regarding the arterial supply of the thyroid.
    (a) The superior thyroid artery is a proximal branch of the external carotid. It courses parallel to the superior laryngeal nerve in part of its course.
    (b) The vascular supply to the parathyroids is predominantly derived from the inferior thyroid artery.
    (c) The inferior thyroid artery comes from the thyrocervical trunk. It crosses the recurrent laryngeal nerve.
    (d) The middle thyroid artery accompanies the middle thyroid vein.
    (e) The thyroid ima artery ascends parallel to the midline and may be injured during a tracheostomy.

Comments The blood supply of the parathyroid glands may be compromised during thyroid surgery. This is especially true if the inferior thyroid artery (and to the lesser extent the superior thyroid artery) is ligated away from the gland, before they have given off the branches for the parathyroid. To avoid this complication, the thyroid blood vessels should be ligated on the surface of the gland. Even though the inferior thyroid artery is the predominant supply to both parathyroid glands in over 80 % of cases, communicating vessels exists between the superior and inferior thyroid artery.

There is no middle thyroid artery accompanying the middle thyroid vein. During the mobilization of the thyroid, it is imperative to localize the middle thyroid vein. Avulsion of this vessel can cause significant bleeding from the internal jugular vein. The middle thyroid vein is inconsistent in its presence and can be doubled (Fig. 1.13).

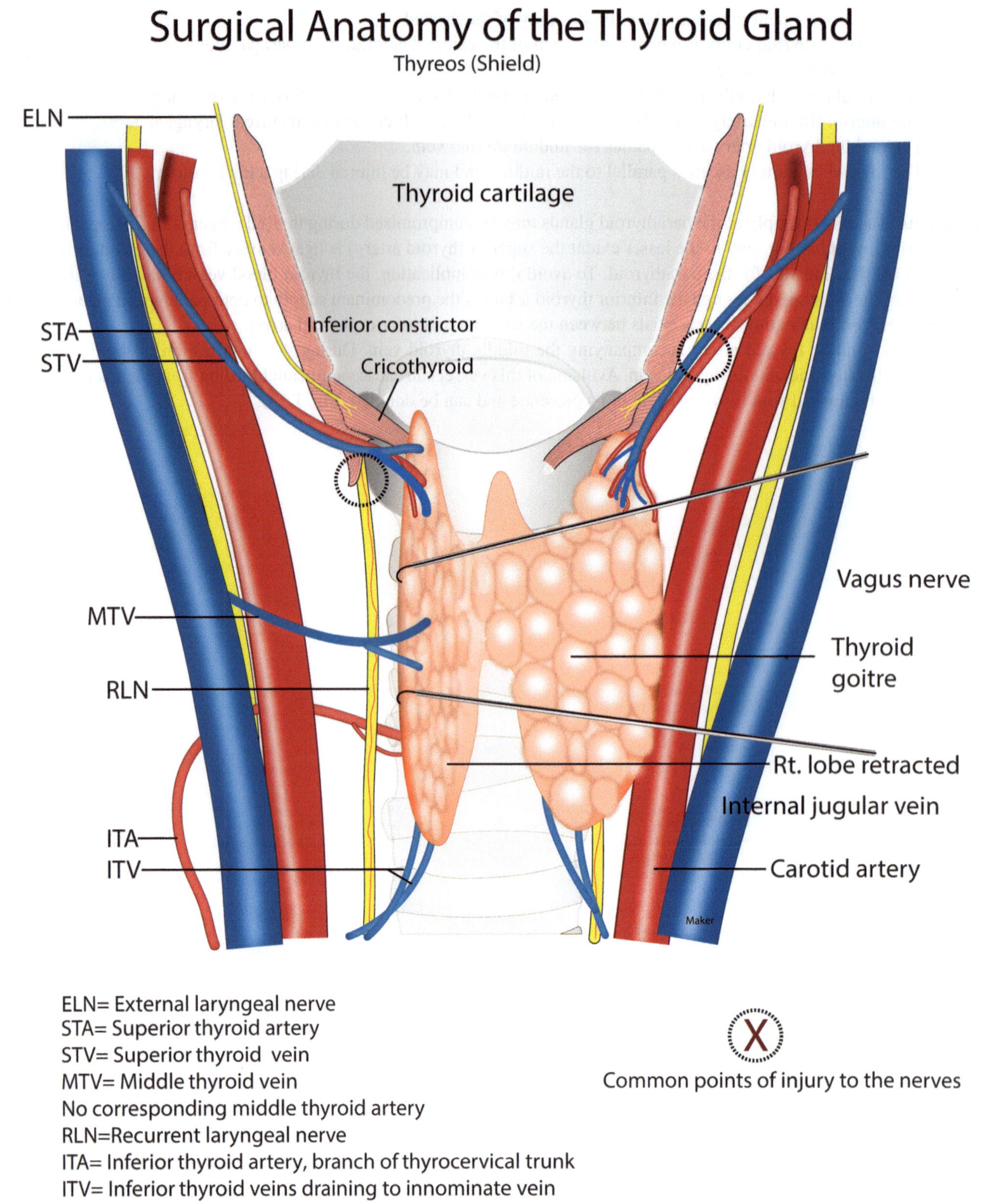

Fig. 1.13 The external laryngeal nerve is prone to injury during ligation of the superior thyroid pedicle. The recurrent laryngeal nerve is most vulnerable to injury in the last 2 cm of its extra laryngeal course

Answer

d

13. Mark the *incorrect* statement regarding the venous and lymphatic drainage of the thyroid.
    (a) The anterior jugular vein receives both the superior and middle thyroid veins.
    (b) The inferior thyroid vein drains into the brachiocephalic veins.
    (c) The thyroid ima vein is a rare variation resulting from the midline confluence of the inferior thyroid veins. It drains into the left brachiocephalic vein.
    (d) The lymphatic spread of the thyroid cancer can involve any of the six lymphatic zones of the neck.
    (e) The most commonly affected lymph nodes in thyroid malignancy belong to the central compartment (zone 6).

Comments There are several differences between the arterial and venous vessels of the thyroid. As mentioned before, the middle thyroid vein is not accompanied by a homologous artery. Whereas the superior thyroid artery arises from the *external* carotid artery, the superior and middle thyroid veins drain into the *internal* jugular. The inferior thyroid artery arises from the thyrocervical trunk, which is a branch of the subclavian artery. In contrast, the inferior thyroid veins drain more medially into the brachiocephalic vein.

The anterior jugular veins (not to be confused with the external jugular veins) are superficial blood vessels running subcutaneously on either side of the trachea. They are the vessel most commonly injured during tracheostomy.

Lymphatic drainage of the thyroid is discussed in question 24.

Answer
a

14. Mark the *false* statement regarding the innervation of the larynx.
    (a) The right recurrent laryngeal nerve loops from anterior to posterior around the right subclavian.
    (b) The nonrecurrent recurrent laryngeal nerves are rare anatomical variations *not* associated with other anomalies.
    (c) The recurrent laryngeal nerves most often cross the inferior thyroid artery posteriorly.
    (d) The cricothyroid junction is a relatively constant landmark to identify the recurrent laryngeal nerve.
    (e) The external branch of the superior laryngeal nerve crosses the superior thyroid artery before entering the larynx. It may do so in front of the thyroid gland.

Comments During early embryogenesis the recurrent laryngeal nerve does not recur. It arises from the vagus and follows a straight course under the sixth aortic arch to reach the sixth pharyngeal arch that will latter give origin to the larynx. As development continues, the sixth pharyngeal arch ascends in relation to the sixth aortic arch, and in doing so it "pulls" the nerve with it, with the sixth aortic arch serving as a turning point.

On the left side, the sixth aortic arch persists, ultimately becoming the ductus arteriosus, which marks the lowermost point in the trajectory of the recurrent nerve on that side. On the right, the sixth and fifth arches disappear, allowing the lowermost aspect of the recurrent laryngeal nerve to ascend, until it reaches the fourth aortic arch, which will give rise to the right subclavian artery.

In contrast to the circuitous route of the recurrent laryngeal nerve, the superior laryngeal nerve follows a fairly direct course to the larynx, where its external branch will provide motor nerve supply to the cricothyroid muscle, the only muscle of phonation not controlled by the recurrent laryngeal nerve. The said muscle tilts the thyroid cartilage anteriorly, putting tension on the vocal cords, in a manner akin to an orchestra director that calls his musicians to attention prior to initiating the performance (Fig. 1.14).

Nonrecurrence of the laryngeal nerve on either side is associated with arterial anomalies (Fig. 1.15). On the right side, the most common is the presence of a subclavian artery originating from the descending aorta. This anomaly leaves the nerve without a fulcrum. At the same time, since the artery has to cross behind the esophagus to reach the right side, it may cause extrinsic compression of the latter, producing dysphagia lusoria (Fig. 1.16). Nonrecurrence of the left laryngeal nerve is most often associated with a right aortic arch.

Nerves of Speech

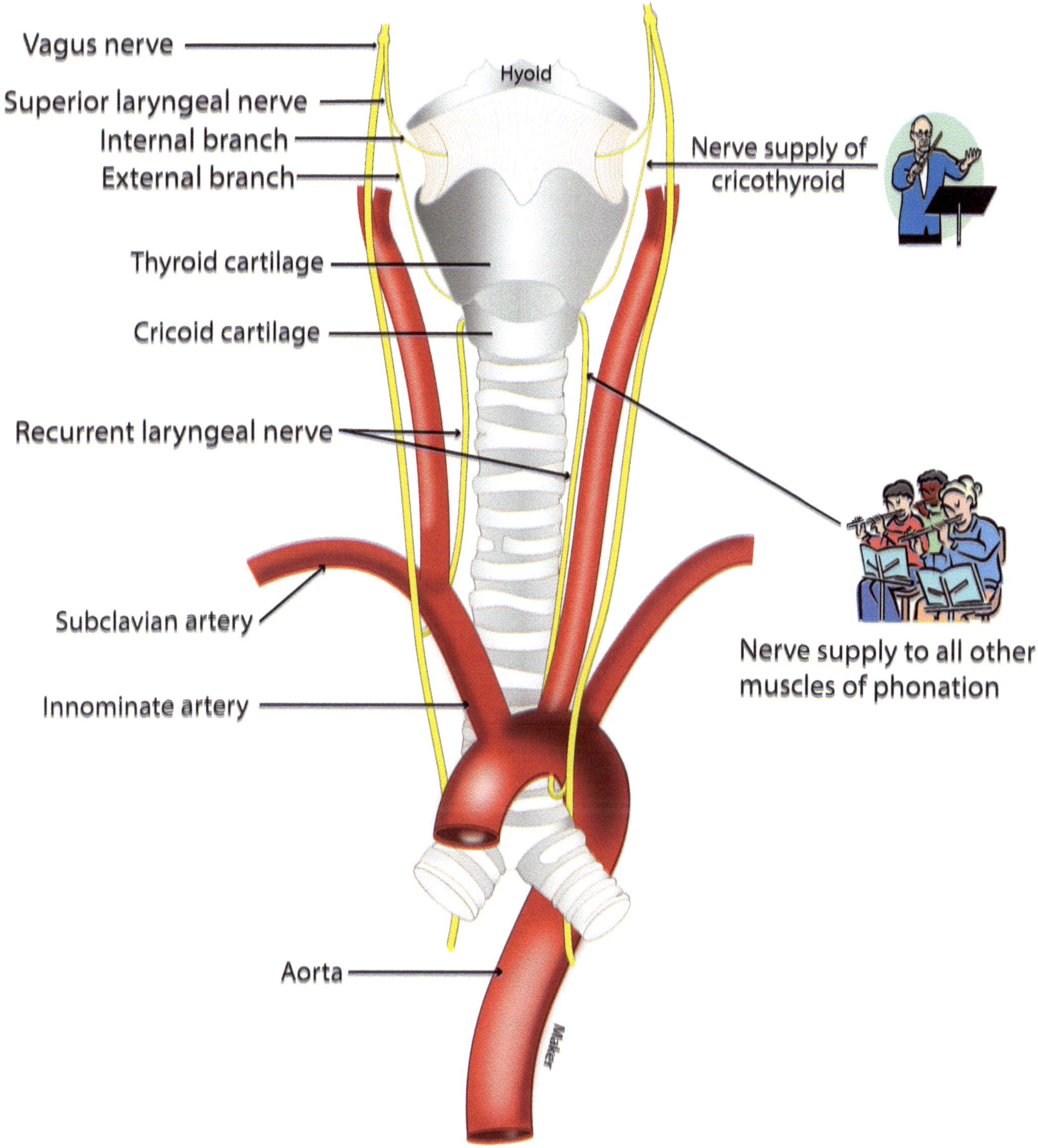

Fig. 1.14 The external branch of the superior laryngeal nerve is the conductor that prepares the orchestra by tensing the vocal cords. A few microseconds later the recurrent laryngeal nerve starts the orchestra playing music through all the other muscles of phonation

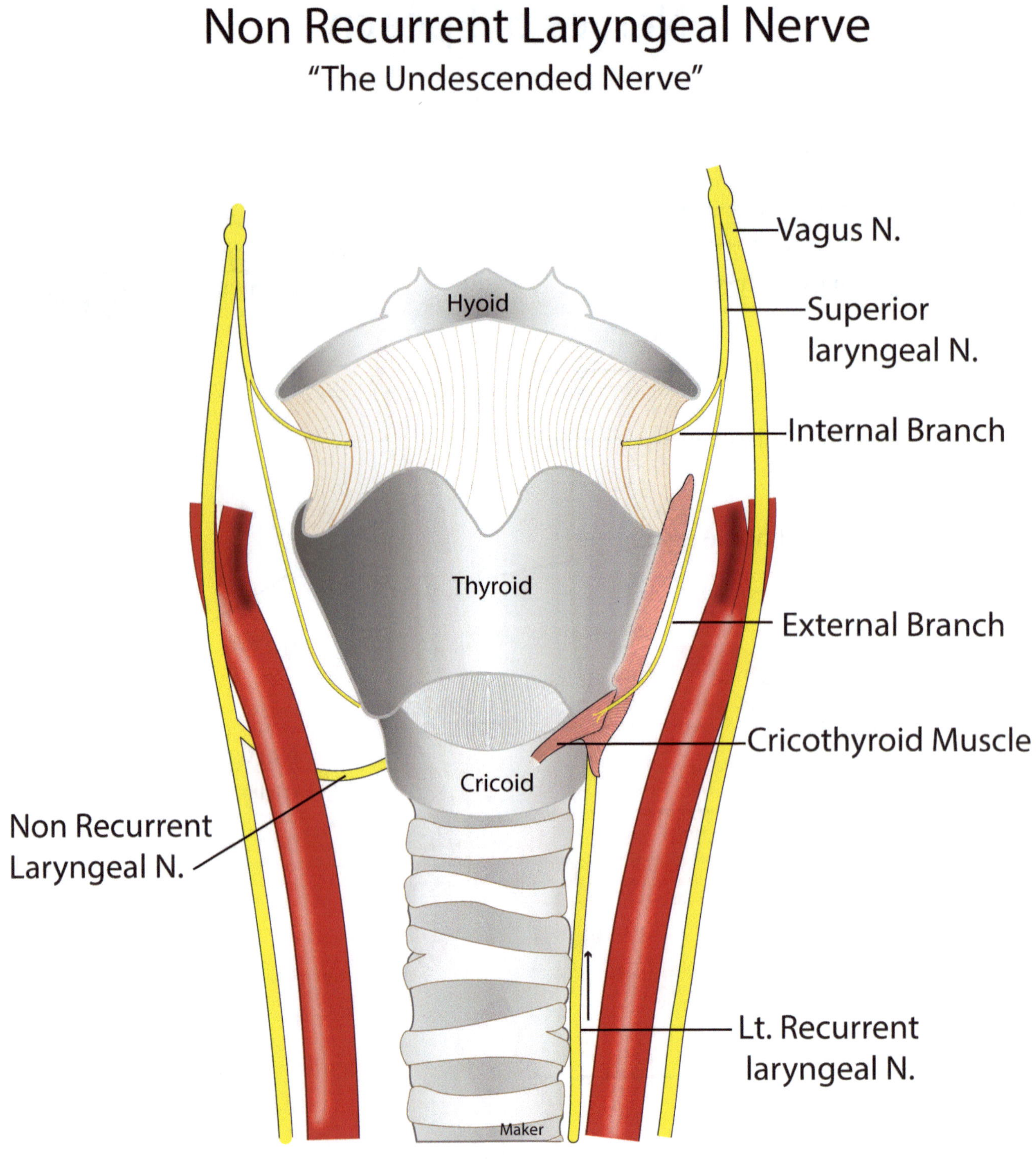

Fig. 1.15 The nonrecurrent laryngeal nerve is rare and seen mostly on the right side. Its "undescended course" is often transverse and posterior to the right carotid artery and associated with aortic arch anomalies

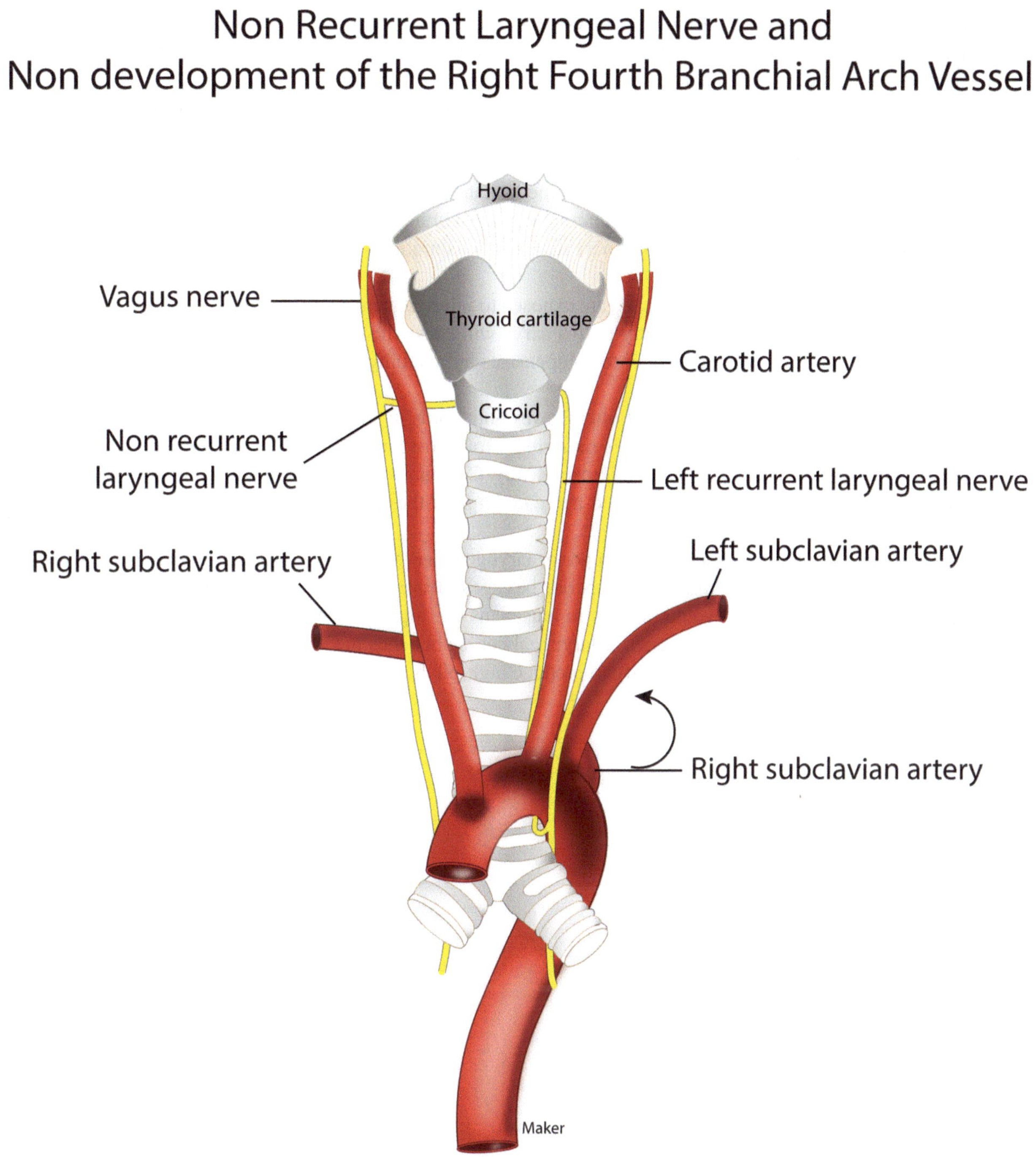

Fig. 1.16 The nonrecurrent laryngeal nerve is most often associated with nondevelopment of the right fourth branchial vascular arch. In these cases, the right subclavian originates from the dorsal aorta after the origin of the left subclavian and crosses to the right behind the trachea and esophagus

Answer

b

15. Regarding thyroid surgery all of the following are correct *except*:
    (a) When the recurrent laryngeal nerve passes between the branches of the inferior thyroid artery, such branches must be individually ligated and divided.
    (b) Inadvertent injury to the vagus nerve may cause symptoms mimicking those of recurrent laryngeal nerve injury.
    (c) Most recurrent laryngeal nerve injuries occur at the point where it passes below the inferior constrictor muscle to become intralaryngeal.
    (d) An injury to the recurrent laryngeal nerve leaves the ipsilateral cord in a median position.
    (e) Injury to the superior laryngeal nerve or its internal laryngeal branch leaves the larynx and piriform recess insensate, resulting in a loss of the cough reflex and increased risk of aspiration.

Comments The vagus nerve and all of its branches are exposed to injury during neck surgery. The recurrent laryngeal nerve is primarily an abductor of the vocal cords. Injury to this nerve will cause the cord to be in a slightly paramedian position, with inability to abduct. The contralateral vocal cord compensates in breathing by abduction and in voice by overadduction, crossing over the midline.

Bilateral recurrent laryngeal nerve injury most often leaves both cords in slightly paramedian position, unable to abduct and hence producing respiratory problems, at times requiring a tracheostomy. When identified intraoperatively, injuries to the recurrent laryngeal nerve should be repaired microsurgically. Constant vasa nervorum are found on the recurrent laryngeal nerve; its presence is useful to align the severed nerve endings. If there is tissue loss, a graft from the great auricular nerve may be used to bridge the defect [16] (Fig. 1.17).

It has been postulated that the recurrence of the superior laryngeal nerve serves to introduce a delay in the signal carried by this nerve. This delay would allow time for the superior laryngeal nerve to tense the vocal cords prior to their apposition by the recurrent laryngeal nerve. This would be akin to musicians tensing the strings on their instruments before playing. Isolated injury to the external branch of the superior laryngeal nerve abolishes the tensing of the vocal cords by contraction of the cricothyroid muscle, which leads to inability to produce high-pitch sounds and leads to quick vocal fatigue.

Vasa Nervorum and Recurrent Laryngeal Nerve

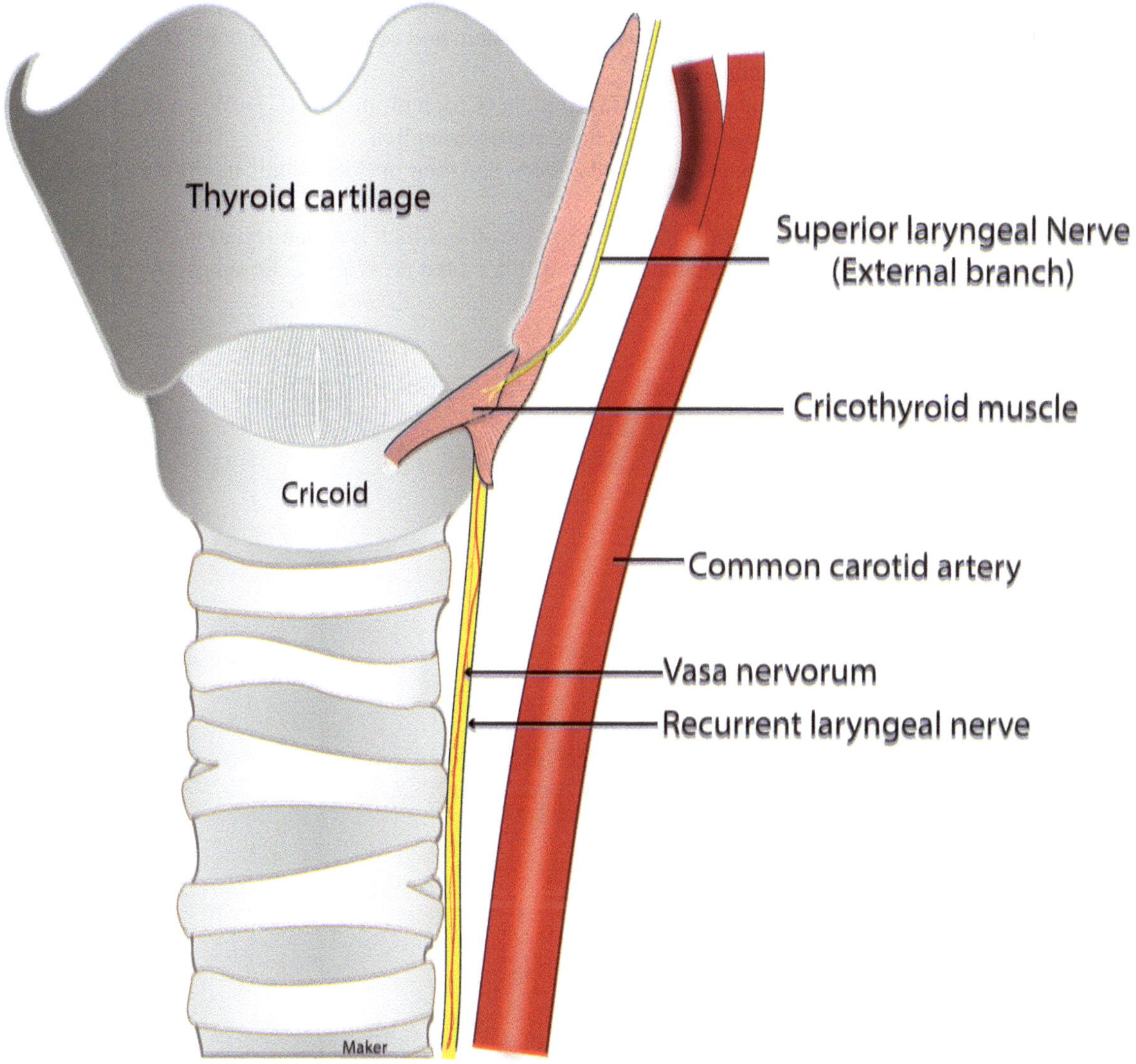

Fig. 1.17 The vasa nervorum are constant small blood vessels present on the recurrent laryngeal nerve and one of the assuring signs of the identification of this nerve. It can be used to orient appropriate approximation of the nerve in case of injury

Answer
d

16. Mark the element which is *not* part of Horner's syndrome.
    (a) Constriction of the pupil
    (b) Partial ptosis of the upper eyelid
    (c) Apparent exophthalmos
    (d) Dilatation of the retinal vessels
    (e) Flushing and dryness of the facial skin

Comments The preganglionic fibers of the sympathetic system supplying the head and neck arise from the posterolateral hypothalamus. They follow a descending course through the brain stem and cervical spinal cord, from which they depart to synapse with the cervical sympathetic ganglia.

There are three sympathetic ganglia: superior (C2–C3), middle (C6), and inferior (C7). When the inferior sympathetic ganglion fuses with the superior thoracic ganglion, it is named stellate ganglion.

These ganglia are connected by a network of sympathetic fibers, and their postganglionic neurons distribute following the distribution of the carotid artery.

Injury to the cervical sympathetic chain results in Horner's syndrome, which is a manifestation of unopposed parasympathetic activity. Some of the cranial nerves carry parasympathetic fibers, but no sympathetic supply. Apparent enophthalmos, not exophthalmos, is observed.

Answer
c

17. Mark the *incorrect* statement pertaining to parathyroid embryology and anatomy.
    (a) The third pharyngeal pouch gives rise to the inferior parathyroids and thymus.
    (b) The fourth pharyngeal pouch gives rise to the superior parathyroids.
    (c) The superior parathyroids are not involved in DiGeorge syndrome, as this syndrome represents isolated absence of the thymus gland.
    (d) The majority of superior parathyroids can be found within one inch of the entrance of the inferior thyroid artery into the thyroid.
    (e) The majority of inferior parathyroids can be found within half an inch of the entrance of the inferior thyroid artery into the thyroid.

Comments The embryology of the parathyroid glands is analogous to that of the lateral thyroid anlagen. While the classical teaching that they derive from the third and fourth pharyngeal pouch is true, the corollary that they are of endodermal origin is not. What occurs is that the third and fourth pharyngeal pouches are invaded by neuroectodermal cells, which will later differentiate into C cells and parathyroid cells. This concept is supported by multiple bodies of evidence. C cells and parathyroid cells express neuroectodermal markers such as S-100 and neuron-specific enolase [17, 18]. Furthermore, the expression of these markers is upregulated in adenomas and carcinomas, illustrating the "regression" of transformed cells [19].

As mentioned previously, the superior parathyroids are derived from the fourth branchial pouch, together with the lateral thyroid. The inferior parathyroids are derived from the third pouch in conjunction with the thymus. Both structures migrate caudally (Fig. 1.18).

The multiple mechanisms responsible for the presence of DiGeorge syndrome share a common denominator: the failure of neuroectodermal cells to migrate towards the pharyngeal pouches, leading to parathyroid agenesis as well as faulty development of C cells. Of more clinical relevance is the unification of MEN-2 syndromes as a group of neuroectodermal neoplasms carrying a RET (*re*arranged during *t*ransfection) mutation. This gene codes for a tyrosine kinase specific to neural crest cells.

Embryological Switch of the Parathyroids

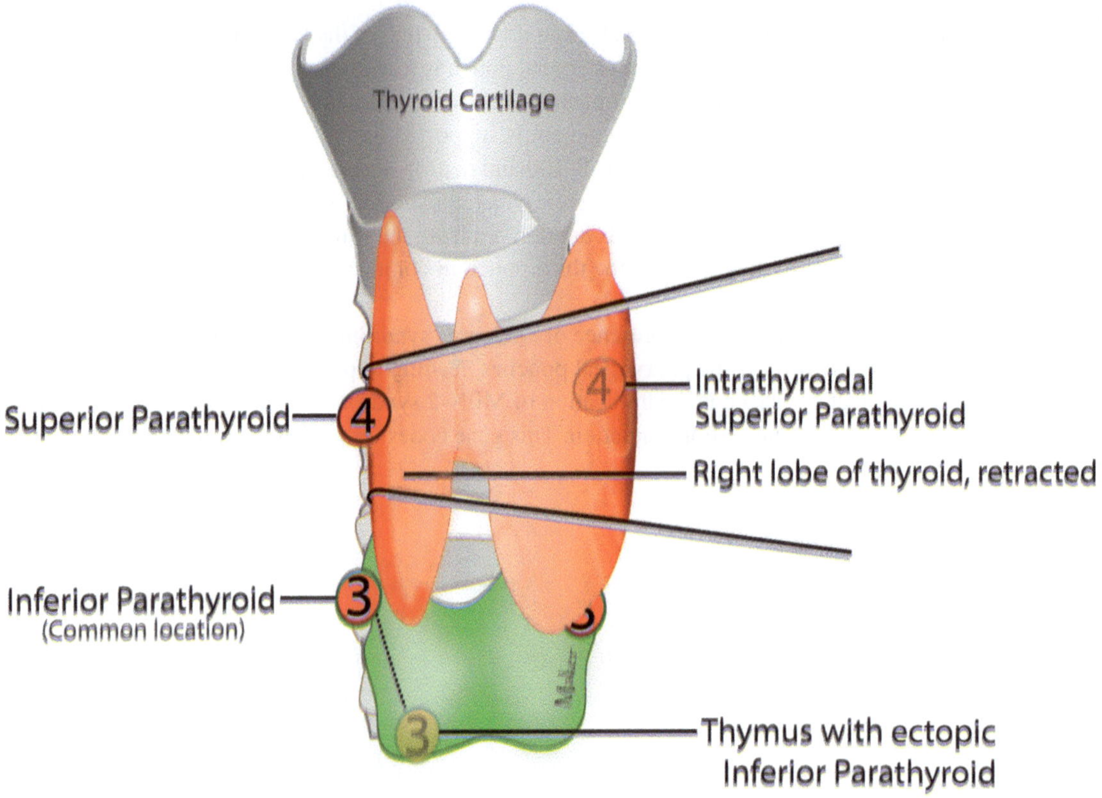

Fig. 1.18 *1* Inferior parathyroids and the thymus develop from the third branchial pouch and descend further than the fourth branchial pouch to occupy the lower position during the embryologic development. *2* The inferior parathyroid, when not found in the usual position, can be in the thymus. *3* The superior parathyroid and lateral lobes of the thyroid develop from the fourth branchial pouch. They have a shorter descent than the inferior parathyroids and hence, end up in the embryologically switched position at a higher level in the posterior and medial part of the thyroid gland. *4* The superior parathyroid, when not found in other aberrant locations, may be intrathyroidal and require ipsilateral thyroid lobectomy for removal

Answer

c

18. Regarding parathyroid anatomy and physiology, all of the following are correct *except*:
    (a) Both the superior and inferior parathyroids are most commonly supplied by the inferior thyroid artery.
    (b) In the absence of an inferior thyroid artery, all parathyroids are most commonly supplied by the superior thyroid artery.
    (c) Parathyroid adenomas may continue their abnormal production of PTH in spite of devascularization.
    (d) The main types of cells found in the parathyroids are chief and oxyphilic.
    (e) Elevated calcium levels increase PTH secretion.

Comments As discussed previously [12] the blood supply for both superior and inferior parathyroids is mainly derived from the inferior thyroid artery. The parathyroid glands have the capability to survive in the absence of direct arterial supply. This feature makes autotransplantation possible. Parathyroid autotransplantation is carried out by dividing the gland into very thin slices with the purpose of increasing its angiogenic area. These slices are placed into a vascular bed such as the muscle. Parathyroid adenomas hypersecrete PTH because they have lost the negative feedback induced by calcium.

Answer
e

19. All of the following are correct *except*:
    (a) The usual site of a tracheostomy is the third or fourth tracheal ring.
    (b) The thyroid isthmus may be elevated but not divided to facilitate tracheal exposure.
    (c) In emergent cricothyroidotomy a vertical skin incision should be used, but the cricothyroid membrane is incised horizontally.
    (d) Injury to the brachiocephalic vessels can occur secondary to a tracheostomy.
    (e) An inadequate curvature in the tracheostomy tube may lead to erosion into the tracheal wall and into other structures.

Comments The incisions performed during an emergent cricothyroidotomy are thought out to minimize bleeding. A vertical skin incision in the midline offers the fastest exposure and allows extension if necessary. The cricothyroid membrane is best incised horizontally in its lower aspect to minimize the likelihood of injury to the cricothyroid artery, which runs horizontally along its superior aspect.

During elective tracheostomy the thyroid isthmus can be safely divided to expose the trachea. Delayed complications of tracheostomy include erosion into adjacent structures like the esophagus and innominate vein.

Answer
b

20. All of the following are correct *except*:
    (a) The salivary glands are of endodermal origin, starting as outgrowths of the oral epithelium.
    (b) Stensen's duct drains the parotid gland and enters the mouth at the level of the second upper molar.
    (c) The facial nerve has multiple branches innervating the parotid gland.
    (d) The parotid gland is supplied by the external carotid artery.
    (e) Regarding the structures embedded in the parotid parenchyma, the facial nerve is superficial, the artery is deep, and the veins are intermediate.

Comments Even though the facial nerve is embedded within the parotid parenchyma, it does not innervate this gland. It enters the gland from its posterior aspect, and within one centimeter from this entry point, it divides into its five branches. The facial nerve divides the gland in a superficial and a deep portion.

Answer
c

21. All of the following are correct *except*:
    (a) The majority of parotid tumors are malignant, whereas tumors in the submandibular gland tend to be benign.
    (b) Benign tumors of the parotid should be treated by nerve-preserving lobectomy.
    (c) Frey's syndrome is caused by injury to intraparotid branches of the auriculotemporal nerve.
    (d) The most important anatomical landmark for identifying the facial nerve trunk during parotidectomy is the tympanomastoid suture.
    (e) The most common tumor of the parotid gland is a pleomorphic adenoma.

Comments Most tumors of the parotid gland are benign. Superficial parotidectomy with sparing of the facial nerve is the treatment of choice in these instances. This operation is also indicated for the treatment of melanoma of the temporal and zygomatic areas, which may spread through lymph nodes into the superficial parotid. The parotid gland has both intra- and extraglandular lymphatics which communicate superiorly with the lymphatics of the face above the oral commissure and inferiorly continue into the cervical lymph nodes [20–22] (Fig. 1.19).

The auriculotemporal nerve is a branch of the trigeminal nerve, carrying the parasympathetic fibers to the parotid gland as well as sensory fibers to the external ear canal and the temporomandibular joint. It enters the gland from its posterosuperior aspect. In the course of a superficial parotidectomy, fibers derived from this nerve are exposed on the cut surface of the gland. These fibers may synapse with the sweat glands and vasomotor nerves of the skin overlying the area. When this occurs, stimulation of the parotid gland also triggers sweating and reddening of the area.

The great auricular nerve is derived from C2 and C3. It may be injured in dissections between the angle of the mandible and the ear lobe, area where it courses parallel to the sternocleidomastoid muscle. Its injury causes temporary numbness to the preauricular region and lower ear lobe.

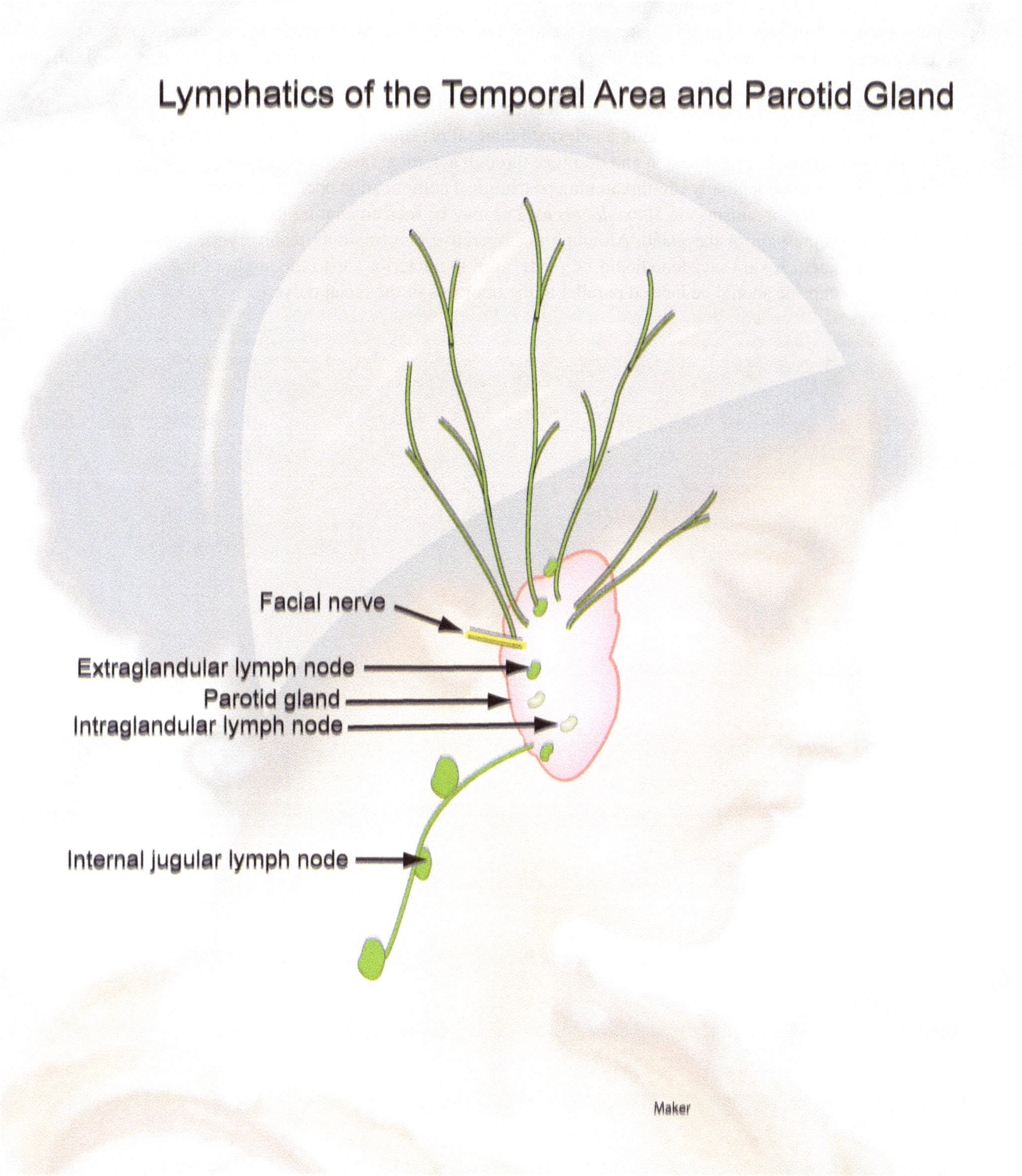

Fig. 1.19 Lymphatics of the temporal area of the scalp often travel through the superficial parotid gland en route to the lymph nodes in the neck. This is particularly relevant to the extent of lymph node dissection during surgery, especially for malignant melanoma of the temporal scalp

Answer
a

22. Mark the incorrect statement regarding postoperative parotitis.
    (a) Inflammation of the parotid gland is intensely painful due to the unyielding nature of the parotid fascia.
    (b) Predisposing factors for this potentially life-threatening complication are debility, dehydration, depressed salivation, and poor oral hygiene.
    (c) The mechanism of infection is the transductal invasion by oral bacteria.
    (d) Parotid abscesses do not fluctuate due to an elevated internal pressure and tense parotid fascia.
    (e) The proper treatment is deep incision and drainage through a vertical incision of the parotid fascia.

Postoperative parotitis is a potentially life-threatening postsurgical complication occurring in debilitated elderly individuals. The most common microorganisms are *Staphylococcus*. Pus may be seen emanating from Stensen's duct, either spontaneously or through compression of the gland. Although postoperative parotitis may resolve with conservative measures, drainage is often indicated. A skin incision should be made from the anterior ear to the angle of the mandible. Once the parotid is exposed, its capsule should be incised parallel to the branches of the facial nerve.

Answer

c

23. Select the *incorrect* statement regarding embryologic remnants of the neck.
    (a) Cervicoauricular fistulas extend from the external auditory canal to the angle of the mouth.
    (b) Cervicoauricular fistulas lie anterior to the facial nerve.
    (c) Lateral cervical fistulas are remnants of the second brachial cleft and pouch, extending to the tonsillar fossa. The fistula courses through the bifurcation of the carotid artery.
    (d) Sinuses are usually found at the anterior border of the sternocleidomastoid.
    (e) Cervical cysts arise from incomplete closure of the brachial clefts or pouches and may lie next to the skin, carotid, jugular, or pharynx.

Comments Cervicoauricular fistulas are remnants of the first branchial cleft, which forms the external auditory canal. They course caudally to open near the angle of the jaw. Although they are intrinsically asymptomatic, manifesting as a skin pit, they may become secondarily infected. In this case, the draining sinus tract must be excised completely.

The second pharyngeal arch gives rise to the muscles of expression. It is innervated by the facial nerve and its blood supply is provided by the external carotid. The third arch is innervated by the glossopharyngeal nerve, and its blood supply comes from the internal carotid. The second branchial cleft is located between these two arches. This explains why fistulas derived from this cleft course between the internal and external carotid arteries.

Answer

a

24. The following structures must be preserved during a classic radical neck dissection *except*:
    (a) Thyroid gland
    (b) Sternocleidomastoid muscle
    (c) Carotid artery
    (d) Subclavian artery
    (e) Mandibular branch of the facial nerve

Comments See question 26.

25. All of the following are correct, in a radical neck dissection, *except*:
    (a) The internal jugular vein is sacrificed.
    (b) The deep cervical fascia must be excised.
    (c) The carotid artery is preserved
    (d) The vagus nerve is sacrificed.
    (e) The platysma muscle is left intact en bloc with the skin flaps.

Comments See question 26.

26. Regarding radical neck dissection all of the following are correct *except*:
    (a) The internal jugular vein should be ligated as proximal as possible.
    (b) After ligation of the internal jugular vein, the main route of collateral flow is the ipsilateral vertebral vein.
    (c) Infiltration of the area around the carotid sinus is used to ameliorate the vasovagal response associated with its manipulation.
    (d) Vigilance should be exercised regarding the possibility of air embolism when manipulating the jugular veins.
    (e) The spinal accessory nerve may be sacrificed without functional or aesthetic consequences.

Comments Radical neck dissection is a procedure that over the years has become more restricted in its indications as well as in the extent of tissue sacrificed. Classically, it involved the removal of the internal jugular vein, the cervical lymph node levels I through V (located along the internal jugular vein), the sternocleidomastoid muscle, and the spinal accessory nerve. In other words, all lymph nodes and associated structures from the angle of the mandible to the clavicle and from the anterior border of the trapezius to (and including) the sternocleidomastoid muscle were removed. Currently, the sternocleidomastoid muscle, internal jugular vein, and spinal accessory nerve may be preserved when not invaded by tumor, constituting a modified radical neck dissection [23] (Fig. 1.20).

The lymph nodes of the neck are grouped as follows [24, 25]:

Level I:
- IA Submental
- IB Submandibular

Level II – Upper jugular group:
- IIA Anteroinferior to the spinal accessory nerve
- IIB Posterosuperior to the spinal accessory nerve

Level III – Middle jugular group

Level IV – Lower jugular group

Level V – Posterior triangle group:
- VA Superior to the cricoid cartilage
- VB Inferior to the cricoid cartilage

Level VI – Central anterior neck group

Level VII – Anterior superior mediastinal nodes (Figs. 1.21 and 1.22)

Level VI is the most commonly involved lymph node basin in thyroid cancer, both papillary and follicular. In this instance, a central neck dissection is indicated. This procedure is always bilateral and includes the pre- and paratracheal, pre-cricoid (Delphian), and perithyroidal nodes. The lateral limits are the carotid arteries, the superior limit is the hyoid bone, and the inferior limit was classically defined as the suprasternal notch [26]. However, due to anatomic continuity in lymphatic drainage and the access afforded from a neck incision, central lymph node dissection is often extended to encompass level IV nodes. In this instance, the innominate and subclavian veins become the inferior marker of the dissection [25]. The presence of the BRAF V600E mutation in biopsy samples of papillary thyroid cancer is predictive of lymph node involvement and may help guide the extent of lymphadenectomy at the time of surgery [27].

Among the structures that are always preserved are the thyroid and parathyroids (unless they are the source of tumor); the common, external, and internal carotids; the subclavian vessels; and the vagus nerve [28].

The sacrifice of the spinal accessory nerve brings about multiple sequelae. There is denervation of the trapezius, which causes inability to elevate the shoulder, limits arm abduction, and induces atrophy of this muscle.

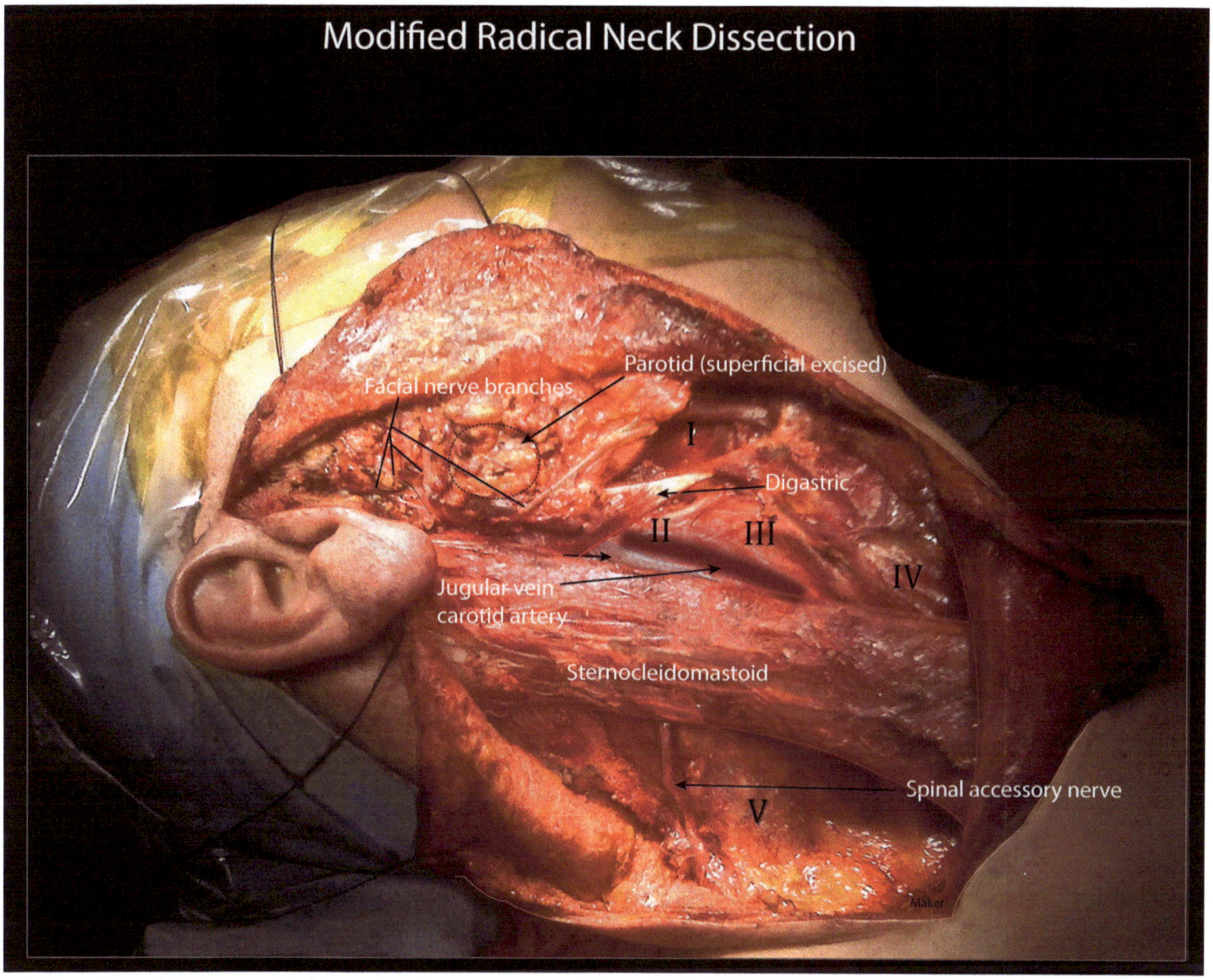

Fig. 1.20 Modified radical neck dissection

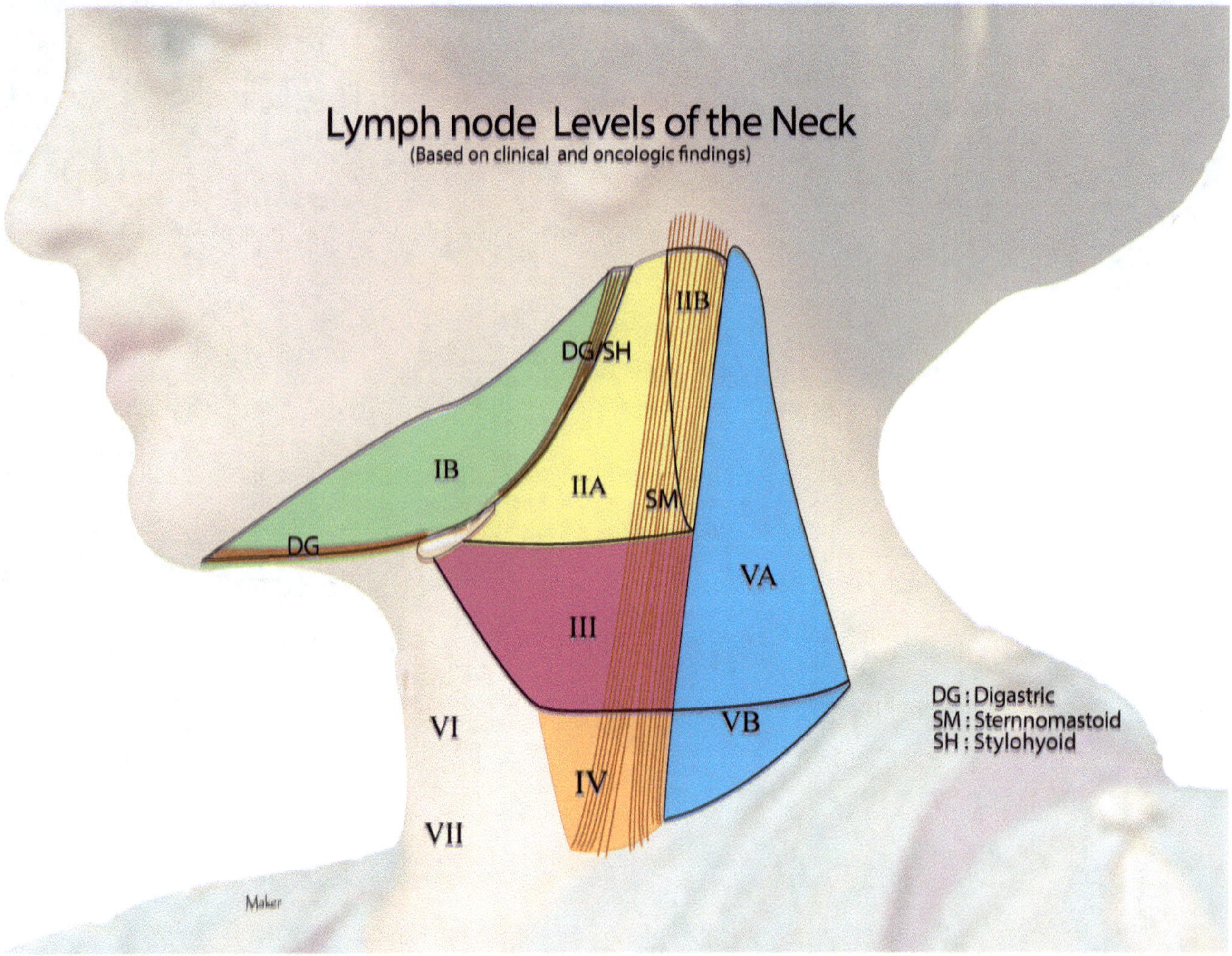

Fig. 1.21 The lateral group of lymph nodes of the neck include levels 1–5. Level 1 is further subdivided into a single level 1a bounded by anterior bellies of the right and left digastric muscle and 1b by the anterior belly of the digastric anteriorly, stylohyoid muscle posteriorly, and the mandible superiorly. Level 2 is subdivided into 2a and 2b by the accessory nerve and level 5 into level 5a and 5b by an axial plane at the level of the cricoid cartilage. The trapezius muscle marks the posterior boundary of level 5. Level 3 represents the middle jugular and level 4 the low jugular lymph nodes. Each of these levels is bounded by the sternohyoid muscle anteriorly and the posterior border of the sternocleidomastoid posteriorly. Transverse axial plane at the level of the cricoid cartilage divides level 3 from level 4. While most lymph nodes in the neck drain head and neck areas, level 4 lymph nodes include lymph drainage from the body below the clavicles, especially on the left side where the thoracic duct drains

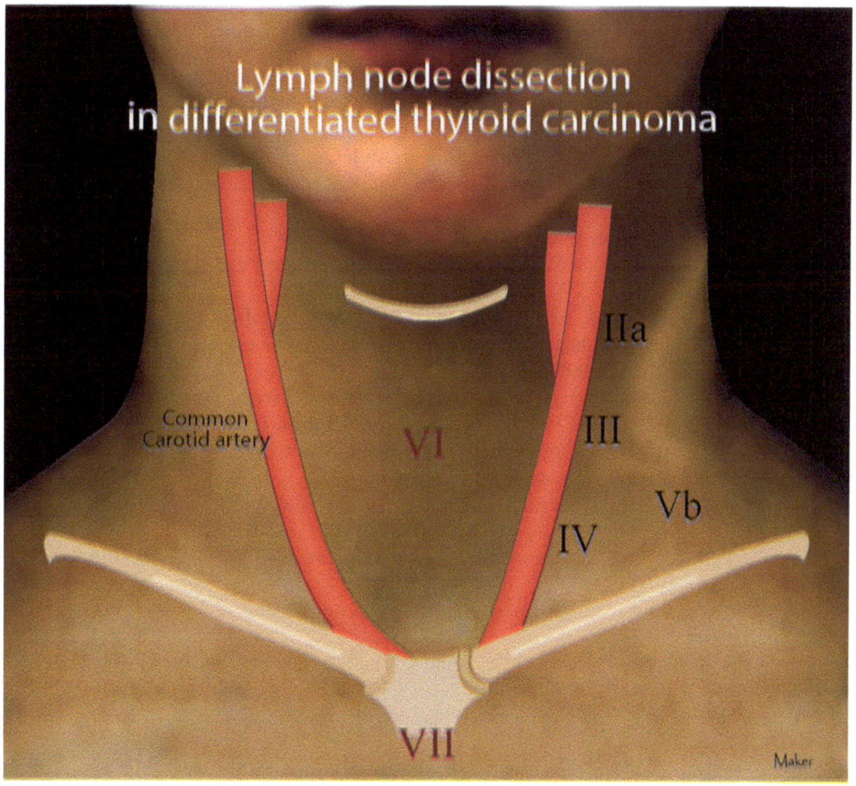

Fig. 1.22 The central compartment of the neck consists of lymph node levels 6 and 7. It is bounded laterally by the carotid arteries, superiorly by the hyoid bone, and inferiorly by the innominate artery on the right and its corresponding axial plane on the left

Answers
Question 24: b
Question 25: d
Question 26: e

References

1. Miller MB, Cohn AS. Case report: fourth branchial pouch sinus. Ear Nose Throat J. 1993;72(5):356–8.
2. Pilarski R, Nagy R. Genetic testing by cancer site: endocrine system. Cancer J. 2012;18(4):364–71.
3. Marple BF. Ludwig angina: a review of current airway management. Arch Otolaryngol Head Neck Surg. 1999;125(5):596–9.
4. Shockley WW. Ludwig angina: a review of current airway management. Arch Otolaryngol Head Neck Surg. 1999;125(5):600.
5. Knight Jr TT, Gonzalez JA, Rary JM, Rush DS. Current concepts for the surgical management of carotid body tumor. Am J Surg. 2006;191(1):104–10.
6. Ferrante MA. The thoracic outlet syndromes. Muscle Nerve. 2012;45(6):780–95.
7. Lee JT, Karwowski JK, Harris EJ, Haukoos JS, Olcott C. Long-term thrombotic recurrence after nonoperative management of Paget-Schroetter syndrome. J Vasc Surg. 2006;43(6):1236–43.
8. Philpott CM, Selvadurai D, Banerjee AR. Paediatric retropharyngeal abscess. J Laryngol Otol. 2004;118(12):919–26.
9. Sato K, Izumi T, Toshima M, Nagai T, Muroi K, Komatsu N, et al. Retropharyngeal abscess due to methicillin-resistant Staphylococcus aureus in a case of acute myeloid leukemia. Intern Med. 2005;44(4):346–9.
10. Larawin V, Naipao J, Dubey SP. Head and neck space infections. Otolaryngol Head Neck Surg. 2006;135(6):889–93.
11. McGovern Jr PJ, Swan KG. Management of bilateral internal jugular venous injuries. Injury. 1985;16(4):259–60.
12. Wen Y, Zhou S, Wang C. Compensation of external jugular vein to the reflux of cerebral blood after bilateral ligation of the internal jugular vein. Zhonghua Kou Qiang Yi Xue Za Zhi. 2000;35(1):64–6.
13. Maves MD, Bruns MD, Keenan MJ. Carotid artery resection for head and neck cancer. Ann Otol Rhinol Laryngol. 1992;101(9):778–81.
14. Amedee RG, Dhurandhar NR. Fine-needle aspiration biopsy. Laryngoscope. 2001;111(9):1551–7.
15. Wahl RA, Vorlander C, Kriener S, Pedall J, Spitza M, Hansmann ML. Isthmus-preserving total bilobectomy: an adequate operation for C-cell hyperplasia. World J Surg. 2006;30(5):860–71.
16. Yumoto E, Sanuki T, Kumai Y. Immediate recurrent laryngeal nerve reconstruction and vocal outcome. Laryngoscope. 2006;116(9):1657–61.
17. Weber CJ, Marangos PJ, Richardson S, LoGerfo P, Hardy MA, Feind C, et al. Presence of neuron-specific enolase and somatostatin in human parathyroid tissues. Surgery. 1985;98(6):1008–12.
18. Zabel M, Dietel M. S-100 protein and neuron-specific enolase in parathyroid glands and C-cells of the thyroid. Histochemistry. 1987;86(4):389–92.
19. Machens A, Dralle H. Multiple endocrine neoplasia type 2 and the RET protooncogene: from bedside to bench to bedside. Mol Cell Endocrinol. 2006;247(1–2):34–40.
20. Lin D, Franc BL, Kashani-Sabet M, Singer MI. Lymphatic drainage patterns of head and neck cutaneous melanoma observed on lymphoscintigraphy and sentinel lymph node biopsy. Head Neck. 2006;28(3):249–55.
21. O'Brien CJ, Uren RF, Thompson JF, Howman-Giles RB, Petersen-Schaefer K, Shaw HM, et al. Prediction of potential metastatic sites in cutaneous head and neck melanoma using lymphoscintigraphy. Am J Surg. 1995;170(5):461–6.
22. Storm FK, Eilber FR, Sparks FC, Morton DL. A prospective study of parotid metastases from head and neck cancer. Am J Surg. 1977;134(1):115–9.
23. Patel KN, Shah JP. Neck dissection: past, present, future. Surg Oncol Clin N Am. 2005;14(3):461–77, vi.
24. Carty SE, Cooper DS, Doherty GM, Duh QY, Kloos RT, Mandel SJ, et al. Consensus statement on the terminology and classification of central neck dissection for thyroid cancer. Thyroid. 2009;19(11):1153–8.
25. Stack Jr BC, Ferris RL, Goldenberg D, Haymart M, Shaha A, Sheth S, et al. American Thyroid Association consensus review and statement regarding the anatomy, terminology, and rationale for lateral neck dissection in differentiated thyroid cancer. Thyroid. 2012;22(5):501–8.
26. Shaha AR. TNM classification of thyroid carcinoma. World J Surg. 2007;31(5):879–87.
27. Howell GM, Nikiforova MN, Carty SE, Armstrong MJ, Hodak SP, Stang MT, et al. BRAF V600E mutation independently predicts central compartment lymph node metastasis in patients with papillary thyroid cancer. Ann Surg Oncol. 2013;20(1):47–52.
28. Ferlito A, Rinaldo A, Silver CE, Shah JP, Suarez C, Medina JE, et al. Neck dissection: then and now. Auris Nasus Larynx. 2006;33(4):365–74.

2 Thoracic Wall and Pleura

1. All of the following are correct *except*
   (a) The ribs, sternum, and intercostal musculature arise from the mesoderm.
   (b) The ribs develop from processes arising from the sternum.
   (c) The sternum develops from two independent ventral mesenchymal condensations known as sternal bars.
   (d) The sternal bars are originally paired, but later in development they "zipper" together in craniocaudal direction.
   (e) Complete rib ossification is achieved at age 20–25.

Comments The muscular and bony elements of the thoracic wall are of mesodermal origin. The ribs arise from the vertebra and extend to the anterior midline following a curvilinear course, joining the sternum through costal cartilages. Anomalies of this developmental process are thought to be the cause of pectus excavatum, which is the most common chest wall deformity (1:400 children).

The sternum is derived from paired sternal bars in the anterior midline. These structures fuse in craniocaudal direction and articulate with the first seven ribs. When this process fails to occur, the separation left in the anterior midline creates aesthetic deformity (bifid sternum) and may allow herniation of the mediastinal structures as well as of the lungs. Association of this pathology with cardiac anomalies has been reported [1, 2].

Answer
b

V.K. Maker, E.D. Guzman-Arrieta, *Cognitive Pearls in General Surgery*,
DOI 10.1007/978-1-4939-1850-8_2,

2. The angle of Louis, corresponding to T4–T5, marks the following *except*:
   (a) Division of the mediastinum into superior and inferior
   (b) Beginning and end of the aortic arch
   (c) Bifurcation of the trachea
   (d) Origin of the superior vena cava
   (e) Positioning of the thoracic duct to the right of the spine

Comments The angle of Louis represents the junction of the sternal manubrium and sternal body. It is a key landmark in thoracic anatomy. While it is true that the thoracic duct starts to the right of the spine at its origin in the cisterna chyli, it crosses the midline towards the left starting at T6 level, to reach the left subclavian vein [3] (Fig. 2.1).

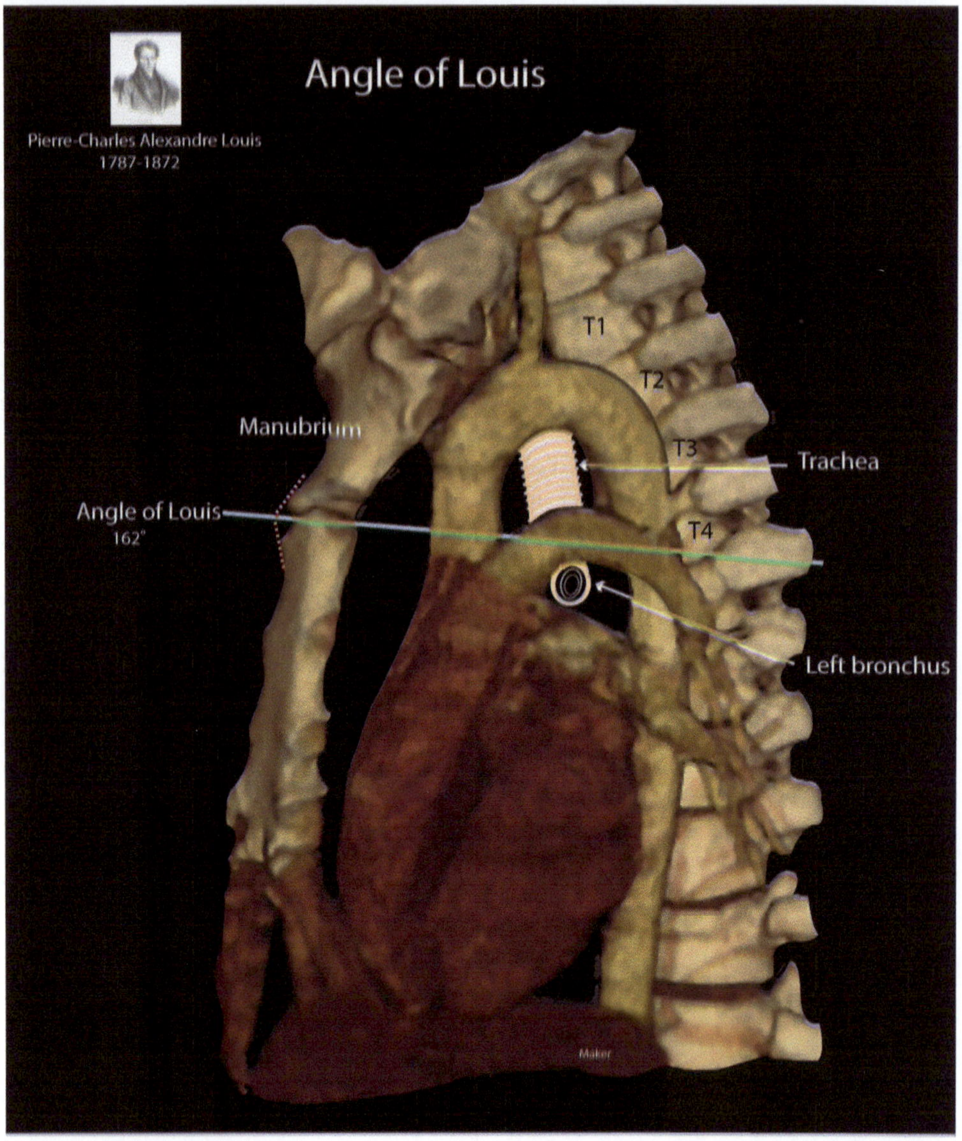

Fig. 2.1 Angle of Louis. Pierre-Charles-Alexandre Louis, a nineteenth century French physician, was of the first to bring mathematics to medicine. The angle of Louis is approximately 162° in males and marks a plane from the second costal cartilage to the lower border of T4 vertebra posteriorly. This is an important anatomical landmark in the chest and represents division of the superior from the inferior mediastinum

Answer

e

3. All of the following are correct *except*:
   (a) The ribs are classified into seven true ribs, five false ribs, and two floating ribs.
   (b) The ribs are staggered between the thoracic vertebrae, articulating with two of them at the same time, superiorly and inferiorly.
   (c) Cervical ribs are found in 1 % of the population, causing symptoms in 10 % of affected individuals.
   (d) The costal groove, running along the inferior border of the rib, contains intercostal neurovascular bundle.
   (e) In the newborn, the intercostal muscles play a key role during breathing.

Comments Ribs are classified into three categories. True ribs are joined to the sternum by the costal cartilages. False ribs are joined to superior ribs by cartilages that in conjunction form the costal arch. Floating ribs do not articulate anteriorly, but are stabilized by the intercostal muscles. In adults, the ribs are placed in a fashion similar to bucket handles, where upon contraction of the intercostals muscles, they are pulled superiorly and anteriorly increasing the diameter of the thoracic cavity and contributing to the negative intrathoracic pressure resulting in inspiration. In contrast, newborns exhibit a nearly horizontal orientation of the ribs. They are unable to generate further radial expansion of the thoracic cavity and rely on craniocaudal expansion through diaphragmatic action for ventilation [4].

The relationship of the intercostal neurovascular bundle to the rib largely dictates the technique for tube thoracostomy and intercostal blocks. Given that the bundle runs along the lower margin of the rib, it is safest to access the pleural cavity along the upper margin of the rib, thus avoiding vascular laceration and subsequent bleeding [5] (Fig. 2.2).

The elements of the neurovascular bundle are arranged with the vein in cranial position, the nerve in caudal position, and the artery in between. They originate posteriorly, at a level more caudal than that of the inferior border of the rib and thus follow an ascending diagonal course towards the rib, making them more accessible posteriorly for an intercostal block. Once they join the rib, they follow a discretely spiral course towards the inferior inner margin of the rib. The neurovascular bundle is deep to the intercostal muscles and immediately adjacent to the pleura [6] (Fig. 2.3).

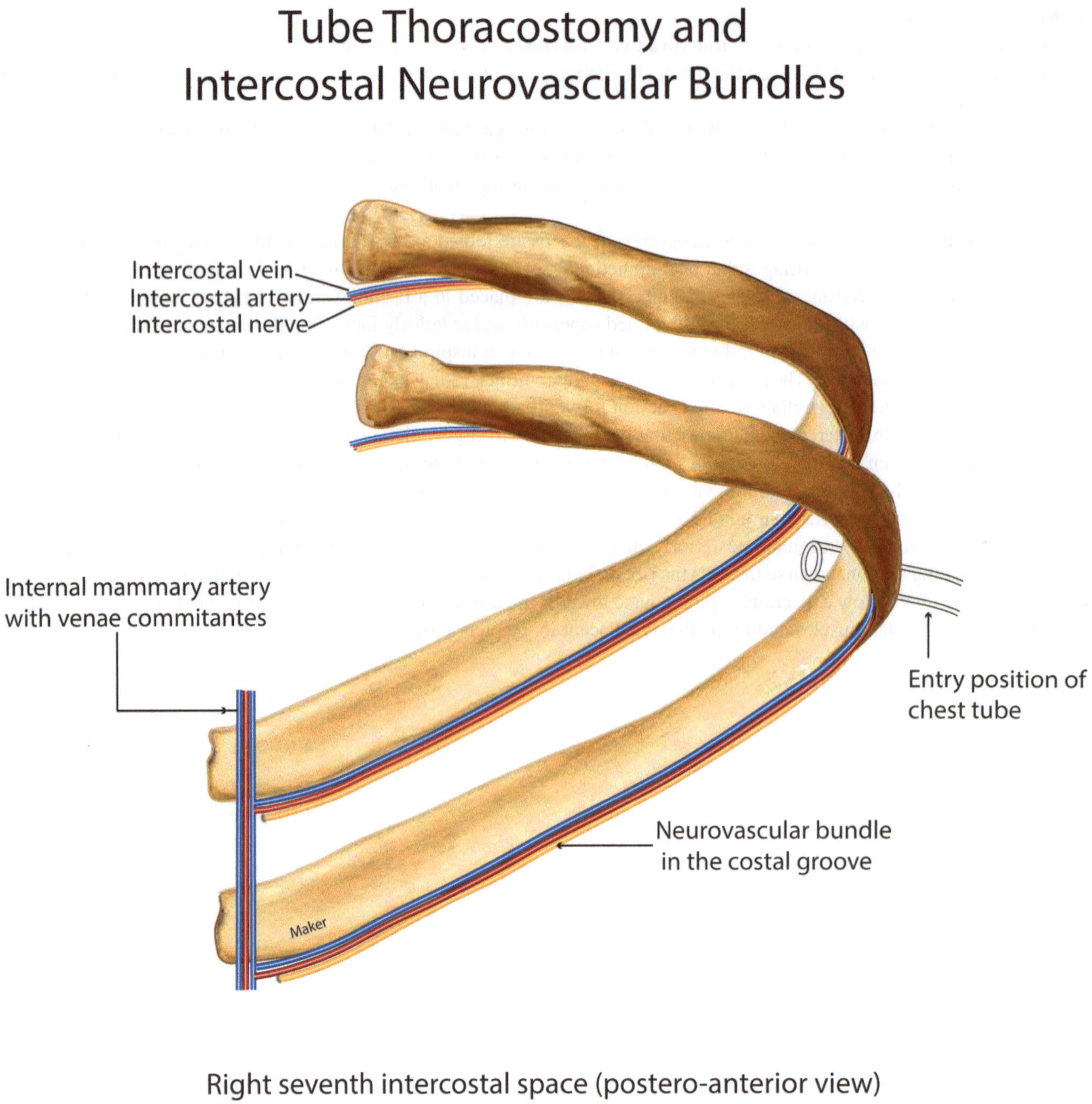

Fig. 2.2 Tube thoracostomy. A chest tube (tube thoracostomy) is typically inserted to drain air or fluid from the pleural cavity. The safest point of entry into the chest cavity is just above the upper border of a rib in the intercostal space. In this location, there is the least chance of injury to the neurovascular bundle. For fluid drainage, a chest tube is inserted laterally near the anterior axillary line and in the safest lower intercostal space for dependent drainage

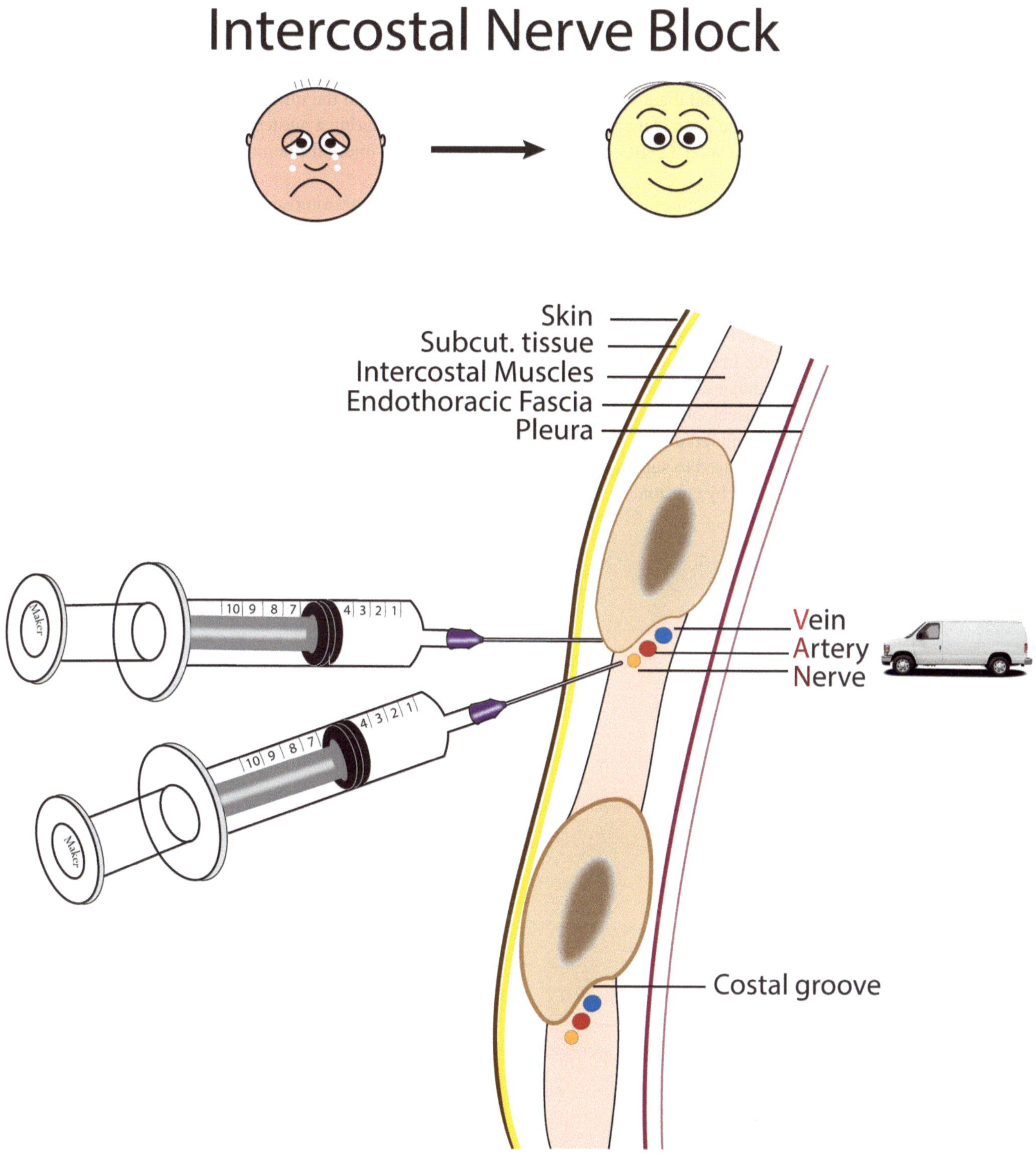

Fig. 2.3 Intercostal block. Two to three inches lateral to the post midline, intercostal nerves are in the ideal location for an intercostal nerve block. The needle is advanced until it approaches the lower border of the rib. Gradually, the needle is walked down the lower border of the rib until it advances. Here, the needle is tilted up to the neurovascular bundle. It is aspirated, and if no blood is aspirated, long-acting local anesthetic is infiltrated. For fractured ribs, two intercostal nerves above and below the fracture are blocked for excellent pain relief and avoidance of atelectasis

Answer

e

4. All of the following are correct *except*:
   (a) The internal mammary artery gives the anterior intercostals, which anastomose with the posterior intercostals arising from the thoracic aorta.
   (b) The distal branches of the internal mammary are the superior epigastric and the musculophrenic arteries.
   (c) The perforating branches of the internal mammary artery may be injured during a mastectomy and retract into the chest.
   (d) Sternal wound complications after CABG are similar when either the internal mammary artery or saphenous vein grafts are used.
   (e) The superior epigastric artery supplies the rectus abdominis muscle and anastomoses with the larger inferior epigastric artery, a branch of the iliac artery.

Comments The internal mammary artery represents the main blood supply to the sternum. Its use in the course of CABG procedures (specially when bilateral) increases the risk of sternal wound infection, mediastinitis, and wound dehiscence. Diabetic patients are at greater risk for this complication [7].

The perforating branches of the internal mammary artery emerge through the six upper intercostal spaces and supply the medial aspects of the pectoralis major and breast. When transected during mastectomy, it is possible for them to retract and bleed into the chest cavity. The musculophrenic artery, one of the terminal branches of the internal mammary artery, supplies the anterior diaphragm. It may be injured during mobilization of the liver and esophageal hiatus.

The superior epigastric artery is used to supply the transverse rectus abdominis myocutaneous flap (TRAM). The blood supply of this flap may be enhanced by anastomosing the inferior epigastric to the axillary vessels (supercharging) [8].

Answer
d

5. Select the false alternative regarding the posterior intercostal vessels.
   (a) The posterior intercostals are dorsal to the esophagus, azygos, and thoracic duct.
   (b) The posterior intercostals give a dorsal branch, responsible for the irrigation of the paraspinal muscles as well as the spinal cord (spinal artery).
   (c) The most significant of the spinal arteries is known as the great radicular artery of Adamkiewicz and is constant in its location at T6 level on the left.
   (d) It is often the only source of spinal perfusion below T10.
   (e) Cross clamping of the aorta above the artery of Adamkiewicz may result in paraplegia.

Comments The blood supply to the spinal cord is provided by three main sources, the vertebral arteries, the posterior intercostal arteries (giving rise to segmental spinal arteries), and branches of the internal iliac arteries. Together these sources supply a rich vascular plexus that surrounds the spinal cord. This plexus has three main axial trunks: a single anterior spinal artery and two posterior spinal arteries, with the former supplying the anterior 2/3 and the latter the posterior 1/3. These three vessels anastomose at the conus medullaris creating a "spinal circle of Willis" [9–12].

The great radicular artery of Adamkiewicz is an important source of blood supply to the lower spinal cord. This large segmental spinal artery has a variable origin, arising anywhere from the 6th to 12th intercostal arteries. Aortic cross clamping above this artery may induce ischemic injury to the spinal cord causing paraplegia, most often presenting as anterior spinal cord syndrome [11] (Fig. 2.4).

Artery of Adamkiewicz

Surgeon's Nightmare of Postoperative Paraplegia

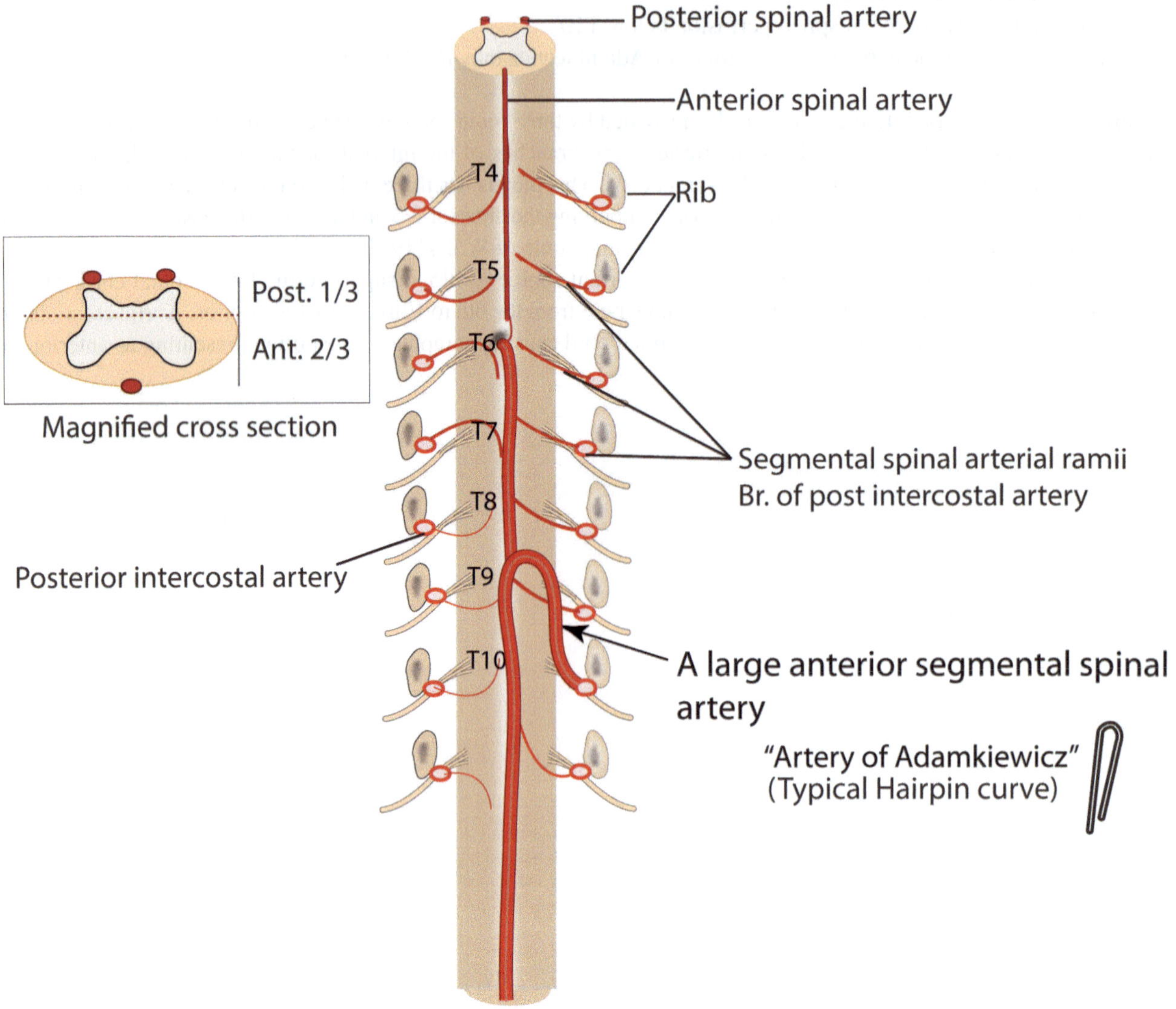

Anterior view of the Spinal cord

Fig. 2.4 Artery of Adamkiewicz. The spinal cord is supplied by a single anterior spinal artery and paired posterior spinal arteries. All three are descending branches of the vertebral arteries. Segmental spinal arterial rami enter through the intervertebral foramina and feed longitudinal anterior and posterior spinal arteries. The artery of Adamkiewicz is typically a large anterior segmental artery, which enters from the left side in a low thoracic or high lumbar intervertebral foramen and connects to the anterior spinal artery. Occlusion of this artery causes paraplegia (anterior spinal cord syndrome) from ischemia of the anterior two thirds of the spinal cord. This is a surgeon's nightmare in surgery of this part of the aorta. Newer techniques have been developed to identify this artery and prevent this injury

Answer

c

6. Select the false alternative regarding chest trauma.
   (a) Fractures of the first three ribs may be associated with brachial plexus and thoracic outlet vascular injuries.
   (b) Fractures of the lower three ribs may be associated with intra-abdominal injury.
   (c) Fractures of ribs three to eight are often associated with significant underlying lung injury
   (d) Paradoxical chest wall movement is the primary mechanism for respiratory failure in flail chest.
   (e) Preexisting pulmonary compromise is an important prognostic factor in chest wall trauma.

Comments As with any bony injury, injury to the surrounding tissues is of the outmost consideration and often determines the central problem, rather than the fracture itself. In the case of rib fractures, injury to the lung may result in pneumothorax and hemothorax, as well as pulmonary contusion, all contributing to respiratory compromise (Fig. 2.5).

Flail chest occurs when there are at least four consecutive ribs with multiple fractures. This creates instability of a segment of chest wall, resulting in paradoxical respiratory movement. The high energy associated with this type of injury also causes significant pulmonary contusion, which is the main determinant of respiratory failure. Pain and hypoventilation also contribute to further respiratory compromise. Management consists of two complementary strategies: pneumatic stabilization and respiratory support via positive pressure ventilation and surgical reconstruction of chest wall stability. Important adjunctive measures include management of respiratory secretions and adequate pain control [13] (Fig. 2.6).

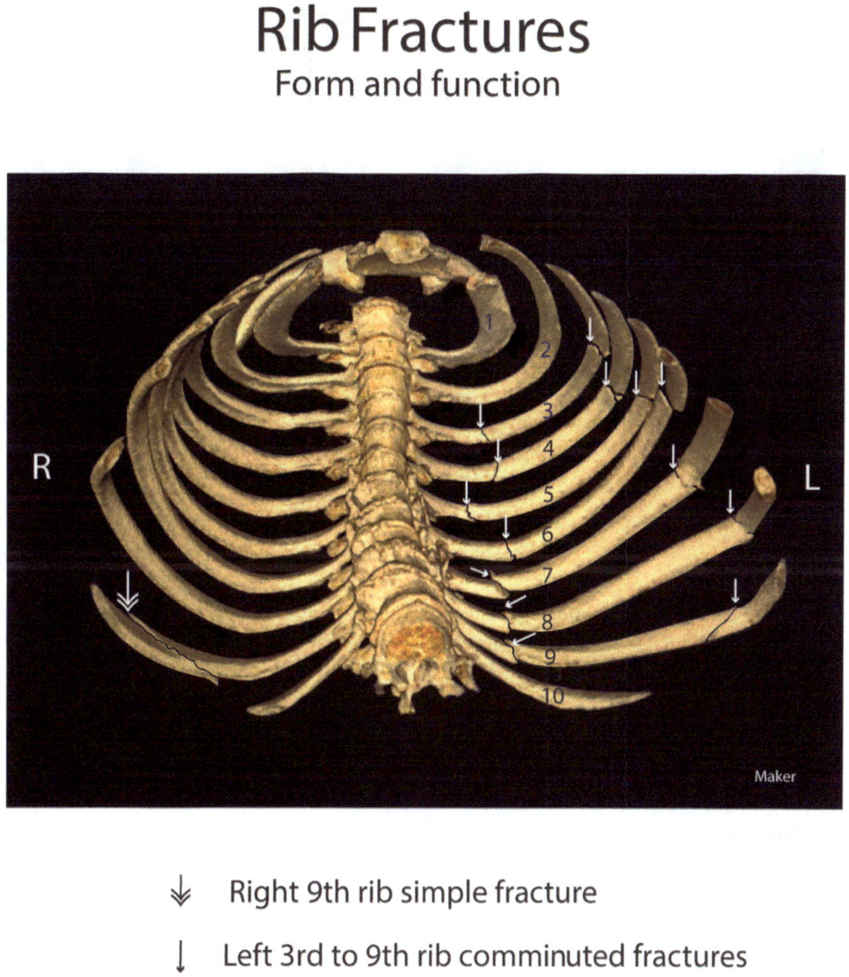

Fig. 2.5 Fractured ribs. All fractured ribs have the potential to cause pain, atelectasis, lung contusion, pneumothorax, and hemothorax. Large segments of comminuted fractured ribs may produce an unstable flail chest. These unstable segments can produce functional problems with respiratory physiology. During inspiration, flail segments move in from the negative intrapleural pressure and move out during expiration causing paradoxical motion

Flail Chest

Pulmonary Contusion

3D CT Scan Lungs Rendition

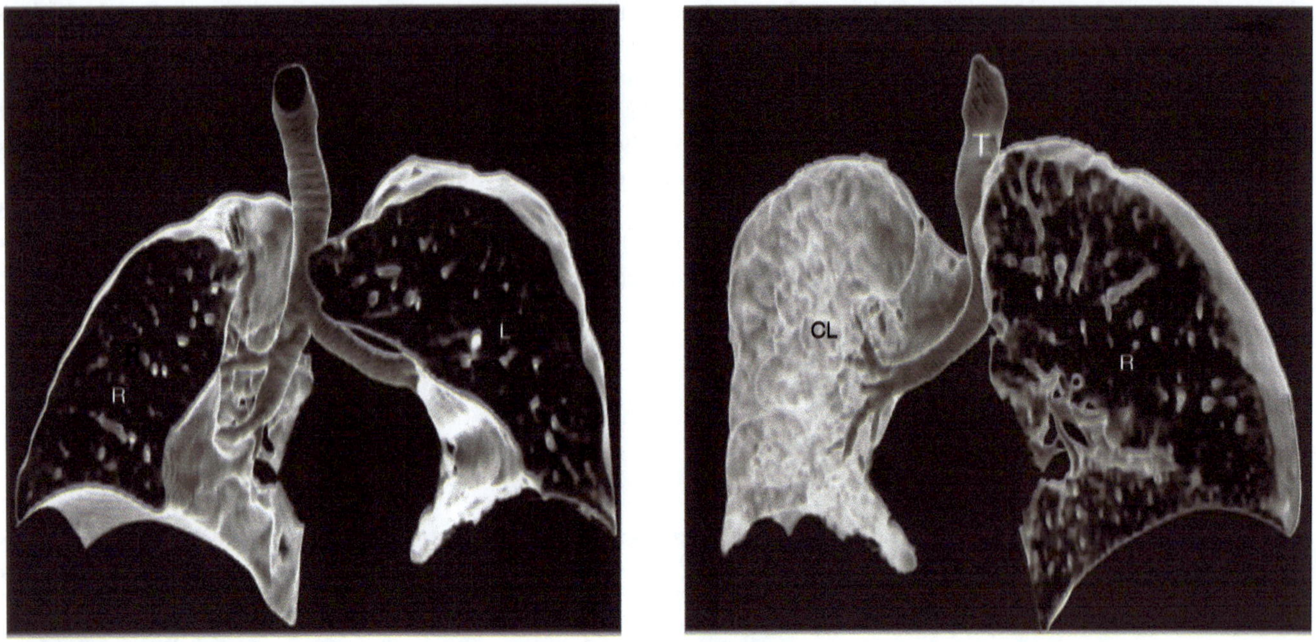

Anterior View Posterior View

T: Trachea and Bronchi
R: Right Lung with normal aeration
L: Left Lung with normal aeration on the anterior part of the Lung
CL: Severe contusion of Left lung with no aeration on its post. aspect

Fig. 2.6 Flail chest and pulmonary contusion. This 50-year-old male sustained multiple fractures to the left second to ninth ribs posteriorly. All of the eight fractured ribs were broken at more than one site producing a flail segment. The admission CT scan was rendered with a 3D software (Vitrea©). The trachea and bronchi are seen with air bronchograms. Posterior rotation of the 3D rendering, reveals a significant contusion of the left lung with a normal bronchus entering the lung but without aeration of alveoli. A pulmonary contusion can result in a ventilation–perfusion mismatch that only exaserbates pain-associated hypoventilation

Answer

d

References

1. Luthra S, Dhaliwal RS, Singh H. Sternal cleft – a natural absurdity or a surgical opportunity. J Pediatr Surg. 2007;42(3):582–4.
2. Padalino MA, Zanon GF, Migneco F, Rubino MG, Fusaro F, Stellin G. Surgical repair of incomplete cleft sternum and cardiac anomalies in early infancy. Ann Thorac Surg. 2006;81(6):2291–4.
3. Skandalakis JE, Skandalakis LJ, Skandalakis PN. Anatomy of the lymphatics. Surg Oncol Clin N Am. 2007;16(1):1–16.
4. Gaultier C. Respiratory muscle function in infants. Eur Respir J. 1995;8(1):150–3.
5. Tomlinson MA, Treasure T. Insertion of a chest drain: how to do it. Br J Hosp Med. 1997;58(6):248–52.
6. Ho AM, Karmakar MK, Critchley LA. Acute pain management of patients with multiple fractured ribs: a focus on regional techniques. Curr Opin Crit Care. 2011;17(4):323–7.
7. Grossi EA, Esposito R, Harris LJ, Crooke GA, Galloway AC, Colvin SB, et al. Sternal wound infections and use of internal mammary artery grafts. J Thorac Cardiovasc Surg. 1991;102(3):342–6.
8. Tachi M, Yamada A. Choice of flaps for breast reconstruction. Int J Clin Oncol. 2005;10(5):289–97.
9. Augoustides JG, Stone ME, Drenger B. Novel approaches to spinal cord protection during thoracoabdominal aortic interventions. Curr Opin Anaesthesiol. 2014;27(1):98–105.
10. Bosmia AN, Hogan E, Loukas M, Tubbs RS, Cohen-Gadol AA. Blood supply to the human spinal cord. I. Anatomy and hemodynamics. Clin Anat. 2013. doi:10.1002/ca.22284. [Epub ahead of print].
11. Tabayashi K. Spinal cord protection during thoracoabdominal aneurysm repair. Surg Today. 2005;35(1):1–6.
12. Brockstein B, Johns L, Gewertz BL. Blood supply to the spinal cord: anatomic and physiologic correlations. Ann Vasc Surg. 1994;8(4):394–9.
13. Molnar TF. Surgical management of chest wall trauma. Thorac Surg Clin. 2010;20(4):475–85.

3 Breast

1. Select the *incorrect* statement regarding the embryogenesis of the breast:
   (a) The glandular tissue of the breast is a modified sebaceous gland; it is of ectodermal origin.
   (b) The stromal tissue of the breast is derived from the mesoderm.
   (c) The nipple is a proliferation of the stratum spinosum.
   (d) The milk lines extend along the thorax and abdomen along the midclavicular line.
   (e) Amastia is often accompanied by absence of the underlying pectoralis major muscle.

Comments During the second month of gestation, two bands of thickened ectoderm develop in the ventral body wall, extending from the axillae to the groins. These are the milk lines and give origin to the breast and nipple. In humans, the pectoral portion gives rise to two mature breasts. However, it is possible for other portions of the milk line to give rise to accessory breast tissue (polymastia), accessory nipples (polythelia), or both. Accessory breast tissue is most common in the axilla. In animals, the milk lines give rise to multiple breasts that are proportional to the size of the litters (Fig. 3.1).

Poland's syndrome consists of absence or hypoplasia of the breast with concurrent underdevelopment or absence of the associated subcutaneous tissue and pectoralis major muscle. The pectoralis minor and ribs 2 through 5 may also be involved. The extensive nature of this defect often requires complex, staged reconstruction [1]. Poland's syndrome is three times more common in boys than girls and affects the right side of the body twice as often as the left. The reasons for these differences are unknown, as is the cause [2].

V.K. Maker, E.D. Guzman-Arrieta, *Cognitive Pearls in General Surgery*,
DOI 10.1007/978-1-4939-1850-8_3, © Springer Science+Business Media New York 2015

Milk Line and Accessory Breast

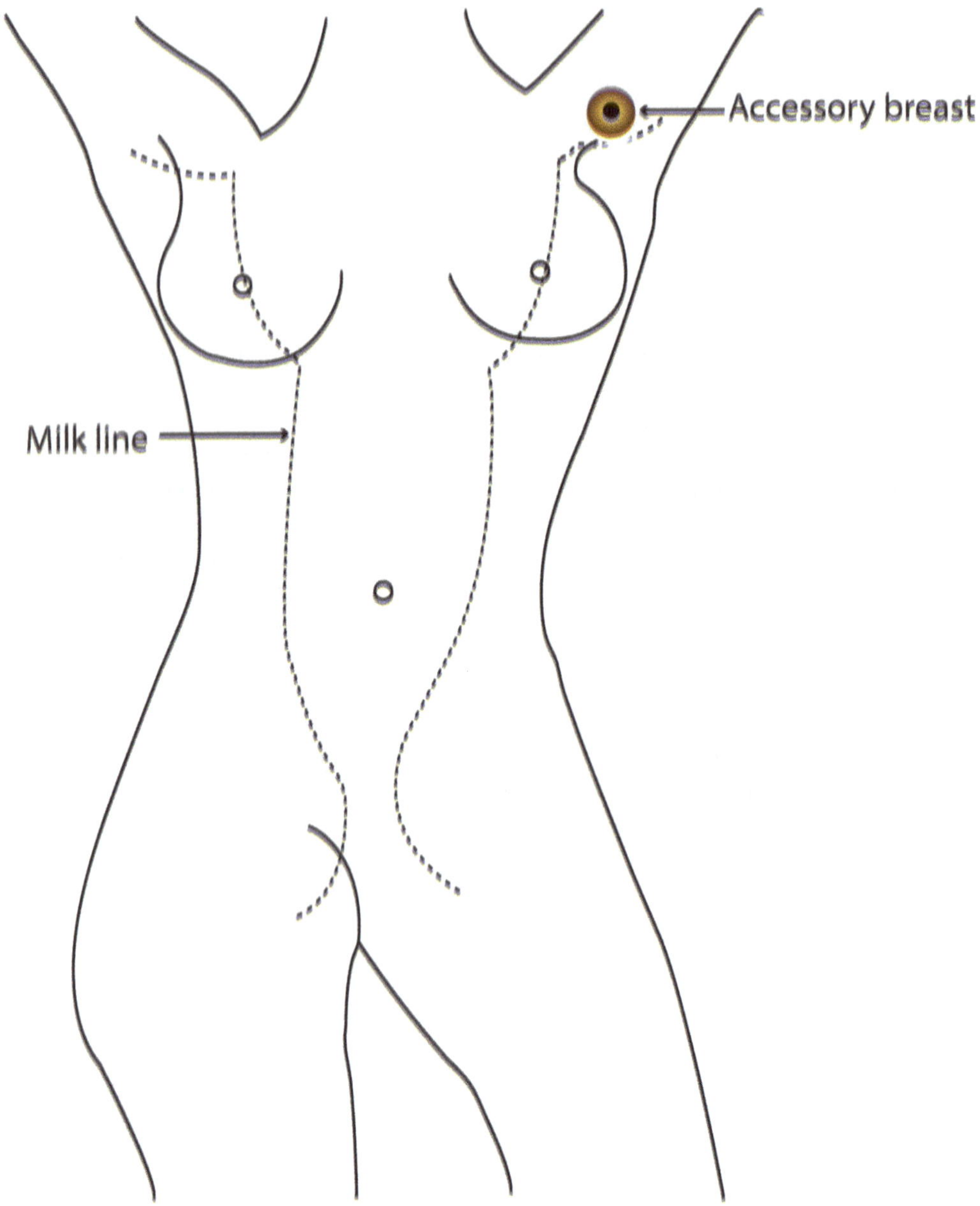

Fig. 3.1 Milk line. Accessory breast tissue in the axilla is the most common ectopic location. Changes with menstruation and pregnancy are diagnostic. Accessory breasts rarely have benign or malignant diseases of the breast. The milk line is an embryologic remnant of the animal kingdom, and extends from the axilla to the groin. It may demonstrate polythelia or polymastia

Answer
d

2. Select the *incorrect* statement regarding the anatomy of the chest wall and axilla.
   (a) The superficial fascia of the breast is continuous with Camper's fascia and the superficial cervical fascia.
   (b) The deep pectoral fascia envelops the pectoralis major.
   (c) The clavipectoral fascia envelops the latissimus dorsi and inserts in the clavicle.
   (d) The clavipectoral fascia is pierced by the cephalic vein.
   (e) The axillary sheath, enveloping the axillary vessels, is an extension of the prevertebral fascia.

Comments The clavipectoral fascia is attached superiorly to the inferior border of the clavicle, surrounding the subclavius muscle. Inferior to the subclavius muscle, the anterior and posterior layers fuse and form the costocoracoid membrane as they travel towards the pectoralis minor muscle. Upon reaching it, the layers once again divide to envelop this muscle. The clavipectoral fascia forms part the anterior wall of the axilla and fuses with the axillary fascia. It must be incised to gain access to the axillary space. This is done along the lateral border of the pectoralis minor, extending into the roof of the axilla along the axillary vein for an excellent exposure to the axilla.

Answer
c

3. All of the following are correct *except*:
   (a) The posterior boundary of an axillary dissection is the latissimus dorsi muscle, which forms the posterior axillary fold.
   (b) The pectoralis minor muscle lies anterior to the axillary vessels and attaches to the coracoid process of the scapula.
   (c) The nerves to the latissimus dorsi and serratus anterior should be preserved in an axillary node dissection, unless involved by tumor.
   (d) The medial and lateral pectoral nerves should be preserved, as they supply the pectoralis major and minor.
   (e) The intercostobrachial nerve is a purely motor nerve.

Comments The axilla is described as pyramidal space with an apex, four walls, and a base. Its contents are lymph nodes and the axillary sheath containing the blood vessels and nerves to the arm. The pectoralis minor muscle is a fan-shaped muscle, which crosses the axillary vessels and divides the axillary lymph nodes into three levels. Level 1 is lateral to the pectoralis minor, level 2 underlies the pectoralis minor, and level 3 is medial to it (Fig. 3.2).

Five nerves are encountered in the course of an axillary node dissection. Some branches of the medial and lateral pectoral nerves run along the lateral edge of the pectoralis minor, innervating it. From there, they travel medially to innervate the pectoralis major. Injury to these nerves may cause muscular atrophy of these muscles.

The long thoracic nerve runs along the midaxillary line and supplies the serratus anterior muscle. Section of this nerve produces winged scapula. The thoracodorsal nerve travels on the anterior edge of the latissimus dorsi muscle, along with the lateral thoracic vessels. Injury to this nerve produces atrophy of said muscle. These four nerves must be preserved, unless directly invaded by cancer. Finally, the intercostobrachial nerve travels parallel to the axillary vessels to reach the skin of the inner arm. It is a purely sensory nerve that may be sacrificed [3–5] (Fig. 3.3).

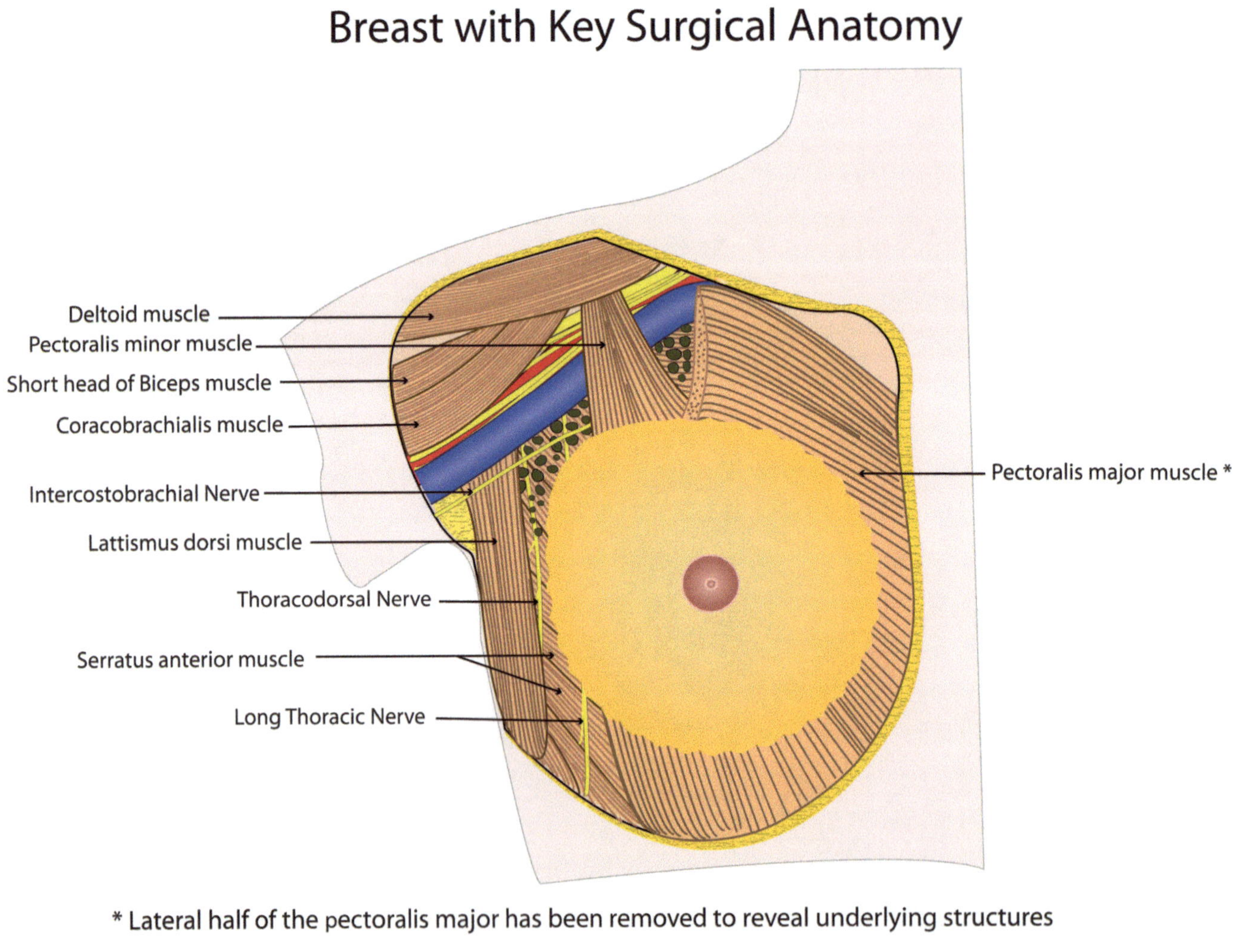

Fig. 3.2 The breast with key surgical anatomy. The applied surgical anatomy of the breast is illustrated demonstrating the muscles, nerves, and blood vessels of the chest wall. The subscapular vessels that accompany the thoracodorsal nerve and the nerves to the pectoralis muscles are not shown

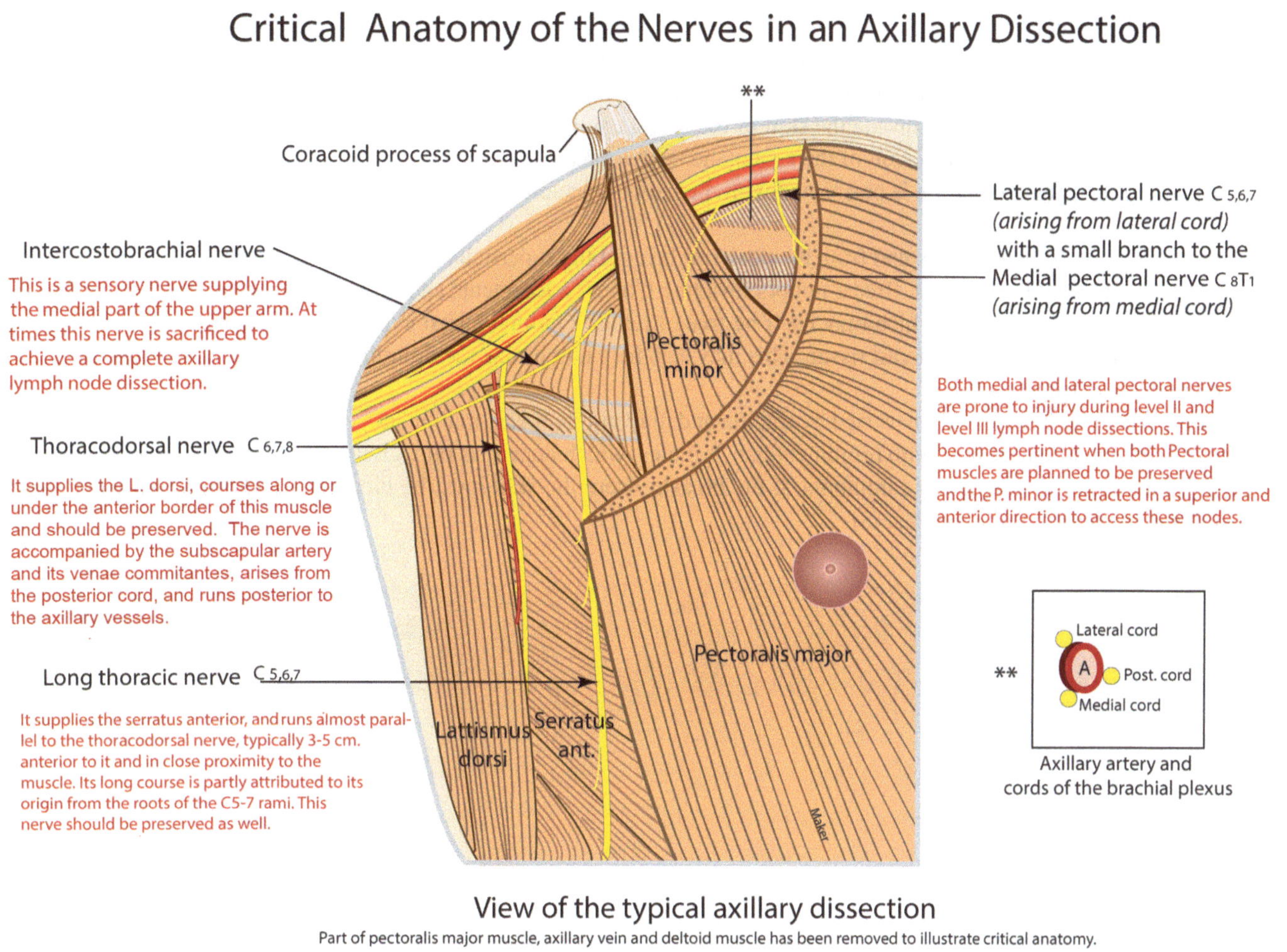

Fig. 3.3 Critical anatomy of the nerves of the axilla. The extent of the axillary lymph node dissection varies depending on the type of cancer and whether it is for diagnostic sampling or therapeutic excision. In either case, extensive knowledge of the exact anatomical location and relative relationships, as described above, is critical. When muscles are being spared or used for flap reconstructions, their nerve supply must be preserved. The nerve supply to the pectoral muscles are specifically at risk

Answer

e

4. Mark the false statement.
   (a) Fat necrosis of the breast may manifest itself as skin dimpling.
   (b) Skin dimpling may be caused by invasion of Cooper's ligaments.
   (c) Breast cancer may directly invade the skin of the breast causing skin dimpling.
   (d) Peau d'orange signifies invasion of the subcutaneous lymphatics.
   (e) Optimal breast examination is performed with the patient in supine position only.

Comments Cooper's ligaments extend from the posterior layer of the superficial pectoral fascia towards the dermis, forming a suspensory network of septations. Breast tumors invading Cooper's ligaments cause them to shorten. This in turn induces retraction of the mammary skin, which may itself be free of tumor. Optimal breast examination is performed in at least two positions so as to examine all the breast tissue. This may also help emphasize the dimpling of the skin as the breast moves in relation to deeper structures [6].

Fat necrosis of the breast is often caused by trauma and may mimic breast malignancy, including skin retraction [7]. Peau d'orange is edema of the dermis, with prominent hair follicles, which appear as pits, giving an orange-peel appearance. This sign is often seen in inflammatory carcinoma of the breast, where the skin must be biopsied in addition to the underlying breast tissue to confirm this diagnosis [8].

Answer

e

5. Mark the incorrect statement regarding the lymphatic drainage of the breast.
   (a) The subareolar plexus of Sappey collects the lymph from most of the breast, which is in its majority directed towards the axilla.
   (b) Rotter's nodes lie between the pectoralis major and minor.
   (c) Breast cancer invasion of the internal mammary lymph nodes should be considered M1 disease.
   (d) Sentinel node(s) is the first node(s) to receive the lymphatic drainage from any given anatomical territory.
   (e) Skip metastasis to the axilla affecting level III nodes without involvement of lower levels is anatomically unlikely.

Comments Reflecting their common ectodermal origin, the breast tissue and the overlying skin share a common lymphatic drainage. Lymphatic drainage of the breast flows centripetally towards the subareolar plexus of Sappey. From this location several lymphatic trunks emerge, coursing parallel to the edge of the pectoralis major to reach the axilla. These two anatomic facts allow the subcutaneous periareolar injection of dye to map the lymphatic drainage of most of the breast tissue (sentinel node mapping) [9]. Additionally, this anatomical distribution of lymphatic flow minimizes the impact of previous breast tissue resection on the accuracy of sentinel node mapping, provided that the lymphatic structures communicating the plexus of Sappey with the axillary nodes were preserved in previous interventions. Most breast neoplasms drain into one to three lymph nodes located in the axilla, rarely are they located in the internal mammary chain [10].

Rotter's nodes are also called interpectoral nodes. While in the past their excision was advocated by some, this approach has fallen out of favor in present times.

Cancer invasion of the internal mammary nodes is an unfavorable finding that is classified as N3, placing the patient in stage IIIb. Invasion of supraclavicular lymph nodes is considered as M1 disease, placing the patient in stage IV [11] (Fig. 3.4).

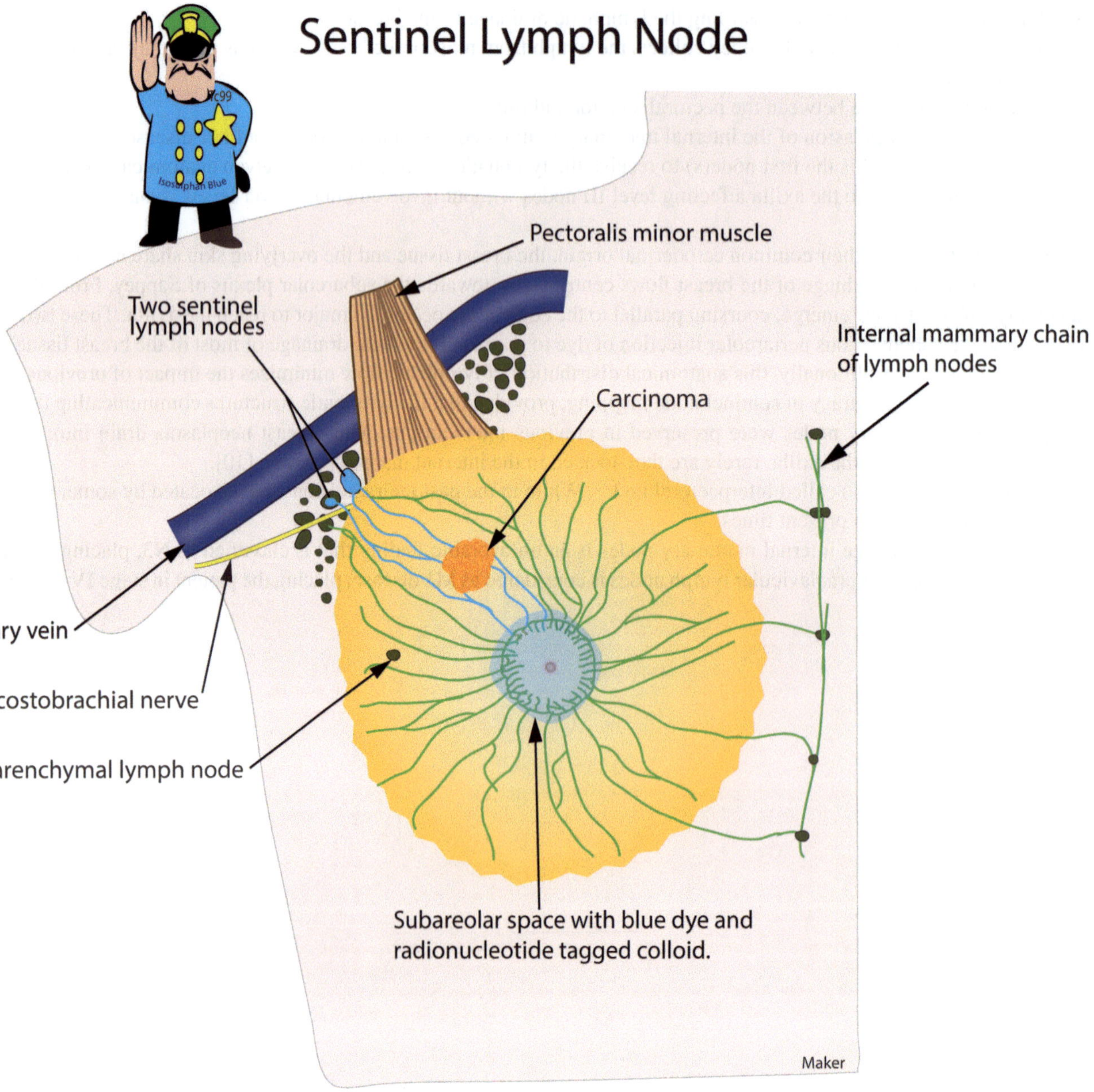

Fig. 3.4 Sentinel lymph node. Sentinel lymph node(s) are like a "sentry" and are most likely the first lymph nodes to drain cancer cells from a primary malignancy. Sentinel lymph nodes are typically identified by a peri-tumoral or subareolar injection of a dye, e.g., isosulfan blue. Most often, as is illustrated, blue dye is used in combination with a radiotagged colloid like technetium-99m-labeled sulfur colloid. Two blue sentinel lymph nodes and their feeding blue lymphatics are illustrated in the diagram as trapping the highest amount of dye and radiotagged colloid. The intercostobrachial nerve runs through the axillary pad of fat and lymph nodes

Answer

c

6. Mark the *incorrect* description of a breast surgical procedure.
   (a) A classical Halsted radical mastectomy involves the excision of the breast, pectoralis major, and minor and axillary nodes.
   (b) A typical radical mastectomy consists of removal of the breast and axillary lymph nodes.
   (c) Simple or total mastectomy comprises excision of the breast only.
   (d) Subcutaneous mastectomy takes approximately 95 % of the breast tissue but preserves the overlying skin completely.
   (e) Lumpectomy is the anatomic excision of a breast lobule.

Comments In the 1960s a supra-radical mastectomy (Urban procedure) was described. It added en bloc dissection of the internal mammary lymph nodes to the classical Halsted mastectomy. These two procedures were abandoned due to increased morbidity without added survival benefit. A modified radical mastectomy at times includes division of pectoralis minor muscles to obtain an adequate axillary dissection, but the pectoralis major is always spared. Simple or total mastectomies as well as subcutaneous mastectomies may leave up to 10 % of the breast tissue intact. Lumpectomy does not follow anatomical lobules; rather, it is based on excision of neoplasm with at least 1 cm margins [12, 13].

Answer

e

7. All of the following are correct *except*:
   (a) Mondor's disease is a superficial thrombophlebitis of the breast.
   (b) Zuska's disease is a chronic draining sinus derived from a mammary duct.
   (c) Batson's plexus allows breast cancers to metastasize to the vertebrae without systemic hematogenous spread.
   (d) Paget's disease of the breast is a primary cancer of the areola.
   (e) Breast cancer may give rise to Krukenberg tumors.

Comments Mondor's disease, also known as superficial thrombophlebitis of the breast, is an uncommon disorder. It is most frequently caused by breast trauma and surgical intervention and is not associated with breast cancer. Pain arises in the affected area, and often, the thrombosed vein may be seen or palpated. Superficial thrombophlebitis of the penis also receives this eponym [14–17] (Fig. 3.5).

In 1951 Zuska described five cases of chronic subareolar breast abscess caused by obstruction of the ductal system characterized by the presence of a chronic draining sinus on the edge of the areola with a tract towards the base of the nipple. His initial case series included his wife. The excision of the fistulous tract he described continues to be the standard of care [18–20] (Fig. 3.6a, b).

The craniospinal venous system, also known as Batson's plexus, is a complex valveless bidirectional venous network spanning the intracranial cortical veins, cavernous sinuses, and vertebral veins, communicating with the sacral and prostatic veins. Its physiologic role is to drain the vertebral bone marrow and provide an alternate pathway for venous drainage of the brain. However, it is better known for its pathologic ability to allow venous spread of disease processes. The association with the prostatic venous plexus allows metastatic cells from the prostate to reach the spine. Breast cancer metastasis may reach Batson's plexus in retrograde fashion through the intercostal veins. Lung cancer and medullary carcinoma of the thyroid are also known to use this route. The hallmark of metastasis through this route is that the vertebrae are affected without any systemic hematogenous spread [21].

There has been controversy on whether Paget's disease represents a primary cutaneous phenomenon or an expression of an underlying process. Together with a 90 % association with breast cancer, recent immunohistochemical studies support the latter hypothesis. Heregulin-α, an HER2/NEU ligand produced by keratinocytes, has been postulated as chemoattractant factor responsible for inducing the migration of underlying tumor cells towards the nipple. It is interesting to note that extramammary Paget's disease may arise from apocrine sweat glands, sharing a common embryologic origin with Paget's disease of the breast [22, 23].

While Krukenberg tumors were traditionally described as metastatic implants on the ovary by signet cell gastric carcinoma, the term is now used for ovarian metastasis from any site. In the breast, lobular carcinomas are the most likely to give intra-abdominal metastasis. However, in the setting of breast cancer, synchronous primary ovarian cancers are up to ten times more common than metastatic ovarian neoplasms [24].

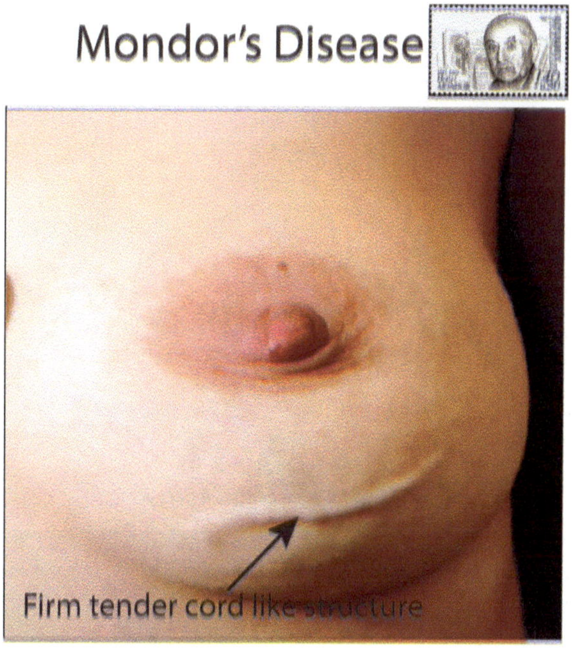

Fig. 3.5 Mondor's disease. Patient presents with a tender, firm, cord-like structure, which can often be traced to a superficial vein. Henri Mondor (1885–1962) a famous French surgeon and a clinical professor of surgery in Paris described this condition (With permission from Soler-Gonzalez and Ruiz [17])

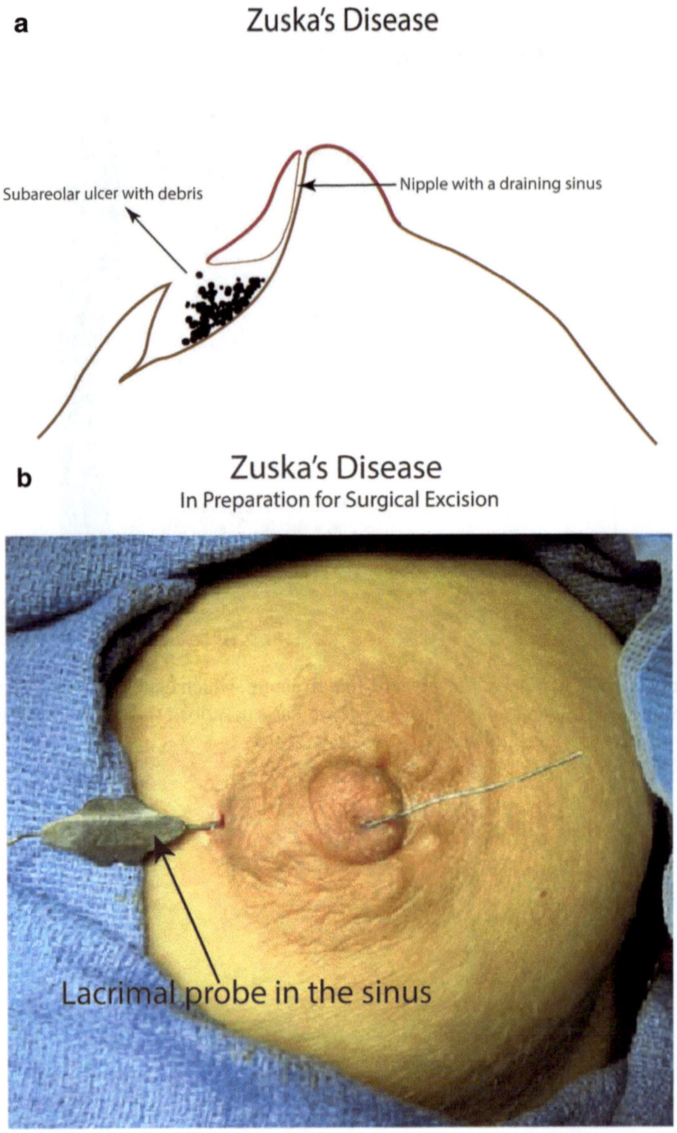

Fig. 3.6 (**a**) Zuska's disease. Illustration shows a lacrimal probe inserted from the draining sinus in the nipple through a subareolar inflammatory collection into a periareolar sinus, in preparation for excision; (**b**) Zuzka's disease excision. Subareolar recurrent abscess with a draining sinus in the nipple is an uncommon benign condition but a difficult disease to treat. It is often quoted with different names including lactiferous fistula, chronic periareolar mastitis, ductal mastitis, etc. Resultant deformity of the nipple adds to the differential diagnosis of malignancy (With permission from Komenka et al. [19])

Answer

d

References

1. Garcia Jr O. Reconstruction of total absence of the breast. Ann Plast Surg. 2007;58(1):12–7.
2. Urschel Jr HC. Poland's syndrome. Chest Surg Clin N Am. 2000;10(2):393–403, viii.
3. Benson JR, della Rovere GQ. Management of the axilla in women with breast cancer. Lancet Oncol. 2007;8(4):331–48.
4. Blichert-Toft M. Axillary surgery in breast cancer management–background, incidence and extent of nodal spread, extent of surgery and accurate axillary staging, surgical procedures. Acta Oncol. 2000;39(3):269–75.
5. Ung O, Tan M, Chua B, Barraclough B. Complete axillary dissection: a technique that still has relevance in contemporary management of breast cancer. ANZ J Surg. 2006;76(6):518–21.
6. Kolb TM, Lichy J, Newhouse JH. Comparison of the performance of screening mammography, physical examination, and breast US and evaluation of factors that influence them: an analysis of 27,825 patient evaluations. Radiology. 2002;225(1):165–75.
7. Tan PH, Lai LM, Carrington EV, Opaluwa AS, Ravikumar KH, Chetty N, et al. Fat necrosis of the breast–a review. Breast. 2006;15(3):313–8.
8. Bristol IJ, Buchholz TA. Inflammatory breast cancer: current concepts in local management. Breast Dis. 2005;22:75–83.
9. Mignotte H, Treilleux I, Chassagne-Clement C, Bem C, Lopez R, Martin X, et al. Interest of periareolar injection for colorimetric detection of sentinel node in breast cancer. Bull Cancer. 2000;87(7–8):600–3.
10. Mabry H, Giuliano AE. Sentinel node mapping for breast cancer: progress to date and prospects for the future. Surg Oncol Clin N Am. 2007;16(1):55–70.
11. Carlson RW, Anderson BO, Burstein HJ, Carter WB, Edge SB, Farrar WB, et al. Invasive breast cancer. J Natl Compr Canc Netw. 2007; 5(3):246–312.
12. Winchester DP, Trabanino L, Lopez MJ. The evolution of surgery for breast cancer. Surg Oncol Clin N Am. 2005;14(3):479–98, vi.
13. Fitzal F, Gnant M. Breast conservation: evolution of surgical strategies. Breast J. 2006;12(5 Suppl 2):S165–73.
14. Kraus S, Ludecke G, Weidner W. Mondor's disease of the penis. Urol Int. 2000;64(2):99–100.
15. Markopoulos C, Kouskos E, Mantas D, Kakisis J, Antonopoulou Z, Kontzoglou K, et al. Mondor's disease of the breast: is there any relation to breast cancer? Eur J Gynaecol Oncol. 2005;26(2):213–4.
16. Pugh CM, DeWitty RL. Mondor's disease. J Natl Med Assoc. 1996;88(6):359–63.
17. Soler-Gonzalez J, Ruiz MC. Images in clinical medicine. Mondor's disease. N Engl J Med. 2005;352(10):1024.
18. Zuska JJ, Crile G, Ayres Jr WW. Fistulas of lactifierous ducts. Am J Surg. 1951;81(3):312–7.
19. Komenaka IK, Pennington Jr RE, Bowling MW, Clare SE, Goulet Jr RJ. A technique to prevent recurrence of lactiferous duct fistula. J Am Coll Surg. 2006;203(2):253–6.
20. Maull KI. Technique to prevent recurrence of lactiferous duct fistula. J Am Coll Surg. 2007;204(1):189–90.
21. Pearce JM. The craniospinal venous system. Eur Neurol. 2006;56(2):136–8.
22. Schelfhout VR, Coene ED, Delaey B, Thys S, Page DL, De Potter CR. Pathogenesis of Paget's disease: epidermal heregulin-alpha, motility factor, and the HER receptor family. J Natl Cancer Inst. 2000;92(8):622–8.
23. Liegl B, Leibl S, Gogg-Kamerer M, Tessaro B, Horn LC, Moinfar F. Mammary and extramammary Paget's disease: an immunohistochemical study of 83 cases. Histopathology. 2007;50(4):439–47.
24. Young RH. From Krukenberg to today: the ever present problems posed by metastatic tumors in the ovary. Part II. Adv Anat Pathol. 2007; 14(3):149–77.

Larynx and Respiratory System

4

1. All of the following are correct *except*
   (a) The larynx arises from a diverticulum in the anterior aspect of the pharynx.
   (b) The cartilages and muscles of the larynx are of mesodermal origin, derived from the fourth and sixth branchial arches.
   (c) Laryngeal atresia requires immediate tracheostomy.
   (d) Congenital laryngomalacia requires surgical correction.
   (e) Congenital subglottic stenosis is due to abnormal development of the cricoid cartilage.

Comments Like the trachea and lungs, the larynx is derived from the foregut (endoderm). However, the endodermal tissues are reinforced by mesodermal derivatives from the fourth and sixth branchial arches, which give rise to the muscular and cartilaginous elements of the larynx. Reflecting the pattern of foregut development, the larynx is at one point obliterated by epithelial proliferation, which subsequently recanalizes. Failure of this developmental step leads to laryngeal atresia, which constitutes a neonatal airway emergency [1].

Laryngomalacia is the most common congenital malformation of the larynx. It is thought to represent a delay in the development of the laryngeal cartilages, which are found to be weak and pliable. During inspiration the cartilages collapse due to the negative intraluminal pressure, causing various degrees of airway obstruction. Fortunately, the degree of obstruction is not overly severe, and watchful waiting is recommended for most cases. This pathology usually resolves within the first 2 years of life. However, severe cases may require tracheostomy or laryngoplasty [2]. In the adult, laryngomalacia may occur from prolonged intubation, as well as from long-standing massive thyroid goiters.

Answer
d

V.K. Maker, E.D. Guzman-Arrieta, *Cognitive Pearls in General Surgery*,
DOI 10.1007/978-1-4939-1850-8_4, © Springer Science+Business Media New York 2015

2. The anatomic relations of the thyroid are as described below *except*:
   (a) At rest, the thyroid cartilage lies from C3 to C6.
   (b) The larynx is suspended from the hyoid bone by the thyrohyoid membrane.
   (c) The hyoid bone is suspended from the base of the skull by ligaments and muscles.
   (d) The thyroid isthmus covers the cricoid cartilage and the cricothyroid membrane.
   (e) The strap muscles (sternothyroid, sternohyoid, thyrohyoid, and omohyoid) cover the thyroid cartilage.

Comments The larynx does not articulate with any fixed bony structures; rather, it is suspended by ligaments from the hyoid bone, which is in turn suspended from the base of the skull. This lack of firm attachment allows the larynx to move cephalad in order to protect the airway during swallowing. Furthermore, the movement of the larynx changes the dimensions of the supraglottic resonant chamber, contributing to changes in voice pitch [3].

The thyroid gland is caudal in relation to the thyroid cartilage; only the superior thyroid poles and pyramidal lobe of the gland make contact with the cartilage. The thyroid isthmus covers the 2nd and 3rd tracheal rings. This anatomical position puts the thyroid out of the surgical field of cricothyroidotomy for emergency airway. It is often necessary to divide the thyroid isthmus during the course of a tracheostomy (Fig. 4.1).

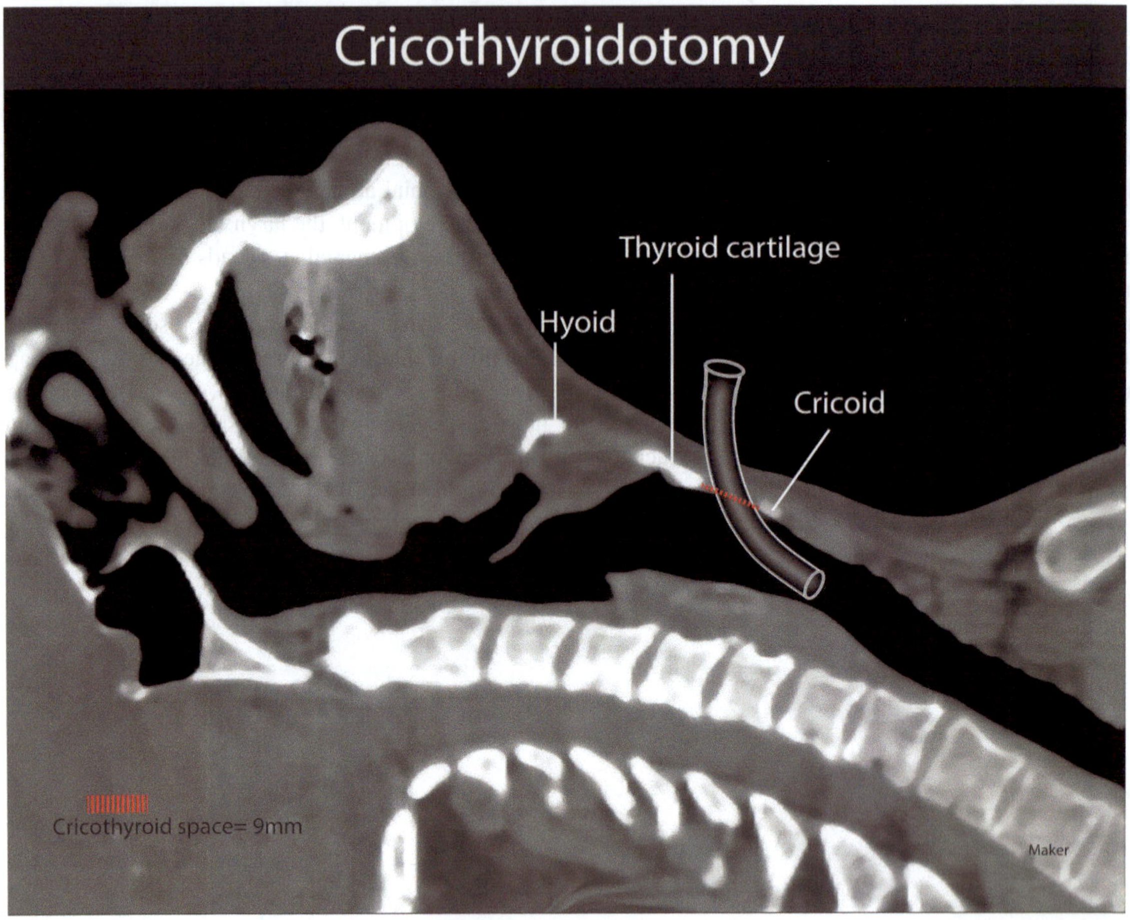

Fig. 4.1 Cricothyroidotomy is the surgical procedure of choice for an acute emergency airway when orotracheal or nasotracheal intubation fails or is not available. The cricothyroid space in the adult is limited to 9 mm and typically a #4 Shiley™ tracheostomy tube is inserted

Answer
d

3. All of the following are correct *except:*
   (a) The first step in management of a tracheoinnominate fistula is securing the airway with an orotracheal tube.
   (b) Herald bleeding is present in 50 % of cases.
   (c) Low-lying tracheostomy (below the 3rd or 4th tracheal ring) is an important risk factor.
   (d) Endovascular repair is an emerging treatment modality.
   (e) Open surgical repair requires median sternotomy.

Comments Tracheoinnominate fistulas are an infrequent but lethal complication of tracheostomies. The chief risk factors are a low-lying tracheostomy, hyperinflated cuff, neck or chest deformity, and prolonged presence of this form of airway.

The anatomical substrate is the proximity between the anterior wall of the trachea and the posterior wall of the innominate artery. Fistulization occurs through a decubitus mechanism and herald bleeding is present in up to 50 % of cases. This makes careful evaluation of bleeding from a tracheostomy site mandatory. Bronchoscopy is the modality of choice [4] (Fig. 4.2).

Emergency management consists of hyperinflation of the tracheostomy cuff to tamponade the bleeding and digital pressure over the tracheostomy. Bronchoscopy is useful in clearing the airway of blood. Manipulation of the tracheostomy tube or exchange of the airway is contraindicated, as it may precipitate massive hemorrhage.

Classically, surgical repair consisted of median sternotomy with resection of the innominate artery without vascular reconstruction [4, 5]. More recently, endovascular stent grafting and coiling have emerged as useful treatment modalities [6, 7] (Fig. 4.3).

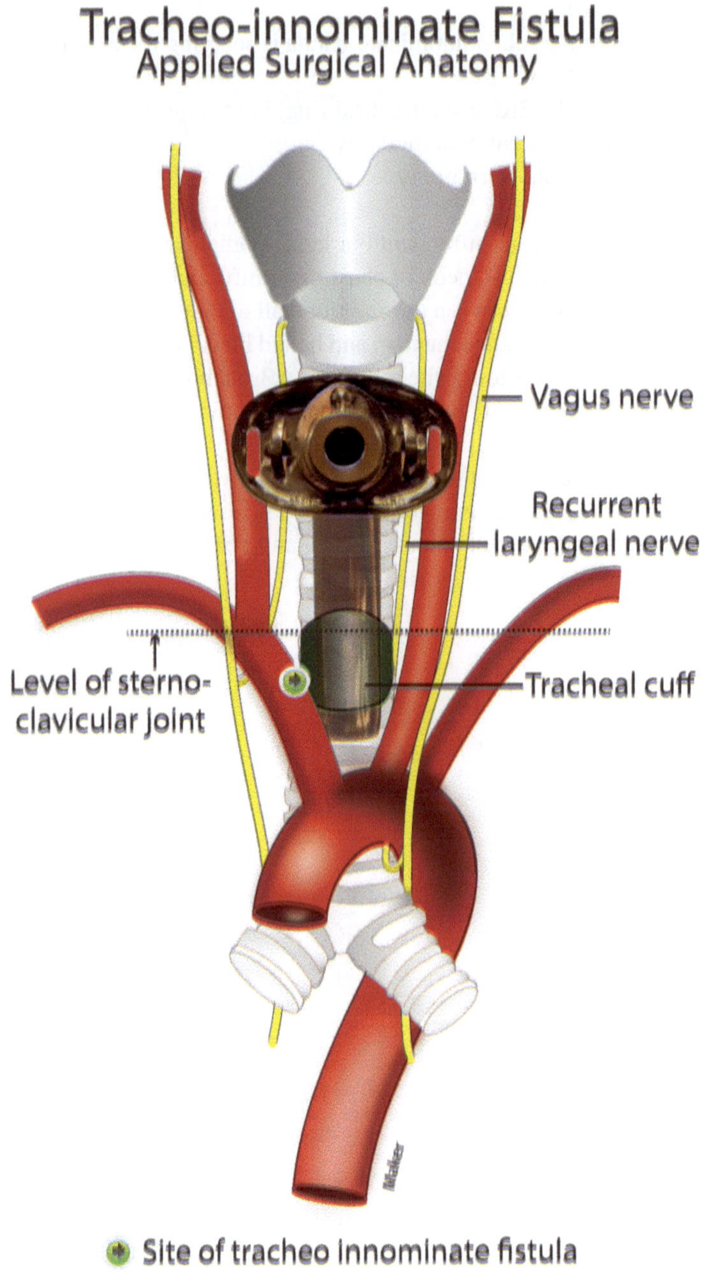

Fig. 4.2 The innominate trunk is the first branch of the aortic arch and divides into the rt. common carotid and subclavian arteries, just posterior to the rt. sternoclavicular joint. In its course it lies on the rt. anterior surface of the trachea. This area is prone to pressure necrosis from the angle of the tracheostomy tube and the pressure from the inflated tracheal cuff, which can cause a delayed tracheoinnominate fistula

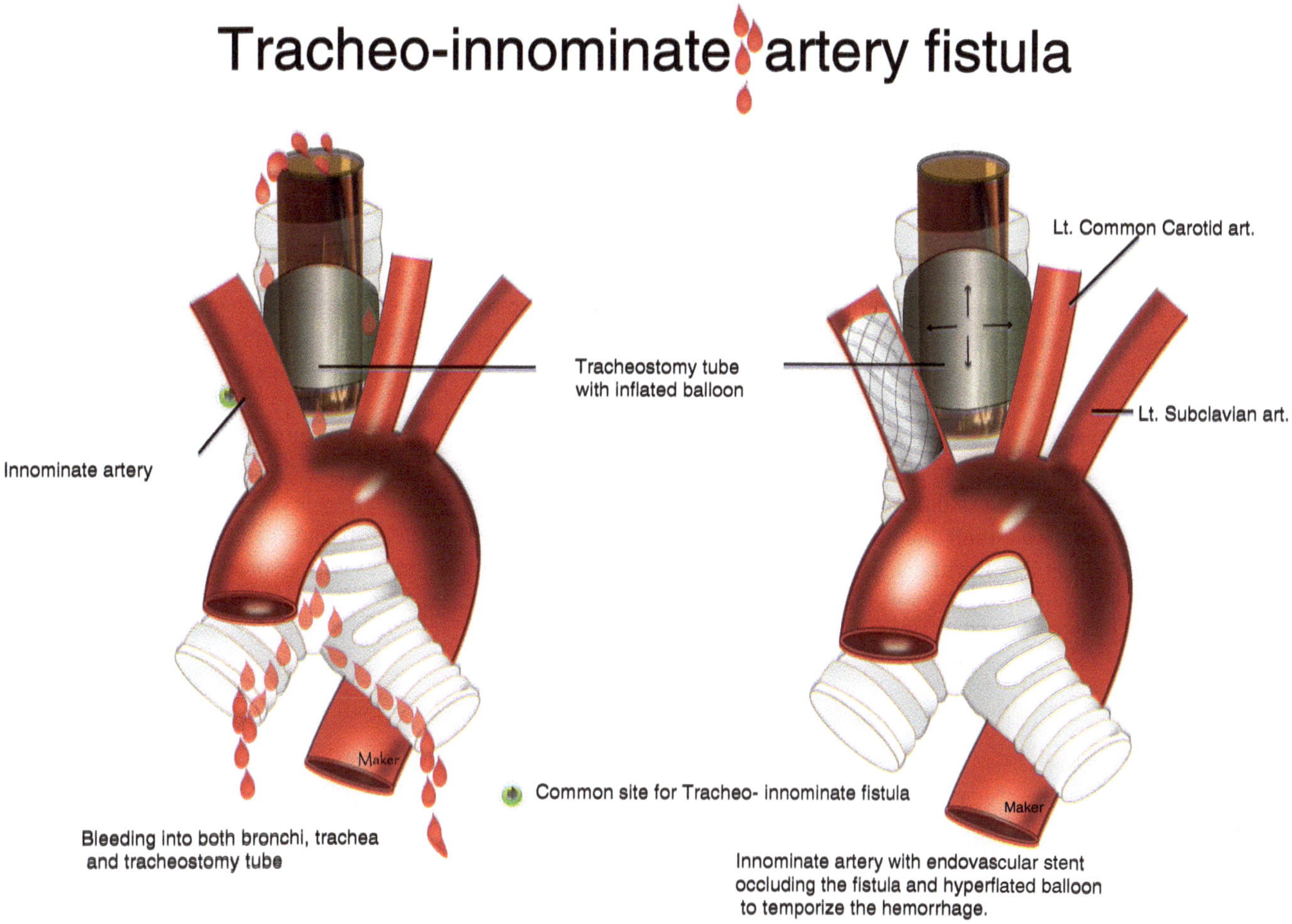

Fig. 4.3 Massive hemorrhage from an indwelling tracheostomy is most likely from a tracheoinnominate artery fistula. Massive aspiration of blood contributes to this life-threatening complication. Pressure necrosis from the curve of the tracheostomy tube and inflated cuff is the likely etiology. Ironically, further hyperinflating the cuff is the initial step in tamponading the bleeding. Endovascular stenting of the innominate artery is now considered the treatment of choice. Long-term results are still awaited as the endovascular stent lies adjacent to the open contaminated trachea

Answer

a

4. All of the following are correct *except*:
   (a) Acute epiglottitis may cause upper airway obstruction in children.
   (b) Newborns are more susceptible than adults to subglottic stenosis secondary to intubation.
   (c) The neonatal larynx is more cranial than in the adult, and the cricothyroid membrane is hard to find, contraindicating emergency cricothyroidotomy.
   (d) A cricothyroidotomy should be converted to a tracheostomy as soon as possible.
   (e) Neonatal endotracheal tubes are unable to deliver PEEP.

Comments Although acute epiglottitis has become less common since the widespread use of *Haemophilus influenzae* vaccines, it should still be considered in the workup of children with acute respiratory distress. It is noteworthy that in this scenario attempts to examine the larynx may lead to worsening of the obstruction. Hence, the recommended diagnostic test is a lateral neck X-ray, which shows a thickened epiglottis. Intubation is then carried out bronchoscopically under general anesthesia [8].

The neonatal larynx is located more cranially than that of the adult; this protects it from trauma, but makes it less accessible for surgical access. It is funnel shaped and much narrower than that of the adult. This determines that comparable increases in epithelial thickness due to edema result in a proportionally greater loss of cross-sectional area in the newborn and young child. Due to its small diameter and shape, the neonatal larynx provides a seal around cuffless endotracheal tubes, allowing the delivery of PEEP without an inflatable cuff. Unfortunately, this tight fit makes it more prone to pressure necrosis leading to the development of subglottic stenosis [9].

Answer
e

5. All of the following are correct *except*:
   (a) The false vocal cords play a role in closing the airway but do not participate in phonation.
   (b) The larynx participates in defecation, urination, and labor.
   (c) The epithelium of the edge of the true vocal cords has abundant lymphatics.
   (d) The extrinsic muscles of the larynx participate in airway protection and phonation.
   (e) The motor innervation of the larynx is derived from the vagus nerve.

Comments The false vocal cords (also named vestibular folds) are folds of pseudostratified epithelium with a core of connective tissue and glands. They lie cephalad to the true vocal cords. Traditionally, the false vocal cords were considered to be rather passive structures, contributing mainly to the lubrication of the larynx through their mucus glands. More recently, this view has been modified to an active role during phonation, airway protection, and the Valsalva maneuver [10].

The muscles of the larynx are divided into intrinsic and extrinsic, based on whether they begin and end on the larynx or beyond it. The intrinsic muscles are responsible for the movements of the vocal cords as well as that of the laryngeal cartilages. The extrinsic muscles elevate or depress the larynx as a whole. The epithelium of the edge of the vocal cords lacks lymphatics, which makes metastatic spread of early malignancies unlikely and allows limited resections. However, lateral to this edge there are lymphatic networks that could allow the spread of malignancy [11].

Answer

c

6. The following statements correctly describe lung development *except*:
   (a) Embryologically, the lung shares a common origin with the esophagus arising from the endodermal foregut.
   (b) Early in its development, the right lung is segmented into three lobes and ten segments, while the left divides into two lobes and eight segments.
   (c) Type 2 pneumocytes, responsible for the formation of surfactant, are not sufficient to prevent alveolar collapse until 7 months of gestation.
   (d) Pulmonary hamartomas are fast-growing tumors.
   (e) Paraneoplastic syndromes seen in lung cancer arise from the neuroendocrine cells of the lung.

Comments The respiratory tract develops as an outgrowth of the anterior aspect of the foregut. Starting from the primitive trachea, serial divisions lead to the arborizing pattern of the mature lung. Recent studies have shown that development of the lung is a highly integrated pattern, involving the interaction of the endoderm-derived primitive lung parenchyma, the mesodermal vasculature, the surrounding mesenchyme, and neural crest-derived cells. Several highly preserved genes have been identified as serving an important role in this process [12, 13]. Resembling gut development, the lung and airways are originally solid, recanalizing at a later stage. Their common origin is also reflected by the existence of tracheoesophageal fistulas, which constitute a failure in the separation from a common origin [14].

Benign tumors of the lung are rare. Among them, hamartomas are the most common (75 %). Although they are most commonly diagnosed in late adulthood, they are developmental anomalies. Hamartomas are slow-growing tumors, containing disorganized, but otherwise normal, cells. The most common feature is the presence of disorganized cartilage appearing as popcorn calcifications on X-ray studies [15] (Fig. 4.4).

The neuroendocrine cells of the lung share the capacity to produce hormones and neurotransmitters with other members of the amine precursor uptake and decarboxylation (APUD) system. This is reflected in two malignancies to which they give origin. Small-cell lung cancers are well known for their propensity to cause paraneoplastic syndromes, through the production of arginine vasopressin (AVP), atrial natriuretic peptide, adrenocorticotropic hormone (ACTH), and growth hormone. Carcinoid tumors, while considered a low-grade malignancy, can cause significant morbidity through the production of serotonin, histamine, and catecholamines [16, 17].

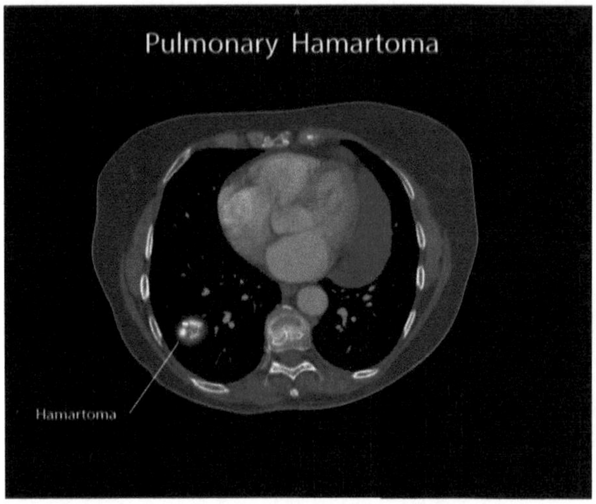

Fig. 4.4 Chest radiograph of this 60-year-old male reveals a classic coin lesion with popcorn calcifications in the right lung. Identical findings were reported in an old radiograph, 10 years earlier, consistent with a hamartoma arising from a benign embryonic rest

Answer
d

7. Mark the *incorrect* statement pertaining pulmonary anatomic anomalies.
   (a) The azygos lobe is a true accessory lobe.
   (b) True accessory lobes have independent bronchial and arterial supply.
   (c) The "tracheal bronchus" consists of a right upper lobe bronchus arising directly from the trachea.
   (d) Pulmonary sequestration is diagnosed during angiographic studies.
   (e) The most common tracheoesophageal fistula consists of a proximal esophageal blind pouch and a fistula communicating the distal esophagus with the trachea (type C).

Comments The azygos lobe is not a true accessory lobe. It is a portion of the apical lung parenchyma partially separated from the remainder of the lung by an anomalous azygos or hemiazygos vein. Its incidence is up to 1 % of autopsy series and 0.4 % of chest X-ray series. It can be an obstacle to the completion of thoracoscopic sympathectomies [18]. Tracheal bronchi may also occur on either side, with the right being more commonly affected. These structures provide ventilation to portions of the upper lobes and have been associated with recurrent pneumonias, atelectasis, and bronchitis [19].

Pulmonary sequestration is defined as a segment of the lung parenchyma lacking a normal connection to the airway and receiving blood from a branch of the aorta, which makes them evident in angiography. They are classified as extralobar or intralobar, based on the presence or absence of an independent pleural envelope. The former drain into systemic veins, whereas the latter do so into the pulmonary veins. They are often a site of recurrent pneumonia [20].

Gross and Vogt classified tracheoesophageal fistulas into five types, as illustrated below. Multiple congenital deformities are often associated. VACTERL is a common acronym uses standing for *v*ertebral defects, *a*nal atresia, *c*ardiac anomalies, *t*racheo*e*sophageal fistulas, *r*enal malformations, and *l*imb deformities [21] (Fig. 4.5).

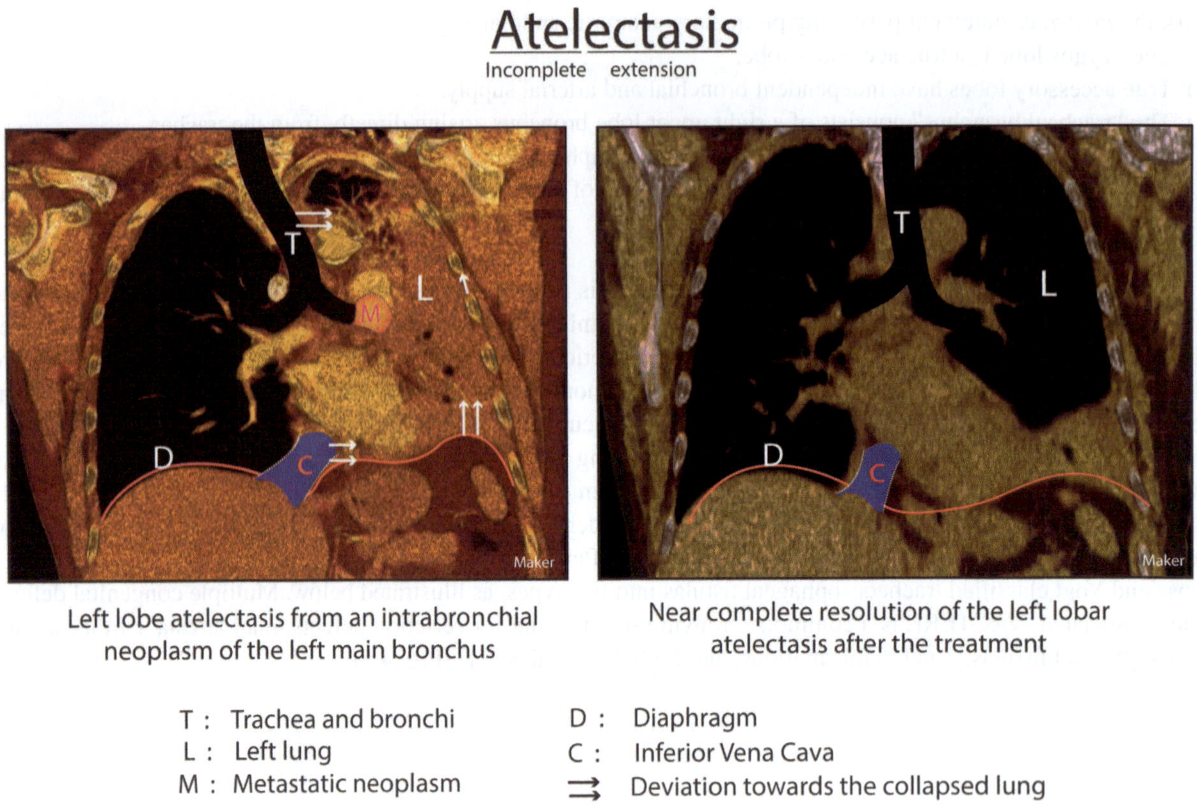

Fig. 4.5 This 50-year-old male presented with near complete left lobe atelectasis secondary to a metastatic malignant melanoma blocking the left main bronchus as seen above in the 3D rendition of his CAT scan. 2 months later, after endobronchial laser ablation of the tumor followed by radiation therapy, most of the left lobe has re-expanded. Note the characteristic findings of the elevated diaphragm, tracheal deviation, narrowing of intercostal spaces, and the deviation of the inferior vena cava on the affected left side. All of these are corrected in the posttreatment images

Answer

a

8. Mark the *false* statement regarding lung anatomy and physiology.
   (a) Airway resistance through a tracheostomy is less than that of an endotracheal tube.
   (b) Negative intrathoracic pressure is greatest in the lung apices in supine position.
   (c) Negative intrathoracic pressure decreases venous return to the left heart.
   (d) Negative intrathoracic pressure decreases venous return to the right heart.
   (e) All modern ventilators are based on positive pressure breathing.

Comments Tracheostomy tubes offer less resistance to air flow than endotracheal tubes by virtue of their shorter length with an equivalent diameter. In addition, tracheostomy tubes also decrease the work of breathing by reducing dead space by 100 ml over the natural airway [22].

Negative intrathoracic pressure varies inside the thorax, achieving the most negative values in the lung apices. This greater pressure differential places the apices under stretch, which renders them more susceptible to the formation and ruptures of blebs. Negative intrathoracic pressure has different effects on the left- and right-sided circulation. On the right, the accentuation of negative intrathoracic pressure leads to an increase in the transmural pressure gradient of the right ventricle, leading to an increase in venous return. In contrast, the same negative pressure sequesters blood in the lungs, reducing venous return to the left ventricle [23].

Unlike spontaneous breathing (negative pressure), contemporary mechanical ventilation is based on positive pressure breathing. As a consequence, the increase intrathoracic pressure (especially when high positive end-expiratory pressure (PEEP) settings are used) decreases intrathoracic return to the right heart and brings about an overall decrease in cardiac output.

Answer

d

9. The following are correct *except*:
   (a) Pulmonary segments are independent anatomical units.
   (b) The pulmonary segments have discrete bronchial and arterial supply with minimal anastomosis between them.
   (c) Pulmonary veins are of use as landmarks demarcating the pulmonary segments.
   (d) The lung has a dual blood supply, from both ventricles of the heart.
   (e) Bronchial veins drain exclusively into the right heart.

Comments Pulmonary segments are portions of the lung parenchyma ventilated by a tertiary bronchus. Following a pattern similar to that found in the liver, the branches of the pulmonary artery follow the bronchi in a central location in each segment, while the branches of the pulmonary veins are located between segments.

Again, in resemblance to the liver, the lung has dual circulation. The pulmonary artery carries venous blood to be oxygenated in the lung, while the bronchial arteries (arising from the aorta) provide nutrition to the lung. Bronchial arteries are the most common source of hemoptysis [24]. Like the name implies, bronchial vessels run along the bronchi and hence are located centrally within lung segments. Bronchial veins are the counterpart to the bronchial arteries. Although part of the venous blood they carry empties into the azygos system, they also empty into the pulmonary veins. This contribution of deoxygenated blood lowers the oxygen saturation of arterial blood.

Answer

e

10. In relation to subclavian and internal jugular central venous catheters, all of the following are correct *except:*
    (a) The internal jugular approach for central venous catheter insertion is associated with the highest tip misplacement rate.
    (b) Placement of subclavian central venous catheters carries the greatest risk of pneumothorax.
    (c) The risk of pneumothorax during central line insertion is greater in mechanically ventilated patients.
    (d) Pneumothorax during central line insertion is most likely to occur on the left.
    (e) Arterial injuries are more common with internal jugular catheters than with subclavian catheters.

Comments

Due to its angle of nearly 90° in relation to the innominate vein, catheters placed in the subclavian vein are more likely to advance towards the contralateral subclavian vein or internal jugular, an event that happens in up to 15 % of insertion attempts. Pneumothorax occurs in 1–1.5 % of line placements. It is more common with subclavian vein cannulation than with the internal jugular approach. However, some series show the opposite. Delayed pneumothorax occurs in up to 4 % of cases. Perhaps the more important point is that the internal jugular approach is not immune to this complication. Additionally, the risk of pneumothorax is greater with left-sided insertions, where the pleural cupola is higher. There is controversy on which side of insertion is safer. The right side is thought to carry a lesser risk of caval perforation, but a higher risk of arterial injury. The left side has a reverse risk profile, but offers less technical difficulty [25, 26].

Answer

a

11. All of the following are correct *except*:
    (a) Atelectasis is an important cause of postoperative respiratory failure.
    (b) Gas resorption distal to an occlusion is the classical mechanism of atelectasis.
    (c) Tension pneumothorax causes circulatory collapse by inhibiting venous return.
    (d) The initial step in the management of tension pneumothorax is positive pressure ventilation.
    (e) Definitive management consists of tube thoracostomy.

Comments Atelectasis is defined as the loss of aerated lung space. It is a common postoperative complication. The classical mechanism consists of gas resorption distal to a segment of occluded airway. Given the greater diffusing capacity of oxygen in relation to nitrogen, increases in the inspired fraction of oxygen facilitate the occurrence of atelectasis. Compression and impairment of surfactant production or distribution also play a role.

Atelectasis results in a loss of gas exchange area, potentially leading to hypoxemia, decreases in pulmonary compliance increasing the work of breathing, and increased pulmonary resistance causing right heart strain. In addition, the repetitive opening and closing of the distal airways and alveoli potentiate lung injury

Treatment of atelectasis consists of resolution of airway occlusions and facilitation of alveolar re-expansion, either via positive pressure ventilation or encouragement of deep breathing [27] (Fig. 4.6).

Tension pneumothorax is a life-threatening event, resulting in circulatory collapse as the venous return to the heart is compressed and angulated by mediastinal shifting. Positive pressure ventilation aggravates this condition by increasing the pressure and volume of air entering the pleural cavity. Initial treatment consists of rapid decompressions, either by needle thoracostomy or simply opening the chest wall in the process of inserting a definitive tube thoracostomy [28, 29] (Fig. 4.7).

Tension Pneumothorax

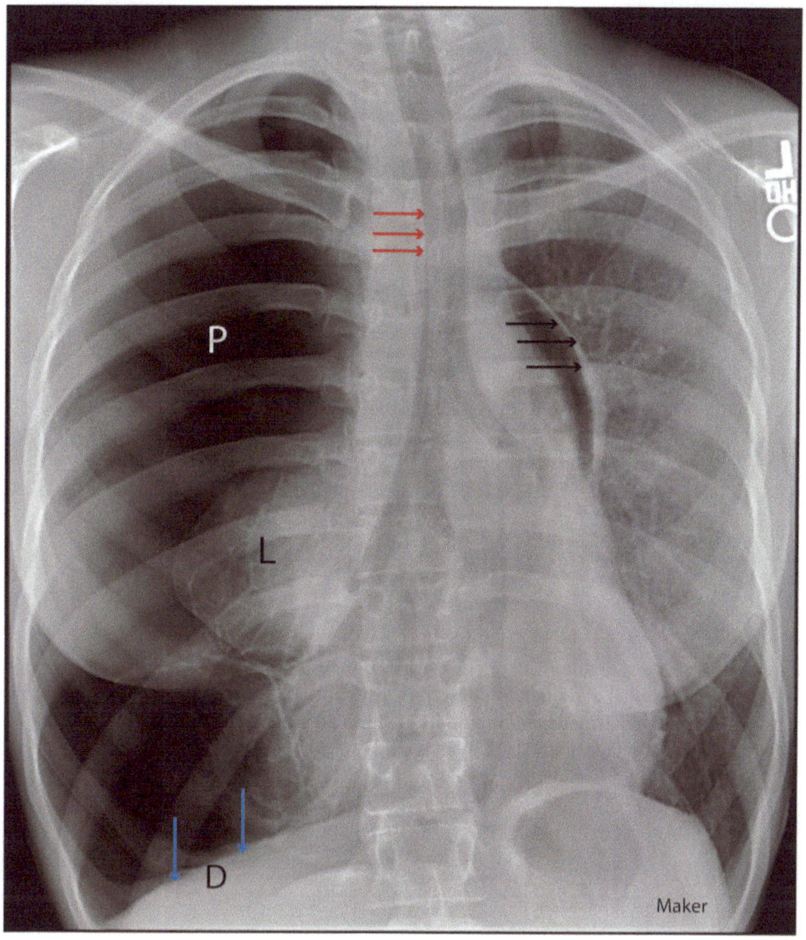

P: Air with absent lung markings

L: Collapsed lung

D: Diaphragm

Trachea pushed to the left

Tension Pnemothorax pushing the opposite lung

Diaphragm pushed down

Fig. 4.6 Tension pneumothorax is a surgical emergency and needs urgent decompression with needle or chest tube thoracostomy prior to the chest radiograph. The radiograph demonstrates a right-sided tension pneumothorax with a collapsed right lung pushing the entire mediastinum and the normal left lung. The affected ipsilateral diaphragm is pushed down and there is widening of the intercostal spaces

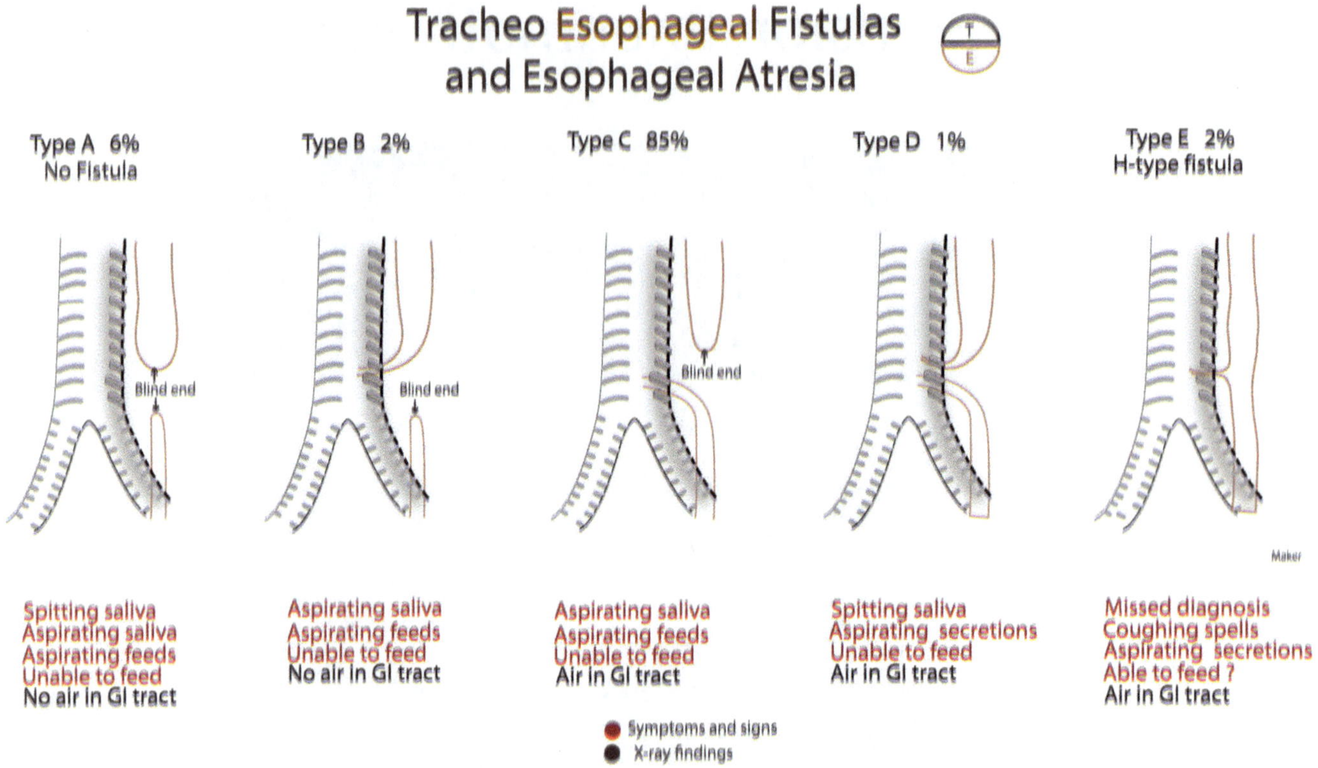

Fig. 4.7 Classification of tracheoesophageal fistulas is based on the location of esophageal atresia and the associated fistula. The illustration above represents a gross modification of the original classification described by Vogt. Each variant has classic clinical diagnostic features and the presence or absence of the air in the GI tract on X-ray depending on its anatomical site of communication with the trachea. Type A has no associated fistula, while Type E has no associated esophageal atresia. Understanding of the variants is critical to aid in medical and surgical management

Answer

d

References

1. Ahmad SM, Soliman AM. Congenital anomalies of the larynx. Otolaryngol Clin North Am. 2007;40(1):177–91, viii.
2. Daniel SJ. The upper airway: congenital malformations. Paediatr Respir Rev. 2006;7 Suppl 1:S260–3.
3. Noordzij JP, Ossoff RH. Anatomy and physiology of the larynx. Otolaryngol Clin North Am. 2006;39(1):1–10.
4. Komatsu T, Sowa T, Fujinaga T, Handa N, Watanabe H. Tracheo-innominate artery fistula: two case reports and a clinical review. Ann Thorac Cardiovasc Surg. 2013;19(1):60–2.
5. Furukawa K, Kamohara K, Itoh M, Morokuma H, Morita S. Operative technique for tracheo-innominate artery fistula repair. J Vasc Surg. 2014;59(4):1163–7.
6. Deguchi J, Furuya T, Tanaka N, Nobori M, Seki Y, Nomura Y, et al. Successful management of tracheo-innominate artery fistula with endovascular stent graft repair. J Vasc Surg. 2001;33(6):1280–2.
7. Hamaguchi S, Nakajima Y. Two cases of tracheoinnominate artery fistula following tracheostomy treated successfully by endovascular embolization of the innominate artery. J Vasc Surg. 2012;55(2):545–7.
8. Loftis L. Acute infectious upper airway obstructions in children. Semin Pediatr Infect Dis. 2006;17(1):5–10.
9. Walner DL, Loewen MS, Kimura RE. Neonatal subglottic stenosis – incidence and trends. Laryngoscope. 2001;111(1):48–51.
10. Chan RW, Fu M, Tirunagari N. Elasticity of the human false vocal fold. Ann Otol Rhinol Laryngol. 2006;115(5):370–81.
11. Liu YH, Xu SC, Tu LL, Zhang KL, Lu DH, Zhang M. A rich lymphatic network exists in the inferior surface of the vocal cord. Surg Radiol Anat. 2006;28(2):125–8.
12. Copland I, Post M. Lung development and fetal lung growth. Paediatr Respir Rev. 2004;5(Suppl A):S259–64.
13. Warburton D, Schwarz M, Tefft D, Flores-Delgado G, Anderson KD, Cardoso WV. The molecular basis of lung morphogenesis. Mech Dev. 2000;92(1):55–81.
14. Girosi D, Bellodi S, Sabatini F, Rossi GA. The lung and the gut: common origins, close links. Paediatr Respir Rev. 2006;7 Suppl 1:S235–9.
15. Hansen CP, Holtveg H, Francis D, Rasch L, Bertelsen S. Pulmonary hamartoma. J Thorac Cardiovasc Surg. 1992;104(3):674–8.
16. Linnoila RI. Functional facets of the pulmonary neuroendocrine system. Lab Invest. 2006;86(5):425–44.
17. Jackman DM, Johnson BE. Small-cell lung cancer. Lancet. 2005;366(9494):1385–96.
18. Cimen M, Erdil H, Karatepe T. A cadaver with azygos lobe and its clinical significance. Anat Sci Int. 2005;80(4):235–7.
19. Sandu K, Monnier P. Congenital tracheal anomalies. Otolaryngol Clin North Am. 2007;40(1):193–217, viii.
20. Gezer S, Tastepe I, Sirmali M, Findik G, Turut H, Kaya S, et al. Pulmonary sequestration: a single-institutional series composed of 27 cases. J Thorac Cardiovasc Surg. 2007;133(4):955–9.
21. Pinheiro PF, Simoes e, Silva AC, Pereira RM. Current knowledge on esophageal atresia. World J Gastroenterol. 2012;18(28):3662–72.
22. Epstein SK. Anatomy and physiology of tracheostomy. Respir Care. 2005;50(4):476–82.
23. Swami A, Spodick DH. Pulsus paradoxus in cardiac tamponade: a pathophysiologic continuum. Clin Cardiol. 2003;26(5):215–7.
24. Mal H, Rullon I, Mellot F, Brugiere O, Sleiman C, Menu Y, et al. Immediate and long-term results of bronchial artery embolization for life-threatening hemoptysis. Chest. 1999;115(4):996–1001.
25. Taylor RW, Palagiri AV. Central venous catheterization. Crit Care Med. 2007;35(5):1390–6.
26. Kusminsky RE. Complications of central venous catheterization. J Am Coll Surg. 2007;204(4):681–96.
27. Duggan M, Kavanagh BP. Atelectasis in the perioperative patient. Curr Opin Anaesthesiol. 2007;20(1):37–42.
28. Haynes D, Baumann MH. Management of pneumothorax. Semin Respir Crit Care Med. 2010;31(6):769–80.
29. Kaneda H, Nakano T, Taniguchi Y, Saito T, Konobu T, Saito Y. Three-step management of pneumothorax: time for a re-think on initial management. Interact Cardiovasc Thorac Surg. 2013;16(2):186–92.

Mediastinum, Heart, and Great Vessels in the Thorax

5

1. Mark the *false* statement:
   (a) The superior mediastinum contains from anterior to posterior the internal mammary vessels, thymus, great vessels, trachea, esophagus, and sympathetic trunks.
   (b) The trachea occupies the anterior mediastinum.
   (c) The middle mediastinum contains the pericardium, phrenic nerves, heart, and roots of the great vessels.
   (d) The posterior mediastinum contains the descending aorta, esophagus, thoracic duct, sympathetic chains, azygos system, and vagus nerves.
   (e) The posterior mediastinum is continuous with the retropharyngeal space.

Comments The mediastinum is a space with the following boundaries:
Anterior – Sternum
Posterior – Thoracic vertebrae and ribs
Lateral – Mediastinal pleura
Superior – Thoracic outlet
Inferior – Diaphragm

An imaginary plane drawn from the angle of Louis to the T4–T5 junction divides the mediastinum into superior and inferior. In turn, the inferior mediastinum is divided by the pericardial sac into anterior, middle, and posterior. The anterior mediastinum contains the caudal aspects of the thymus, lymph nodes, and connective tissue. The trachea is located in the posterior aspect of the superior mediastinum. It divides at the angle of Louis and hence does not reach into the inferior mediastinum (Fig. 5.1).

V.K. Maker, E.D. Guzman-Arrieta, *Cognitive Pearls in General Surgery*,
DOI 10.1007/978-1-4939-1850-8_5,

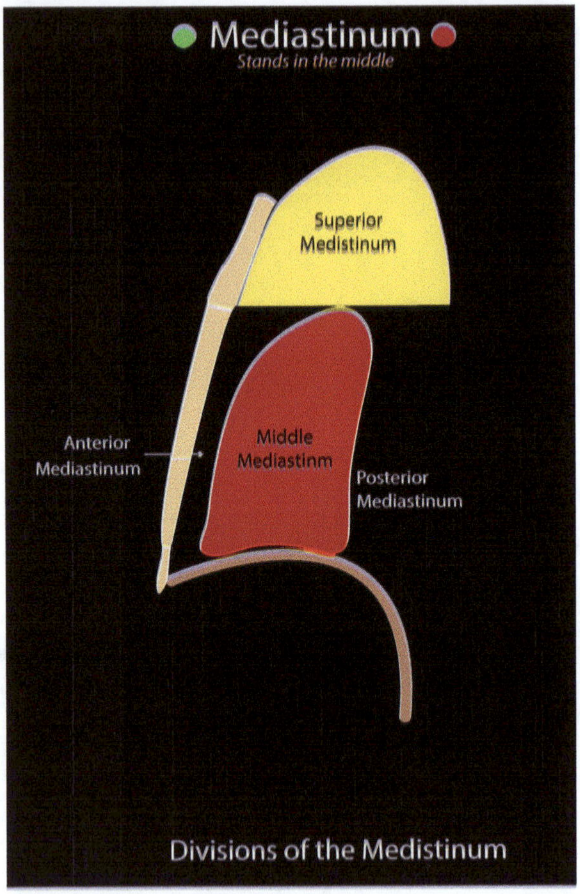

Fig. 5.1 As the name states, the mediastinum is a partition which "stands in the middle" of the two hemithoraces. In the embryo, major cardiac, vascular, lymphatic, and solid organ transitions occur at the level of T4. A line drawn between the lower end of the manubrium and T4/T5 divides the mediastinum into a superior and inferior compartment. The pericardial sac divides the inferior mediastinum into anterior, middle, and posterior divisions, each with characteristic pathology

Answer

b

2. Mark the *incorrect* statement.
   (a) The posterior intercostal arteries are longer on the right than the left side.
   (b) The posterior intercostal arteries are posterior to the azygos, hemiazygos, and the sympathetic trunks.
   (c) The thoracic duct starts crossing from right to left at the level of T6 as it courses cephalad.
   (d) The thoracic duct collects the lymph from the upper right hemithorax and right arm.
   (e) The cisterna chyli collects all the lymph from the abdomen and lower extremities.

Comments The position of the descending aorta, to the left of the vertebral column, determines that the posterior intercostal arteries arising from it are longer on the left than on the right. The relationship of the sympathetic trunks with the vasculature becomes relevant during thoracoscopic or open sympathectomies.

The thoracic duct is often exposed to injuries during thoracic and mediastinal procedures. It arises from the cisterna chyli and carries the lymph from the abdomen and the lower extremities. As it courses towards the left subclavian vein, it receives lymph from the left hemithorax, left upper extremity, and left jugular territory. The upper right hemithorax, upper extremity, and head drain into the right thoracic duct, which starts in the thorax and empties into the right subclavian vein [1]. This distribution of lymphatic drainage often determines the route of cancer spread (Figs. 5.2 and 5.3).

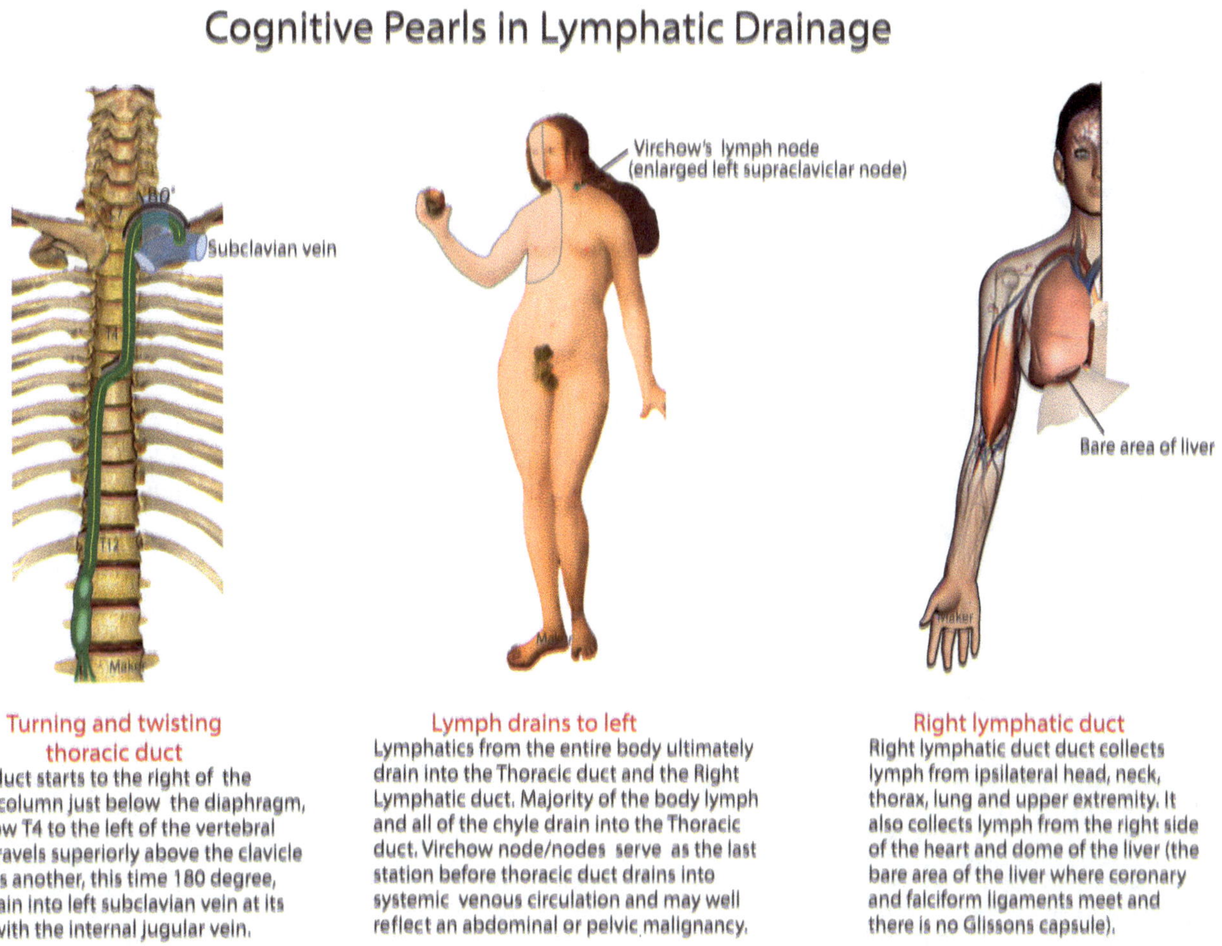

Fig. 5.2 Cognitive pearls in lymphatic drainage. The thoracic duct begins to the right of the vertebral column, just below the diaphragm and starts its turning and twisting course up the thorax into the left side of the neck. The thoracic duct is the major lymphatic channel draining lymph and chyle from most of the body into the systemic circulation at the junction of the left subclavian and the internal jugular veins. Virhcow's lymph node is the last lymph node station in this course. An abnormal and or enlarged Virchow's node may represent an advanced abdominal/pelvic malignancy. The right lymphatic duct collects the lymph from the ipsilateral head, neck, thorax, lung, and upper extremity. It also collects lymph from the right side of the heart and the bare area of the liver. The bare area of the liver is at its dome where all the ligaments reflect away from the liver leaving an area without a covering of Glisson's capsule

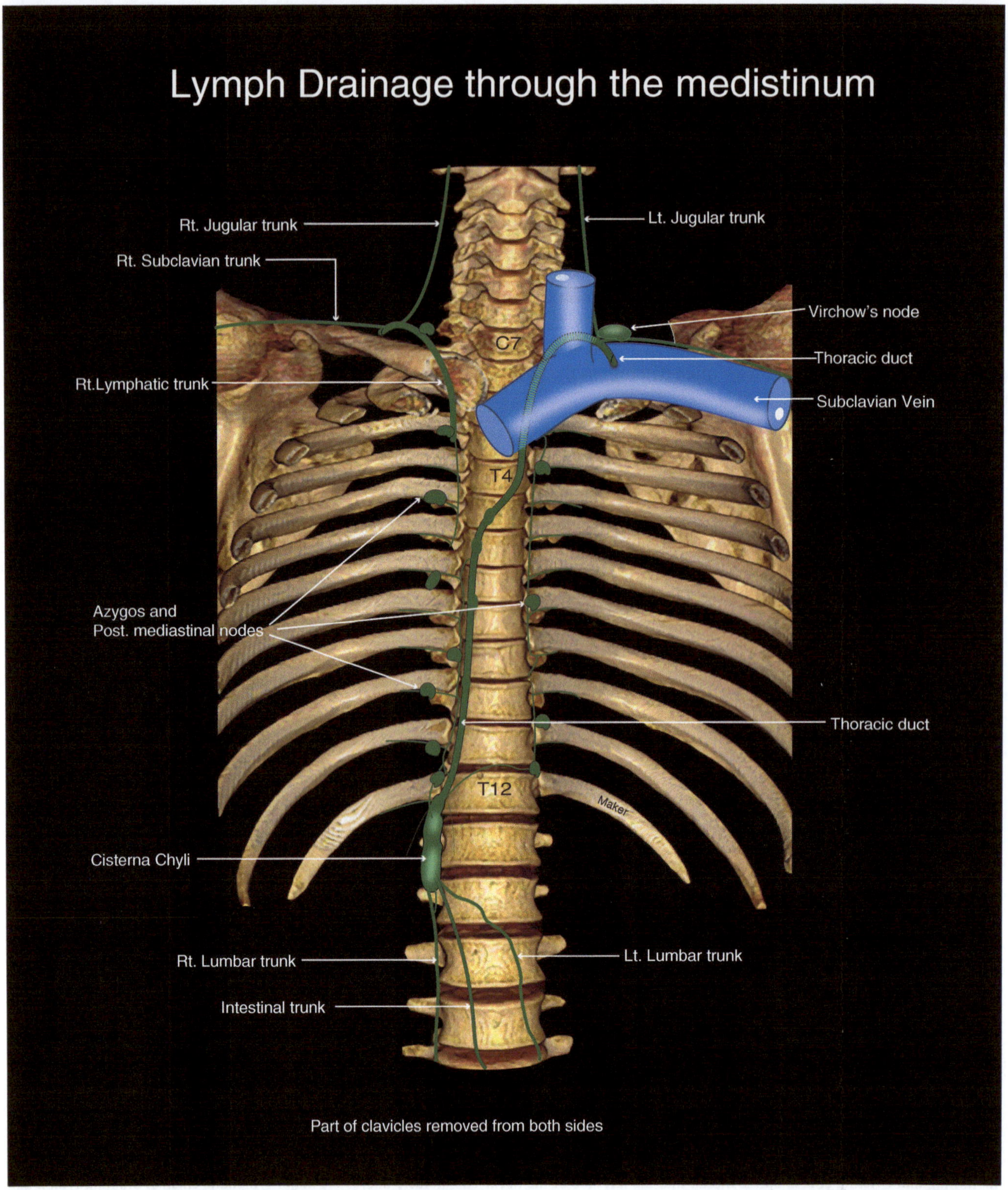

Fig. 5.3 Lymphatics generally follow the veins but as opposed to veins have the physiologic ability to drain large protein molecules. The thoracic duct additionally drains fatty acid-rich chyle from the intestinal trunk to the cisterna chyli. The lymph from the right and the left side of the head, neck, and upper extremities drains through the jugular and subclavian trunks into the right lymphatic duct and the thoracic duct, respectively. Lumbar trunks drain the lower extremities into the cisterna chyli. Tumors that spread through the lymphatics will therefore metastasize to similar locations if they drain through the same channels

Answer
d

3. Mark the *false* statement.
   (a) The anterior scalene node (Virchow's node) may harbor metastasis from the mediastinum, thorax, breasts, and abdominal organs.
   (b) Mediastinal masses are most often symptomatic.
   (c) Indirect signs of mediastinal masses are displacement of the apical heartbeat and tracheal deviation.
   (d) The most common tumors of the superior mediastinum are thymomas, lymphomas, thyroid tumors, and parathyroid adenomas.
   (e) The most common tumors of the posterior mediastinum are neurogenic tumors and enteric cysts.

Comments Rudolf Virchow (1821–1902), considered the father of pathology, described that enlarged left-sided supraclavicular nodes were harbingers of intra-abdominal malignancy. This node, later named after Virchow, is the highest in the bronchomediastinal chain. It is located at the confluence of the thoracic duct and the left subclavian vein. When enlarged, it can be palpated in the left supraclavicular fossa, just above the middle third of the clavicle [2, 3].

Mediastinal tumors are most often asymptomatic and discovered incidentally. When they cause symptoms these tend to be due to compression of adjacent structures. Mediastinal tumors are derived from the structures normally found in its compartments or from their embryologic forebears. For example, the preponderance of neurogenic and enteric cysts in the posterior mediastinum reflects the posterior location of the neural crest and foregut, respectively. The middle mediastinum gives rise to mesenchymal tumors (pericardial cysts, lipomas, liposarcomas, fibromas, and fibrosarcomas). The superior mediastinum may present any of the tumors found in the compartments of the inferior mediastinum, as well as tumors extending from the neck (e.g., retrosternal goiter) [4–7] (Fig. 5.4).

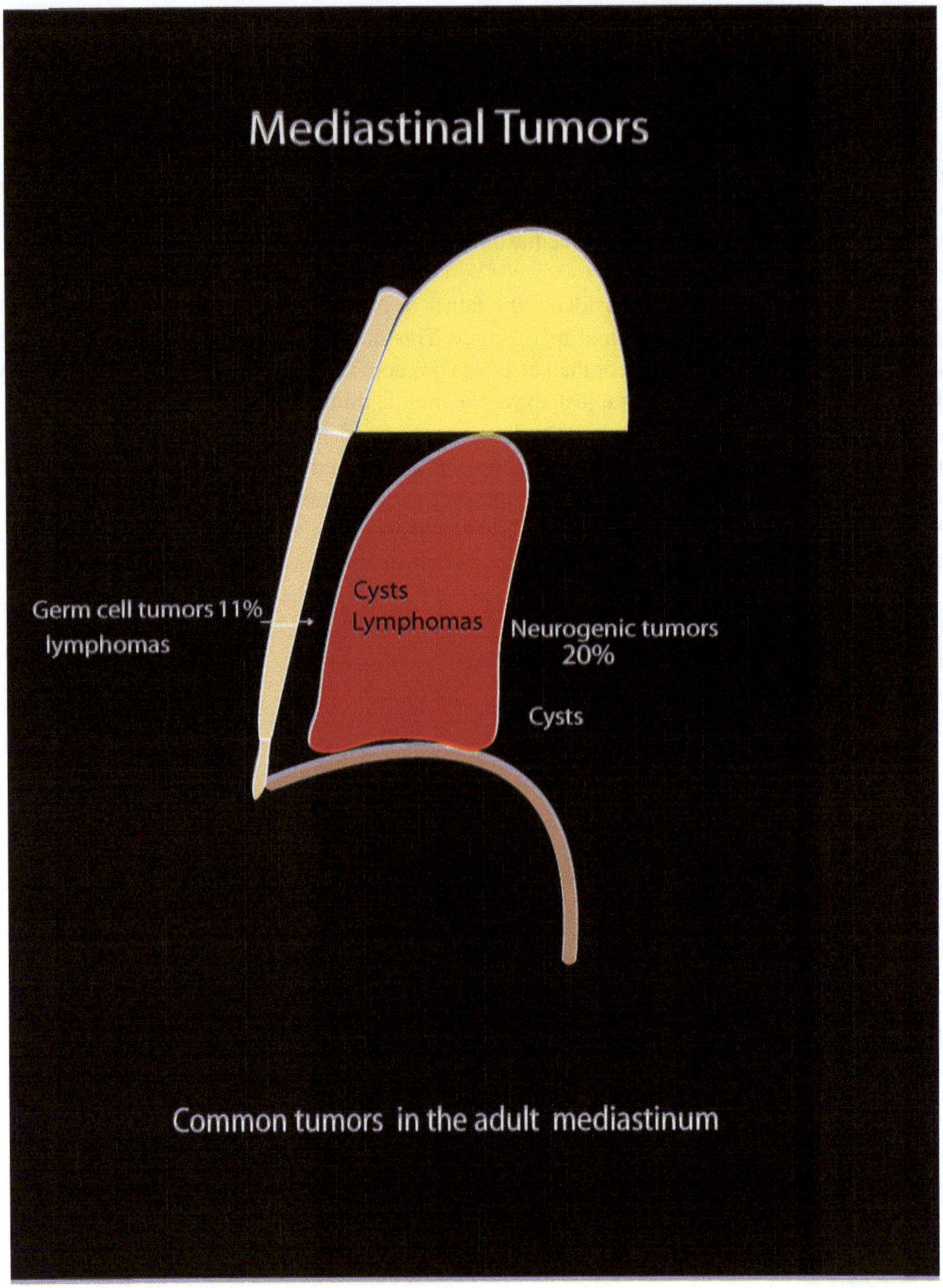

Fig. 5.4 Tumors in the mediastinum are formed of the embyological tissue that developed in the corresponding compartment. The most common tumors of the superior mediastinum are retrosternal goiters. These are often accessed through the neck. The posterior mediastinum harbors tumors from neural crest cells and foregut-derived cysts. Lymph node-derived neoplasms, primary and metastatic, dominate the middle mediastinum. The trachea is located in the superior mediastinum and bifurcates below the T4 vertebra into the posterior mediastinum. This area is surrounded by hilar lymph nodes draining the lungs as well as other mediastinal structures. The anterior mediastinum is the most common site for extragonadal germ cell tumors. 50–70 % of these tumors are found in this location

Answer
b

4. The following statements regarding the thymus are correct *except:*
   (a) The thymus shares a common origin with the superior parathyroids.
   (b) Hassall's corpuscles are the histological hallmark of the thymus.
   (c) The main blood supply to the thymus comes from the inferior thyroid arteries and the internal mammary arteries.
   (d) The thymic veins drain to the SVC on the right and the brachiocephalic vein on the left.
   (e) The thymus lacks efferent lymphatics.

Comments The thymus shares a common origin with the inferior parathyroids. Both are derived from the third branchial pouch. When inferior parathyroids cannot be found, the thymus is often searched for and removed. Hassall's corpuscles represent concentric layers of medullary epithelial cells surrounding an eosinophilic, partially keratinized core. Their function is thought to be related to the selection and maturation of thymocytes. Their numbers have been found to increase with age. Unlike what occurs in lymph nodes, lymphocytes exit the thymus through veins [8].

Answer
a

5. Mark the *false* statement regarding heart development
   (a) A common mesodermal atrium and ventricle undergo septation.
   (b) The aorta and pulmonary artery are derived from two independent arterial trunks.
   (c) Neural crest-derived cells contribute to the formation of the cardiac conduction system.
   (d) Pericardial defects may lead to congenital cardiac herniation.
   (e) Pericardial cysts represent remnants of the pleuropericardial canal.

Comments During the first 3 weeks of gestation, the human embryo obtains its nutrients by diffusion. At this time, paired mesoderm-derived endocardial tubes fuse to form the primitive heart. This single chamber structure already has contractile properties. The primitive heart then folds upon itself. In this process the atria, which were originally caudal, take a postero-cephalic location, whereas the ventricles become anterior and caudal.

As the folding of the primitive heart occurs, septations form within it, under the influence of neural crest-derived cells [9]. Failure in this septation process results in abnormal communication between chambers, the most common of which are atrial septal defect and ventricular septal defect. The common ventricular outflow tract also undergoes division to form the aorta and pulmonary artery. Defects in this process lead to the transposition of great vessel and persistence of the truncus arteriosus [10, 11].

Defects in the formation of the pericardium may form orifices through which the heart (most commonly the left atria) can herniate. While largely asymptomatic, these defects may cause paroxysmal chest pain. The herniated heart may become incarcerated and compromise of coronary circulation may occur. Treatment of this pathology is surgical and involves attempts to close the defect or enlarge it to a size in which strangulation no longer occurs [12, 13].

Pericardial cysts, along with bronchial and enteric cysts, are embryologic remnants found in the mediastinum.

Answer

b

6. Mark the *incorrect* statement in relation to congenital heart malformations.
   (a) Cyanotic cardiac malformations involve right to left shunting.
   (b) Eisenmenger's syndrome consists of secondary left to right shunting due to increases in pulmonary vascular resistance.
   (c) Left to right shunting allows survival in the presence of transposition of the great vessels.
   (d) When present, a left persistent superior vena cava drains into the left atrium.
   (e) Ventricular septal defects are the most common congenital cardiac anomaly.

Comments Congenital cardiac malformations may be classified into cyanotic and noncyanotic, with the former being more severe. Cyanotic cardiac malformations cause blood to shunt from the right heart to the left heart, bypassing the lungs and creating desaturation that does not respond to oxygen therapy. Some examples are the tetralogy of Fallot, truncus arteriosus, and transposition of the great vessels. In noncyanotic cardiac malformations oxygenated blood is shunted from the left heart to the right, causing an increased load for the latter. This shunting occurs across atrial and ventricular defects as well as a patent ductus arteriosus. Over time, the right heart hypertrophies to compensate for the increased workload and comes to generate pressures greater than those found in the left heart. At this point, a reversal in flow occurs, and right to left shunting takes place. This is known as Eisenmenger's syndrome [14, 15].

Transposition of the great vessels generates two independent parallel circulatory circuits. In this scenario, venous blood returning from the systemic circulation is sent back to the systemic arteries without passing through the lungs. A patent ductus arteriosus allows oxygenated blood to cross into the arterial circulation sustaining life.

Answer

b

7. Mark the *incorrect* statement about pericardial anatomy.
   (a) A rim of air seen around the pericardium, continuing along the diaphragmatic surface, is radiologically indicative of esophageal perforation.
   (b) Pericardiotomy should be performed in transverse fashion.
   (c) The pericardium has a common origin with the pleurae and the peritoneum.
   (d) Subxiphoid pericardiostomy is the classical surgical treatment for malignant pericardial effusions.
   (e) The central tendon of the diaphragm and the inferior aspect of the pericardium have a common origin in the septum transversum.

Comments The pericardial pleura continues as the diaphragmatic pleura; hence, air on the left side of the mediastinum will dissect along the diaphragmatic pleura as well. This is one of the early signs of Boerhaave syndrome. When present on chest X-ray, it is called the V sign of Naclerio [16, 17] (Fig. 5.5).

The phrenic nerve runs along the posterior aspect of the pericardium. This dictates that pericardiectomy should be carried out in longitudinal fashion (Fig. 5.6).

There are several options to relieve pericardial effusion. In emergent situations where hemodynamically significant tamponade exists, needle pericardiocentesis is the initial procedure of choice prior to formal exploration. When ongoing drainage is expected, a subxiphoid pericardiectomy is indicated to allow ongoing drainage [18] (Fig. 5.7).

The septum transversum originates in the neck region and descends to occupy the lower thorax as the developing lungs and heart occupy the space above it. In the process, the phrenic nerve (C3–C5) is pulled down in a longitudinal fashion. This explains why diaphragmatic or pericardial irritation (e.g., basal pneumonia, inferior myocardial infarction, subphrenic abscess, and free air) causes referred pain to the neck and shoulder region.

V-sign of Naclerio

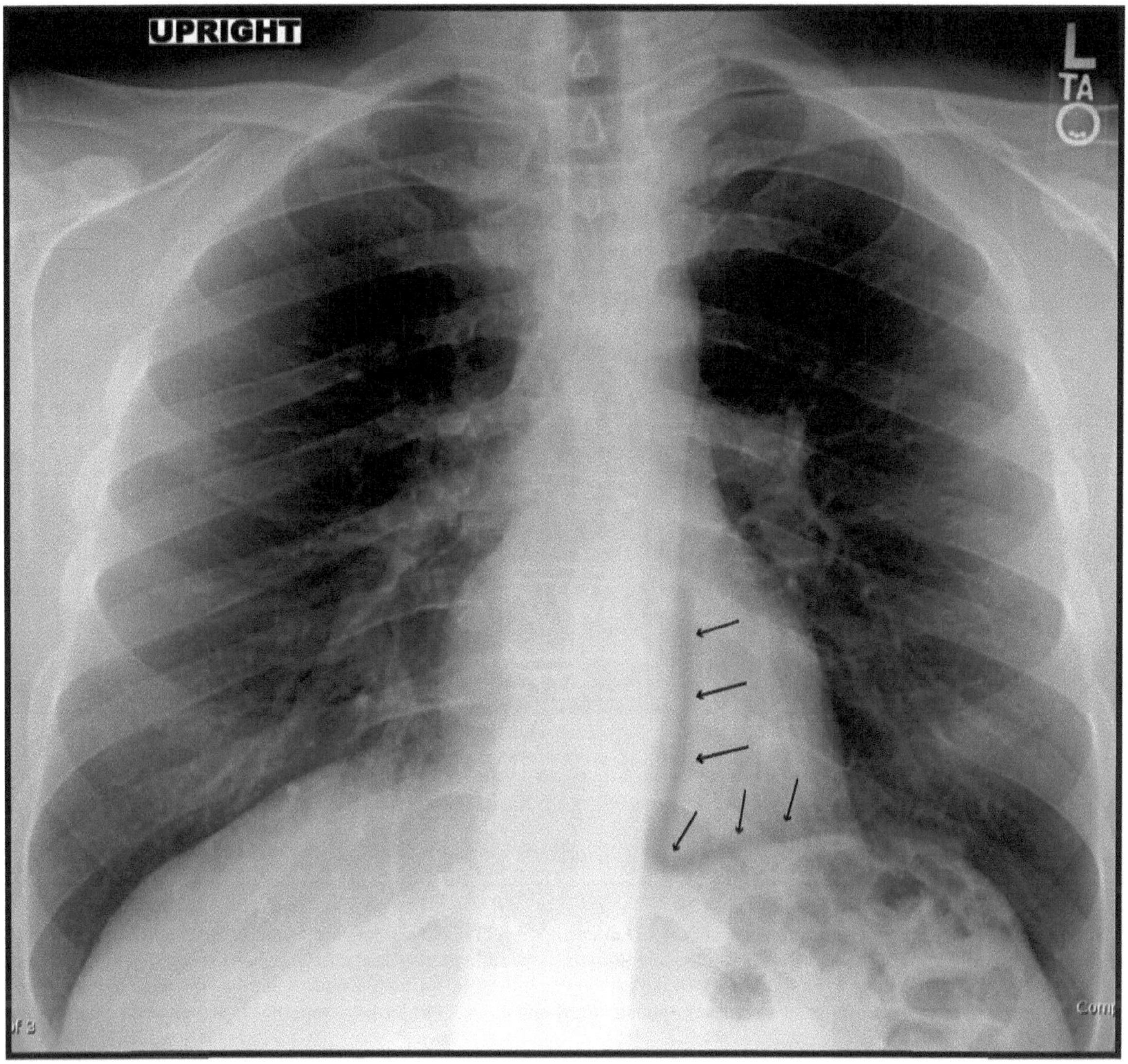

Arrowsare pointing at the pneumomediastinum outlining the thoracic and mediastinal pleura

Fig. 5.5 Dr. Emil A. Naclerio from New York described the "V sign" as an early warning sign on a plain radiograph of the abdomen for spontaneous rupture of the esophagus. Free air from the rupture outlines the thoracic and the mediastinal pleura over the left hemidiaphragm

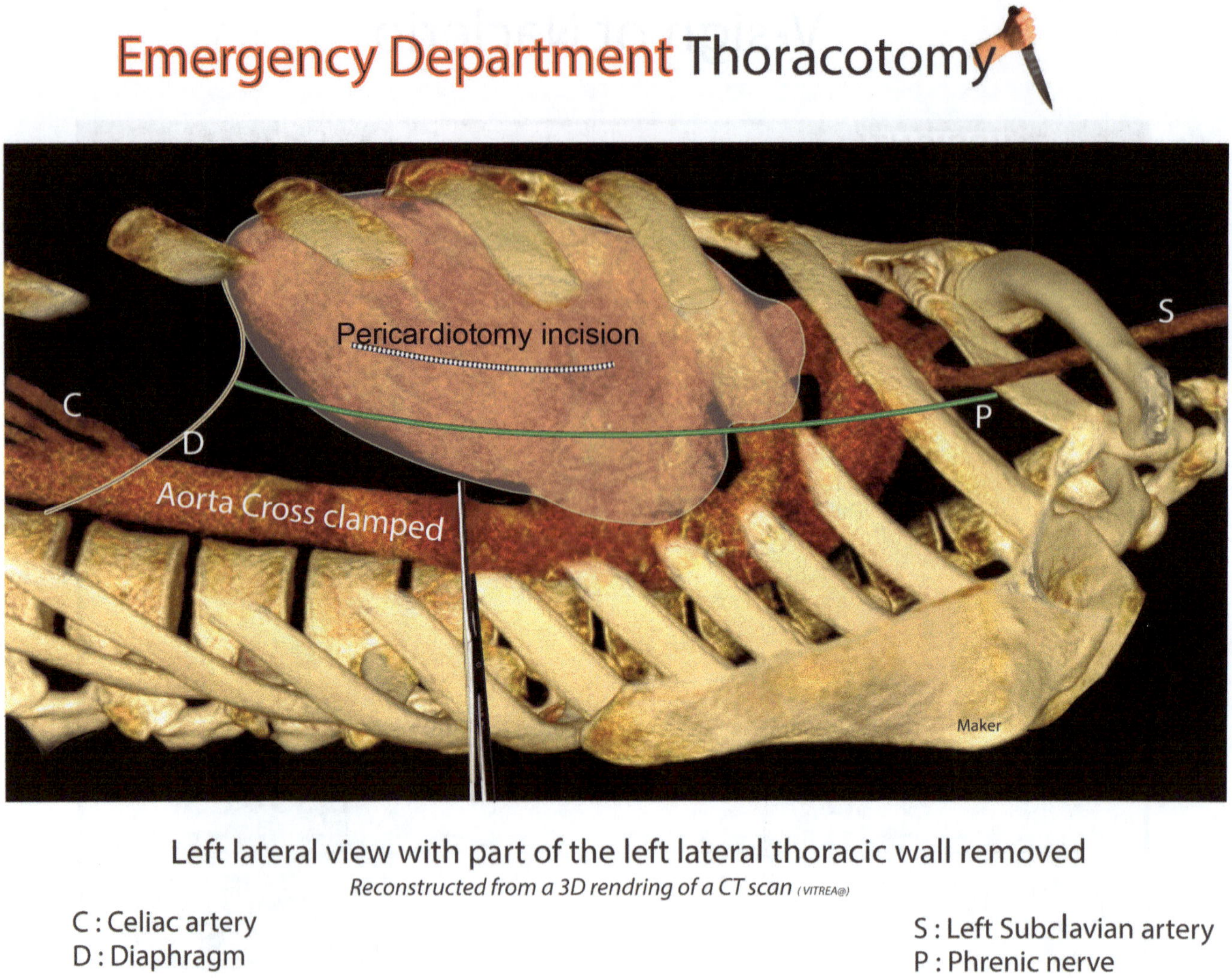

Fig. 5.6 This illustration depicts four clear components of the ED thoracotomy. (1) Pericardiotomy incision is placed anterior to the phrenic nerve for quick relief of pericardial tamponade and control of bleeding from the penetrating injury to the heart, when present. (2) Cross clamping of the thoracic aorta to preferentially increase cerebral perfusion of the patient in extremis. (3) Effective internal cardiac massage in hypovolemic shock. (4) Fast access to the thoracic cavity through an anterolateral thoracotomy and control of bleeding from the chest wall and/or the left lung

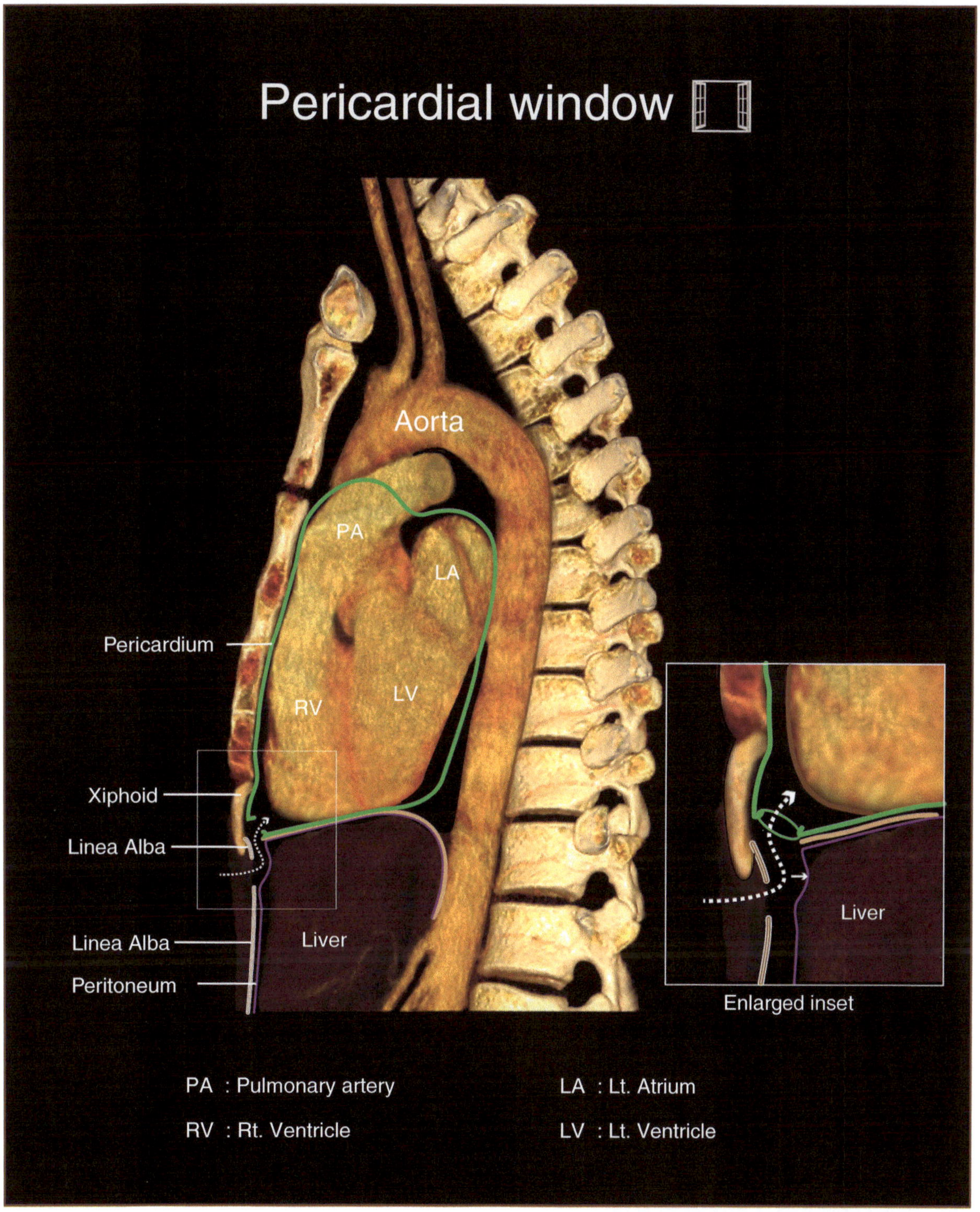

Fig. 5.7 Pericardial window, as the name signifies, provides a window to the pericardial cavity for the therapeutic drainage of pericardial fluid. It can also be a diagnostic modality when a small part of the pericardium is biopsied for pathogenesis. The subxiphoid approach illustrated here with a *dotted arrow* shows midline entry through an incision in the linea alba entering the preperitoneal space. The midline diaphragm is entered to gain access to the pericardium. The inferior wall of the pericardium and the tendinous part of the diaphragm are closely related embryologically; both arising from the septum transversum in the neck with the phrenic nerve supply of cervical 3, 4, and 5 nerve roots

Answer
b

8. All of the following are correct *except*:
   (a) The coronary sulcus demarcates the atria from the ventricles. It houses the right coronary artery as well as the circumflex branch of the left coronary artery.
   (b) The coronary arteries arise from the aorta, 2 cm distal to the aortic valve.
   (c) The interventricular sulcus parallels the interventricular septum. It contains the anterior descending (branch of the left coronary) and the posterior descending (branch of the right coronary).
   (d) Left coronary dominance occurs when the posterior descending artery arises from the circumflex artery instead of the right coronary.
   (e) In the absence of left coronary dominance, anastomoses occur between the right coronary and left coronary systems along the interventricular septum.

Comments Occasionally, a general surgeon is faced with repairing a penetrating wound of the heart as an emergency. Classical repair is performed with the surgeon's finger tamponading the heart while nonabsorbable sutures with pledgets are placed. Basic knowledge of the location of major coronary vessels becomes critical during this repair.

Answer

b

9. Mark the *false* statement.
   (a) The atria are electrically isolated from the ventricles by the fibrous cardiac skeleton.
   (b) The atrioventricular node specializes in the delay of electrical signals transmitted from the atrial node.
   (c) The accessory bundles of Kent cause Wolff–Parkinson–White syndrome.
   (d) The Cox maze procedure is designed to interrupt the communications between the atrial and atrioventricular nodes in order to treat chronic atrial fibrillation.
   (e) Cardiac nerves are carefully preserved and anastomosed during cardiac transplant.

Comments Optimal functioning of the heart requires that the atria contract while the ventricles are relaxed, in order to create a pressure gradient that allows ventricular filling. The fibrous cardiac skeleton prevents nonspecific propagation of depolarization from the atria to the ventricles. Instead, conduction occurs through specialized fibers communicating the atrial node with the atrioventricular node. The latter further delays the electrical signal that will eventually depolarize the ventricles [19, 20]. In Wolff–Parkinson–White syndrome the above order is disrupted by the bundles of Kent, which are anomalous muscle fibers that bypass the fibrous skeleton, constituting alternative pathways for electrical impulse transmission leading to premature ventricular contraction (PVC) [21]. This syndrome is surgically correctable and was the first of many arrhythmias to be treated in this manner [22].

While it is true that the heart is under neural control by the sympathetic and parasympathetic nerves, its intrinsic contractility allows it to function independently, albeit regulatory function is lacking. Parasympathetic denervation causes an increased in resting heart rate to 90–100 beats per minute as well as increased contractility. Sympathetic denervation manifests itself as a failure to increase heart rate and contractility in response to exercise. There is, however, a delayed and partial compensation mediated by epinephrine released by the adrenal medulla. Over time, these defects improve. It is thought that this is due to some degree of spontaneous reinnervation [23].

Answer
e

10. Mark the *incorrect* statement.
    (a) The most common tumors of the heart are metastatic.
    (b) Myxomas are the most common primary tumors of the heart.
    (c) Sarcomas are the most common primary malignant tumors of the heart.
    (d) A paradoxical embolus starts from the venous side of the heart and ends up on the arterial side.
    (e) Carcinoid syndrome most often affects the mitral valve.

Comments The abundant blood supply of the heart likely explains that metastatic tumors are 100–1,000 times more common than primary tumors in end-stage malignancies [24]. Among the primary tumors myxomas are the most common, with 75 % of them arising from the rim of the fossa ovalis in the left atrium. This may be due to the abundance of myxoid material that closes the atrial septum. Reflecting its mesodermal origin, it's no surprise that sarcomas are the most common primary malignancies of the heart [25].

An abnormal communication between the atria or ventricles is not sufficient to cause paradoxical embolism; there is also need for right to left shunting to be present [26].

The cardiac valves, per se, do not have a blood supply; they solely depend on diffusion of nutrients from the blood inside the heart [27]. In carcinoid syndrome liver metastasis produces large amounts of serotonin overwhelming the detoxifying capacities of mono amino oxidase (MAO). These vasoactive amines follow the hepatic veins into the right heart, producing swelling of the tricuspid valve cusps, a finding referred to as banana valves. As the disease progresses, edema gives way to fibrosis. The pulmonary valve is the second most common involved valve. Following the outflow from the ventricle, serotonin enters the lungs, which are also a site of MAO activity preventing the development of left-sided lesions. However, when carcinoid syndrome arises from the lungs, left valvular lesions may occur, affecting primarily the mitral valve [28].

Answer
e

11. All of the following are correct *except*:
    (a) During central venous access procedures, PVC is often a sign of ventricular cannulation.
    (b) Arterial cannulation is necessary for placement of left ventricular pacemaker leads.
    (c) In atrial fibrillation single-chamber pacemakers are placed in the right ventricle.
    (d) AV sequential pacemakers have atrial and ventricular leads.
    (e) Pacemakers and ventricular defibrillators are now placed transvenously.

Comments When PVC is noticed during central venous catheter insertion, the catheter is usually withdrawn with disappearance of this arrhythmia.

The majority of pacemakers introduced today are transvenous AV sequential pacemakers, with leads in both the right atrium and right ventricle. These pacemakers recreate the physiologic atrial contraction augmenting cardiac output. The coronary sinus is located in the right atrium, just above the inferior vena cava. It drains the coronary veins and provides an excellent access to the left ventricle. This access is used to place left ventricular pacemaker leads transvenously for biventricular pacing [29].

Answer
b

12. All of the following are correct *except*:
    (a) A trapdoor thoracotomy exposes the carina.
    (b) A median sternotomy provides fast access to the structures of the middle mediastinum.
    (c) Posterolateral thoracotomies are classically used for surgery of the lung and esophagus.
    (d) Left anterolateral thoracotomy provides emergent access to the heart and descending aorta.
    (e) Clamshell thoracotomy is performed in emergent situations to access both thoracic cavities.

Comments Trapdoor thoracotomy classically consists of a median sternotomy extending laterally along the clavicle. A portion of the clavicle can be resected. The clavicle and sternum are then elevated from the underlying tissue, providing access to the subclavian vessels, pleural apex, and aortic arch (on the left).

Median sternotomy is the traditional incision used for cardiac surgery. It provides broad exposure and excellent access to the anterior and middle mediastinum. The lungs and mid-esophagus are best exposed through posterolateral thoracotomies.

In witnessed traumatic arrest secondary to penetrating wounds, emergency anterolateral thoracotomy may be lifesaving. This approach is carried out on the fourth rib space on the left side. It approaches the pericardial sac and descending aorta, with the goal of relieving tamponade, providing internal cardiac massage and defibrillation, and redirecting aortic blood flow to the heart and brain by cross clamping the aorta. On occasion after performing this incision, it becomes evident that there are right-sided injuries that require emergent care. In this scenario, the left anterolateral thoracotomy is extended across the sternum to the right side. The sternum is then elevated anteriorly and cephalad providing a clamshell-like exposure (Fig. 5.8).

Approaches to the Chest

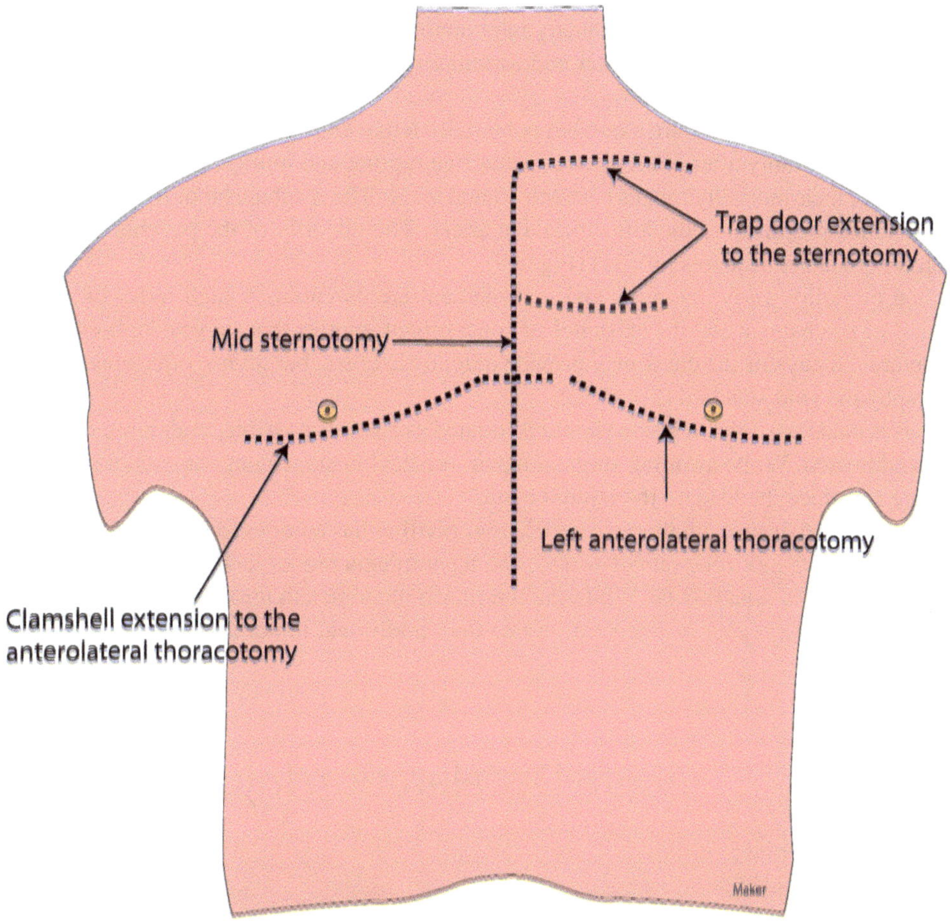

Fig. 5.8 Classic approaches to the anterior chest are through a midline sternotomy or an anterolateral thoracotomy. In case of an emergency, a clamshell extension through the sternum can be done to explore and expose both sides of the chest. In an emergency or for access to the innominate or subclavian vessels, a trapdoor extension can be added to the midsternotomy on either side of the chest

Answer

a

13. All of the following are correct *except*:
    (a) Blunt thoracic aortic injuries result from deceleration mechanisms.
    (b) Plain X-rays are effective in ruling out thoracic dissection.
    (c) Endovascular repair has emerged as the treatment modality of choice.
    (d) Open repair has a lower incidence of secondary intervention than endovascular repair.
    (e) Lifelong surveillance is recommended after endovascular repair.

Comments Blunt thoracic aortic injuries are a rare but potentially lethal entity. It is thought that these lesions are one of the main causes of immediate mortality after blunt trauma, when free rupture and immediate exsanguination occur. While their incidence is less than 1 %, their mortality ranges between 75 and 90 %. The mechanism of this injury is deceleration causing a tear at the aortic isthmus, just distal to the left subclavian artery. The majority of the patients that survive long enough to reach the hospital have contained ruptures [30, 31] (Fig. 5.9).

Given the elevated mortality, early diagnosis and management are essential. A high index of suspicion for this injury should be on the basis of mechanism and the existence of concomitant injuries that suggest high-energy trauma (e.g., 1st rib fracture, sternal fracture). X-rays of the chest may provide diagnostic clues, but do not offer great sensitivity or specificity, making CT angiography the gold standard (Fig. 5.10).

Once the diagnosis is made, significant lesion should be treated as early as possible, after more immediate life-threatening problems have been addressed. While awaiting surgical repair, medical management consists of reducing the heart rate and mean arterial pressure to reduce the load on the injured aorta.

Currently, endovascular repair through thoracic aortic stent grafting has emerged as the treatment of choice. Open repair had a mortality rate of 15–20 %, a stroke rate of 4–6 %, and a paraplegia rate of 2–10 %. Endovascular repair has lowered these numbers to 8–13 %, <1 %, and 0–3 %. While the long-term outcomes in terms of mortality for both approaches are similar, stent graft therapy has a higher re-intervention rate than traditional repair and requires close lifelong surveillance [32, 33] (Fig. 5.11).

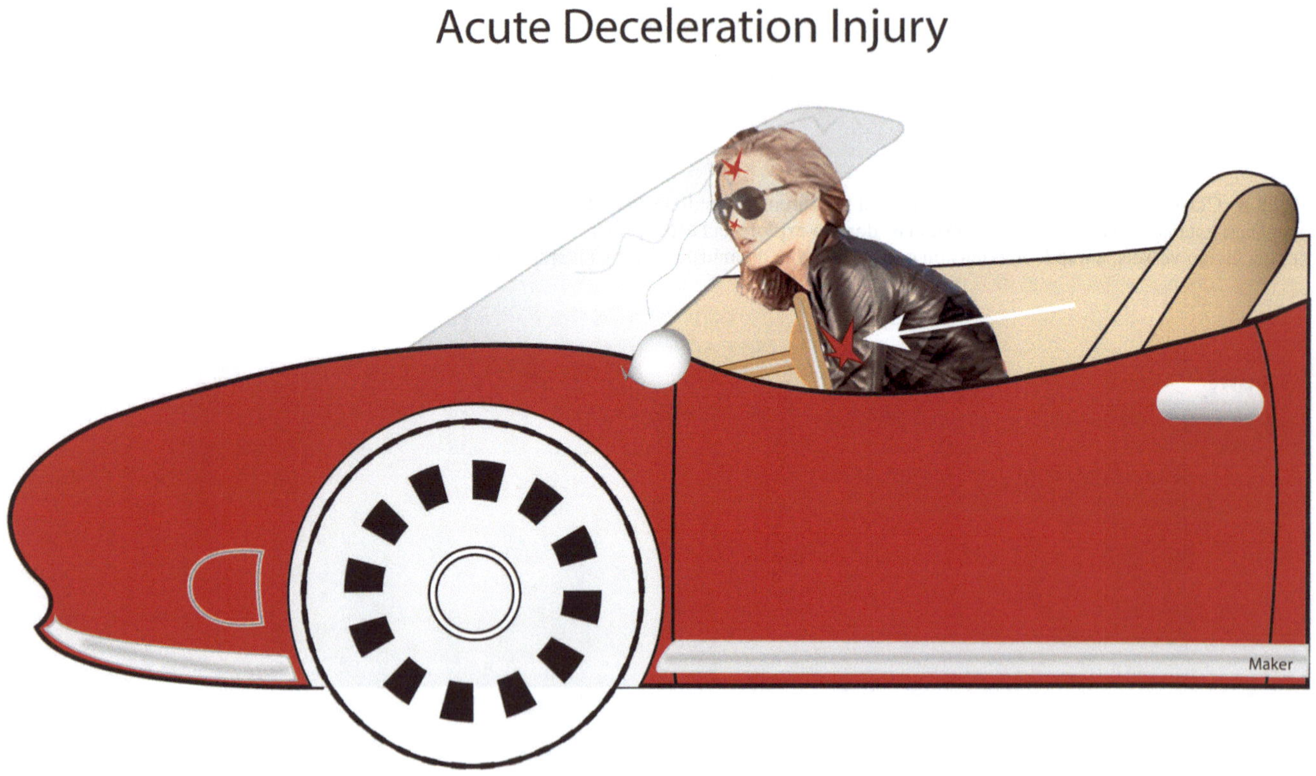

Fig. 5.9 Acute deceleration injury. Driver side collisions and head on collisions are common causes of traumatic shear injury to the thoracic aorta

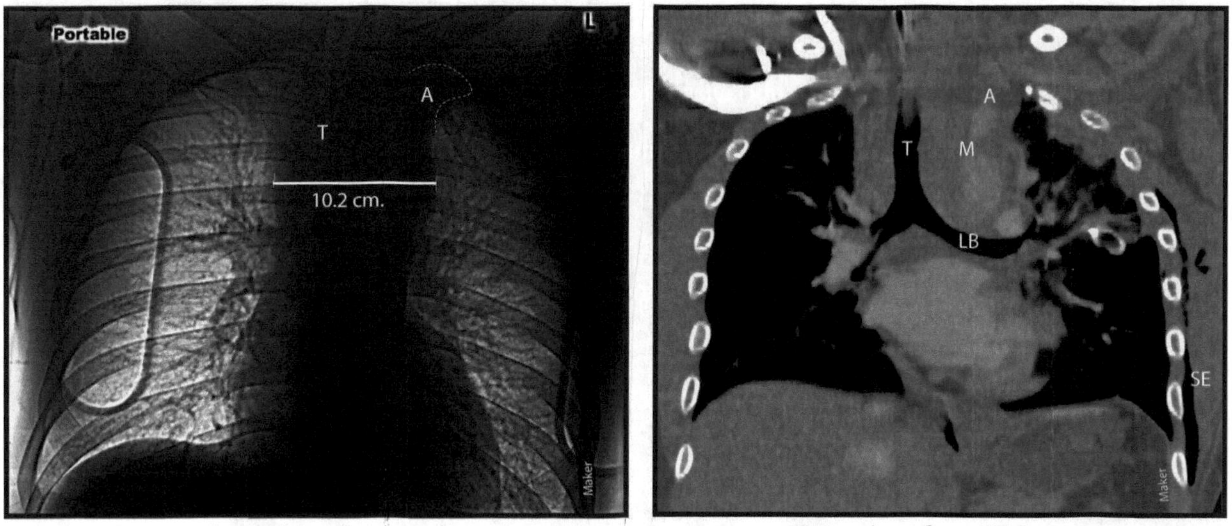

Fig. 5.10 Widened mediastinum has a width greater than 6 cm on an upright PA film of chest X-ray or a width more than 8 cm on a supine AP chest. In acute blunt trauma, traumatic rupture of the aorta is one of the most urgent diagnostic challenges. Shifting of the trachea to the right and the left bronchus inferiorly is commonly seen. An apical cap is formed by a hematoma dissecting above the left pleura. Depending on the nature and extent of the trauma, sternal and rib fractures, lung contusions, and hemothorax are commonly associated injuries

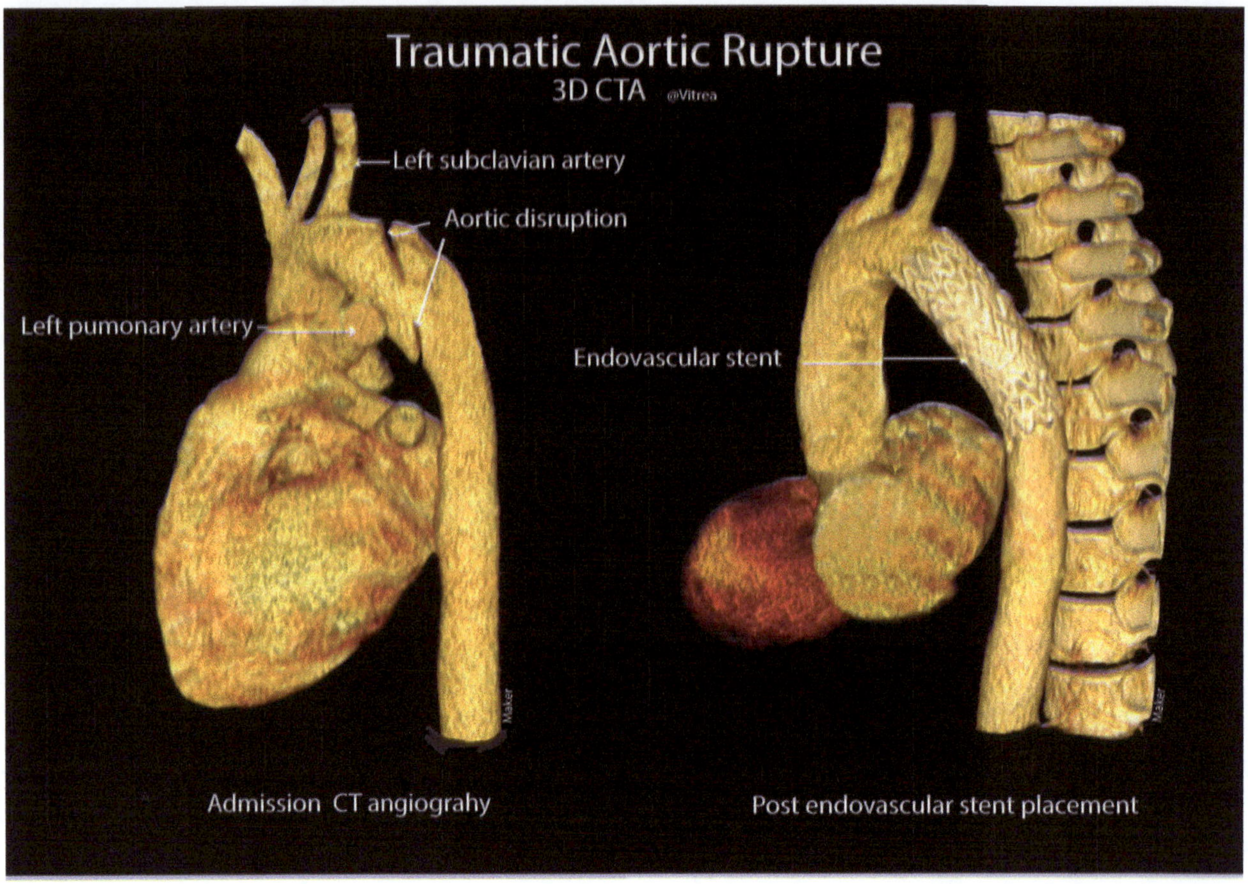

Fig. 5.11 This 31-year-old male car driver was admitted after a motor vehicle accident with a head-on collision of the two cars. He was hypotensive with fractured left 4th and 5th ribs, fractured left humerus, and a left lung contusion. 3-dimensional CTA revealed classic traumatic avulsion of the aorta right past the take-off the left subclavian artery and at the point of where the left pulmonary artery crosses under the aorta. The patient was stabilized and an endovascular stent was placed. Recovery was uneventful

Answer

a

References

1. Skandalakis JE, Skandalakis LJ, Skandalakis PN. Anatomy of the lymphatics. Surg Oncol Clin N Am. 2007;16(1):1–16.
2. Cervin JR, Silverman JF, Loggie BW, Geisinger KR. Virchow's node revisited. Analysis with clinicopathologic correlation of 152 fine-needle aspiration biopsies of supraclavicular lymph nodes. Arch Pathol Lab Med. 1995;119(8):727–30.
3. Mizutani M, Nawata S, Hirai I, Murakami G, Kimura W. Anatomy and histology of Virchow's node. Anat Sci Int. 2005;80(4):193–8.
4. Jaggers J, Balsara K. Mediastinal masses in children. Semin Thorac Cardiovasc Surg. 2004;16(3):201–8.
5. Priola AM, Priola SM, Cardinale L, Cataldi A, Fava C. The anterior mediastinum: diseases. Radiol Med (Torino). 2006;111(3):312–42.
6. Strollo DC, Rosado de Christenson ML, Jett JR. Primary mediastinal tumors. Part 1: tumors of the anterior mediastinum. Chest. 1997;112(2):511–22.
7. Strollo DC, Rosado-de-Christenson ML, Jett JR. Primary mediastinal tumors: part II. Tumors of the middle and posterior mediastinum. Chest. 1997;112(5):1344–57.
8. Raica M, Encica S, Motoc A, Cimpean AM, Scridon T, Barsan M. Structural heterogeneity and immunohistochemical profile of Hassall corpuscles in normal human thymus. Ann Anat. 2006;188(4):345–52.
9. Brown CB, Baldwin HS. Neural crest contribution to the cardiovascular system. Adv Exp Med Biol. 2006;589:134–54.
10. Restivo A, Piacentini G, Placidi S, Saffirio C, Marino B. Cardiac outflow tract: a review of some embryogenetic aspects of the conotruncal region of the heart. Anat Rec A Discov Mol Cell Evol Biol. 2006;288(9):936–43.
11. Gittenberger-de Groot AC, Bartelings MM, Deruiter MC, Poelmann RE. Basics of cardiac development for the understanding of congenital heart malformations. Pediatr Res. 2005;57(2):169–76.
12. Bennett KR. Congenital foramen of the left pericardium. Ann Thorac Surg. 2000;70(3):993–8.
13. Gatzoulis MA, Munk MD, Merchant N, Van Arsdell GS, McCrindle BW, Webb GD. Isolated congenital absence of the pericardium: clinical presentation, diagnosis, and management. Ann Thorac Surg. 2000;69(4):1209–15.
14. Hopkins WE. Severe pulmonary hypertension in congenital heart disease: a review of Eisenmenger syndrome. Curr Opin Cardiol. 1995;10(5):517–23.
15. Minette MS, Sahn DJ. Ventricular septal defects. Circulation. 2006;114(20):2190–7.
16. Bejvan SM, Godwin JD. Pneumomediastinum: old signs and new signs. AJR Am J Roentgenol. 1996;166(5):1041–8.
17. Naclerio EA. The V, sign in the diagnosis of spontaneous rupture of the esophagus (an early roentgen clue). Am J Surg. 1957;93(2):291–8.
18. Moores DW, Dziuban Jr SW. Pericardial drainage procedures. Chest Surg Clin N Am. 1995;5(2):359–73.
19. Mikawa T, Hurtado R. Development of the cardiac conduction system. Semin Cell Dev Biol. 2007;18(1):90–100.
20. Perry RS, Illsley SS. Basic cardiac electrophysiology and mechanisms of antiarrhythmic agents. Am J Hosp Pharm. 1986;43(4):957–74.
21. Al Khatib SM, Pritchett EL. Clinical features of Wolff-Parkinson-White syndrome. Am Heart J. 1999;138(3 Pt 1):403–13.
22. Cox JL. Cardiac surgery for arrhythmias. J Cardiovasc Electrophysiol. 2004;15(2):250–62.
23. Boettger R, Lee J, Rifkin C, Kayser S. Heart transplantation and altered drug response, part I: heart transplantation and innervation. Prog Cardiovasc Nurs. 2006;21(2):100–3.
24. Bussani R, De Giorgio F, Abbate A, Silvestri F. Cardiac metastases. J Clin Pathol. 2007;60(1):27–34.
25. Butany J, Nair V, Naseemuddin A, Nair GM, Catton C, Yau T. Cardiac tumours: diagnosis and management. Lancet Oncol. 2005;6(4): 219–28.
26. Holmes Jr DR, Cohen H, Katz WE, Reeder GS. Patent foramen ovale, systemic embolization and closure. Curr Probl Cardiol. 2004; 29(2):56–94.
27. Harper WF. The blood supply of heart valves in relation to endocarditis. J Anat. 1938;73(Pt 1):94–111.
28. van der Horst-Schrivers AN, Wymenga AN, Links TP, Willemse PH, Kema IP, de Vries EG. Complications of midgut carcinoid tumors and carcinoid syndrome. Neuroendocrinology. 2004;80 Suppl 1:28–32.
29. Allen M. Pacemakers and implantable cardioverter defibrillators. Anaesthesia. 2006;61(9):883–90.
30. Callcut RA, Mell MW. Modern advances in vascular trauma. Surg Clin North Am. 2013;93(4):941–61, ix.
31. Kwolek CJ, Blazick E. Current management of traumatic thoracic aortic injury. Semin Vasc Surg. 2010;23(4):215–20.
32. Naughton PA, Park MS, Morasch MD, Rodriguez HE, Garcia-Toca M, Wang CE, et al. Emergent repair of acute thoracic aortic catastrophes: a comparative analysis. Arch Surg. 2012;147(3):243–9.
33. Weidenhagen R, Bombien R, Meimarakis G, Geisler G, Koeppel TA. Management of thoracic aortic lesions – the future is endovascular. Vasa. 2012;41(3):163–76.

6 Diaphragm

1. All of the following contribute to the formation of the diaphragm *except*
   (a) Septum transversum
   (b) Glisson's capsule
   (c) Visceral peritoneum
   (d) Pleuroperitoneal membranes
   (e) Dermatomes from T6 to T12

Comments The septum transversum forms the central part of the diaphragm in the adult. This mesodermal structure originates in the neck at C3 level. From there, it descends bringing its innervation from C3 to C5, forming the phrenic nerve. In fish, the diaphragm is immediately below the gills and heart, at a level that would correspond to the human neck. As the lungs developed in evolution, the septum transversum was displaced caudally. This migration explains referred pain to the neck from diaphragmatic irritation, inferior wall myocardial infarctions, and basal pneumonia (Fig. 6.1).

The septum transversum does not completely separate the abdomen from the thorax. Posterolateral to it are the pleuroperitoneal canals, which are obliterated by the pleuroperitoneal membranes. During the 8th week of gestation, the diaphragmatic descent is complete. The central portion of the diaphragm joins, the body wall circumferentially (T6 anteriorly to T12 posteriorly). The mesodermal body wall contributes muscular tissue to the peripheral diaphragm. This component of the diaphragmatic musculature receives segmental innervation. Irritation to the peripheral diaphragm may produce referred pain along the T6–T12 dermatomes. Lastly, the dorsal mesentery provides connective tissue to the posterior midline of the diaphragm.

The parietal peritoneum lines the entire peritoneal cavity, including the diaphragmatic cupola. It reflects on the liver through the hepatophrenic attachments, forming Glisson's capsule of the liver, which does not contribute to the diaphragm [1–3].

V.K. Maker, E.D. Guzman-Arrieta, *Cognitive Pearls in General Surgery*,
DOI 10.1007/978-1-4939-1850-8_6, © Springer Science+Business Media New York 2015

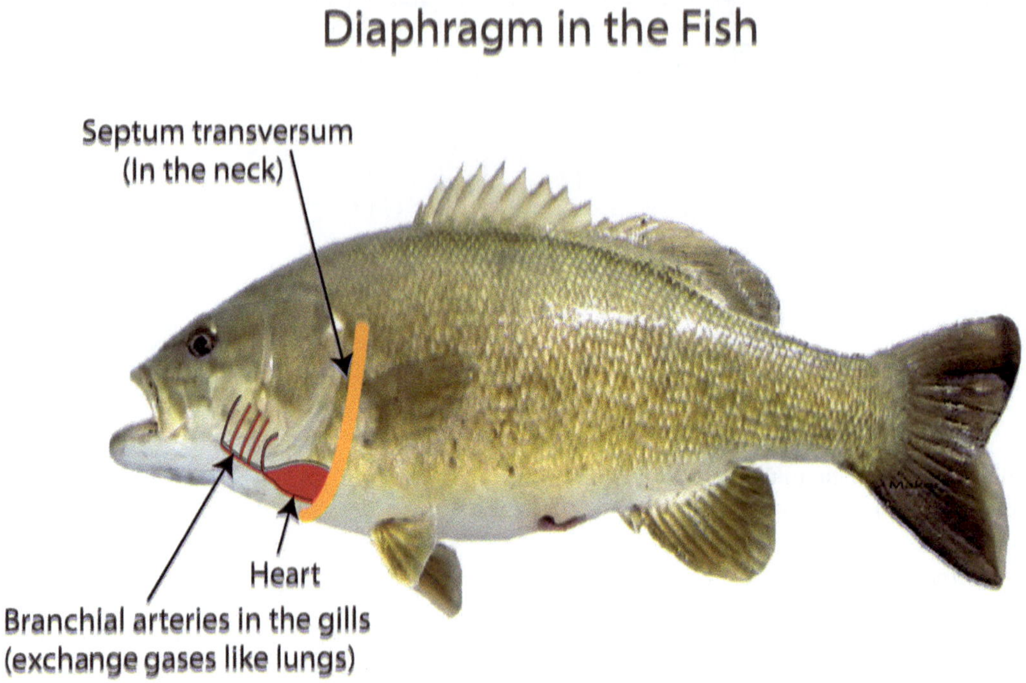

Fig. 6.1 Gills (branchium) of the fish act as the lungs. The septum transversum of the fish lies in the neck distal to the heart. During evolution, the septum transversum remained below the developing lungs and maintained innervation by the cervical nerves. This explains why pain from a myocardial infarction, or from diseases effecting the diaphragm are referred to the neck and shoulder

Answer
b

2. Mark the *incorrect* statement:
   (a) Morgagni hernias occur anteriorly, through the attachments of the diaphragm to the xiphoid process.
   (b) Bochdalek hernias occur posterolaterally, representing a defect of the pleuroperitoneal membranes.
   (c) Diaphragmatic eventration consists of pathologic elevation of the diaphragm, without a loss in continuity.
   (d) Pulmonary hypoplasia is commonly associated with congenital diaphragmatic hernias.
   (e) Congenital short esophagus is a common anomaly present in children.

Comments Diaphragmatic hernias may occur through any of the normal orifices of the diaphragm as well as through abnormal orifices. The most significant congenital diaphragmatic hernias are Bochdalek hernias, which occur through a defect in the contribution of the pleuroperitoneal membranes to the posterolateral diaphragm. In this pathology, invasion of the thorax by abdominal contents prevents normal lung development which may lead to neonatal hypoxemia. These hernias are more frequent and symptomatic on the left, due to the presence of the liver on the right [2, 4].

Morgagni–Larrey hernias occur in the central part of the anterior diaphragm, where the internal mammaries exit the chest. They are not very large and are not associated with lung hypoplasia. They are diagnosed later in life due to their tendency to incarcerate [5]. Of note, Bochdalek and Morgagni–Larrey hernias are unique in that the sac has two serosal layers, derived from the peritoneum and pleura [6] (Fig. 6.2).

Diaphragmatic eventration occurs due to the lack of muscularization of the diaphragm (congenital) or phrenic nerve injury (acquired) [7]. True congenitally short esophagus is a rare entity in the newborn. The esophagus is normal; there is a supradiaphragmatic stomach with no hernial sac, no displacement of the left gastric artery, and normal phrenoesophageal ligament. There is considerable debate surrounding its true congenital origin [8].

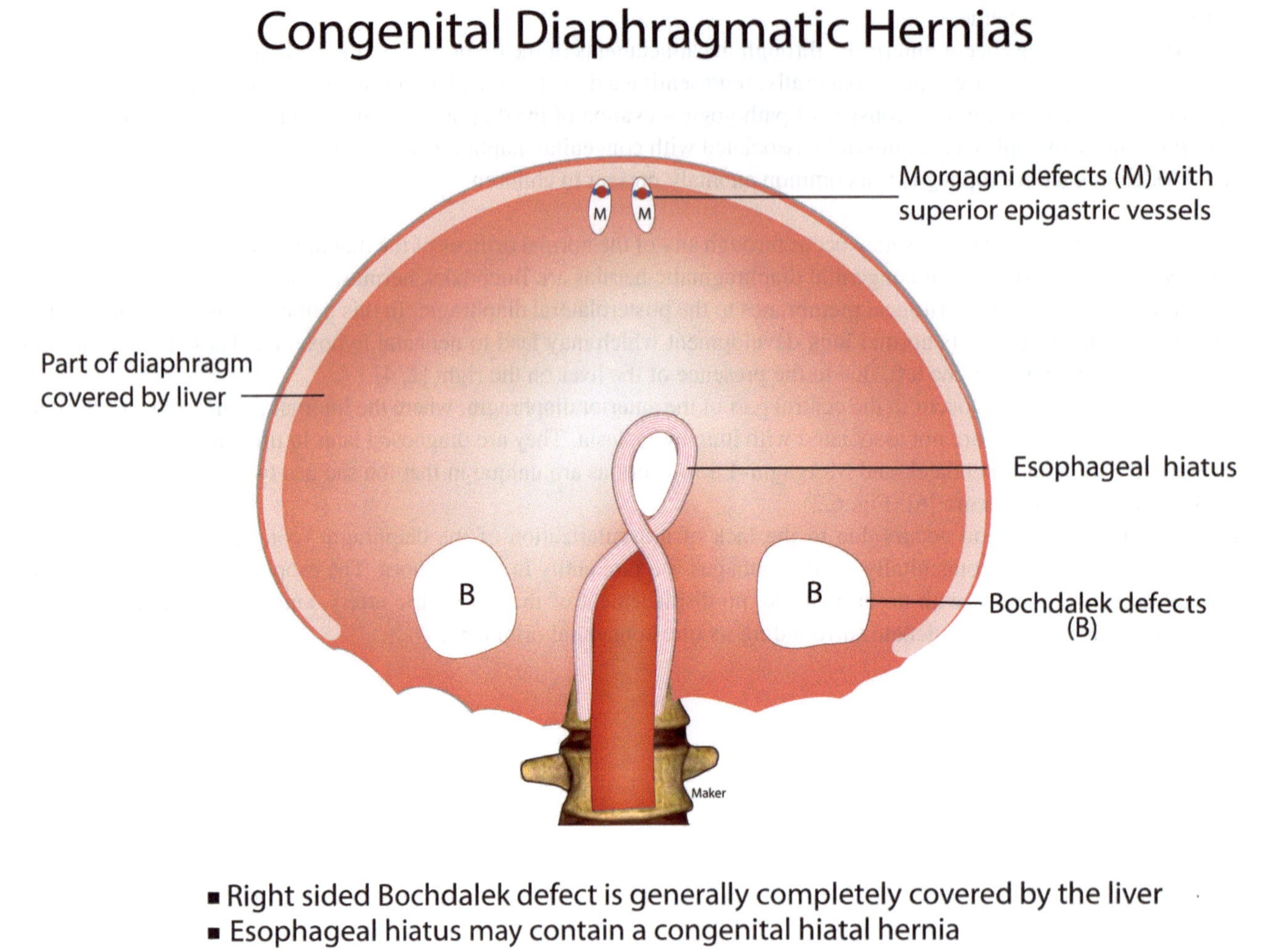

Fig. 6.2 Congenital diaphragmatic hernias (CDH) result from the improper or delayed fusion of the central tendon (septum transversum), posterolateral pleuroperitoneal canals, and peripheral T6–T12 somites. Other associated congenital anomalies, especially cardiac, may lead to severe morbidity and mortality. Non-closure of the pleuroperitoneal canals results in the Bochdalek hernia which is often associated with pulmonary hypoplasia. These hernias are common on the left side as the large neonatal liver often covers right-sided defects. In neonates, this hernia presents as a surgical emergency. Morgagni hernias are anterior and between the fusion of sternocostal somites. Diagnosis of CDH is today largely made during prenatal ultrasound. Modern surgical treatment has shifted from emergency to semi-elective after stabilization

Answer

e

3. In relation to hiatal hernias, all of the following are correct *except*:
   (a) An enlarged esophageal hiatus and a weak phrenoesophageal ligament favor the occurrence of a sliding esophageal hernia.
   (b) Sliding hernias are so named because the stomach forms part of the hernial sac.
   (c) Symptomatic paraesophageal hernias may be treated nonoperatively.
   (d) Paraesophageal hiatal hernias do not disturb the position of the GE junction.
   (e) Combined hiatal hernias behave as sliding hiatal hernias.

Comments Hiatal hernias are classified into [9]:

- Sliding, where the esophagogastric junction is above the diaphragm
- Paraesophageal or rolling, occurring through the esophageal hiatus but with the GE junction in its normal location
- Combined, which has a sliding and rolling component (the most frequent)
- Complex, when organs other than the esophagus or stomach herniate (Fig. 6.3)

The normal esophagogastric junction lies to the left of the midline, with a 2–3 cm segment of intra-abdominal esophagus. The existence of the abdominal esophagus is fundamental in avoiding gastroesophageal reflux. Even though there is no anatomic lower esophageal sphincter, there is surely a functional sphincter. Positive intra-abdominal pressure exerted on the intra-abdominal diaphragm causes its collapse and prevents reflux [10]. The treatment of sliding hiatal hernias for all intents and purposes is that of reflux esophagitis, rather than the correction of the anatomic defect per se. The same concept applies to combined hiatal hernias.

In the past, there was agreement on the need to repair all paraesophageal hernias promptly. More recently, this belief has been challenged, and watchful waiting of asymptomatic or minimally symptomatic hernias is a viable alternative. Controversy also exists regarding the best method of repair: open vs. laparoscopic, transthoracic vs. transabdominal and with or without antireflux procedure. There is also discussion regarding the benefits or using mesh for the repair and performing esophageal lengthening procedures. While paraesophageal hernias classically present after the fifth decade of life, this hernias may occur due to traumatic diaphragmatic injury at any age. Very often the history of trauma may be absent or remote [11, 12].

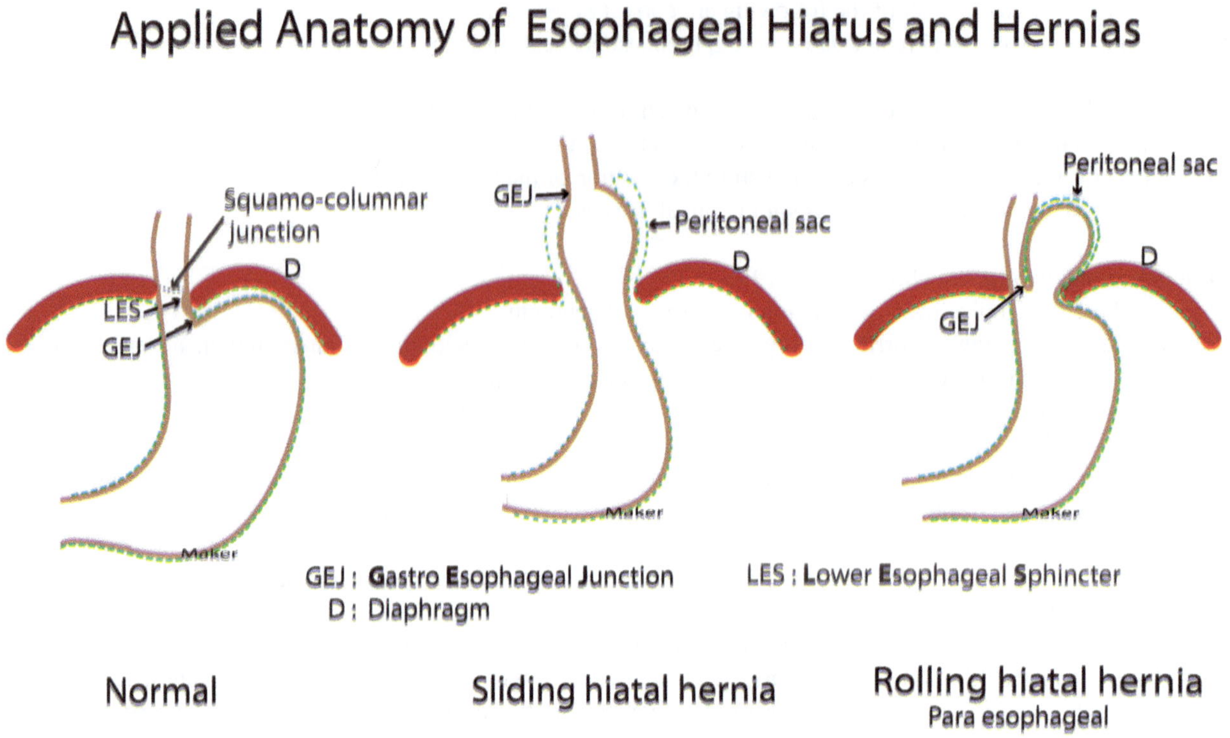

Fig. 6.3 The normal gastroesophageal junction (GEJ) is below the diaphragm. A functional lower esophageal sphincter (LES), external sphincter function provided by the crura, and an intra-abdominal esophagus are the key factors in preventing esophageal reflux. In a sliding hernia, the GEJ and LES are both above the diaphragm, and a part of the stomach is covered by the hernia sac. In paraesophageal hernia, the GEJ and LES are in the anatomical position, but a part of the stomach herniates into the chest covered with the hernia sac. Depending on the size of the hernia and the size of the defect, paraesophageal hernias may strangulate in the chest producing a serious surgical emergency.

Answer

c

4. All of the following are correct *except*:
   (a) The foramen of Morgagni allows the passage of the internal mammary arteries.
   (b) The inferior vena cava courses with the vagus nerves.
   (c) The esophageal hiatus contains the esophagus and esophageal vessels.
   (d) The aortic opening gives passage to the aorta, azygos and hemiazygos veins, and thoracic duct.
   (e) The median arcuate ligament joins the left and right crura anterior to the aorta.

Comments The diaphragm has three major orifices [1, 3]:

- The esophageal hiatus, which also accommodates the left (anterior) and right (posterior) vagus nerves on their way to supply the foregut and midgut
- The aortic hiatus, shared by the cisterna chyli and azygos and hemiazygos veins
- The caval hiatus, providing a conduit for the suprahepatic inferior vena cava to the right atrium

Anteriorly and in paramedian position, the foramina of Morgagni can be found, allowing the passage of the internal mammary on either side of the midline. The internal mammary artery divides into the superior epigastric and musculophrenic arteries.

The median arcuate ligament is a fibrous communication between the two crura as they cross anterior to the aortic hiatus. The median arcuate ligament may compress an abnormally high celiac trunk, causing ischemic symptoms of postprandial pain (Dunbar's syndrome) [13].

The caval foramen pierces the central tendon. It may also give passage to the right phrenic nerve and lymphatic vessels. The left phrenic nerve pierces the diaphragm by itself in a position mirroring the caval hiatus.

Answer

b

5. All of the following are correct *except*:
   (a) The phrenic nerve supplies the diaphragm from its abdominal surface.
   (b) The phrenic nerves provide sensory innervation to the diaphragmatic pleura, peritoneum, and pericardium.
   (c) The safest incision in the diaphragm is circumferential and peripheral.
   (d) Injury to the phrenic nerve causes depression of the ipsilateral diaphragm.
   (e) Pain in the left shoulder (Kehr's sign) is seen in splenic injury.

Comments The phrenic nerve, from its origin in the neck, traverses the entire mediastinum on either side to come to the diaphragm and supply it largely from its abdominal surface. Because of its long course, multiple diseases of the neck and mediastinum can irritate the phrenic nerve causing hiccups or paralysis. A paralyzed hemidiaphragm becomes elevated. Irritation of the left diaphragm by a subphrenic abscess, free air, or hematoma may present with referred pain in the left shoulder [1].

After piercing the diaphragm, each nerve divides into an anterior and posterior branch with somewhat variable course, which may be partly intradiaphragmatic. The safest incision in the diaphragm should be placed peripherally, leaving enough diaphragmatic tissue to repair of the incision. Peripheral circumferential incisions take advantage of the fusion plane between the embryologic components derived from the septum transversum and thoracic body wall.

Radial incisions of the diaphragm will end up sacrificing some branches of the phrenic nerve; however, one should attempt to salvage the major branches. The left phrenic nerve pierces the diaphragm anteriorly, giving a short anterior branch and a long posterior one providing lateral branches. A safe radial incision is the left paracrural, which runs from the posterior attachment of the diaphragm, 2 cm lateral to the esophageal hiatus, coming directly anteriorly towards the central tendon, stopping short of the entry of the phrenic nerve across the diaphragm [14].

Answer
d

6. All of the following are correct regarding acquired diaphragmatic hernias *except*:
   (a) Acquired diaphragmatic hernias are most commonly caused by a sudden increase in abdominal pressure.
   (b) Acute herniation with visceral compromise is the most common presentation.
   (c) The obstructive phase of herniation is characterized by obstruction and perforation.
   (d) Surgical repair may be approached from the chest or abdomen.
   (e) The key goal of diaphragmatic repair is to avoid tension.

Comments Acquired diaphragmatic hernias are a relatively rare complication of blunt and penetrating trauma. They are present in 1–6 % of severe thoracoabdominal injuries, where a sudden increase in abdominal pressure causes the diaphragm to rupture into the thorax, most commonly on the left side. The right side is somewhat protected by the liver. Herniation is often delayed, particularly in mechanically ventilated patients. However, over time, negative intrathoracic pressure drives visceral migration into the thorax.

In the acute phase, diaphragmatic hernias may be difficult to diagnose. Chest X-rays have a sensitivity of 34 %. CT scanning improves upon this, offering a 50–78 % detection rate. The most sensitive diagnostic algorithm consists of diagnostic peritoneal lavage followed by laparoscopy or thoracoscopy if positive [15]. The clinical presentation of the acute phase is most often dominated by concomitant injuries.

The acute phase of diaphragmatic rupture, when undiagnosed, evolves into a latent, often asymptomatic phase of variable duration. Over time, as herniation progresses, an obstructive phase appears. During this time, the herniated viscus becomes incarcerated, potentially leading to obstruction, ischemia, and perforation (Fig. 6.4).

Repair of all traumatic diaphragmatic hernias is recommended. The urgency of the repair is largely based on the clinical scenario. Treatment approaches are varied. These lesions may be approached from the chest or the abdomen, either with open or thoracoscopic/laparoscopic instrumentation. On occasion, approaches may be combined.

Given that traumatic hernias lack a peritoneal sac, adhesions between the herniated organs and the lungs are frequent. These may be better addressed from the thorax. In order to avoid tension over the repair, prosthetic material is often used as a patch [16, 17].

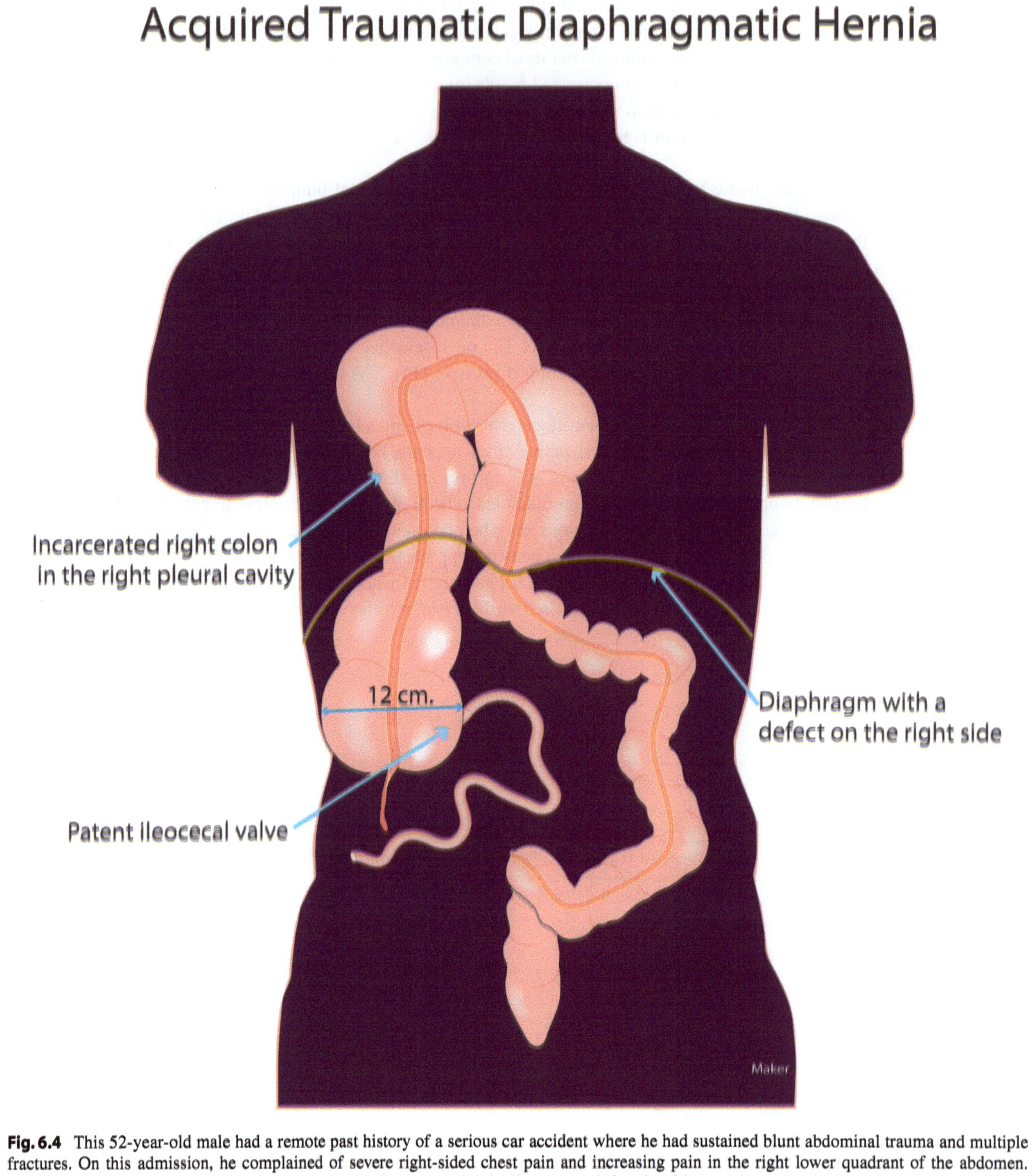

Fig. 6.4 This 52-year-old male had a remote past history of a serious car accident where he had sustained blunt abdominal trauma and multiple fractures. On this admission, he complained of severe right-sided chest pain and increasing pain in the right lower quadrant of the abdomen. CT scan and later surgery confirmed a post-traumatic incarcerated right diaphragmatic hernia with a nearly ruptured cecum. In this case, the distal obstruction combined with a patent ileocecal valve resulted in cecal dilation and pending rupture given the clinical applicability of Laplace's Law.

Answer

b

7. All of the following are correct regarding median arcuate ligament syndrome *except*:
   (a) Median arcuate ligament syndrome is a rare form of chronic mesenteric ischemia.
   (b) Celiac trunk compression by the median arcuate ligament is improved by exhalation.
   (c) Celiac trunk compression is most often asymptomatic.
   (d) The key surgical principle is release of the median arcuate ligament.
   (e) Vascular reconstruction is frequently required after release is complete.

Comments Median arcuate ligament syndrome, also known as celiac artery compression syndrome or Dunbar's syndrome, is an infrequent form of chronic mesenteric ischemia. The existence of this entity continues to be debated, and this entity remains a diagnosis of exclusion. Like the more common atherosclerotic chronic mesenteric ischemia, symptoms consist of chronic postprandial abdominal pain and weight loss.

The anatomical substrate is the caudal compression of the celiac trunk by the median arcuate ligament, often accompanied by a poststenotic dilatation. This compression is dynamic, worsening with exhalation and improving or even disappearing with inhalation [18]. A low insertion or the diaphragm and high takeoff of the celiac trunk are predisposing factors. However, it should be noted that the majority of instances of celiac trunk compression are asymptomatic, owing to the extensive mesenteric collateral pathways [19] (Fig. 6.5a, b).

The key surgical principle in this pathology is the surgical release of the median arcuate ligament syndrome, which may be achieved via laparotomy or laparoscopy. It is often the case that the celiac artery may have developed an intrinsic stenosis that requires further treatment, in the form of patch angioplasty or the creation of an aorto-celiac bypass.

When laparoscopy is used for the release, the underlying celiac artery stenosis may be managed with endovascular balloon angioplasty or stenting.

Primary stenting without surgical release has a high failure rate, with stent compression and fracture being expected outcomes.

In properly selected patients, surgical intervention has good outcomes, with an 85 % rate of symptom resolution, and a 6–7 % rate of late symptom recurrence [20].

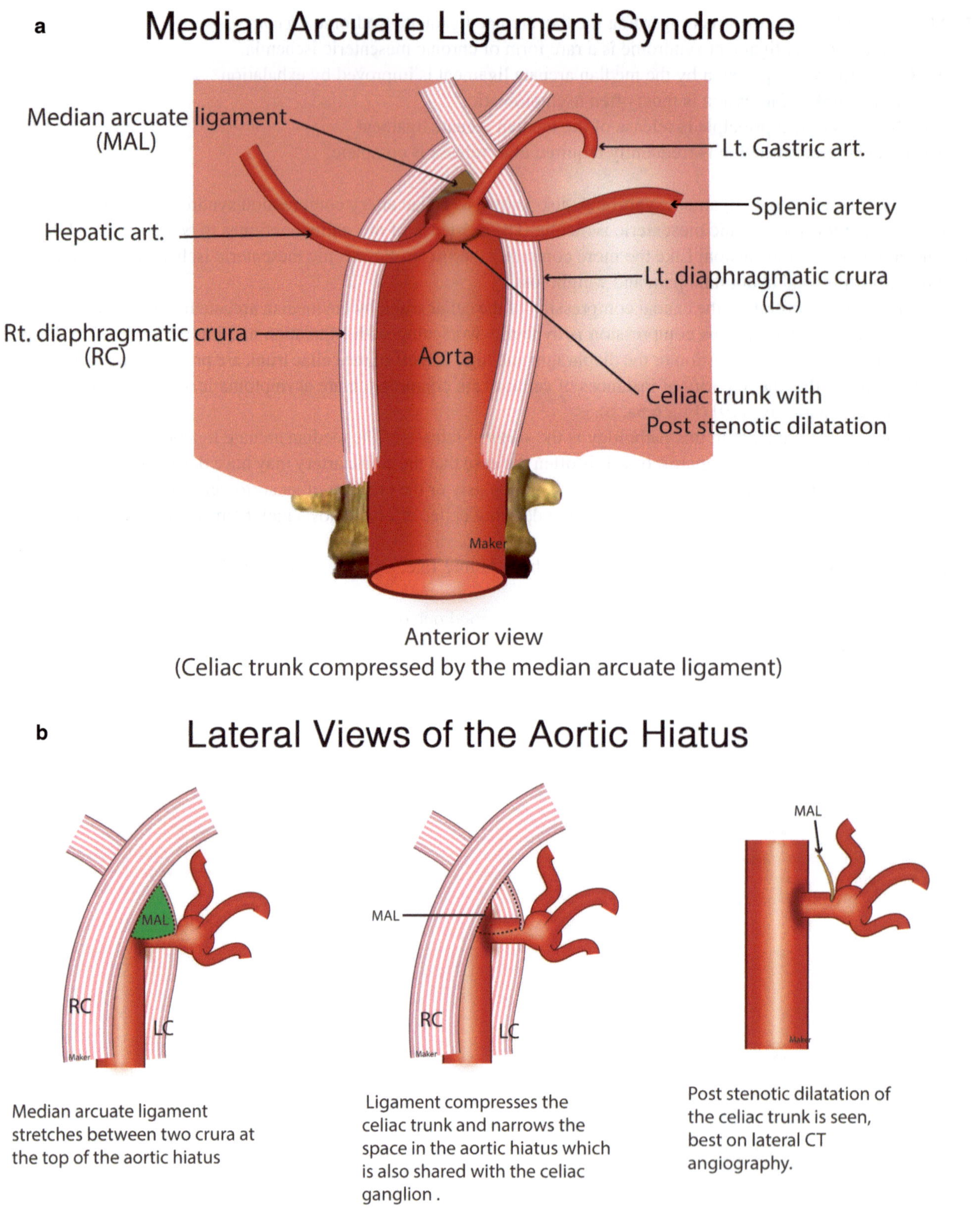

Fig. 6.5 (**a**) Median arcuate ligament syndrome. (**b**) Lateral views of the aortic hiatus

Answer

b

References

1. Fell SC. Surgical anatomy of the diaphragm and the phrenic nerve. Chest Surg Clin N Am. 1998;8(2):281–94.
2. Rottier R, Tibboel D. Fetal lung and diaphragm development in congenital diaphragmatic hernia. Semin Perinatol. 2005;29(2):86–93.
3. Schumpelick V, Steinau G, Schluper I, Prescher A. Surgical embryology and anatomy of the diaphragm with surgical applications. Surg Clin North Am. 2000;80(1):213–39, xi.
4. Clugston RD, Greer JJ. Diaphragm development and congenital diaphragmatic hernia. Semin Pediatr Surg. 2007;16(2):94–100.
5. Loong TP, Kocher HM. Clinical presentation and operative repair of hernia of Morgagni. Postgrad Med J. 2005;81(951):41–4.
6. Haroon J, Chamberlain RS. An evidence-based review of the current treatment of congenital diaphragmatic hernia. Clin Pediatr (Phila). 2013;52(2):115–24.
7. Deslauriers J. Eventration of the diaphragm. Chest Surg Clin N Am. 1998;8(2):315–30.
8. Beningfield S. Hiatus hernia/congenitally short oesophagus. S Afr Med J. 1999;89(8):843.
9. Kavic SM, Segan RD, George IM, Turner PL, Roth JS, Park A. Classification of hiatal hernias using dynamic three-dimensional reconstruction. Surg Innov. 2006;13(1):49–52.
10. Lipan MJ, Reidenberg JS, Laitman JT. Anatomy of reflux: a growing health problem affecting structures of the head and neck. Anat Rec B New Anat. 2006;289(6):261–70.
11. Stylopoulos N, Gazelle GS, Rattner DW. Paraesophageal hernias: operation or observation? Ann Surg. 2002;236(4):492–500.
12. Landreneau RJ, Del Pino M, Santos R. Management of paraesophageal hernias. Surg Clin North Am. 2005;85(3):411–32.
13. De Cecchis L, Risaliti A, Anania G, Donini A, Terrosu G, Cautero N, et al. Dunbar's syndrome: clinical reality or physiopathologic hypothesis? Ann Ital Chir. 1996;67(4):501–5.
14. Perera H, Edwards FR. Intradiaphragmatic course of the left phrenic nerve in relation to diaphragmatic incisions. Lancet. 1957;273(6985):75–7.
15. Wardi G, Lasoff D, Cobb A, Hayden S. Traumatic diaphragmatic hernia. J Emerg Med. 2014;46(1):80–2.
16. Blitz M, Louie BE. Chronic traumatic diaphragmatic hernia. Thorac Surg Clin. 2009;19(4):491–500.
17. Davoodabadi A, Fakharian E, Mohammadzadeh M, Abdorrahim KE, Mirzadeh AS. Blunt traumatic hernia of diaphragm with late presentation. Arch Trauma Res. 2012;1(3):89–92.
18. Bobadilla JL. Mesenteric ischemia. Surg Clin North Am. 2013;93(4):925–40, ix.
19. Gloviczki P, Duncan AA. Treatment of celiac artery compression syndrome: does it really exist? Perspect Vasc Surg Endovasc Ther. 2007;19(3):259–63.
20. Jimenez JC, Harlander-Locke M, Dutson EP. Open and laparoscopic treatment of median arcuate ligament syndrome. J Vasc Surg. 2012;56(3):869–73.

7 Abdominal Pain

1. All of the following are correct *except*
   (a) Visceral pain is commonly felt along midline structures.
   (b) Somatic pain has radicular radiation.
   (c) Visceral pain is always the result of organ injury.
   (d) Somatic pain is often lateralized.
   (e) Visceral pain commonly has an insidious onset.

Comments The clinical presentation of abdominal pain is the result of the complex interaction of pathologic processes stimulating somatic and visceral pain receptors which provide sensory input that the central nervous system interprets, generating autonomic and cognitive responses.

In general, visceral pain is described as ill-defined both in onset and location, dull and nonspecific, often accompanied by autonomic deregulation. Visceral pain is not generated by all viscera such as the liver, kidney, and lung, although their investing layers (Glisson's capsule, Gerota's fascia and pleura) are indeed a source of somatic pain. The perception of visceral pain is not directly linked to injury; for example, cutting of the intestine is painless. Visceral pain is often perceived in the midline, perhaps reflecting the original location of the primitive gut. However, it is often associated with radiation which may be lateralized, but retains a fairly ill-defined nature [1].

In contrast, somatic pain is much better defined in its location and time of onset and tends to lateralize. It is not necessarily accompanied by a visceral response, and it is generally linked to injury. Radiation of visceral pain follows a radicular pattern [2] (Fig. 7.1).

As noted in Fig. 7.1, there is a different perceived location of pain originating from the foregut, midgut, and hindgut, corresponding to the supraumbilical, periumbilical, and infraumbilical areas, which in turn parallels the embryologic location of the vascular supply to either segment and the origin and distribution of visceral pain fibers. Another important clinical feature is that colicky pain originating from obstruction of hollow viscera corresponding to either level has different intervals between spastic episodes, reflecting the baseline peristaltic function of each segment [3] (Fig. 7.2).

In approaching the manifestations of digestive pathology, and the consequences of the surgical interventions to address it, it is useful to liken the GI tract to an internal combustion engine, where the foregut prepares and delivers the fuel, the midgut acts as the engine carrying out the bulk of the work of digestion and absorption, and the hindgut processes the exhaust products (Fig. 7.3).

V.K. Maker, E.D. Guzman-Arrieta, *Cognitive Pearls in General Surgery*,
DOI 10.1007/978-1-4939-1850-8_7, © Springer Science+Business Media New York 2015

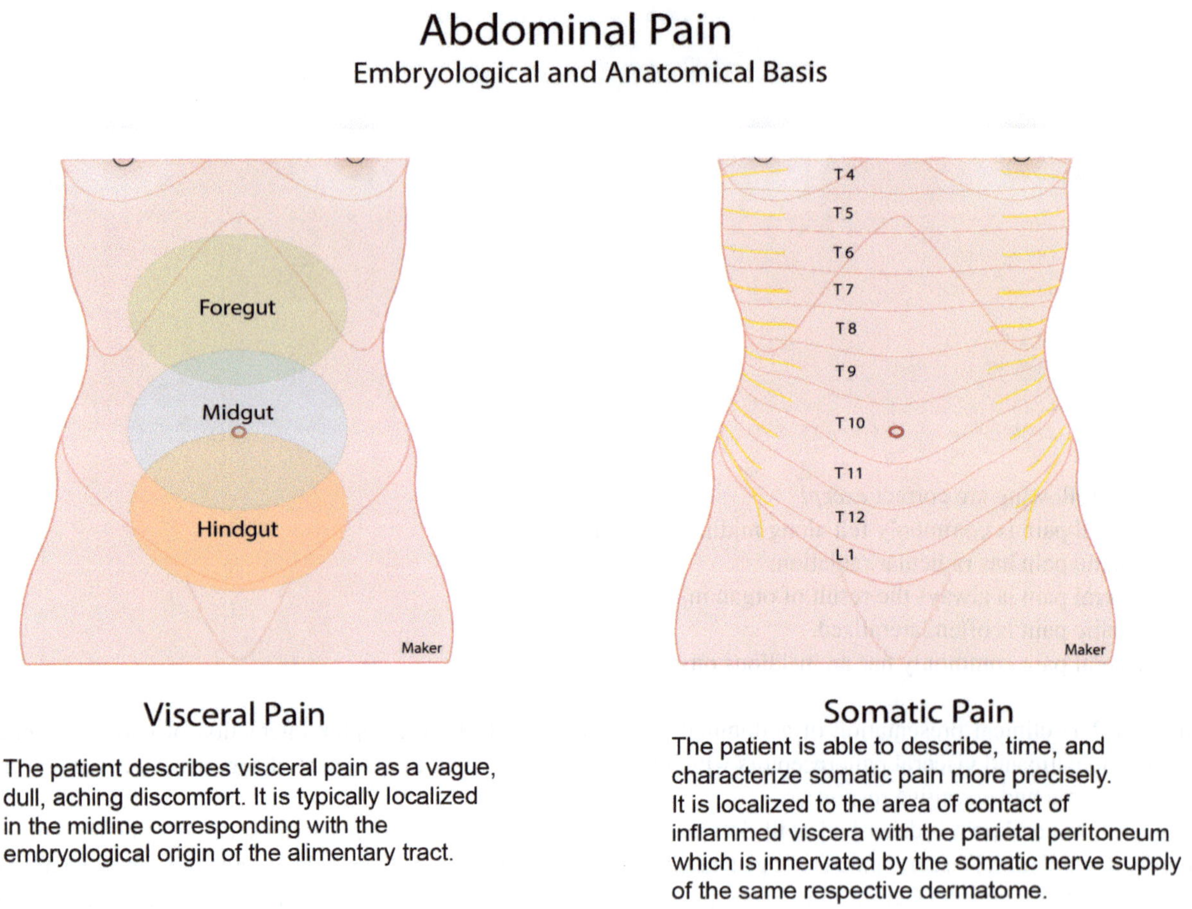

Fig. 7.1 Abdominal pain: embryological and anatomical basis

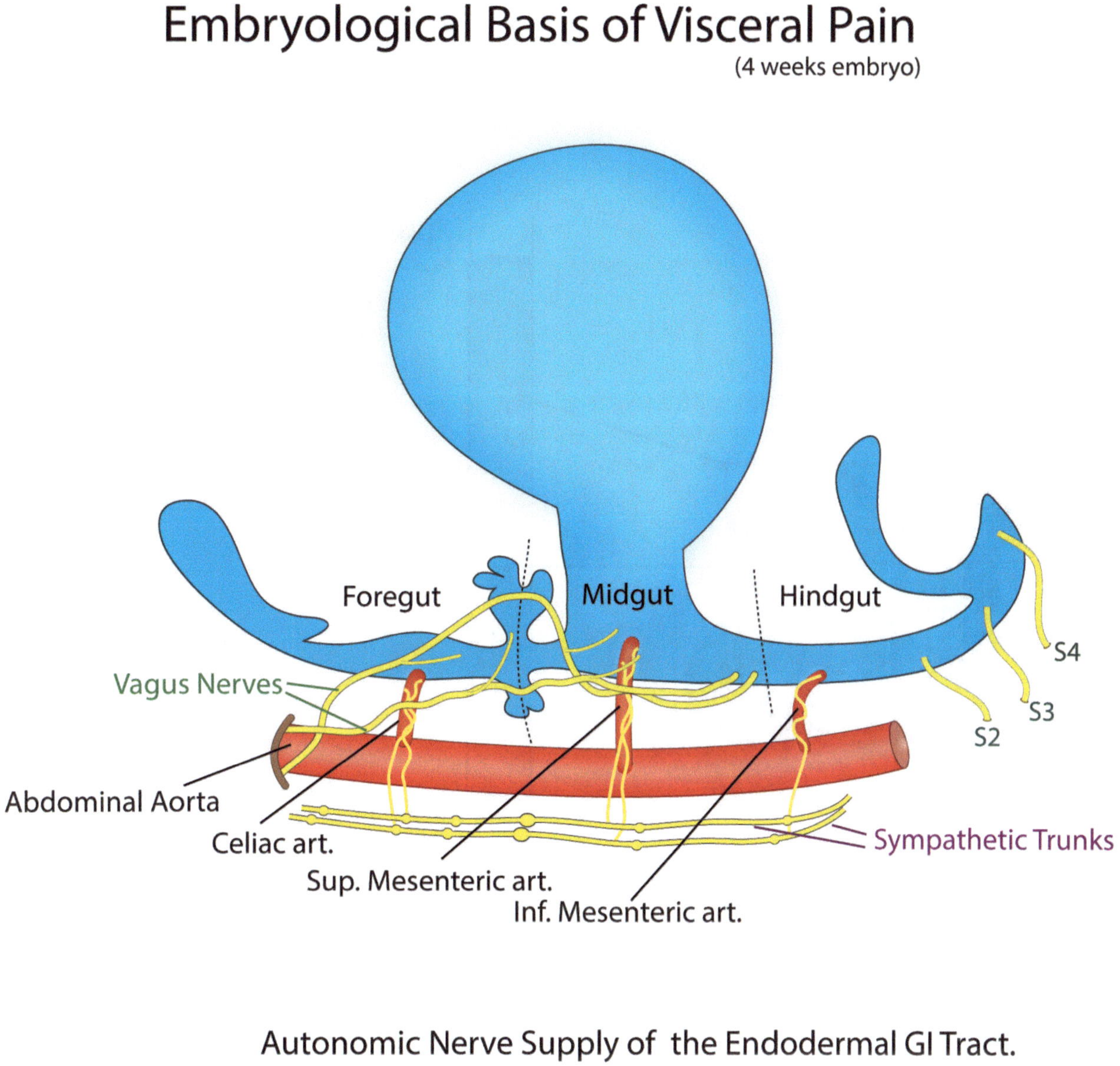

Fig. 7.2 Visceral pain is mediated through parasympathetic and sympathetic systems. Parasympathetic nerves travel through the vagus nerve to the foregut and midgut while sacral 2, 3, and 4 nerves innervate the hindgut. Sympathetic nerves travel with celiac, superior mesenteric, and inferior mesenteric vessels to their respective embryological fore-, mid-, and hindguts

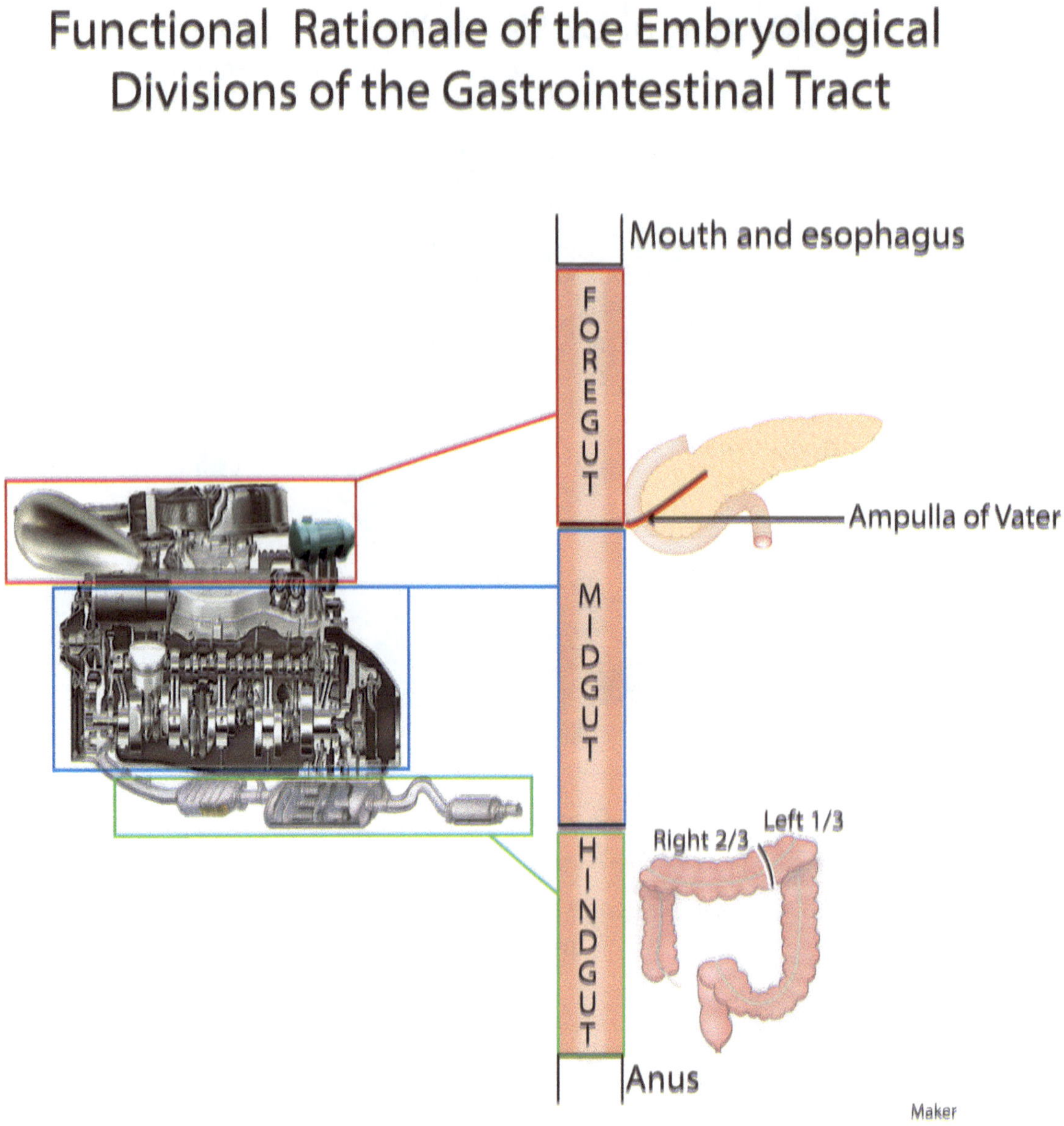

Fig. 7.3 The endodermal derived foregut extends from the esophagus to the ampulla of Vater and, in the big picture of the GI tract, is largely responsible for storing and mixing the ingested food with the saliva, gastric secretions, bile, and pancreatic enzymes. The midgut, on the other hand, is the main digestive engine responsible for digestion and absorption. The midgut extends from the ampulla of Vater and extends to the right two-thirds of the transverse colon including all of the jejunum and the ileum. The hindgut behaves like the muffler of the engine extending from the lateral one-third of the transverse colon to the rectum. Its main function is to store and evacuate the products of digestive "combustion"

Answer

c

2. All of the following are correct *except*:
   (a) The origin and mechanisms of visceral pain are not fully understood.
   (b) Ischemia plays an important role in the transition of visceral to somatic pain.
   (c) The end result of sustained increased intramural pressure is necrosis of the bowel wall.
   (d) Afferent autonomic pain fibers are nonmyelinated.
   (e) There are well-defined visceral pain receptors.

Comments It is often the case that there is an orderly progression of visceral to somatic pain in the natural history of the majority of inflammatory and obstructive abdominal pathologies.

The exact processes and pathways that originate and mediate visceral pain are not fully elucidated, nor are the distribution of specific visceral pain receptors. In that context, we offer the following hypothesis, centered around the role of perineural lymphatics in the nourishment of nonmyelinated visceral afferent fibers [4–6].

In this model, the onset of hollow viscus visceral pain is brought about by increases in intraluminal pressure that in turn generate elevations in mural pressure that exceed the pressure of the perineural lymphatics, thus interrupting the supply of nutrients to the nerve, generating a distress signal interpreted as pain. As the elevated pressure subsides, pain resolves, until the next cycle (Fig. 7.4).

As repeated cycles of increased pressure continue, there is progressive disruption of the normal bowel wall architecture, first with lymphedema, ultimately with an organized inflammatory response, that further enhances pain perception by the delivery of inflammatory mediators that heighten pain perception (Fig. 7.5).

It is at this point where the transition to somatic pain occurs. As the pathologic process continues, a more global ischemic phenomenon occurs. The progressive and sustained rise in intramural pressure results in collapse and functional obstruction of the bowel wall venules, thus generating stagnation of venous return and ischemia in a mechanism similar to that of phlegmasia cerulea dolens. This in turn facilitates the breakdown of the mucosal barrier, resulting in bacterial invasion of the bowel wall, leading to microvascular thrombosis causing further ischemia, that ultimately leads to bowel wall necrosis and perforation with an associated inflammatory response [7] (Fig. 7.6).

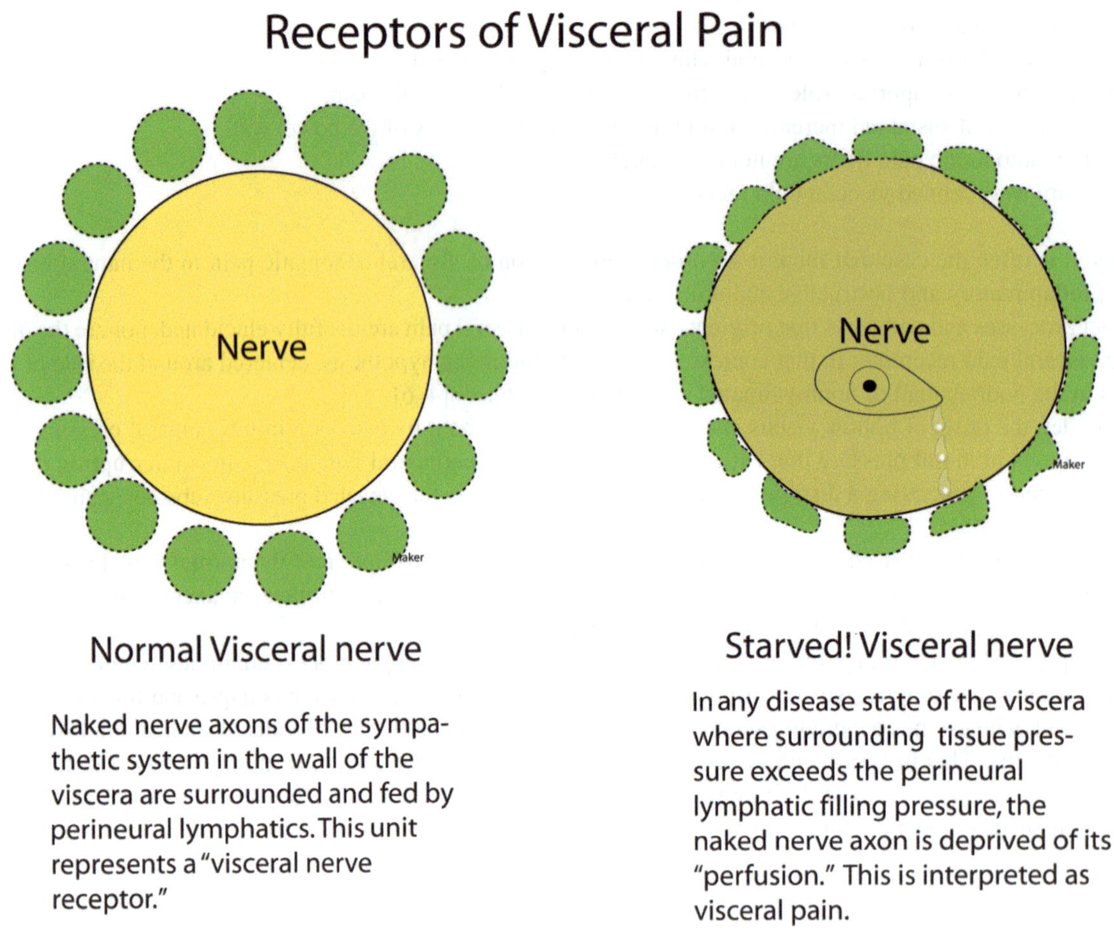

Fig. 7.4 Receptors of visceral pain

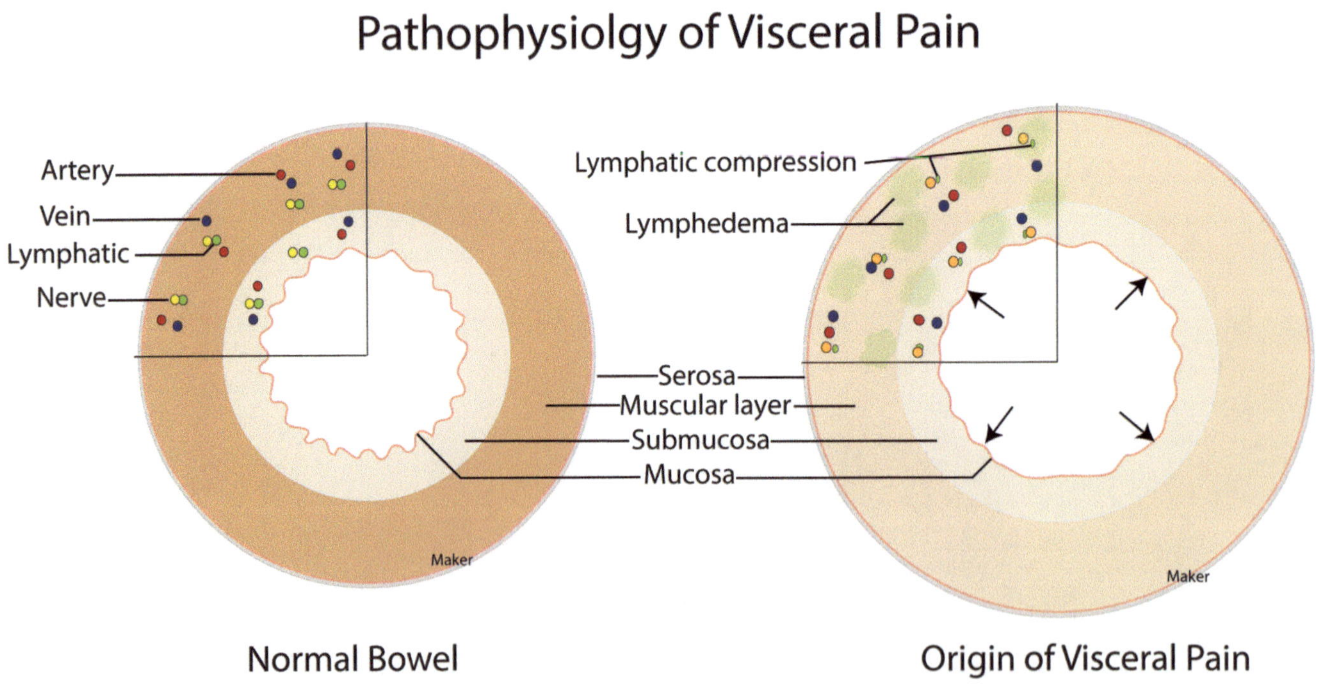

Fig. 7.5 Part I: When increased intraluminal pressure exceeds the low-pressure lymphatic system, we hypothesize that perineural lymphatics are compressed, and that this lack of perineural perfusion to visceral sympathetics manifests as vague, poorly localized visceral pain. The pain will be localized at the embyological origin of the nerve supply along the midline. Clinically, this process results in lymphedema of the wall of the affected viscera producing "woody" edema

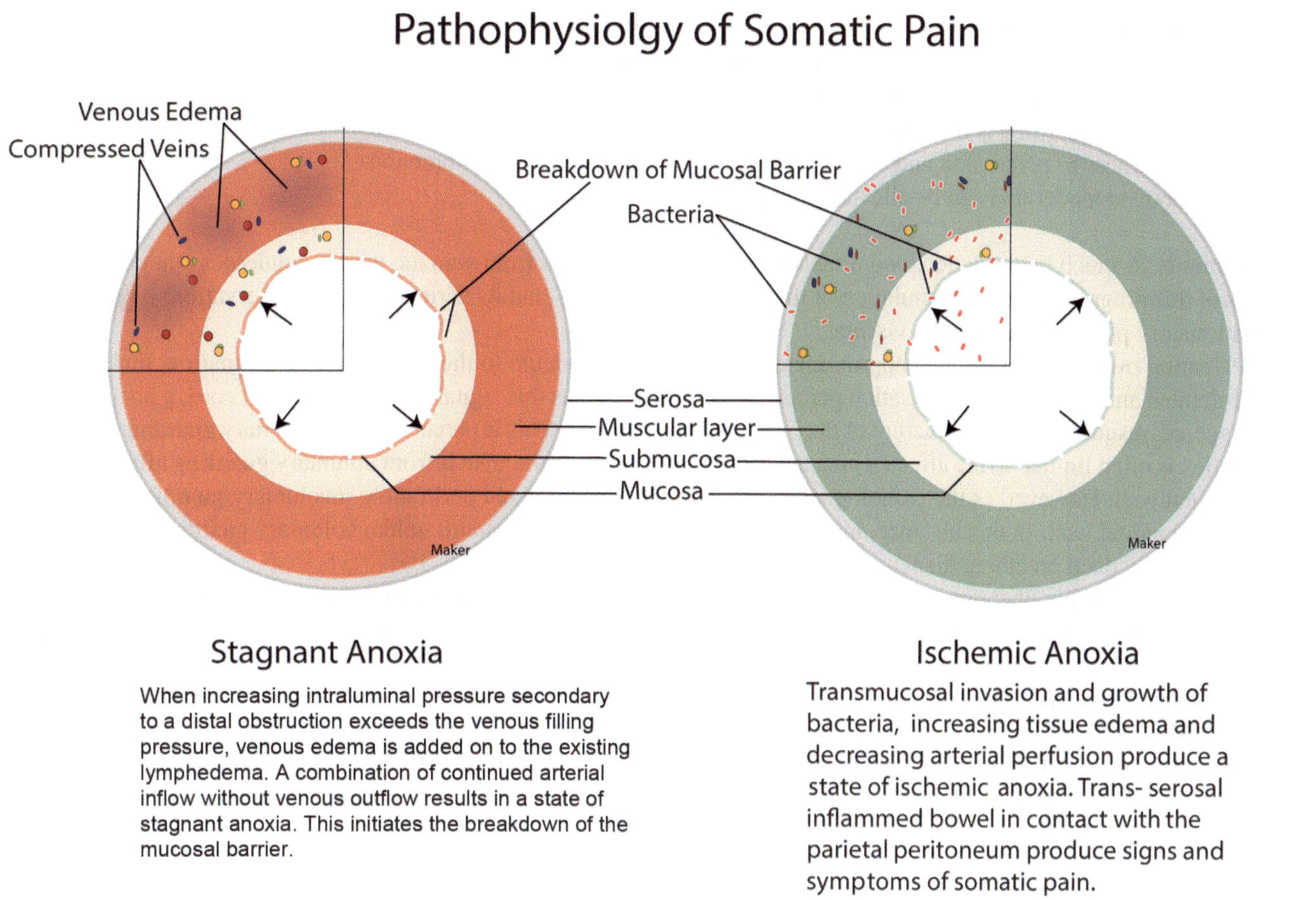

Fig. 7.6 Part II: Pathophysiology of somatic pain results from the breakdown of the mucosal barrier. Transmucosal invasion of intraluminal contents leads to trans-serosal inflammation. It is the contact of inflammed serosa (or the outermost layer of the viscera) to the parietal peritoneum which initiates somatic pain. Since the parietal peritoneum is innervated by somatic sensory nerves, classic well-described and characterized somatic pain ensues

Answer

e

3. All of the following are correct *except*:
   (a) Tenderness to palpation is mediated primarily by the parietal peritoneum.
   (b) Involuntary guarding constitutes a protective nociceptive reflex.
   (c) Voluntary guarding is often limited to the area of pathology.
   (d) Tenderness to percussion and decompression represents the same phenomenon.
   (e) Rebound tenderness can be alleviated by gentle compression.

Comments A much better understood transition is that which occurs from somatic pain to tenderness on palpation. At the basis of this progression is the stimulation of the parietal peritoneum (and its dermatome type innervation) by the underlying inflammatory process affecting the viscera.

Palpation over the affected area approximates the parietal peritoneum to the underlying inflammation, thus generating a well-defined and localized pain sensation perceived as tenderness. As this signal reaches the spinal cord, a nociceptive reflex is triggered, resulting in the contracture of the overlying musculature. This is perceived as involuntary guarding. Interestingly, the reflex is often limited to the affected area and side, which helps distinguish it from voluntary guarding affecting the entire abdominal wall. However, as the pathologic process extends to generalized peritonitis, involuntary guarding may affect the entire abdominal wall. In this instance, involuntary guarding becomes constant, unlike voluntary guarding, which can often be resolved by deep breathing maneuvers or distractors [8, 9] (Fig. 7.7).

A variation of this phenomenon occurs when oscillation of the parietal peritoneum over the underlying inflammatory process is induced. In its gentler form, this can be elicited by gentle percussion over the affected area. A clearer albeit much more painful demonstration may be obtained by rebound tenderness, or tenderness to rapid decompression. In this instance, the pain can be alleviated by compressing the affected area, followed by gentle decompression once the pain has subsided [10, 11] (Fig. 7.8).

The outcome of either maneuver can often be anticipated by a careful clinical history, in which the patient describes sharp abdominal pain due to sudden motions, such as those incurred upon during transportation. In these instances, patients may resort to bracing themselves with their hands or pillows.

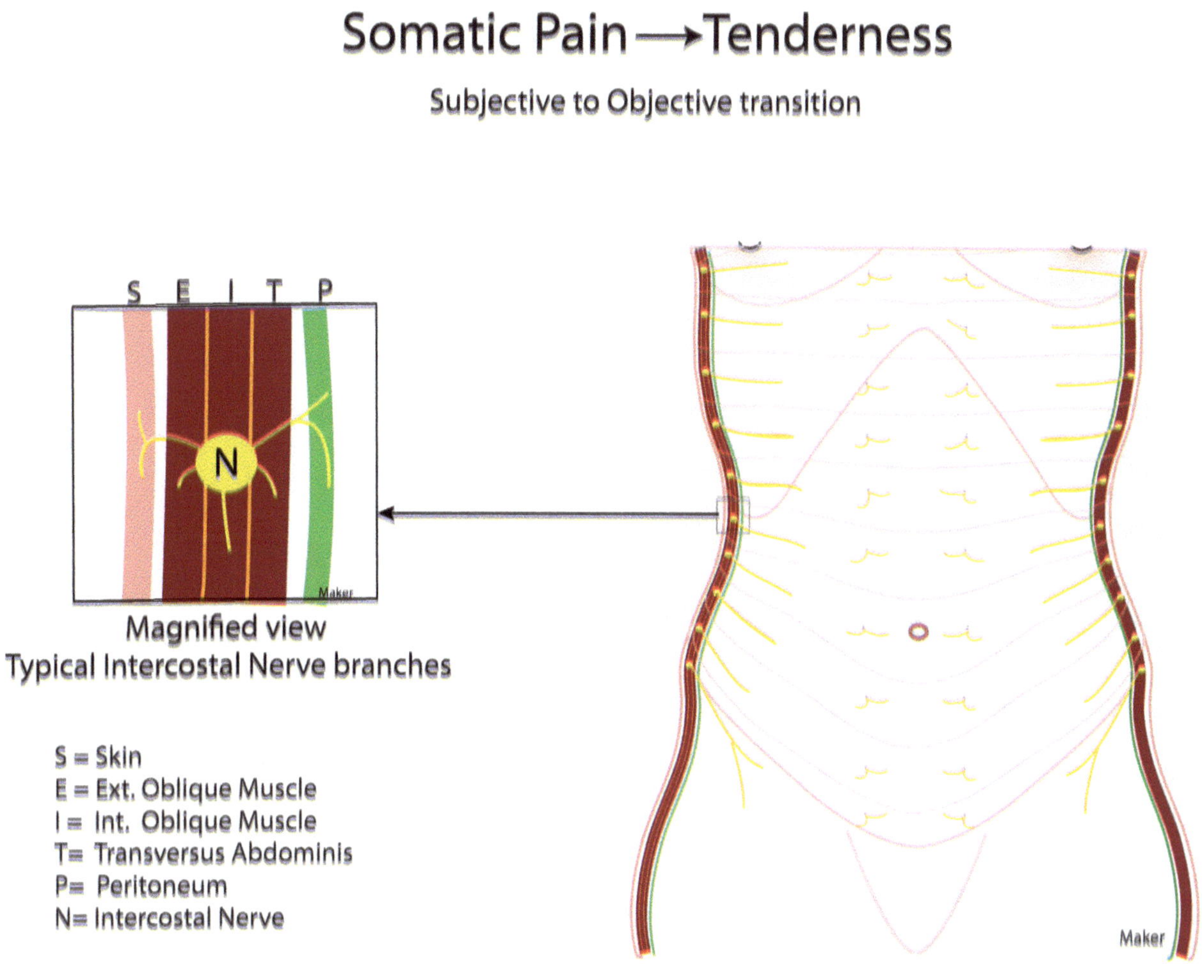

Fig. 7.7 Intercostal spinal nerves are mixed nerves supplying the skin, muscles, and parietal peritoneum of the corresponding dermatome. Inflammed visceral peritoneum (serosa) in contact with the parietal peritoneum initiates the somatic pain. On physical examination, this focuses the area of tenderness, muscle rigidity, and hyperesthesia of the skin to the same dermatome(s)

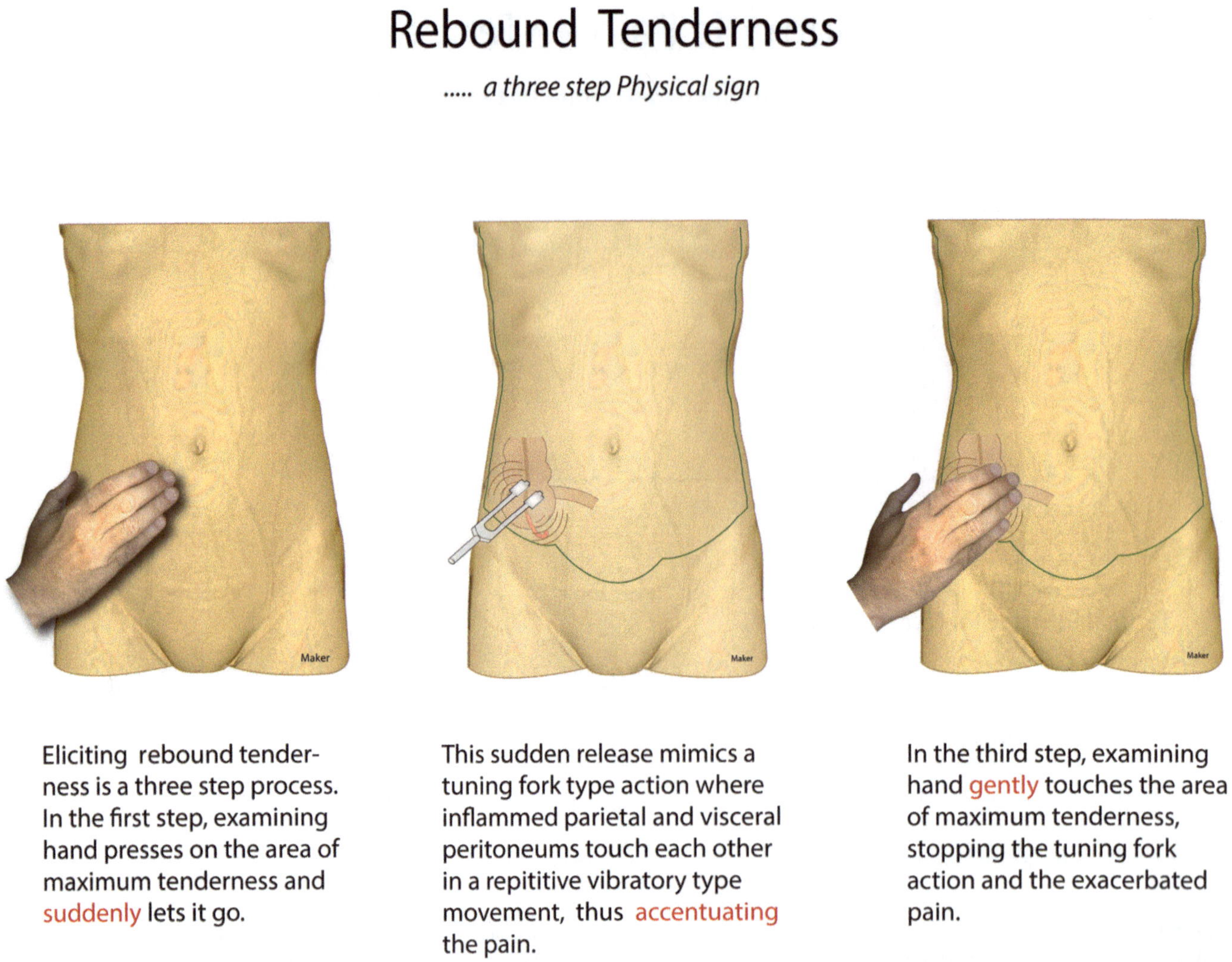

Fig. 7.8 Rebound tenderness: a three-step physical sign

> **Answer**
> c

4. All of the following are correct *except*:
   (a) The psoas sign can be elicited by hip flexion.
   (b) The obturator sign is elicited by internal rotation of the hip.
   (c) The Howship–Romberg sign suggests the presence of an obturator hernia.
   (d) Kehr's sign may be present in cases of lower thoracic pathology.
   (e) Right-sided shoulder pain may result from right-sided diaphragm irritation.

Comments Depending on the location and radiation patterns, the transition from visceral to somatic pain may take fairly specific manifestations, which need to be kept in mind when attempting to diagnose intra-abdominal pathologies. While classically described in the context of appendicitis, the following two signs may occur with other pathologies in those areas [12].

The psoas sign is often associated with retrocecal appendicitis. When the psoas comes into contact with an inflammatory process, the patient will attempt to relieve the pain by relaxing the psoas muscle by flexing the hip. Pain may be elicited by extending the hip, thus generating motion and tension. Ideally, hip extension should be carried back beyond the plane of the body, either in standing position or by allowing the leg to fall back below the level of the exam surface with the patient supine (Fig. 7.9).

The obturator sign consists of pelvic/abdominal pain elicited by internal rotation of the hip joint, with the knee and hip flexed at 90° angles. It is described for pelvic appendicitis, and more commonly obturator hernias. In the case of obturator hernias, the hernia may compress the obturator nerve, causing pain along the inner thigh, a finding termed the Howship–Romberg sign [13] (Fig. 7.10).

Kehr's sign is a manifestation of somatic pain of the diaphragm and consists of ipsilateral shoulder pain. This pattern of radiation reflects the cervical origin of the diaphragm as well as the radicular roots of the phrenic nerve (C3–C5). While typically described in the context of splenic injury, it may become manifest with other pathologies such as splenic abscess and pneumonia. An analogous finding can be found on the right side, as a consequence of hepatic pathology or collections in the suprahepatic space [14, 15] (Fig. 7.11).

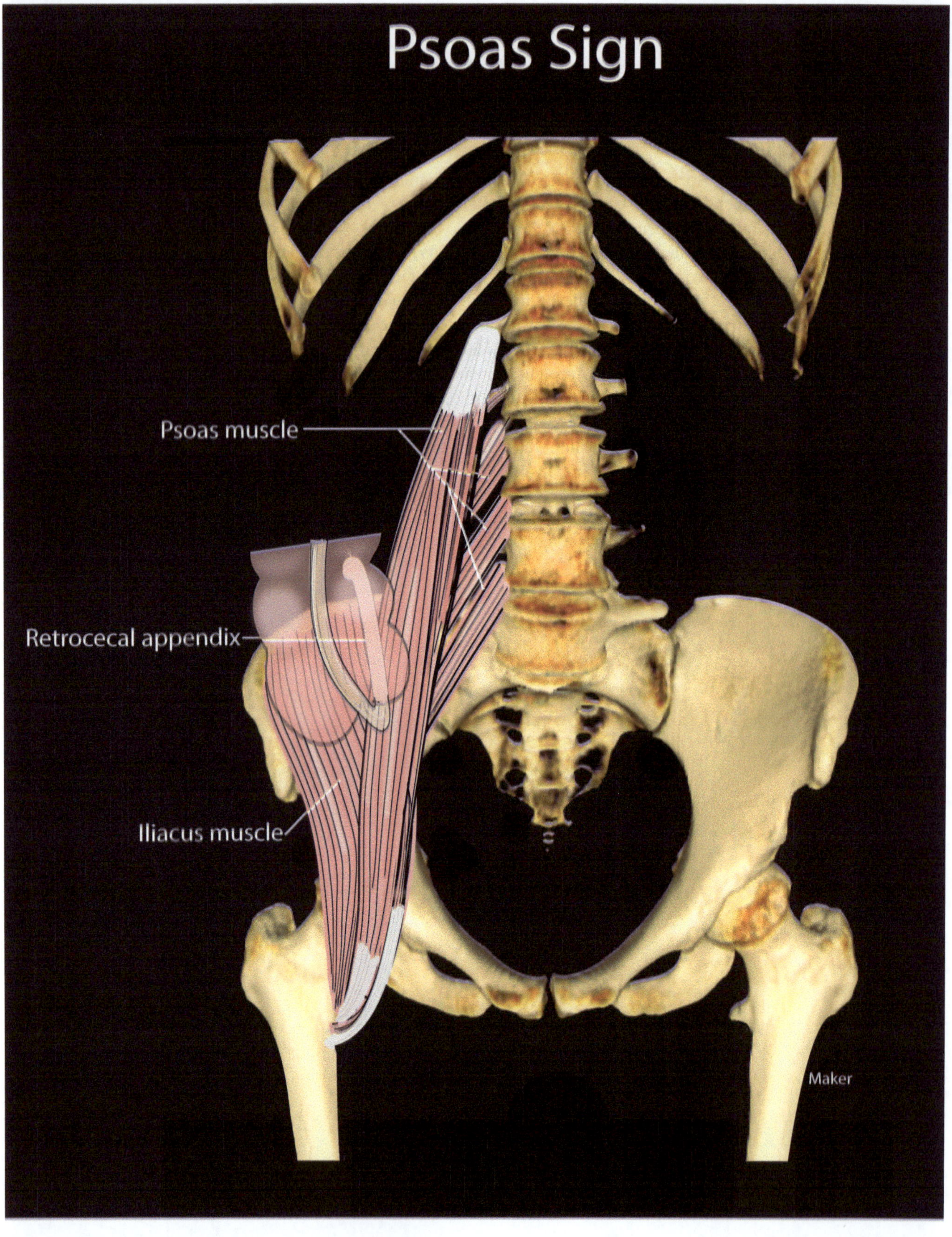

Fig. 7.9 The psoas sign is one of the muscle signs of the acute abdomen where the patient will keep a position or posture to keep the inflammed/injured muscle in its resting position so as to not allow the muscle to be stretched. Any attempt to stretch this muscle produces subjective and objective pain. In case of an inflammed appendix overlying the iliopsoas muscle, the patient often assumes the position of a flexed thigh to relieve the pain. Any attempt to stretch the iliopsoas muscle, i.e., extending the hip, causes pain (positive psoas sign). This is one of the classic muscle signs of acute appendicitis when involving the iliopsoas muscle, but will be true of any condition directly or indirectly involving this muscle in an inflammatory process

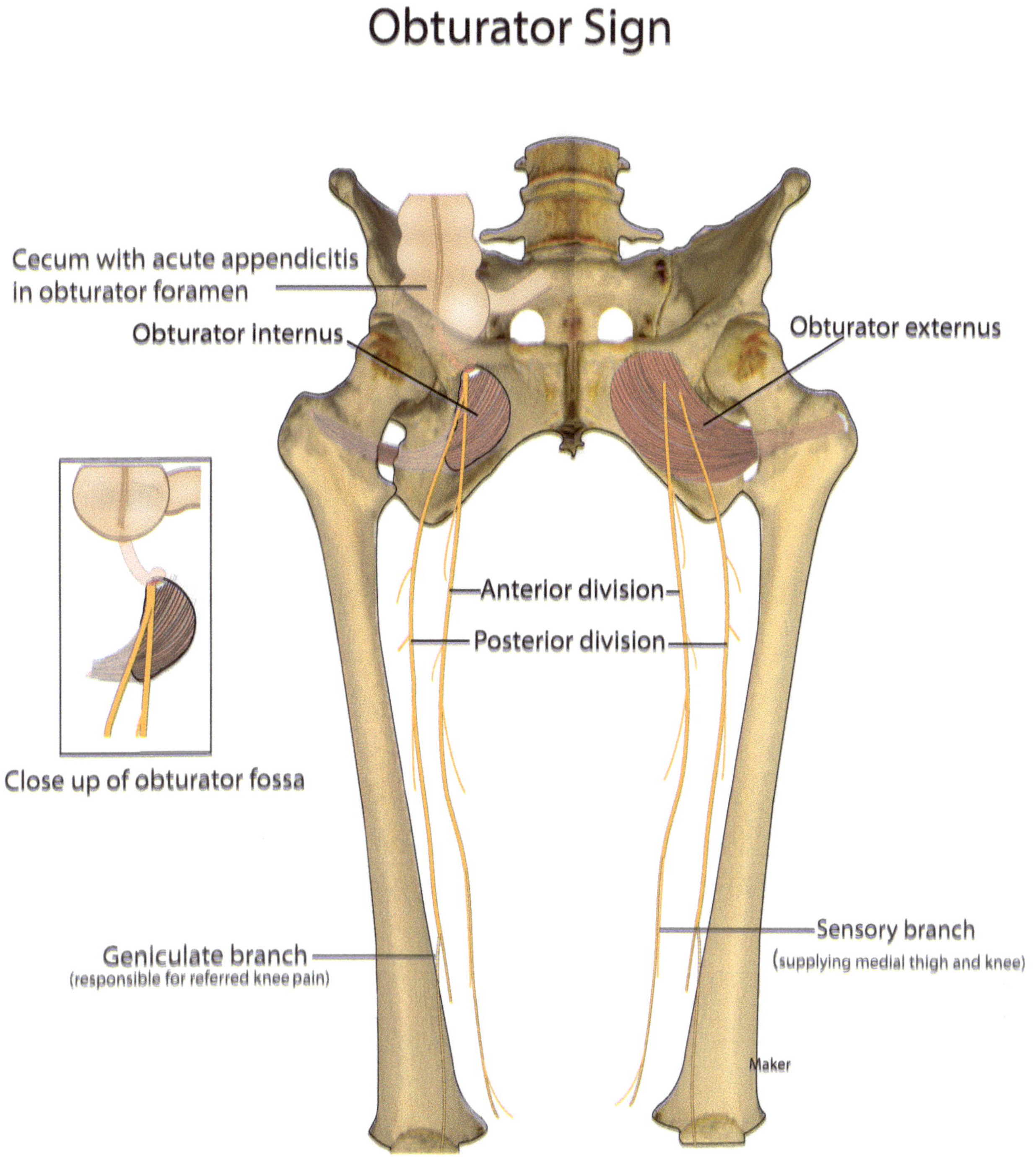

Fig. 7.10 The obturator nerve (L 2, 3, 4) has an interesting anatomical course and supply pattern which forms the basis of a muscle sign and two referred pain scenarios in disease processes involving the obturator foramen, i.e., obturator hernia and an obturator location of appendicitis. The obturator nerve runs over the pelvic fascia deep to the common iliac vessels and exits the pelvis through the obturator foramen running a short course between the obturator internus and externus muscles. During its course between the two muscles, it divides into anterior and posterior divisions. The anterior division supplies the adductor and pectineus muscles, hip joint, and sensory branches to the skin of the medial thigh and knee. The posterior division supplies the obturator externus, adductors, and a geniculate branch to the knee joint. A positive obturator sign is increasing pain on stretching the obturator internus muscle by internally rotating the leg with the hip and knee flexed at 90°. Conditions affecting the obturator nerves can also produce referred pain at the hip or knee, and/or paresthesia on the medial side of the thigh and knee because of the sensory and geniculate nerve distributions

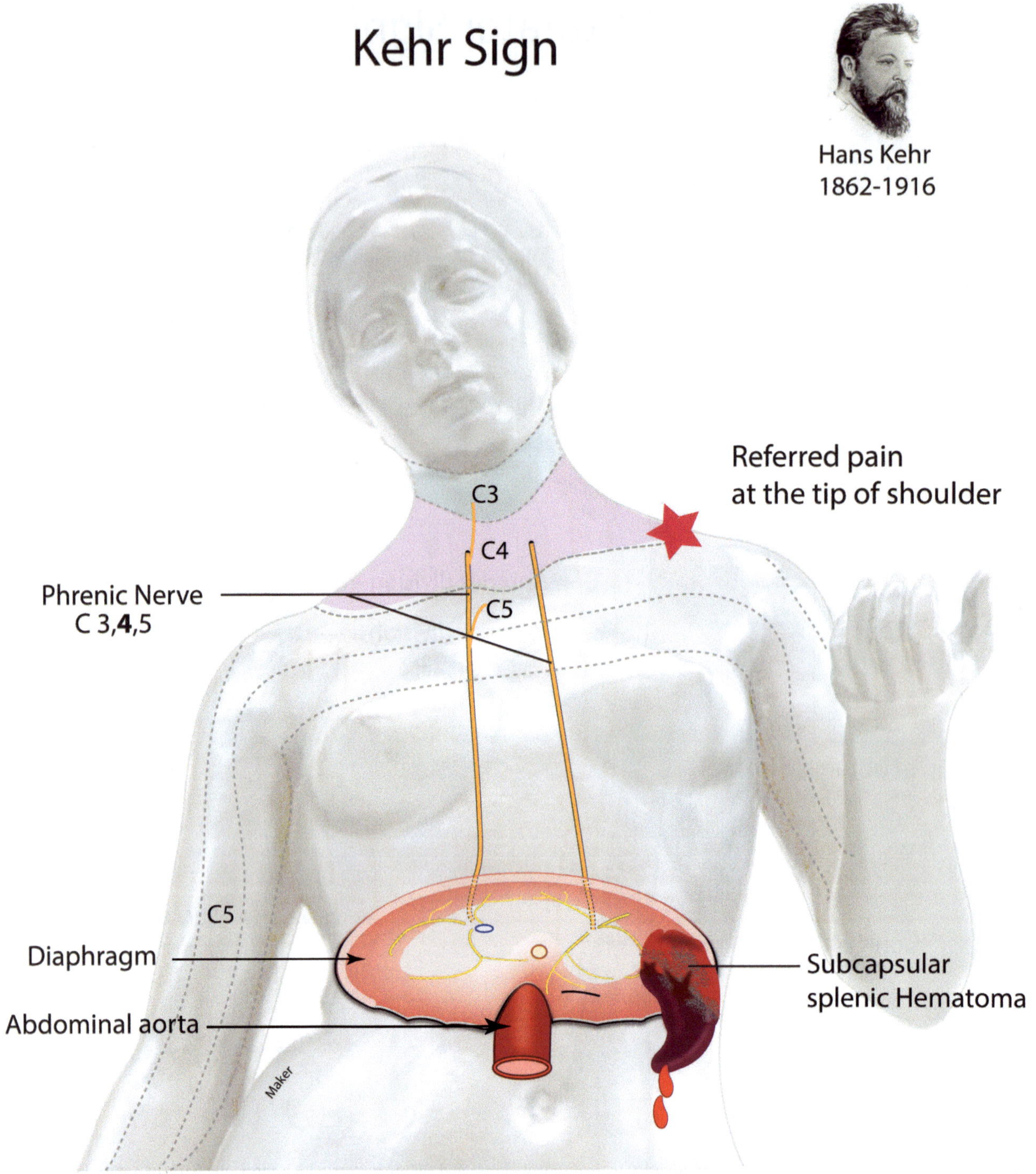

Fig. 7.11 Kehr's sign (now being questioned to be described by Dr. Kehr) is referred pain at the tip of the left shoulder, along the distribution of the phrenic nerve, secondary to subdiaphragmatic irritation from a subcapsular splenic hematoma. Referred pain in either shoulder can be from a variety of disease processes involving the phrenic nerve, including basal pneumonia, subdiaphragmatic abscess, free blood in the abdomen, etc.

Answer
a

References

1. Cervero F, Laird JM. Visceral pain. Lancet. 1999;353(9170):2145–8.
2. Rivero FM, Moreira V, Riesco Lopez V, Rodriguez Gandia JM, Garrido MA, Milicua GE, Salamero JM. Pain originating from the abdominal wall: a forgotten diagnostic option. Gastroenterol Hepatol. 2007;30(4):244–50.
3. Raj PP. Visceral pain. Agri. 2004;16(1):7–20.
4. Sikandar S, Dickenson AH. Visceral pain: the ins and outs, the ups and downs. Curr Opin Support Palliat Care. 2012;6(1):17–26.
5. Mayer EA, Tillisch K. The brain-gut axis in abdominal pain syndromes. Annu Rev Med. 2011;62:381–96.
6. Wood JD. Visceral pain: spinal afferents, enteric mast cells, enteric nervous system and stress. Curr Pharm Des. 2011;17(16):1573–5.
7. Kubikova E, Elfalougy H, Selmeciova P. The bases of the inflammatory acute abdomen. Bratisl Lek Listy. 2012;113(3):172–4.
8. Cartwright SL, Knudson MP. Evaluation of acute abdominal pain in adults. Am Fam Physician. 2008;77(7):971–8.
9. Flasar MH, Goldberg E. Acute abdominal pain. Med Clin North Am. 2006;90(3):481–503.
10. Bemelman WA, Kievit J. Physical examination – rebound tenderness. Ned Tijdschr Geneeskd. 1999;143(6):300–3.
11. Moll VC, de Jongh TO. Physical examination of patients with acute abdominal pain. Ned Tijdschr Geneeskd. 2011;155:A2658.
12. Petroianu A. Diagnosis of acute appendicitis. Int J Surg. 2012;10(3):115–9.
13. Petrie A, Tubbs RS, Matusz P, Shaffer K, Loukas M. Obturator hernia: anatomy, embryology, diagnosis, and treatment. Clin Anat. 2011;24(5):562–9.
14. Soyuncu S, Bektas F, Cete Y. Traditional Kehr's sign: left shoulder pain related to splenic abscess. Ulus Travma Acil Cerrahi Derg. 2012;18(1):87–8.
15. Klimpel V. Does Kehr's sign derive from Hans Kehr? A critical commentary on its documentation? Chirurg. 2004;75(1):80–3.

Abdominal Wall and Hernias

8

1. The following are true statements in relation to the linea alba *except*
   (a) The fibers coming from the oblique and transversus abdominis muscles *do not* cross the midline.
   (b) The linea alba gains considerable strength through the interlocking of collagen fibers.
   (c) The linea alba widens with increasing age.
   (d) The width of the linea alba varies with the angle of the costal arches.
   (e) Transverse incisions have greater bursting strength than vertical incisions.

Comments Among vertical incisions, midline incisions are the strongest by virtue of the anatomy of the linea alba. The linea alba represents the fusion of the aponeurotic envelopes of the external oblique, internal oblique, and transversus abdominis, by decussation, condensation, and interlocking of collagen fibers. The linea alba extends from the xiphoid process to the pubic symphysis. Its extensively decussated collagen fibers are oriented in oblique direction, making it resistant to tension in this plane, and at the same time making it compliant to longitudinal stretching. As one moves away from the linea alba into the rectus sheath, the gridiron of decussating fibers becomes looser, which determines the decreased strength of paramedian incisions [1,2].

The orientation of collagen fibers in the abdominal wall gives transverse incisions the theoretical advantage of minimizing structural damage, lending greater bursting strength when compared to midline incisions. In clinical practice, transverse incisions have been associated with lower incidence of wound dehiscence and incisional hernia, as well as with decreased postoperative pain pulmonary complications when compared to midline incisions [3]. However, more recent meta-analysis challenges these claims [4].

The width of the linea alba can be predicted by the angle of the costal arch. People with wide costal arches generally have a wider linea alba and vice versa.

Answer
a

V.K. Maker, E.D. Guzman-Arrieta, *Cognitive Pearls in General Surgery*,
DOI 10.1007/978-1-4939-1850-8_8, © Springer Science+Business Media New York 2015

2. All of the following are correct *except*:
   (a) The femoral artery provides the blood supply of the anterior aspect of the inferior abdominal wall.
   (b) The lower intercostal and lumbar arteries constitute a deep system supplying the oblique muscles and the transversus abdominis.
   (c) The rectus abdominis muscles receive their blood supply from the superior and inferior epigastric arteries.
   (d) The rectus abdominis muscle has segmental innervation, which allows its transection with subsequent preservation of function.
   (e) The rectus abdominis muscle should be retracted from lateral to medial to avoid disturbing the musculocutaneous nerves.

Comments The blood supply of the abdominal wall is multiple. The descending aorta directly contributes to the blood supply of the abdominal wall through the lower intercostal arteries and the analogous lumbar arteries. The femoral artery contributes to the blood supply of the lower abdominal wall through the superficial circumflex, superficial epigastric, and external pudendal branches.

The rectus abdominis muscles have a dual blood supply that runs posterior to the muscle. Cephalad, the superior epigastrics, which are a continuation of the internal mammaries, travel caudally to anastomose with the inferior epigastrics which branch off the external iliac arteries at the level of the inguinal ligament. Throughout their course, these arteries send branches anteriorly, which enter the substance of the muscle. These branches continue their anterior course through the muscle to supply the skin and subcutaneous tissues of the area, allowing the creation of musculocutaneous flaps based on the epigastric arteries.

The rectus muscle has a complex embryologic origin from multiple dermatomes spanning T6–T12, with the umbilicus at T10 level. It is not clear whether the transverse intersections of the rectus abdominis represent divisions between the myotomes that give origin to the muscle or if they arise independently. In any case, the transverse disposition of nerve fibers allows the muscle to be transected without denervation. In paramedian incisions, the rectus muscle should always be retracted laterally to keep an intact nerve supply [1].

Answer
e

3. Mark the *false* statement in relation to the layers of the abdominal wall and scrotum.
   (a) Scarpa's fascia becomes the dartos layer of the scrotum.
   (b) The external oblique fascia is continuous with the external spermatic fascia.
   (c) The internal oblique muscle fibers are continuous with the cremaster muscle and fascia.
   (d) The transversus abdominis muscle is continuous with the internal spermatic fascia.
   (e) The parietal peritoneum is continuous with the processus vaginalis.

Comments The layers of the scrotum are continuous with the layers of the abdominal wall. These are shown in Table 8.1 and Fig. 8.1.

As can be noted in Table 8.1, the transversus abdominis muscle does not contribute to the layers of the scrotum.

The classical view describes the testicles as arising in the retroperitoneum, without peritoneal coverage. As they descend into the scrotum, the peritoneum evaginates, forming the bilayered tunica vaginalis. This tunica travels anterior to the testicle and eventually surrounds the testicle with exception of its posterior aspect. However, the testicle remains extraperitoneal.

Table 8.1 The layers of the scrotum are continuous with the layers of the abdominal wall

Layer of the abdominal wall	Layer of the scrotum
Skin	Skin
Scarpa's fascia	Dartos
External oblique fascia	External spermatic fascia
Internal oblique muscle	Cremaster
Fascia transversalis	Internal spermatic fascia
Peritoneum	Tunica vaginalis

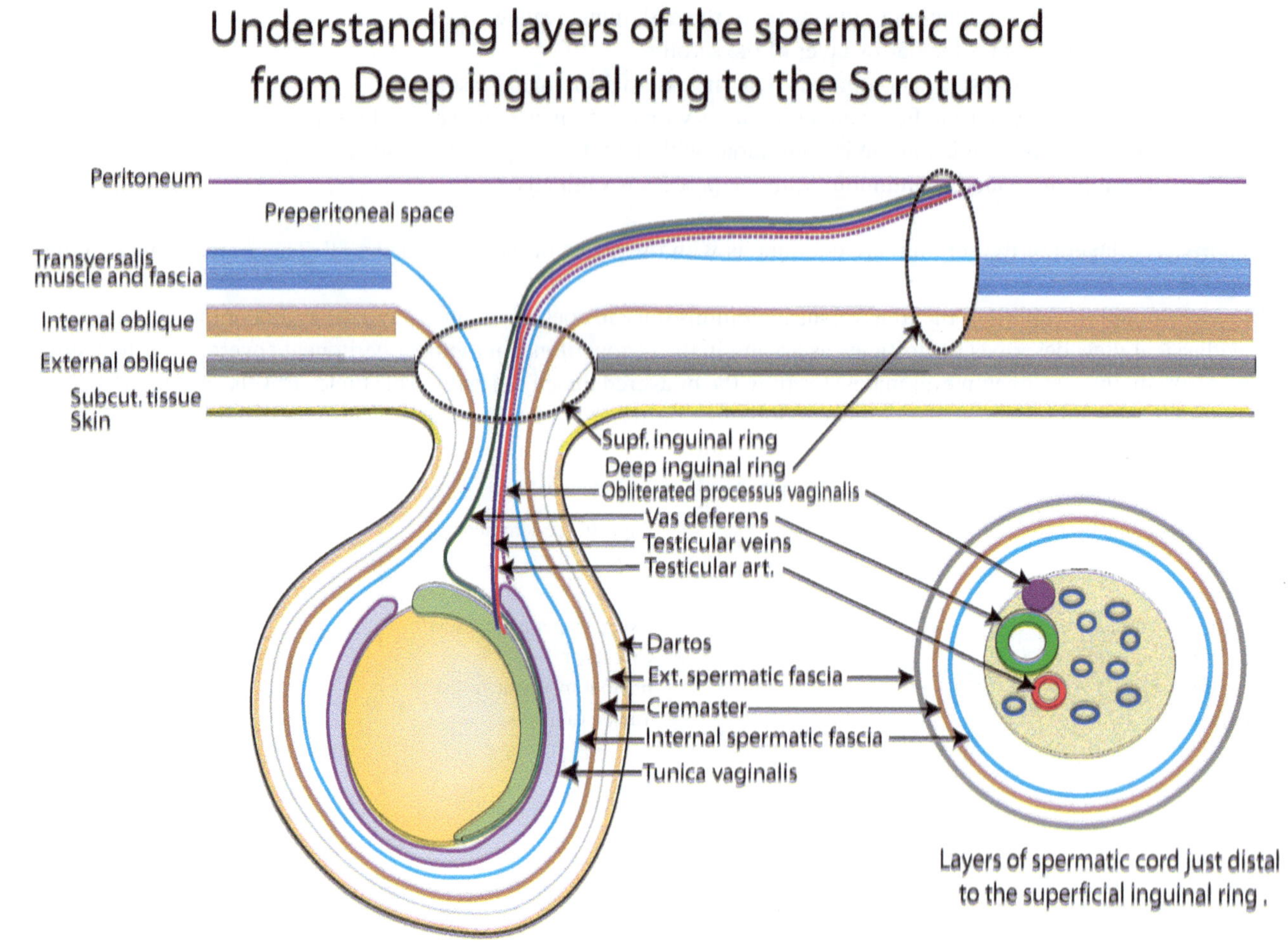

Fig. 8.1 As the normal testicles descend from their retroperitoneal embryonic origin to the anteriorly situated scrotal sac to maintain lower temperature for spermatogenesis, they bring along a thin covering of each layer of the abdominal wall progressively from the deep inguinal ring past the superficial inguinal ring. Testicles, even though enveloped by a knuckle of the double layer of the peritoneum, continue to be extraperitoneal. The vas deferens, spermatic vessels, and lymphatics continue to drain into their respective preperitoneal and retroperitoneal target organs

Answer

d

4. The following structures define the boundaries of the myopectineal orifice *except*:
   (a) Inferior border of the internal oblique
   (b) Inguinal ligament
   (c) Iliopsoas muscle
   (d) Lateral border of the rectus abdominis
   (e) Superior edge of the superior pubic ramus

Comments See question 7.

Answer
b

5. The following structures define the boundaries of the inguinal canal *except*:
   (a) Cooper's ligament
   (b) External oblique aponeurosis
   (c) Transversus abdominis aponeurosis and transversalis fascia
   (d) Inferior edge of the internal oblique
   (e) Inguinal ligament

Comments See question 7.

Answer

a

6. The following statements are correct *except*:
   (a) In laparoscopic and open repair, prosthetic material is ideally placed in the preperitoneal space.
   (b) The inguinal ligament (ligament of Poupart) is the thickened inferior edge of the external oblique aponeurosis.
   (c) Intraparietal hernias should always be sought in an inguinal hernia repair.
   (d) The lacunar ligament (ligament of Gimbernat) joins the medial aspect of the inguinal ligament to the pubic symphysis.
   (e) The pectineal ligament (Cooper's ligament) is the thickened periosteum of the superior pubic ramus.

Comments See question 7.

Answer
d

7. The following structures define the femoral ring *except*:
   (a) Femoral vein
   (b) Cooper's ligament
   (c) Inguinal ligament
   (d) Lacunar ligament
   (e) Pubic tubercle

Comments The myopectineal orifice represents an opening through the anterior abdominal wall that allows the passage of the spermatic cord and of the femoral vessels and nerve. It is limited laterally by the iliopsoas muscle, medially by the edge of the rectus sheath, superiorly by the edge of the internal oblique, and inferiorly by Cooper's ligament. The inguinal ligament divides the myopectineal orifice into the inguinal region superiorly and the femoral region inferiorly.

The inguinal ligament and its shelving edge form the lower boundary of the inguinal canal, with the upper border provided by the free edge of the internal oblique muscle. The roof (ventral) of the inguinal canal is formed by the external oblique aponeurosis, and the floor (dorsal) is formed by the transversus abdominis aponeurosis reinforced by the transversalis fascia [5].

The transversus abdominis aponeurosis is not to be confused with the transversalis fascia, although both structures may be fused together. The former is the fibrous extension of the transversus abdominis muscle, as it extends towards the midline and pubic tubercle, whereas the latter is a part of the endoabdominal fascia, which lines all the walls of the abdomen, including the diaphragm and pelvis [6].

The inguinal canal extends from the internal (deep and lateral) inguinal ring to the external (superficial and medial) inguinal ring. In the newborn, these two rings overlie each other, allowing the passage of the testicle into the scrotum. During growth to adulthood, the two rings separate with the superficial ring overlying the pubic tubercle and the deep ring located at the mid-inguinal point. The deep inguinal ring is located in the transversalis fascia and transversus abdominis muscle. It vests the internal spermatic fascia on the structures traversing it. The superficial ring is located in the external oblique aponeurosis and provides the external spermatic fascia vesting any structure going through this opening [7] (Fig. 8.2).

The variability of the inguinal region has led to some semantic confusion with multiple names attached to the same structures depending on surgical exposure.

The femoral canal lies medial to the femoral vein, normally containing a small amount of fat and the lymph node of Cloquet. Its medial aspect is the lacunar ligament (ligament of Gimbernat), which is a collection of fibers arising from the inguinal ligament, inserting on the medial aspect of the superior pubic ramus, close to the pubic tubercle. These fibers may be incised when attempting to release an incarcerated femoral hernia. Its ventral margin is the inguinal ligament, and its posterior margin is Cooper's ligament. Because of the tight and fixed boundaries of the femoral ring, femoral hernias are more likely to strangulate than inguinal hernias [8].

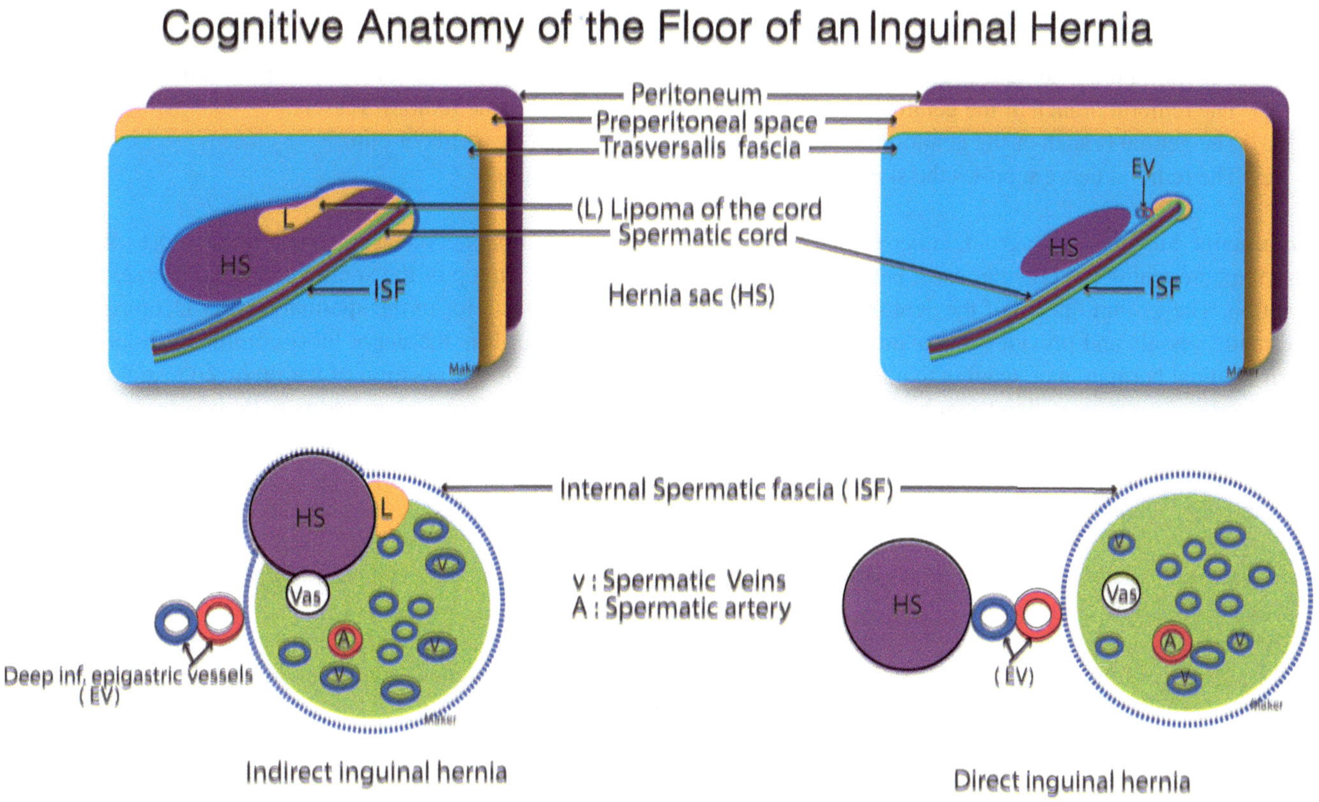

Fig. 8.2 Illustrated is a diagrammatic representation of the floor of the inguinal canal and the cross-sections of the spermatic cord in indirect and direct inguinal hernias. The deep or internal inguinal ring lies in the transversalis fascia, bounded medially by the deep inferior epigastric artery and vein. An indirect hernia sac is often accompanied by herniated fat from the preperitoneal space erroneously called the lipoma of the cord. Any structure which comes through the deep ring is enveloped by the internal spermatic fascia, which is a continuation of a thin fascia from the transversalis that must be incised to get to the hernia sac. Direct hernias protrude directly from the floor of the inguinal canal, medial to the deep inferior epigastric vessels. The preperitoneal space carries varying amounts of fat and continues laterally and posteriorly into the retroperitoneal space

Answer

e

8. Mark the false statement regarding the nerve supply of the inguinal area.
   (a) Entrapment of the lateral femoral cutaneous nerve (L2–L3) causes meralgia paresthetica.
   (b) The ilioinguinal nerve (L1–L2) travels with the spermatic cord to innervate the base of the penis and scrotum.
   (c) The femoral branch of the genitofemoral nerve supplies the skin over the femoral vessels.
   (d) The genital branch of the genitofemoral nerve supplies the glans of the penis or clitoris.
   (e) The femoral nerve supplies the skin and muscles of the anterior thigh.

Comments Surgery of the groin, either open or laparoscopic, places multiple nerves at risk. The nerve most often recognized upon opening the inguinal canal is the ilioinguinal nerve, which lies on top of the spermatic cord. It serves a sensory function. The genital branch of the genitofemoral nerve lies outside and posterior to the spermatic cord accompanying the spermatic vessels and provides motor innervation to the cremaster muscle. It is the nerve most commonly injured during open inguinal hernia repair, leading to a loss of the cremasteric reflex and a lower position of the involved testicle. The iliohypogastric nerve runs within the substance of the internal oblique, near its inferior edge, and may be injured when sutures are placed in this area, especially during mesh fixation. The iliohypogastric nerve may also be injured during the creation of a Pfannenstiel incision; in either case, numbness of the pubic region ensues.

The laparoscopic approach puts at risk additional nerves: the lateral femoral cutaneous nerve (most commonly injured), the anterior femoral cutaneous nerve, the femoral branch of the genitofemoral nerve, and the femoral nerve. These four structures lie in the so-called triangle of pain, limited by the gonadal vessels medially, the iliopubic tract superiorly, and the peritoneal reflection laterally.

Immediately medial to the triangle of pain is the triangle of doom, which contains the femoral vessels and the genital branch of the genitofemoral nerve. This triangle is limited by the vas deferens medially, the gonadal vessels laterally, and the peritoneal reflection inferiorly.

In practical terms, the existence of these two triangles determines that no tacks or sutures are to be placed below the iliopubic tract lateral to the vas deferens during the course of a laparoscopic groin hernia repair [9] (Fig. 8.3).

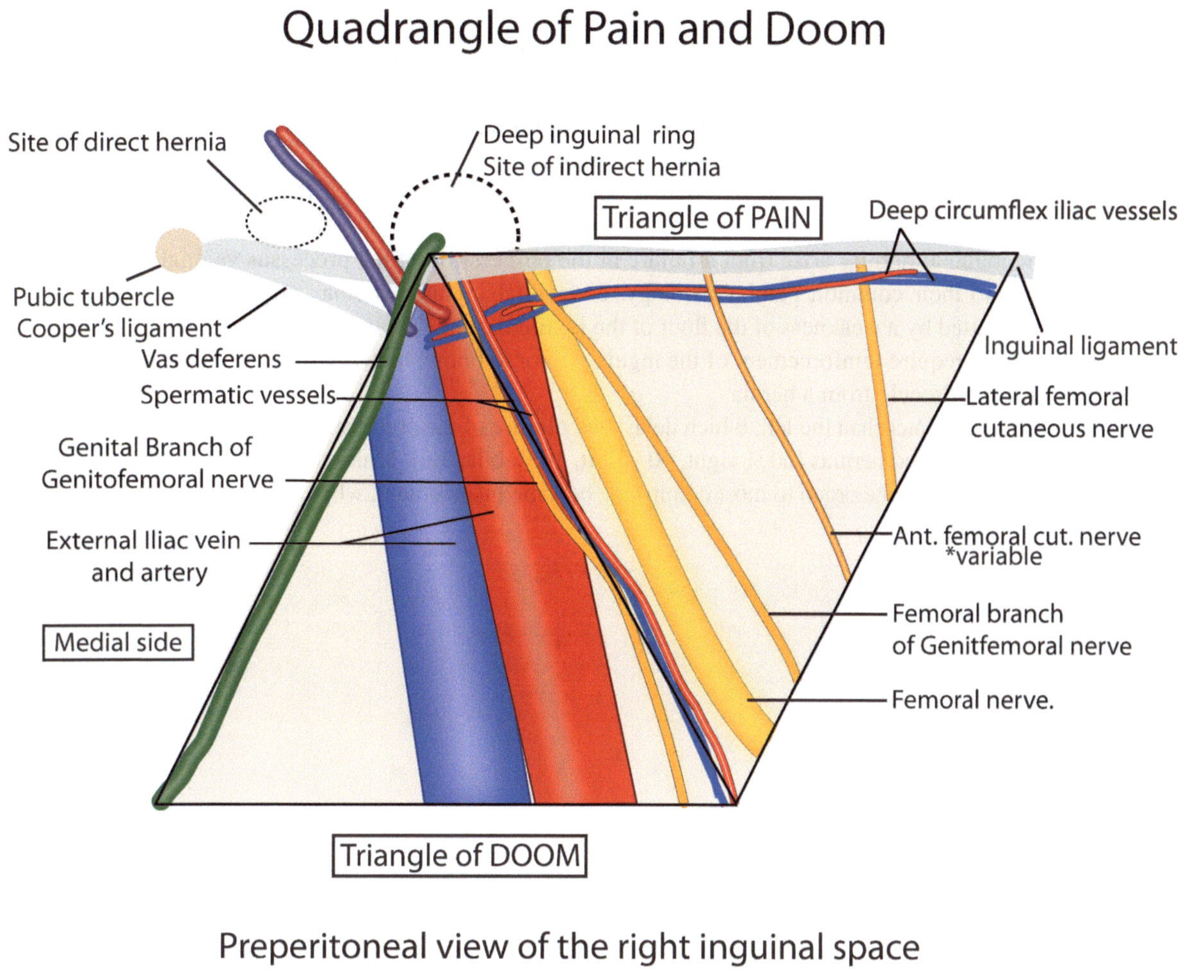

Fig. 8.3 Exposure of the preperitoneal space in laparoscopic surgery presents an inside-out view of the floor of the inguinal canal and presents different challenges in the surgery in this space. The quadrangle of pain and doom represents the combination of the triangle of doom and triangle of pain divided by the anatomical landmark of the spermatic vessels together with the genital branch of genitofemoral nerve and lymphatics coming from the retroperitoneal space en route to the deep inguinal ring. The triangle of doom is bounded by the vas deferens on its medial side with external iliac vessels running through it. At its apex is the deep inguinal ring with deep epigastric vessels arising from the external iliacs. Immediately lateral is the triangle of pain with its apex pointing posteriorly. This triangle is bounded superiorly by the reflected part of the inguinal ligament and deep circumflex iliac vessels also arising from external iliac vessels, just lateral to the entry of deep epigastric vessels. This triangle contains multiple nerves, which, if injured, will be the cause of postop pain and paresthesia. Cooper's ligament is the shiny white strong ligament over the iliopubic area, also called the pectineal ligament (Modified from Colborn and Skandalakis [10])

Answer

d

9. Mark the incorrect answer.
   (a) In the infant, the internal and external inguinal rings are nearly superimposed.
   (b) Newborns with inguinal hernias require repair of the floor of the inguinal canal.
   (c) Inguinal hernias are more common in premature than in full-term newborns.
   (d) Congenital inguinal hernias are more common on the right.
   (e) The most common organ to incarcerate in a female congenital inguinal hernia is the ovary.

Comments Pediatric inguinal hernias arise from a failure in the obliteration of the processus vaginalis, and as such are of the indirect kind. Due to their common pathophysiology, congenital inguinal hernias may coexist with communicating hydroceles. Neither is caused by a weakness of the floor of the inguinal canal. Their treatment consists of closing the processus vaginalis and does not require reinforcement of the inguinal floor. Of note, transillumination of the scrotum is not a reliable test to distinguish a hydrocele from a hernia.

The right testicle descends later than the left, which delays the closure of the processus vaginalis on this side, explaining the increased frequency of right-sided hernias (60 % right, 40 % left, 10 % bilateral). Males are affected six times more often than females. In males, the intestine is the organ to most commonly become incarcerated, whereas in females it is the ovary [11].

Answer

b

10. Mark the incorrect statement.
    (a) The overall incidence of incisional hernia after laparotomy is approximately 10 %.
    (b) Abdominal wall closure using interrupted sutures has the lowest rate of incisional hernia.
    (c) Sutures under excessive tension stimulate an inadequate fibroblast response leading to poor wound healing.
    (d) Obesity, prolonged ileus, bowel obstruction, and infection are risk factors for wound dehiscence.
    (e) Evisceration may be prevented by the placement of retention sutures.

Comments Incisional hernias are a common complication after laparotomy (5–15 % after 1 year). The previously held belief that transverse incisions had a lower incidence of incisional hernia has not been proven to be true. Incidence of incisional hernias is affected by closure techniques. The current consensus states that continuous sutures are superior to interrupted sutures, as they distribute force more evenly along the closure. The material of choice is a slowly absorbable suture such as PDS, which retains its tensile strength for up to 6 weeks. While nonabsorbable sutures have a lesser incidence of incisional hernias, the increased frequency of sinus tract formation and chronic pain make slowly absorbable sutures a better choice. Full-thickness retention sutures do not prevent fascial dehiscence. Currently, their role is to prevent complete evisceration, allowing fascial repair to be delayed or even not performed provided there is adequate coverage of the abdominal contents [12,13].

Answer

b

11. The following statements about hernias are true *except*:
    (a) Spigelian hernias may occur at any point along the semilunar line.
    (b) The superior lumbar triangle (Grynfeltt) is limited by the 12th rib, the paraspinal muscles, and the internal oblique.
    (c) The inferior lumbar triangle (Petit) is limited by the iliac crest, the latissimus dorsi, and the external oblique.
    (d) Epigastric hernias occur through the supraumbilical linea alba.
    (e) Obturator hernias are frequently obvious on physical exam.

Comments Spigelian hernias occur through defects in the semilunar line. They are most frequently located at the intersection of the semilunar line and the semicircular line of Douglas, where the disappearance of the posterior rectus sheath creates a weak spot. However, other weak spots may occur at the fusion points of the dermatomes contributing to the abdominal wall, allowing for other sites of herniation. Spigelian hernias are classical examples of intraparietal hernias, where the hernial sac dissects between the layers of the abdominal wall [14].

Lumbar hernias occur through two distinct weak spots in the dorsal abdominal wall. They are more frequently of the Grynfeltt variety, where a near horizontal position of the 12th rib is a predisposing factor. Since the lumbar triangles each have a fixed, bony boundary, primary closure of the hernial defect is often difficult and under tension; due to this, underlay mesh repair is preferred. Currently, laparoscopy is emerging as the preferred surgical modality [15].

Epigastric hernias were originally considered to be a congenital defect of the linea alba. Currently, they are thought to be acquired, with a component of congenital linea alba weakness, related to poor fiber decussation or vascular lacunae. These hernias affect 3–5 % of the population and are the most common in young men [16].

Obturator hernias have been called "skinny old lady hernias." They affect women almost exclusively. Bulging in the obturator region is hardly ever seen, and the most common presentation is bowel obstruction. The protrusion of the hernial sac through the obturator canal often causes compression of the obturator nerve. This compression becomes clinically apparent through pain in the medial thigh (Howship–Romberg sign) as well as through the absence of the obturator reflex in the affected side (Hannington-Kiff sign). Diagnosis is most often confirmed through CT scanning [17].

Answer
e

12. Mark the *incorrect* answer.
    (a) Fibrosis of the vas deferens manifests itself as groin pain made worse with ejaculation.
    (b) The most common nerve injured during laparoscopic hernia repair is the lateral femoral cutaneous nerve.
    (c) The initial treatment of osteitis pubis is surgery.
    (d) Recurrence rates are similar for laparoscopic and open inguinal hernia repairs.
    (e) Testicular atrophy is associated with excessive dissection around the spermatic cord.

Comments The vas deferens is exposed to injury during inguinal hernia repair. Transection should be treated by immediate reanastomosis. More often, blunt trauma to the spermatic cord during dissection leads to fibrosis. This reaction may also be induced by the presence of mesh.

Nerve injuries are an important complication of inguinal herniorrhaphy often causing intense and prolonged pain. During surgery, both open and laparoscopic, attempts should be made to identify and preserve the nerves. When a nerve injury is identified, the proximal end of the nerve should be ligated and buried within muscle tissue. Chronic post-herniorrhaphy pain should be initially managed nonoperatively. If this approach fails, triple neurectomy (ilioinguinal, genitofemoral, and iliohypogastric nerves) should be undertaken. In similar fashion, pain arising from sutures or tacks placed on the pubic periosteum (osteitis pubis) should be initially approached nonoperatively. If this approach fails, removal of the foreign material may be indicated.

Aggressive dissection of the hernial sac from the spermatic cord, especially when carried beyond the pubic tubercle may injure the pampiniform plexus, leading to venous congestion and stagnant hypoxemia of the testicle resulting in delayed atrophy. Occasionally, this process is severe enough to create ischemic orchitis in the immediate postoperative period [18].

Answer

c

13. The following statements regarding congenital pathology of the abdominal wall are true *except*:
    (a) Infantile umbilical hernias require prompt surgical repair.
    (b) Cardiac malformations are the most common defect associated with omphalocele.
    (c) Omphalocele represents the failure of the developing intestines to return to the abdominal cavity.
    (d) Malrotation and incomplete fixation of the intestine are common in the setting of omphalocele.
    (e) Loss of domain may occur in both omphalocele and gastroschisis.

Comments See question 14.

Answer

a

14. The following statements about gastroschisis are correct *except*:
    (a) Children with gastroschisis often have multiple associated malformations.
    (b) Gastroschisis is due to defective development of the muscles of the abdominal wall.
    (c) Gastroschisis does not have a hernial sac.
    (d) Gastroschisis occurs in a paramedian position.
    (e) Gastroschisis may be accompanied by small bowel atresia.

Comments Infantile umbilical hernias represent a failure of fascial closure of the umbilical ring, formerly occupied by the omphalomesenteric duct. They are more frequent in premature infants. The fact that up to 80 % of infantile umbilical hernias close spontaneously combined with a low incarceration rate makes observation the preferred management strategy. However, for defects larger than 2 cm, repair is recommended due to a low probability of spontaneous closure. Surgery should also be performed if complications arise or if the hernia has not closed until age 3–5 [16].

Omphalocele represents persistence of the omphalomesenteric duct, whereas gastroschisis is related to an abnormal involution of the right umbilical vein (defects are on the right of the umbilical cord) leading to abnormal development of the muscles of the abdominal wall.

While omphalocele is associated with multiple congenital defects (cardiac; musculoskeletal; GI; genitourinary; trisomies 13, 18, and 21; and Beckwith–Wiedemann syndrome), gastroschisis is not. The intestinal atresia seen with gastroschisis does not represent a true congenital defect, rather it is caused by exposure of the bowel to amniotic fluid due to the lack of a hernial sac. This exposure does not occur in omphalocele, because a hernial sac formed by the amniotic membrane is present [19].

Answer
a

15. Match the eponym on the right with the description on the left.

1. Richter hernia	(a) Inguinal containing the appendix
2. Littre hernia	(b) Strangulating but nonobstructing hernia
3. Pantaloon hernia	(c) Hernia containing Meckel's diverticulum
4. Maydl hernia	(d) Intra-abdominal strangulation of small bowel loop
5. Amyand hernia	(e) Coexisting direct and indirect inguinal hernias

Comments Notwithstanding the large variety of abdominal hernia types and associated eponyms, all hernias share a common structure, formed by a fascial hernial ring or neck that allows the abnormal passage of hernia contents contained by a hernial sac (Fig. 8.4).

Richter hernia, also known as partial enterocele, consists of the protrusion and/or incarceration of part of the bowel wall through a hernia ring. Richter hernias may progress to strangulation and perforation without a significant obstruction [20].

Littre hernia is the protrusion of a Meckel's diverticulum through a hernia orifice, most commonly the inguinal ring, followed by the umbilicus and femoral ring. Occasionally, the diverticulum may be accompanied by the adjacent bowel. Treatment consists of repair of the hernia and diverticulectomy [21].

The first successful appendectomy was performed by Amyand in 1735. During a groin exploration on an 11-year-old boy, he found the cecal appendix that had been perforated by a swallowed pin. Subsequently, inguinal hernias containing the appendix (inflamed or not) have been termed Amyand hernias [22–24].

Pantaloon hernias are the combination of direct and indirect hernial sacs straddling over the inferior epigastric vessels. Maydl hernias involve incarceration of W-shaped loop of the bowel. When strangulation happens, it is the intra-abdominal portion which suffers the most serious consequence (Fig. 8.5).

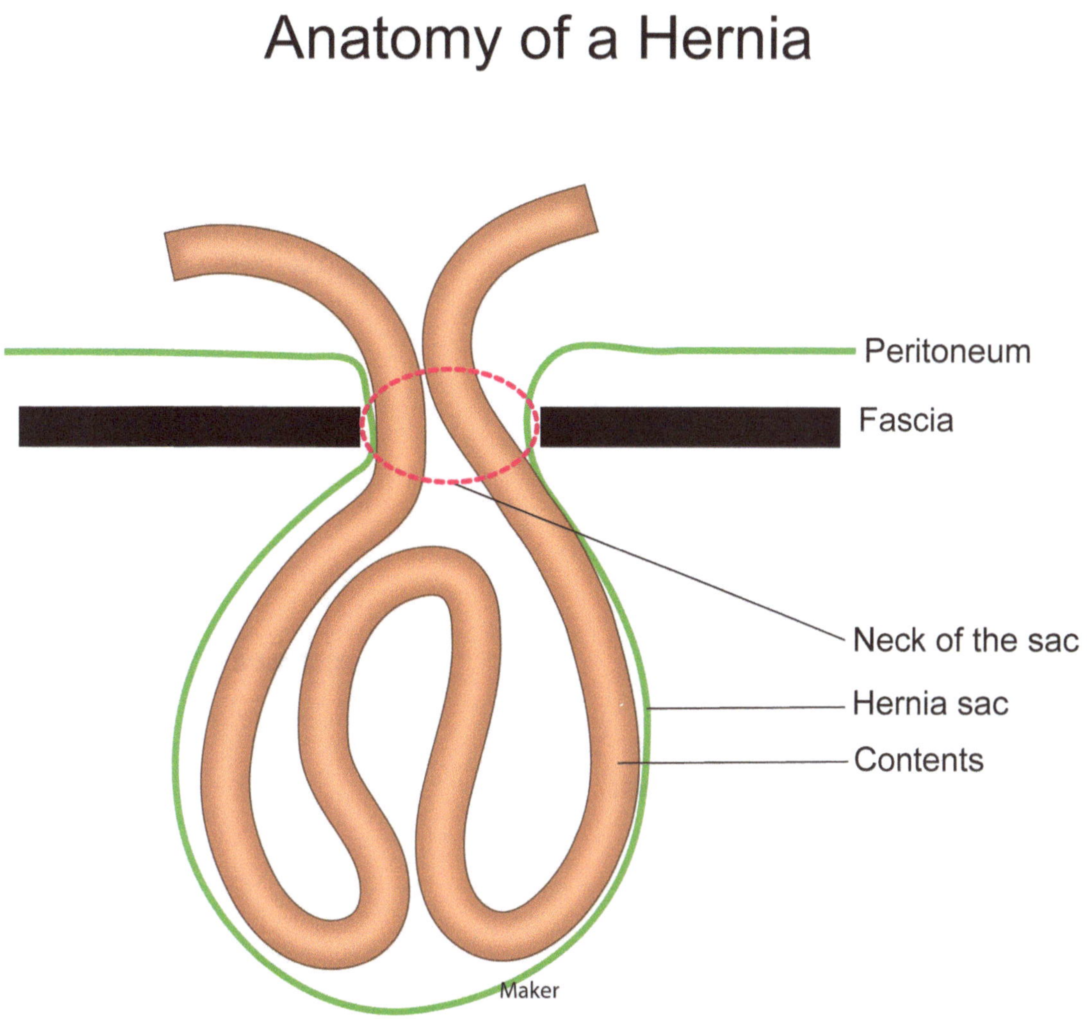

Fig. 8.4 Typically an abdominal hernia protrudes through a normal or an abnormal opening in the fascia. This opening becomes the neck of the hernia and is the tightest or the smallest part of the protrusion. Assessing the size and the anatomy of the neck of the hernia is important as this is the most likely site for strangulation and will need to be widened to reduce the strangulation. The hernia sac is the peritoneal covering of the contents of the hernia

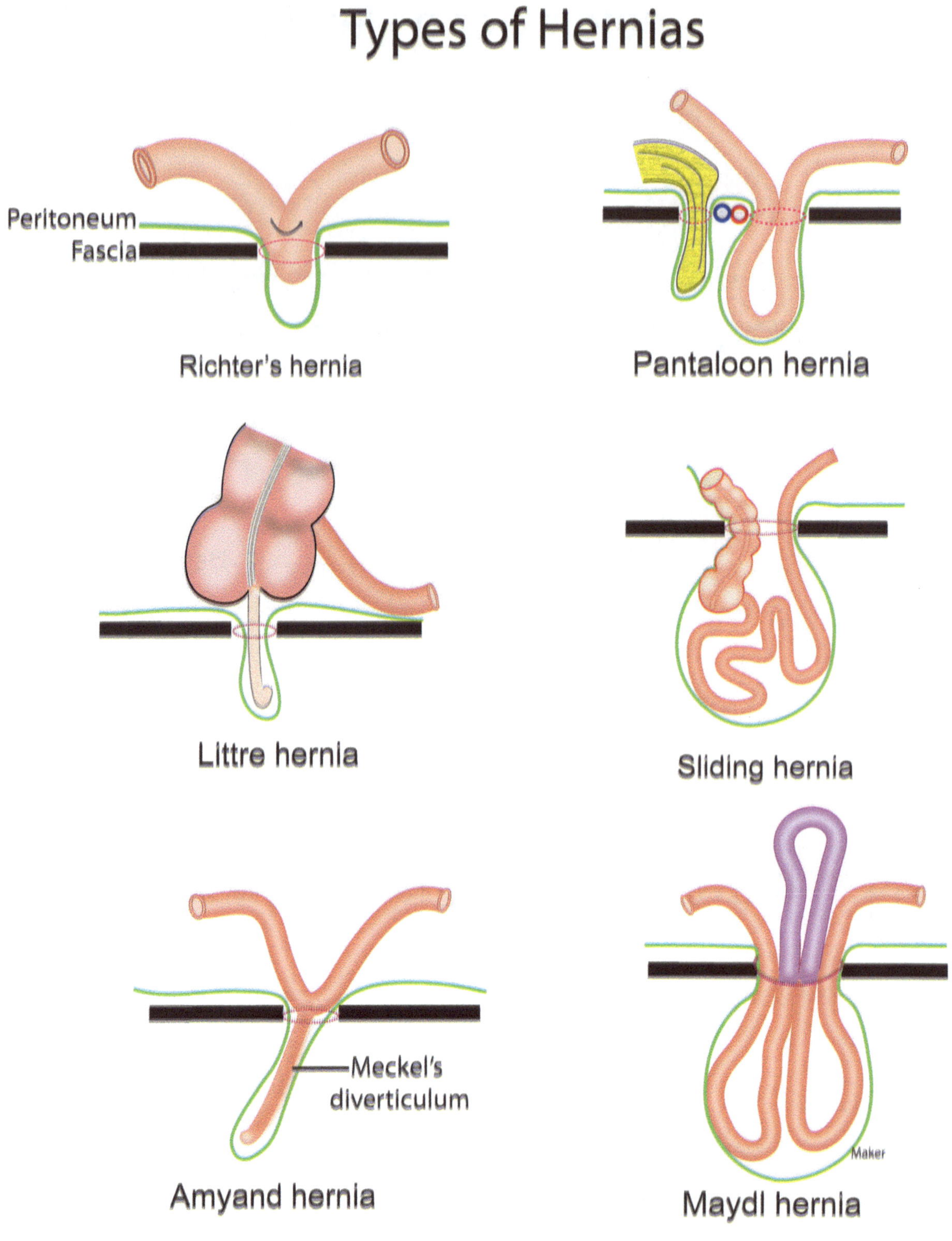

Fig. 8.5 In a Richter's hernia, a part of the wall of the bowel herniates and may strangulate without a complete bowel obstruction. In a sliding hernia, part of the wall of the sac is a viscus. Hence, it is critical to not enter the sac in the area of the viscus. In a pantaloon hernia, there is a direct and indirect inguinal hernia bulging next to each other like pant legs with the deep inferior epigastric vessels in the crotch. In a Maydl hernia, a letter "W"-shaped loop of the bowel herniates. This is very important to establish as the intraperitoneal loop of the bowel will be the first to strangulate being compressed from both sides. In all such cases, it is important to establish continuity of the entering loop in the sac to its exit back from the sac

Answer

1, b; 2, c; 3, e; 4, d; and 5, a.

16. Match the hernia repair on the right with the description on the left.

1. Bassini	(a) Transversalis fascia to Cooper's ligament
2. McVay	(b) Plug and patch
3. Lichtenstein	(c) Layered internal oblique and transversalis fascia to inguinal ligament
4. Shouldice	(d) Conjoint tendon to inguinal ligament
5. Rutkow	(e) Sutured nonabsorbable patch bridging the internal oblique and transversus abdominis to the inguinal ligament

Comments While there are multiple ways to repair inguinal hernias, the gold standard at present is to provide a tension-free repair with a prosthetic graft. This approach has reduced the recurrence rates from 10 % seen with the classical tension repairs to 2 % or less.

Prosthetic material may be placed as an onlay (superficial to the inguinal floor) or as an underlay (deep to the inguinal floor). In the latter case, the prosthetic material is placed in the preperitoneal space. This second location is utilized by laparoscopic repairs as well as by a properly placed hernia plug during open repairs (Fig. 8.6).

As described, it is necessary to gain access into the preperitoneal space in order to place the hernia plug and allow it to "flower," creating a large underlay effectively blocking the hernia ring. This creates a mechanical advantage in that increases in intra-abdominal pressure compress the deployed plug against the pelvic floor providing greater traction and fixation, thus resisting herniation [25,26] (Fig. 8.7).

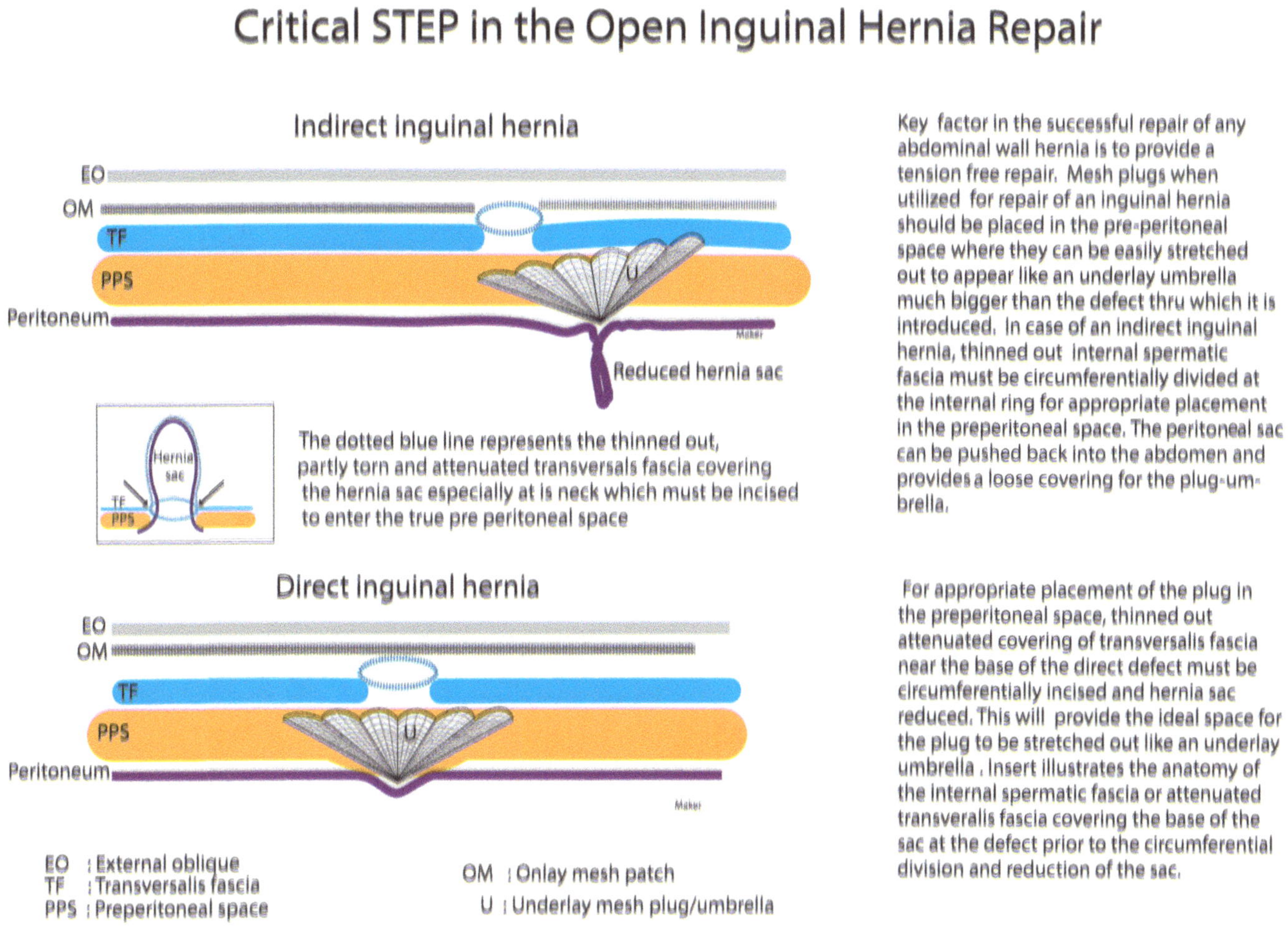

Fig. 8.6 Critical *step* in the open inguinal hernia repair. *EO* external oblique, *TF* transversalis fascia, *PPS* preperitoneal space, *OM* onlay mesh patch, *U* underlay mesh plug/umbrella

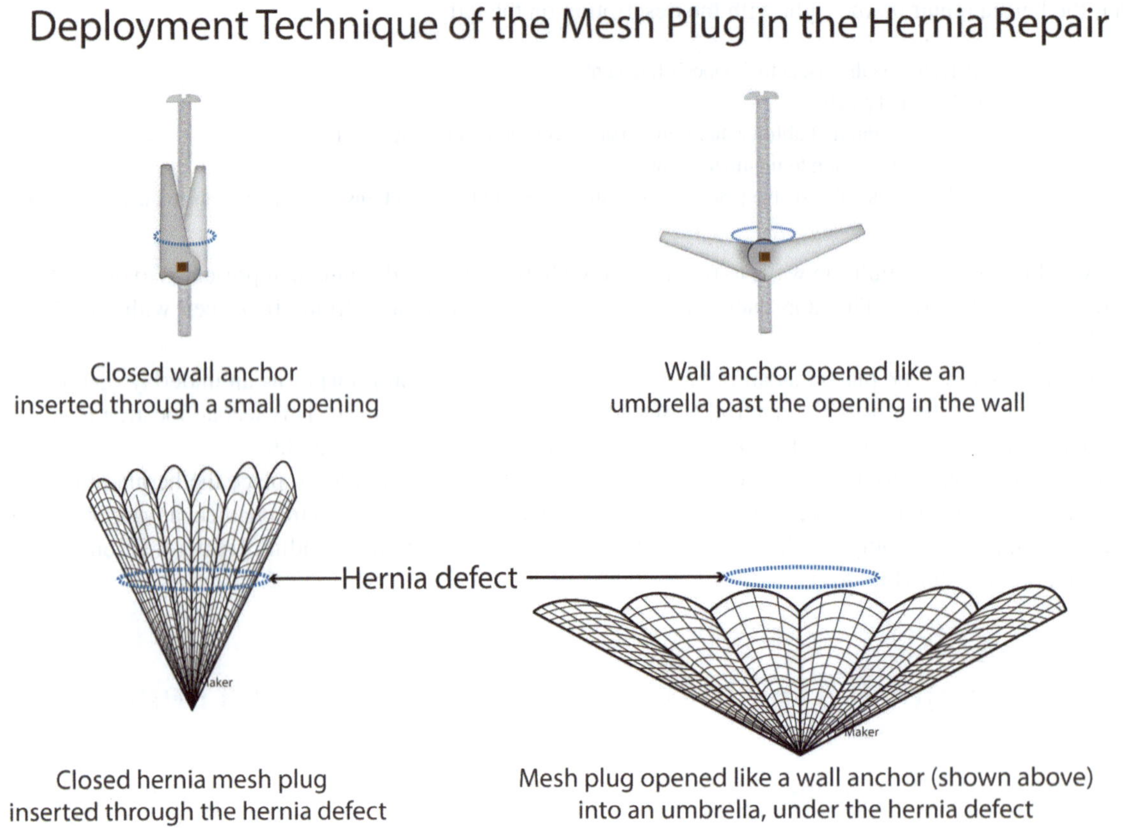

Fig. 8.7 Mesh plugs when used in hernia repairs should be placed in the preperitoneal space where they can be spread out like an umbrella. This is based on the same principle as some of the wall anchors which are inserted through small openings and then open up beyond the wall.

Answer

1, d; 2, a; 3, e; 4, c; and 5, b.

References

1. Grevious MA, Cohen M, Shah SR, Rodriguez P. Structural and functional anatomy of the abdominal wall. Clin Plast Surg. 2006;33(2):169–79, v.
2. Grassel D, Prescher A, Fitzek S, Keyserlingk DG, Axer H. Anisotropy of human linea alba: a biomechanical study. J Surg Res. 2005;124(1):118–25.
3. Grantcharov TP, Rosenberg J. Vertical compared with transverse incisions in abdominal surgery. Eur J Surg. 2001;167(4):260–7.
4. Brown SR, Goodfellow PB. Transverse versus midline incisions for abdominal surgery. Cochrane Database Syst Rev. 2005;4:CD005199.
5. Fagan SP, Awad SS. Abdominal wall anatomy: the key to a successful inguinal hernia repair. Am J Surg. 2004;188(6A Suppl):3S–8.
6. Bendavid R, Howarth D. Transversalis fascia rediscovered. Surg Clin North Am. 2000;80(1):25–33.
7. Avisse C, Delattre JF, Flament JB. The inguinal rings. Surg Clin North Am. 2000;80(1):49–69.
8. Skandalakis JE, Colborn GL, Androulakis JA, Skandalakis LJ, Pemberton LB. Embryologic and anatomic basis of inguinal herniorrhaphy. Surg Clin North Am. 1993;73(4):799–836.
9. Wijsmuller AR, van Veen RN, Bosch JL, Lange JF, Kleinrensink GJ, Jeekel J, et al. Nerve management during open hernia repair. Br J Surg. 2007;94(1):17–22.
10. Colborn GL, Skandalakis JE. Laparoscopic anatomy of the inguinal area. Probl Gen Surg. 1995;12:13–20.
11. Antonoff MB, Kreykes NS, Saltzman DA, Acton RD. American Academy of pediatrics section on surgery hernia survey revisited. J Pediatr Surg. 2005;40(6):1009–14.
12. van 't RM, Steyerberg EW, Nellensteyn J, Bonjer HJ, Jeekel J. Meta-analysis of techniques for closure of midline abdominal incisions. Br J Surg. 2002;89(11):1350–6.
13. O'Dwyer PJ, Courtney CA. Factors involved in abdominal wall closure and subsequent incisional hernia. Surgeon. 2003;1(1):17–22.
14. Skandalakis PN, Zoras O, Skandalakis JE, Mirilas P. Spigelian hernia: surgical anatomy, embryology, and technique of repair. Am Surg. 2006;72(1):42–8.
15. Moreno-Egea A, Baena EG, Calle MC, Martinez JA, Albasini JL. Controversies in the current management of lumbar hernias. Arch Surg. 2007;142(1):82–8.
16. Muschaweck U. Umbilical and epigastric hernia repair. Surg Clin North Am. 2003;83(5):1207–21.
17. Losanoff JE, Richman BW, Jones JW. Obturator hernia. J Am Coll Surg. 2002;194(5):657–63.
18. Bendavid R. Complications of groin hernia surgery. Surg Clin North Am. 1998;78(6):1089–103.
19. Ledbetter DJ. Gastroschisis and omphalocele. Surg Clin North Am. 2006;86(2):249–60, vii.
20. Skandalakis PN, Zoras O, Skandalakis JE, Mirilas P. Richter hernia: surgical anatomy and technique of repair. Am Surg. 2006;72(2):180–4.
21. Skandalakis PN, Zoras O, Skandalakis JE, Mirilas P. Littre hernia: surgical anatomy, embryology, and technique of repair. Am Surg. 2006;72(3):238–43.
22. Sharma H, Gupta A, Shekhawat NS, Memon B, Memon MA. Amyand's hernia: a report of 18 consecutive patients over a 15-year period. Hernia. 2007;11(1):31–5.
23. Akopian G, Alexander M. De Garengeot hernia: appendicitis within a femoral hernia. Am Surg. 2005;71(6):526–7.
24. Rutkow IM. A selective history of groin hernia surgery in the early 19th century. The anatomic atlases of Astley Cooper, Franz Hesselbach, Antonio Scarpa, and Jules-Germain Cloquet. Surg Clin North Am. 1998;78(6):921–40.
25. Cavazzola LT, Rosen MJ. Laparoscopic versus open inguinal hernia repair. Surg Clin North Am. 2013;93(5):1269–79.
26. Bittner R, Schwarz J. Inguinal hernia repair: current surgical techniques. Langenbecks Arch Surg. 2012;397(2):271–82.

9 Peritoneum, Omentum, and Internal Hernias

1. The following are true regarding the embryology of the abdominal cavity *except*:
   (a) Originally the ventral and dorsal mesenteries separate the future peritoneal cavity into the right and left compartments.
   (b) The right compartment becomes the lesser sac.
   (c) The left compartment becomes the general peritoneal cavity or greater sac.
   (d) The midgut and hindgut possess a ventral mesentery.
   (e) The dorsal mesogastrium gives rise to the greater omentum and gastrosplenic ligament.

Comments See question 2.

Answer
d

V.K. Maker, E.D. Guzman-Arrieta, *Cognitive Pearls in General Surgery*,
DOI 10.1007/978-1-4939-1850-8_9,

2. The following are true regarding the embryology of the abdominal cavity *except*:
   (a) The greater omentum is derived from the dorsal mesentery.
   (b) The lesser omentum is derived from the ventral mesentery.
   (c) Congenital omental defects are a common cause of small bowel obstruction.
   (d) The adult transverse mesocolon is the fusion of the transverse mesocolon and dorsal mesogastrium.
   (e) A hernia of Waldeyer is a congenital defect in the mesentery.

Comments In the embryo, the foregut-derived organs are aligned in the anteroposterior axis along the ventral (liver, biliary system, and ventral pancreas) and dorsal (dorsal pancreas and spleen) mesenteries. These mesenteries separate the celomic cavity (future peritoneal cavity) into the right and left compartments. The adult disposition of abdominal contents comes about through a combination of two motions.

First, there is a clockwise rotation along the longitudinal axis. This rotation displaces the liver, biliary tree, and ventral pancreas from their anterior position to the right and the spleen and dorsal pancreas from their posterior position to the left. In turn, the left compartment becomes the anterior greater sac, while the right compartment becomes the posterior lesser sac. Secondly, the greater curvature of the stomach grows at a faster pace than the lesser curvature, with the distal stomach and duodenum shifting towards the right [1].

The motions that the foregut undergoes during its development correlate with the course of the vagi. The right vagus becomes posterior in the abdominal esophagus, while the left nerve is more anteriorly located (Los Angeles = Left vagus Anterior). The entire parasympathetic nerve supply to the stomach comes from the lesser curvature through the nerves of Latarjet (anterior and posterior gastric nerves) [2].

All three segments of the gut possess a dorsal mesentery, while only the foregut is endowed with a ventral mesentery. The ventral mesentery gives rise to the falciform ligament, which splits to envelop the liver as Glisson's capsule and comes together along its inferior left edge to form the lesser omentum, which connects the liver with the stomach. The dorsal mesentery unites the stomach with the spleen and the spleen with the body wall. Elongation and redundancy of the dorsal mesentery give rise to the greater omentum, which later fuses with the transverse mesocolon, derived from the dorsal mesentery of the midgut. These two structures can be surgically separated, creating an access point to the lesser sac [3, 4] (Fig. 9.1).

Through the development of the mesentery and omenta, defects can occur, creating potential areas of herniation and strangulation. These internal hernias are rare, and most commonly these defects are asymptomatic.

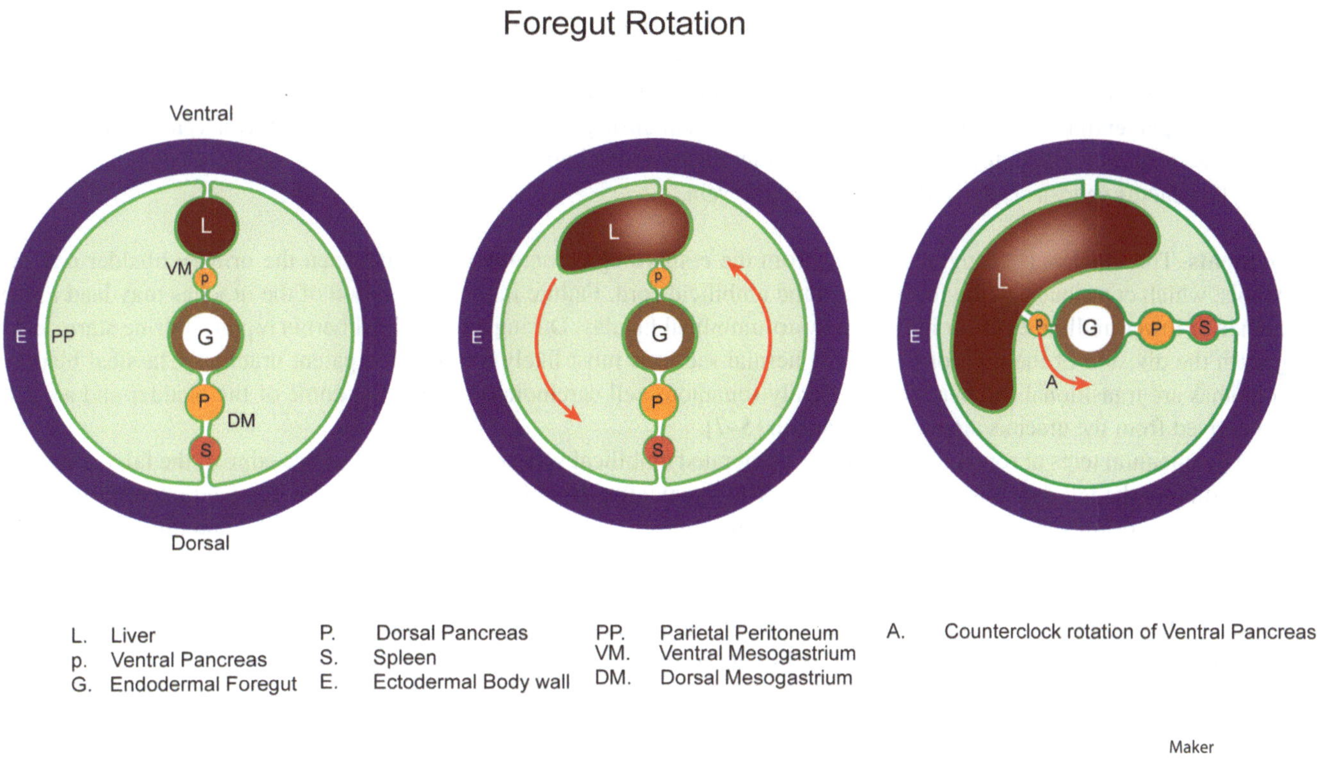

Fig. 9.1 Embryological rotation of the midline foregut in a counterclockwise fashion for 90° explains the adult location of all foregut related solid organs, mesenteries, and ligaments as well as the final adult anatomy of the pancreas. The entire liver and biliary tract, pancreas, and spleen develop in the midline suspended by the mesodermal ventral and dorsal mesogastria. As this mesodermal partition rotates to the right with the enlarging liver, the general peritoneal cavity becomes an anterior structure and the dorsal two layers fuse to form the retroperitoneum. The ventral pancreas rotates around the duodenum to form the uncus and part of the head of the pancreas. The ventral mesogastrium becomes Glisson's capsule of the liver and the gastrohepatic ligament, while the dorsal mesogastrium forms the multiple ligaments attaching the stomach, spleen, and pancreas. While some of these ligaments are avascular and division aids in surgical mobilization, others carry the blood supply. *L* liver, *p* ventral pancreas, *P* dorsal pancreas, *G* endodermal foregut, *S* spleen, *E* ectodermal body wall, *PP* parietal peritoneum, *VM* ventral mesogastrium, *DM* dorsal mesogastrium, *A* counterclockwise rotation of the ventral pancreas

Answer

c

3. The following are true regarding the embryology of the abdominal cavity *except*:
   (a) The urachus is the remnant of the obliterated allantois.
   (b) The ligamentum teres represents the obliterated umbilical vein.
   (c) The ligamentum venosum connects the umbilical vein through the left portal vein to the inferior vena cava.
   (d) The medial umbilical folds represent the obliterated umbilical arteries.
   (e) The ductus venosus is derived from the hepatic vein.

Comments The urachus is vestigial structure from the embryologic communication between the urinary bladder and the allantois, which contributes to the formation of the umbilical cord. Failure in the obliteration of the urachus may lead to the presence of lower midline cysts, or if total, to cysto-umbilical fistulas. During an umbilical hernia repair, if urine starts leaking from the division of the inferior part of the hernial sac, it is most likely a transected patent urachus. Classical bladder carcinomas are transitional cell carcinomas. Rarely squamous cell carcinomas arise in the dome of the bladder and are felt to be derived from the urachus/allantois connection [5–7].

The ligamentum teres or round ligament is the obliterated umbilical vein running along the free edge of the falciform ligament, ending in the left division of the portal vein. The ligamentum teres is continuous with the ligamentum venosum. The ligamentum venosum represents the obliterated ductus venosus, which during fetal life allows the shunting of placental blood from the liver to the systemic circulation.

The umbilical arteries are derived from the iliac arteries and run along the lower anterior abdominal wall towards the umbilicus. They obliterate, forming the medial umbilical folds on either side of the midline, constituting an important landmark in laparoscopic abdominal wall hernia [8] (Fig. 9.2).

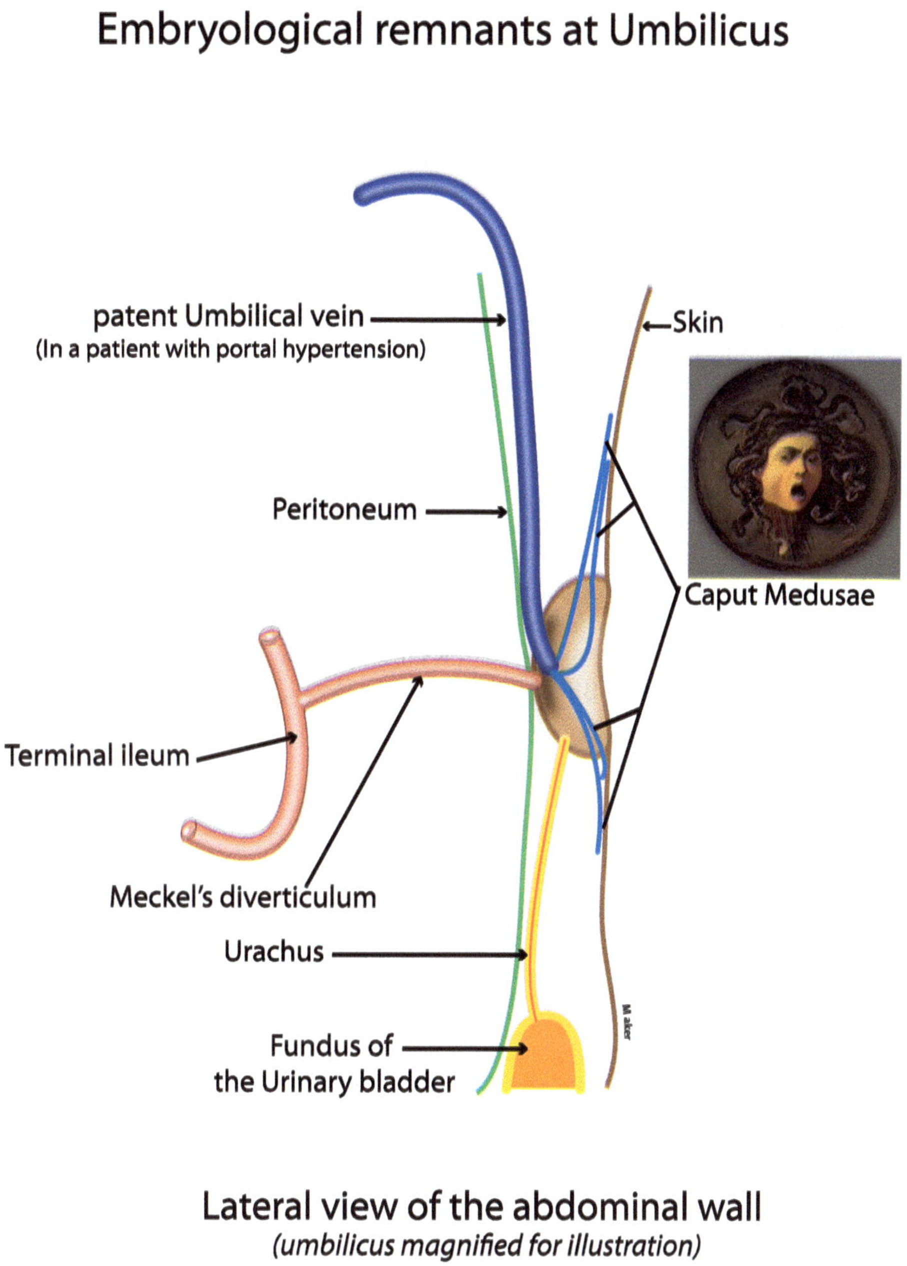

Fig. 9.2 The urachus is the vestigial remnant connecting the fundus of the urinary bladder to the umbilicus and in the fetus continuing into the umbilical cord. With a laparoscopic view of the anterior abdominal wall, the obliterated urachus appears as the median umbilical fold in the anterior preperitoneal space. The inferior epigastric arteries create the lateral umbilical fold, while the medial umbilical fold represents the obliterated umbilical arteries. A patent urachus, among its other presentations, may present as a sinus draining urine at the umbilicus. A patent and enlarged umbilical vein typically represents portal hypertension. It forms a site of portosystemic shunt with the superior and inferior epigastric veins clinically manifested as caput medusae. An enlarged umbilical vein represents the caput (head) of the medusae while collaterals of epigastric veins form a nest of veins resembling Medusa's hair of snakes. The umbilicus may also be the site of draining distal small bowel contents from a patent Meckel's diverticulum, the vestigial remnant of the vitellointestinal duct

Answer

e

4. The following are true regarding the anatomy of the abdominal cavity *except*:
   (a) The retropubic space of Retzius separates the bladder from the pubis.
   (b) The root of the small bowel mesentery attaches from the left of L1 to the right sacroiliac joint.
   (c) The veins of Sappey drain the venous blood from the falciform ligament.
   (d) The male peritoneal cavity is continuous with the environment external to the body.
   (e) Blumer's shelf is a pathologic projection in the anterior wall of the rectum just above the prostate representing the most dependent part of the pouch of Douglas.

Comments The space of Retzius is the extension of the preperitoneum behind the pubis. It is filled by the bladder as urine accumulates. The space of Retzius ends at the umbilicus, which determines that the bladder will never expand past this point. Access to the infraumbilical abdominal cavity should not be attempted with a full bladder [9].

The oblique attachment of the root of the small bowel mesentery works as a baffle directing right-sided perforations to the Morrison pouch and left-sided perforations to the pelvis.

The veins of Sappey are a group of vessels that drain the falciform ligament and also act as conduits for portosystemic shunting. They communicate the portal vein through the umbilical vein with the superior and inferior epigastrics. They branch around the umbilicus and when dilated form the caput medusae seen in portal hypertension [10].

While the male peritoneal cavity is sealed to the outside environment, females have a route of communication through the uterus and fallopian tubes. This determines that local and remote peritoneal seeding may occur from a genital source of infection, and may also explain some cases of benign pneumoperitoneum in females [11].

The pouch of Douglas is the most dependent part of the peritoneal cavity, as such it is the area most often affected by dropped metastatic seeding, which manifests as Blumer's shelf (Fig. 9.3).

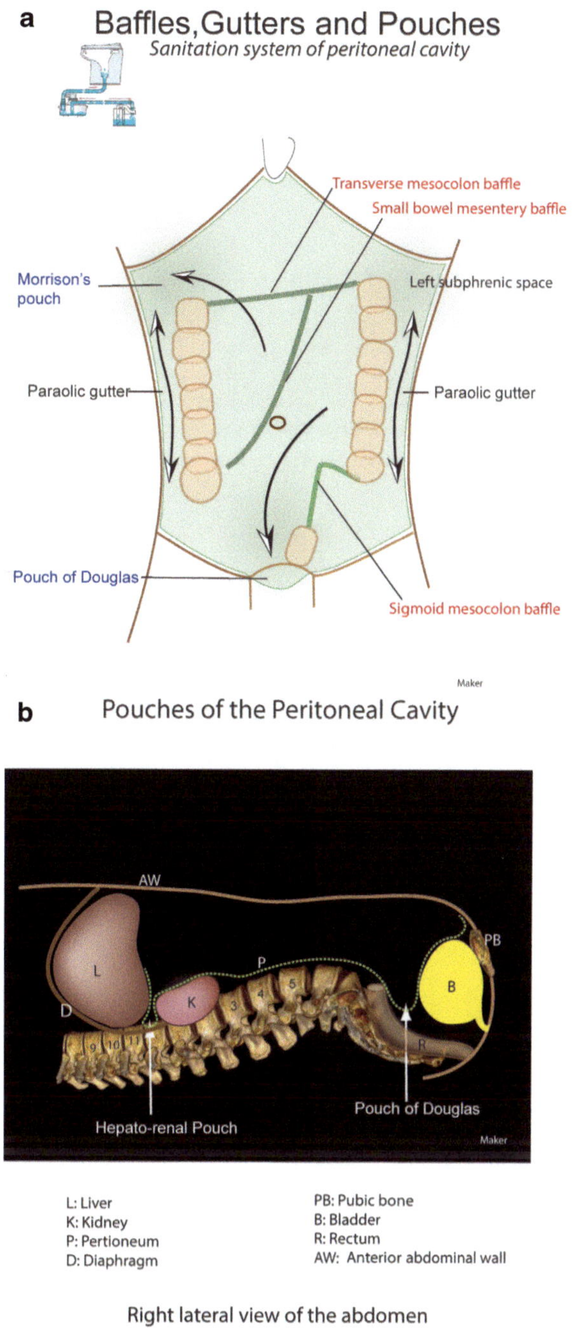

Fig. 9.3 (**a**, **b**) Baffles, gutters, and pouches. (**b**) Pouches of the peritoneal cavity (lateral view). When all of the viscera are removed from the peritoneal cavity, an elegant sanitation system is revealed which helps one to understand the drainage patterns of intra-abdominal diseases. This system consists of three baffles, two gutters, two pouches, and two spaces. The transverse mesocolon baffle separates the supracolic from the infracolic compartment. This shunts drainage of the supracolic compartment to right and left subphrenic spaces or more commonly to the dependent hepatorenal pouch. The right and left paracolic gutters provide lateral pathways to connect the supra- and infracolic compartments. The root of the small bowel mesentery extends from the left of L1 to the right sacroiliac joint and works as an oblique baffle. In concert with the sigmoid mesocolon baffle, it helps to preferentially direct the left infracolic space into the pelvic pouch (pouch of Douglas) the most dependent area of the pelvis. Most perforated diverticular abscesses drain into the pelvis while perforations in the stomach, duodenum, and gallbladder drain into the hepatorenal pouch and/or subphrenic spaces. *L* liver, *K* kidney, *P* peritoneum, *D* diaphragm, *PB* pubic bone, *B* bladder, *R* rectum, *AW* anterior abdominal wall

Answer

d

5. The structures defining the foramen of Winslow are as follow *except*:
   (a) Falciform ligament
   (b) Caudate lobe of the liver
   (c) Hepatoduodenal ligament
   (d) IVC
   (e) First portion of the duodenum

Comments See question 6.

Answer
a

6. The hepatoduodenal ligament contains the following structures *except*:
   (a) Extrahepatic bile ducts
   (b) Portal vein
   (c) Hepatic artery
   (d) Inferior vena cava
   (e) Aberrant right hepatic artery (when present)

Comments The foramen of Winslow communicates the lesser and greater omental sacs. It lies between the liver and duodenum. In cases of pancreatitis, the foramen of Winslow becomes a conduit for draining the lesser sac into the greater sac and may become obliterated. In the latter case, it contributes to the formation of pancreatic pseudocysts. Anteriorly, it is bound by the hepatoduodenal ligament, which contains the portal triad [12] (Fig. 9.4).

During surgery, the foramen of Winslow is of relevance in that vascular control of the liver may be obtained at this level through compression of both the hepatic artery and the portal vein (Pringle maneuver) [13] (Fig. 9.5).

The hepatoduodenal ligament may also contain an aberrant right hepatic artery, stemming from the superior mesenteric artery. When present, this artery lies lateral to the common bile duct and may course to the liver through Calot's triangle.

The hepatoduodenal ligament is right border of the gastrohepatic ligament. The gastrohepatic ligament may contain aberrant left hepatic arteries derived from the celiac trunk. All aberrant blood vessels should be considered replacing vessels as opposed to accessory vessels and should be carefully preserved [14].

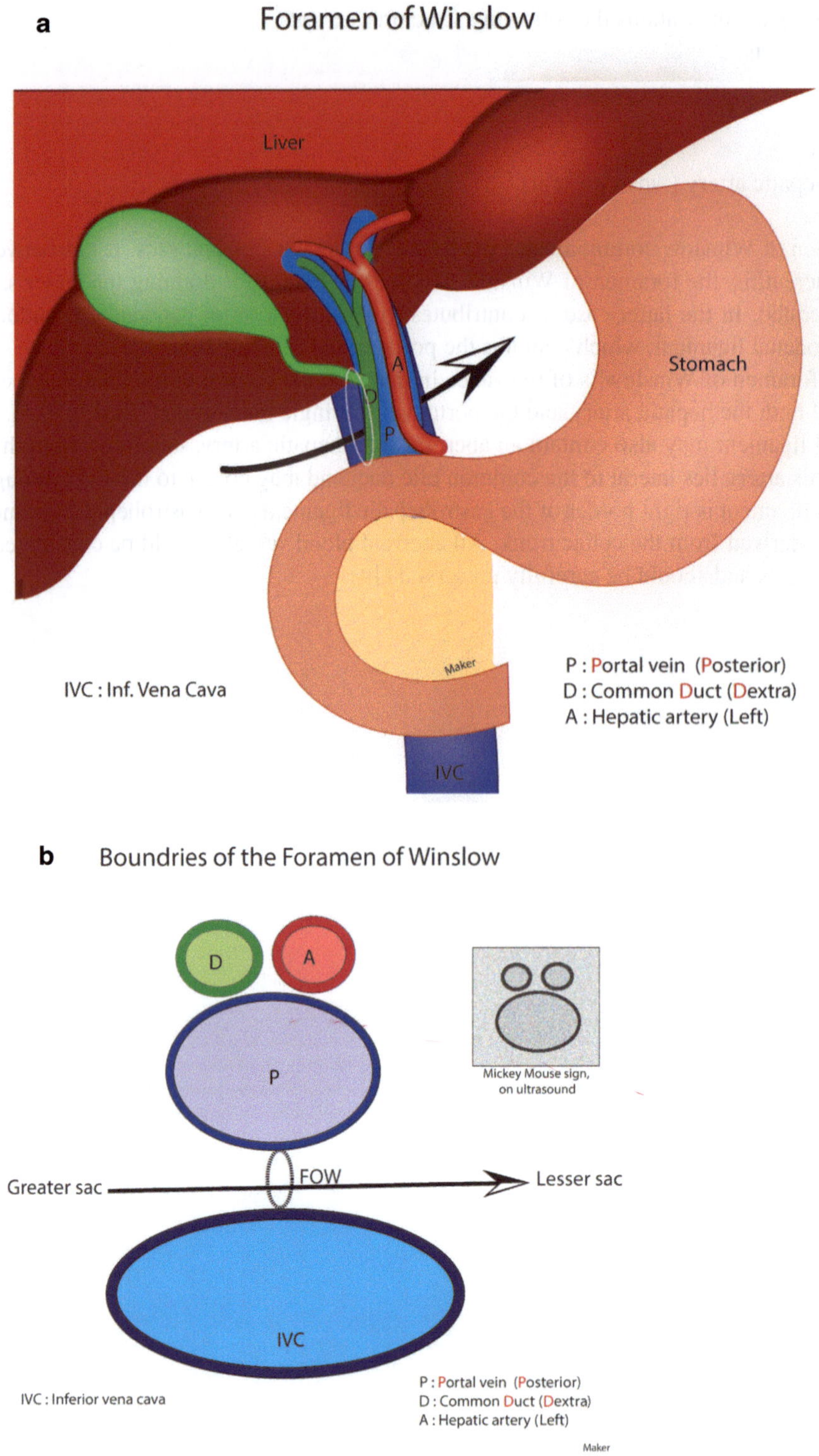

Fig. 9.4 (**a**, **b**) Foramen of Winslow. (**b**) Boundaries of the foramen of Winslow. The foramen of Winslow connects the general peritoneal cavity (greater sac) to the lesser sac. It is ~4 cm opening bounded anteriorly by the three structures of the portal triad, posteriorly by the inferior vena cava, superiorly by the caudate lobe of the liver, and inferiorly by the first part of the duodenum. On intraoperative ultrasound, a classic "Mickey Mouse sign" is produced by the portal vein posteriorly and the hepatic artery and common duct anteriorly. *IVC* inferior vena cava, *P* portal vein (posterior), *D* common duct (dextra = *right*), *A* hepatic artery (*left*)

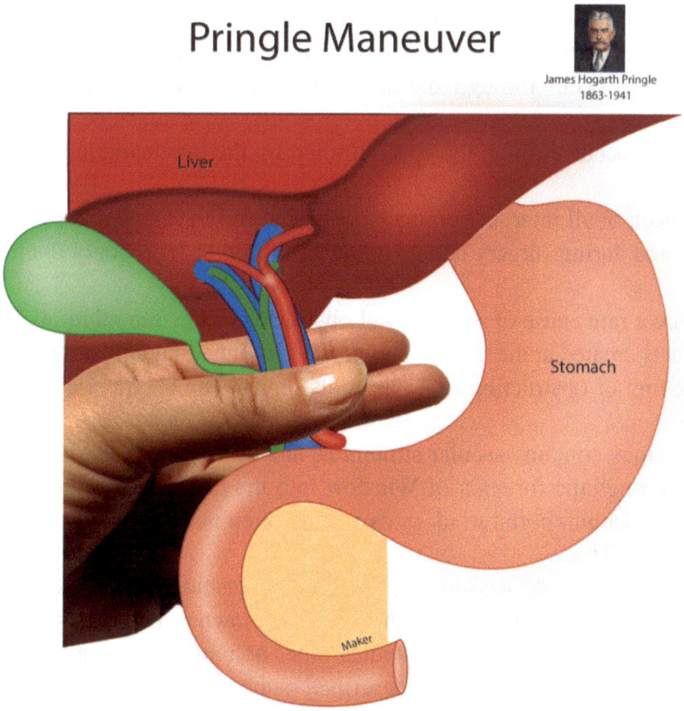

Fig. 9.5 The Pringle maneuver consists of controlling the inflow of the porta to the liver through the foramen of Winslow, as shown above. This can be accomplished by using a vascular clamp or touniquet, as needed. Mobilization of the duodenum prior to the Pringle maneuver is optional

Answer

d

7. The following are correct in relation to internal hernias *except*:
   (a) The most common cause of internal hernias are congenital mesenteric defects.
   (b) Right paraduodenal hernias occur through the space limited by the duodenum, superior mesenteric artery, and vertebrae.
   (c) Left paraduodenal hernias occur through the space limited by the duodenojejunal flexure, inferior mesenteric vein, and left colic artery.
   (d) The boundaries of the neck of all internal hernias must be carefully evaluated before releasing the constricting ring.
   (e) Mesenteric defects created during surgery should either be closed or left widely open.

Comments Internal hernias are a rare cause of small bowel obstruction and strangulation. They are most commonly due to adhesions and mesenteric defects created at the time of surgery, with congenital defect being a rare cause that must nonetheless be kept in mind in the setting of obstruction in a virgin abdomen. The classical congenital hernias are paraduodenal, paracecal, and parasigmoid.

The neck of internal hernias may contain vascular structures, and as such does not lend itself to careless release maneuvers. As an example, hernias through the foramen of Winslow into the lesser sac are not amenable to hernia neck release, which would injure the liver, duodenum, portal triad, or cava. It is often necessary to resect the herniated bowel in order to preserve these structures [15] (Fig. 9.6).

Roux-en-Y gastrojejunostomy, performed in antecolic or retrocolic fashion, generates a potential space between the mesentery of the Roux limb and the transverse mesocolon. This space is known as Petersen's space and may give rise to a hernia bearing the same name. In addition, this operation generates other potential spaces as illustrated below [16]. While these spaces and their corresponding hernias are traditionally described in the context of gastric reconstruction, they may also arise in any situation in which a loop of the small bowel is placed in a supramesocolic location (Figs. 9.7 and 9.8).

When constructing a retrocolic anastomosis, it is useful to note that there is a relatively avascular area to the left of the SMA and caudal and medial to the marginal artery of Drummond (Fig. 9.9).

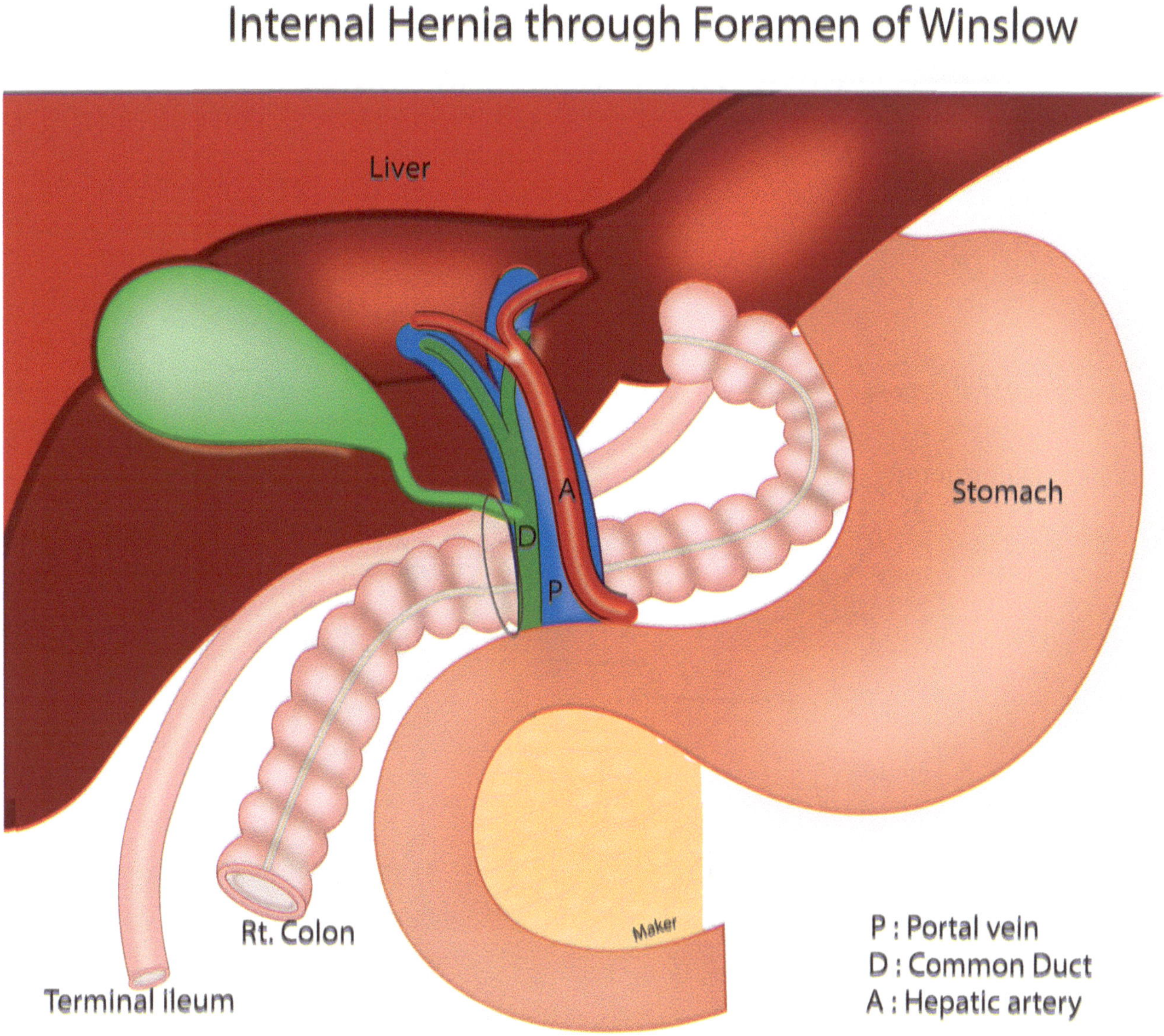

Fig. 9.6 Most internal abdominal hernias are through acquired defects. Congenital internal hernias are rare. Incarcerated or strangulated hernias through the foramen of Winslow (*FOW*) present a very difficult anatomical challenge for reduction and repair. The neck of a hernia is the tightest part and the site of strangulation that usually needs division to reduce the hernia. The neck of the hernia through the FOW has critical boundaries on all aspects, and none of them can be divided. Strangulated hernias through the FOW need to be resected in the lesser sac before reduction and repair. *P* portal vein, *D* common duct, *A* hepatic artery

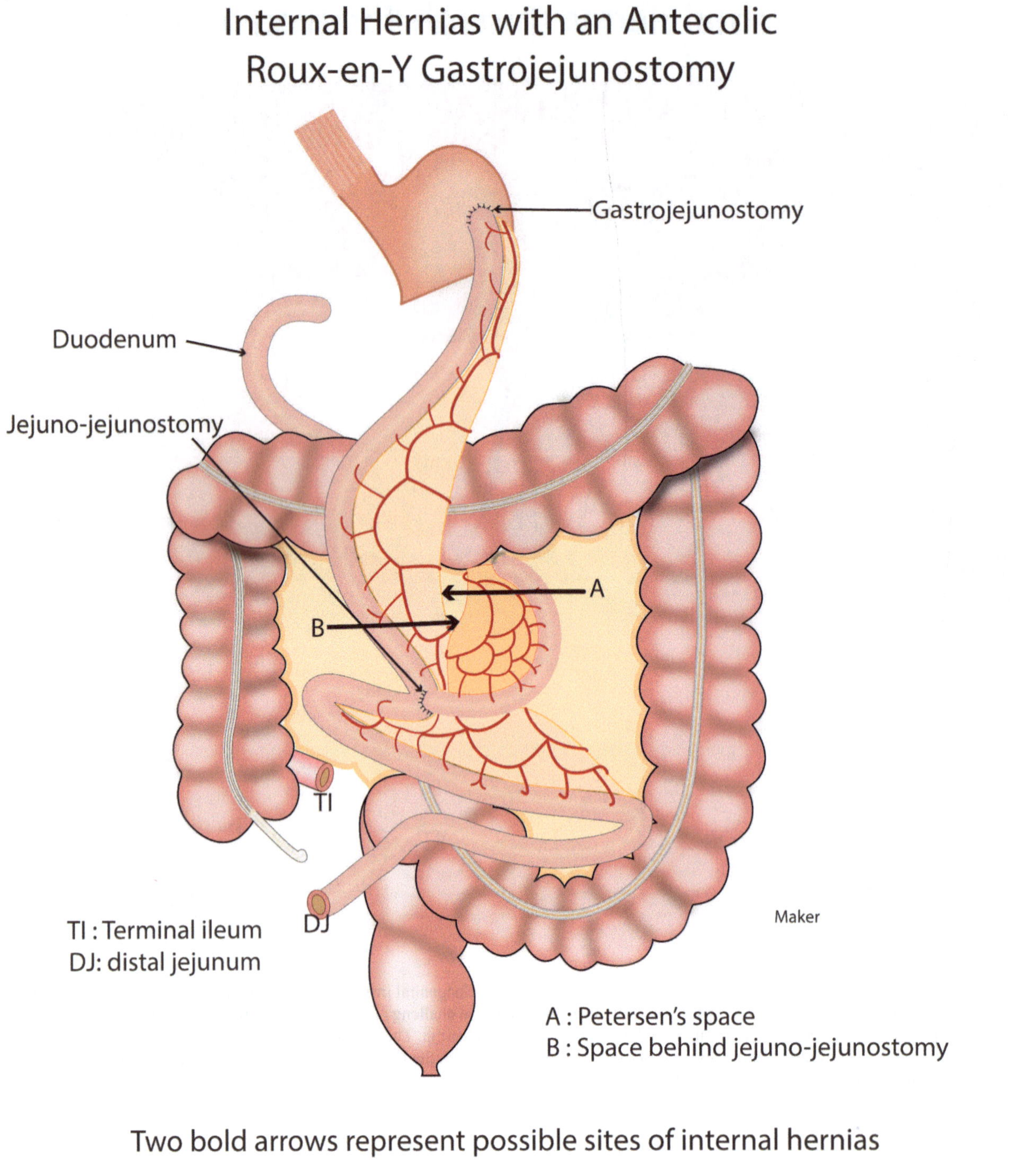

Fig. 9.7 Internal hernias are uncommon, but the incidence has increased after bariatric gastric surgery. After a Roux-en-Y antecolic gastrojejunostomy, a hernia behind the gastrojejunostomy loop and transverse mesocolon is called a Petersen's space hernia even though this is different than the original description by Dr. Petersen in 1900. An internal hernia may also occur behind the loop of the jejunojejunostomy. *TI* terminal ileum, *DJ* distal jejunum, *A* Petersen's space, *B* space behind jejunojejunostomy

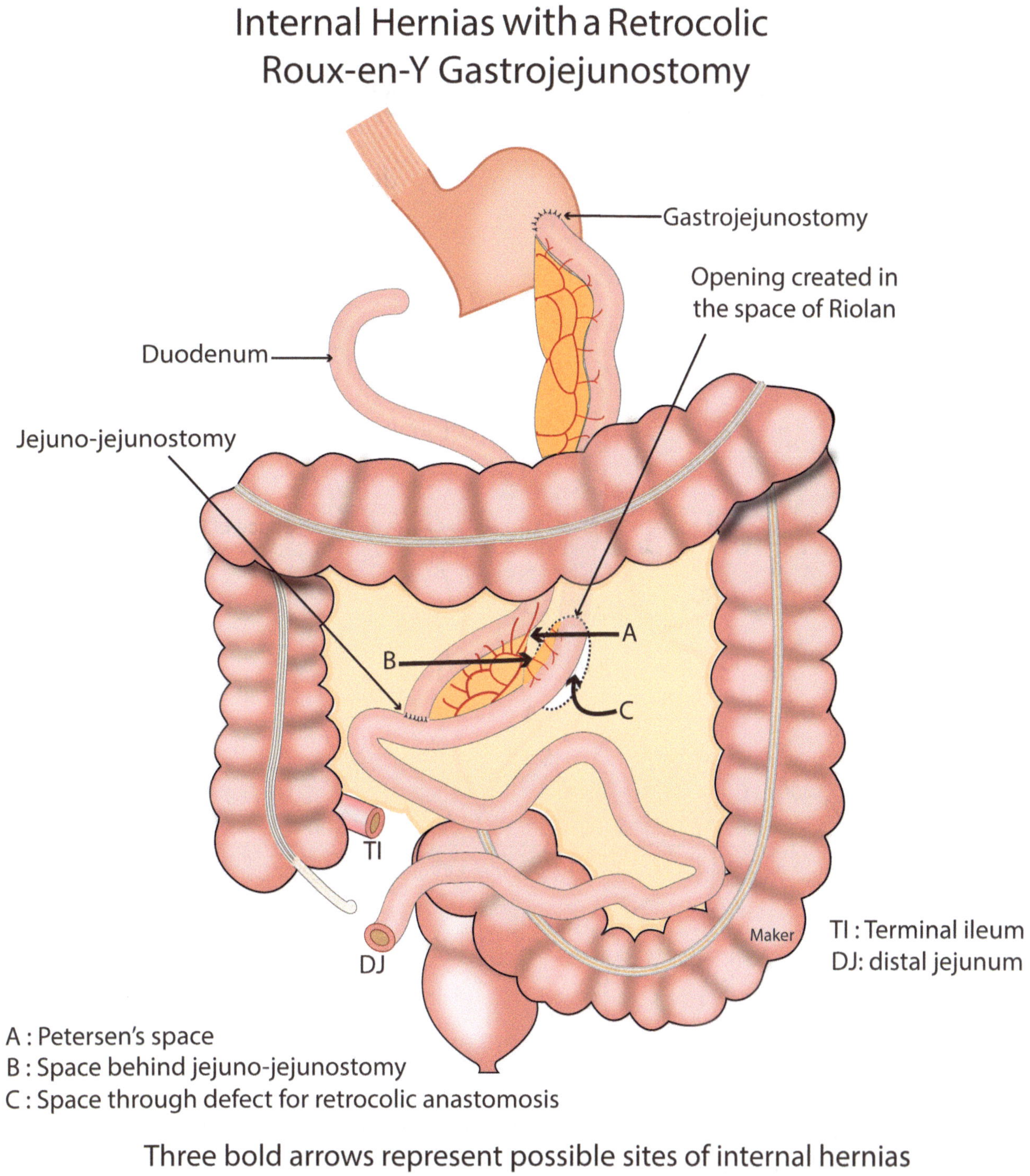

Fig. 9.8 Incidence of internal hernias after laparoscopic bariatric gastric surgery has increased likely secondary to less spontaneous post-op adhesions and subsequent weight loss enlarging the spaces created. After retrocolic gastrojejunostomy, there are three likely sites for the internal hernias. A hernia behind the afferent loop is often referred to as a Petersen's space hernia. Internal hernias may also occur behind the loop of the jejunojejunostomy as well as through the space created in the left mesocolon for the retrocolic anastomosis. *A* Petersen's space, *B* space behind jejunojejunostomy, *C* space through the defect for a retrocolic anastomosis, *TI* terminal ileum, *DJ* distal jejunum

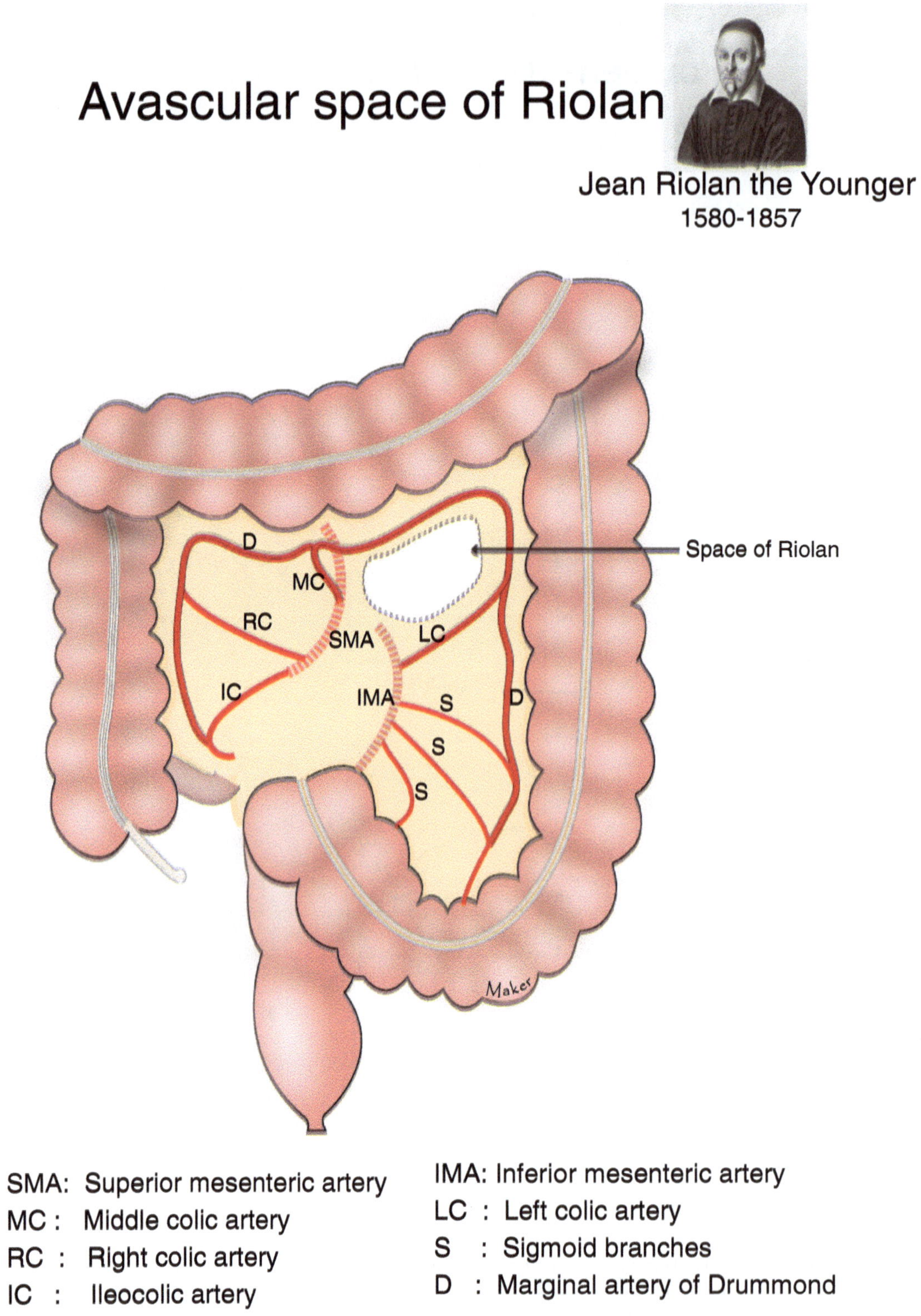

Fig. 9.9 Superior and inferior mesenteric arteries supply the right and left parts of the colon. Their divisions meet at the junction of the right two-thirds to the left one-third of the transverse colon. Corresponding to this division is the avascular zone in the mesocolon attributed to Riolan, a famous French anatomist. This area in the mesocolon is used for providing access to the supracolic compartment for a retrocolic approach. *SMA* superior mesenteric artery, *MC* middle colic artery, *RC* right colic artery, *IC* ileocolic artery, *IMA* inferior mesenteric artery, *LC* left colic artery, *S* sigmoid branches, *D* marginal artery of Drummond

Answer

a

8. All of the following are correct *except*:
   (a) Omental infarction may mimic an acute surgical abdomen.
   (b) Omental neoplasms are most often primary.
   (c) Mesenteric cysts represent the abnormal sequestration of lymphatic tissue.
   (d) Sclerosing mesenteritis may cause bowel obstruction.
   (e) Mesenteric desmoids are a manifestation of familial adenomatous polyposis.

Comments Omental torsion and infarction are an infrequent cause of abdominal pain, which is right sided in 80 % of cases. They are most common in males in the fourth and fifth decades of life and manifest as localized peritonitis with a paucity of systemic symptoms. If found during surgical exploration, resection is indicated. The omentum is often the seat of transperitoneal metastatic invasion, most notably in ovarian and GI cancer. When metastatic involvement is complete, an "omental cake" develops. Primary neoplasms of the omentum are extremely rare [17].

Reflecting their lymphatic origin, mesenteric and omental cysts are filled with chyle or lymph. They may attain great size before causing compressive symptoms, or undergoing complications such as torsion and infarction. While simple aspiration is usually followed by recurrence, excision and internal drainage to the peritoneal cavity are often curative. If part of the cyst wall is left behind, meticulous pathological examination is mandatory, as malignancy may be present in the cyst wall [18].

Sclerosing mesenteritis is the idiopathic inflammation of the mesenteric fat, leading to chronic inflammatory changes of the mesentery. In this pathology, the mesentery becomes shortened, hardened, and nodular, causing abnormal angulations of the bowel that may progress to obstruction requiring surgical management. However, the disease is rarely lethal, manifesting itself through systemic inflammatory signs as well as recurrent abdominal pain [19].

Mesenteric desmoid tumors, associated with FAP, are characterized by their rapid growth and tendency to invade adjacent structures, having the potential to cause significant complications such as bowel obstruction, perforation, hydronephrosis, and even aortic rupture. They are also characterized by a high recurrence rate after resection (60–85 %). However, survival from desmoid tumors is good, with 60–70 % of patients surviving for more than 10 years [20]. Of note, desmoid tumors may precede or follow the development of colonic pathology in patients with FAP.

Answer
b

9. Mark the *correct* statement in relation to the greater omentum.
   (a) The greater omentum is composed of two peritoneal layers.
   (b) The greater omentum is fully developed in children.
   (c) The superior mesenteric artery is the sole vessel responsible for supplying the greater omentum.
   (d) Division of the gastrocolic ligament affords the best approach to the lesser sac.
   (e) The greater omentum is resistant to metastatic seeding.

Comments The greater omentum is derived from the dorsal mesogastrium, which is composed of two peritoneal layers (one on either side). As the dorsal mesentery grows and becomes redundant, it forms a loop-like structure attached to the greater curve anteriorly and the posterior body wall at the level of the pancreas posteriorly. The anterior and posterior aspects of the loop fuse together to form the four-layered greater omentum. In a more cephalad position, the posterior aspect of the above-described loop fuses with the mesentery of the transverse colon, giving four layers to this structure. At the same level, the anterior aspect of the loop remains as the two-layered gastrocolic ligament, which offers the preferred entry to the lesser sac [21].

The greater omentum has a rich blood supply, derived from the right gastroepiploic artery (derived from the superior gastroduodenal–hepatic–celiac) and the left gastroepiploic artery (derived from the splenic–celiac). However, anastomotic networks around the duodenum may allow perfusion from the superior mesenteric artery [4].

The greater omentum is a highly plastic organ, which is not fully developed in children, limiting their ability to localize peritoneal pathology, hence the higher incidence of free appendiceal perforation. In the adult, its fat content is highly variable. The abundance of visceral fat has been linked to the derangements seen in metabolic syndrome, via the production of adipokines. It has been shown that omentectomy in conjunction with adjustable gastric banding does not improve weight loss, but has significant impact on glucose tolerance [22, 23].

Finally, the omentum is subject to implantation of abnormal tissue, both benign (splenosis, endometriosis) and malignant (ovarian cancer and mucinous cystadenocarcinomas and almost any GI cancer). In the latter case, the involved omentum appears thickened on CT, a finding termed "omental caking."

Answer

d

References

1. Androulakis J, Colborn GL, Skandalakis PN, Skandalakis LJ, Skandalakis JE. Embryologic and anatomic basis of duodenal surgery. Surg Clin North Am. 2000;80(1):171–99.
2. Skandalakis LJ, Donahue PE, Skandalakis JE. The vagus nerve and its vagaries. Surg Clin North Am. 1993;73(4):769–84.
3. Liebermann-Meffert D. The greater omentum. Anatomy, embryology, and surgical applications. Surg Clin North Am. 2000;80(1):275–93.
4. Yoo E, Kim JH, Kim MJ, Yu JS, Chung JJ, Yoo HS, et al. Greater and lesser omenta: normal anatomy and pathologic processes. Radiographics. 2007;27(3):707–20.
5. Cothren C, Ferucci P, Harken AH, Veve R, Finlayson CA, Johnson JL. Urachal carcinoma: key points for the general surgeon. Am Surg. 2002;68(2):201–3.
6. McMahon RF, Hunt CR. In situ adenocarcinoma of the bladder: the role of the urachus. Am J Surg Pathol. 2002;26(2):271–2.
7. Snyder CL. Current management of umbilical abnormalities and related anomalies. Semin Pediatr Surg. 2007;16(1):41–9.
8. Auh YH, Rubenstein WA, Markisz JA, Zirinsky K, Whalen JP, Kazam E. Intraperitoneal paravesical spaces: CT delineation with US correlation. Radiology. 1986;159(2):311–7.
9. Mirilas P, Colborn GL, McClusky III DA, Skandalakis LJ, Skandalakis PN, Skandalakis JE. The history of anatomy and surgery of the preperitoneal space. Arch Surg. 2005;140(1):90–4.
10. Yang PM, Chen DS. Images in clinical medicine. Caput medusae. N Engl J Med. 2005;353(21):e19.
11. Jacobs VR, Mundhenke C, Maass N, Hilpert F, Jonat W. Sexual activity as cause for non-surgical pneumoperitoneum. JSLS. 2000;4(4):297–300.
12. Forbes SS, Stephen WJ. Herniation through the foramen of Winslow: radiographic and intraoperative findings. Can J Surg. 2006;49(5):362–3.
13. van Gulik TM, de Graaf W, Dinant S, Busch OR, Gouma DJ. Vascular occlusion techniques during liver resection. Dig Surg. 2007;24(4):274–81.
14. Lopez-Andujar R, Moya A, Montalva E, Berenguer M, De Juan M, San Juan F, et al. Lessons learned from anatomic variants of the hepatic artery in 1,081 transplanted livers. Liver Transpl. 2007;13(10):1401–4.
15. Smith GH, Skipworth RJ, Duff MD, Anderson DN. Red herring: a rare cause of small bowel obstruction. Surgeon. 2006;4(2):107–10.
16. Reiss JE, Garg VK. Bowel gangrene from strangulated Petersen's space hernia after gastric bypass. J Emerg Med. 2014;46(2):e31–4.
17. Breda Vriesman AC, de Mol van Otterloo AJ, Puylaert JB. Epiploic appendagitis and omental infarction. Eur J Surg. 2001;167(10):723–7.
18. Uramatsu M, Saida Y, Nagao J, Takase M, Sai K, Okumura C, et al. Omental cyst: report of a case. Surg Today. 2001;31(12):1104–6.
19. Wat SY, Harish S, Winterbottom A, Choudhary AK, Freeman AH. The CT appearances of sclerosing mesenteritis and associated diseases. Clin Radiol. 2006;61(8):652–8.
20. Jalini L, Hemming D, Bhattacharya V. Intraabdominal desmoid tumour presenting with perforation. Surgeon. 2006;4(2):114–6.
21. Healy JC, Reznek RH. The peritoneum, mesenteries and omenta: normal anatomy and pathological processes. Eur Radiol. 1998;8(6):886–900.
22. Thorne A, Lonnqvist F, Apelman J, Hellers G, Arner P. A pilot study of long-term effects of a novel obesity treatment: omentectomy in connection with adjustable gastric banding. Int J Obes Relat Metab Disord. 2002;26(2):193–9.
23. Iannucci CV, Capoccia D, Calabria M, Leonetti F. Metabolic syndrome and adipose tissue: new clinical aspects and therapeutic targets. Curr Pharm Des. 2007;13(21):2148–68.

Retroperitoneum and Great Vessels in the Abdomen

10

1. All of the following are correct *except*:
   (a) The retroperitoneum is bound by the peritoneum and the posterior body wall.
   (b) The retroperitoneum is continuous with the preperitoneal space.
   (c) Retroperitoneal pathology may extend into the thigh and inguinal area.
   (d) The retroperitoneal space extends anteriorly between the leaves of the mesentery.
   (e) The retroperitoneal space does *not* extend above the diaphragm.

Comments The retroperitoneum is a space containing the kidneys, adrenals, great and gonadal vessels, lymphatics, pancreas, duodenum, ascending and descending colon, and varying amounts of areolar and fatty tissue. While its boundaries are didactically demarcated, this space is in reality continuous with the preperitoneal space. This determines that abscesses, hematomas, and tumors originating in the retroperitoneum may extend away from it along the body wall. Conversely, the retroperitoneal space may be entered through a flank approach to expose the anterior aspect of the vertebra, kidneys, and great vessels. The major advantage of this surgical exposure is that one stays extraperitoneal, decreasing the incidence of postoperative ileus.

The psoas muscle (filet mignon) traverses the entire retroperitoneum from T12 to L5, inserting below the inguinal ligament into the lesser trochanter of the femur, thus creating a route for the spread of infection. Abscesses of the psoas muscle can then present in the medial thigh as well as in the inguinal area [1–3]. Lastly, there is a communication towards the posterior mediastinum, which may become apparent in the case of pancreatic pseudocysts [4]. It is interesting to note that all the mesenteric vessels extend from the aorta towards the bowel between the leaves of the mesentery, which anatomically demarcate an extension of the retroperitoneum.

Answer
e

V.K. Maker, E.D. Guzman-Arrieta, *Cognitive Pearls in General Surgery*,
DOI 10.1007/978-1-4939-1850-8_10, © Springer Science+Business Media New York 2015

2. Mark the *correct* answer.
   (a) The SMA leaves the retroperitoneum at the lower edge of the pancreas.
   (b) The left spermatic artery arises from the left renal artery.
   (c) The right spermatic vein drains into the right renal vein.
   (d) The renal pelvis lies anterior to the renal vasculature.
   (e) The renal artery is anterior to the renal vein.

Comments The disposition of the spermatic vessels, renal vessels, and collecting system is often a source of confusion. Their position can be easily remembered when one considers the location of the vena cava and aorta in relation to the posterior midline. Since the vena cava lies slightly anterior and to the right of the midline, this will determine that the right renal vein will follow a short course to the kidney, while the left renal vein will cross the midline and continue anterior to the aorta to reach the left kidney. The reverse holds true for the aorta and renal arteries (i.e., long right renal artery and short left renal artery). As the left renal vein crosses in front of the aorta, it comes in relation to the superior mesenteric artery, which courses along its superior and anterior aspects.

Since the spermatic veins do not cross the midline, the right spermatic vein drains into the vena cava, whereas the left spermatic vein drains into the left renal vein. Both spermatic arteries arise directly from the aorta [5].

Finally, the collecting structures of the kidney as well as the ureters take a dorsal position in relation to the above-described vascular structures.

Answer

a

3. All of the following are correct *except*:
   (a) Meralgia paresthetica may be a key clinical manifestation of a retroperitoneal tumor.
   (b) The femoral nerve can be injured in the wide excision of locally advanced colon cancer.
   (c) The psoas muscle is unique in that it is enclosed in a stocking-like fascial sheath.
   (d) The ureter, gonadal vessels, and genitofemoral nerve overlie the psoas in the medial to lateral direction.
   (e) The lumbar plexus lies in the substance of the quadratus lumborum.

Comments The lumbar plexus (T12–L4) and the associated sympathetic ganglia are in close relation to the psoas muscle, with fibers passing within its substance or closely behind it. The lumbar plexus innervates the infraumbilical body wall as well as the upper thigh. In the retroperitoneum, four branches of the lumbar plexus are particularly vulnerable to retroperitoneal tumors as well as to surgical injury: the lateral femoral cutaneous nerve, the genitofemoral nerve, the femoral nerve, and the obturator nerve. Retroperitoneal tumors may grow to large sizes as they displace the peritoneal contents anteriorly and laterally.

The lateral femoral cutaneous nerve is responsible for meralgia paresthetica (numbness and paresthesias of the lateral thigh). This nerve is frequently compressed at the level of the superior anterior iliac spine by tight or heavy belts as well as by redundant adipose tissue. In the absence of these sources of compression, retroperitoneal pathology must be suspected [6, 7]. While the genitofemoral nerve is most often injured during inguinal surgery, it is also prone to injury during surgery for retroperitoneal neoplasms, as it follows a long course along the anterior surface of the psoas muscle, laterally to the ureters and in immediate relation to the gonadal vessels (Fig. 10.1).

The femoral nerve may be injured as it becomes lateral to the psoas muscle. This may occur in the setting of cecal or sigmoid colon carcinoma, extending into the retroperitoneum, as well as extensive primary retroperitoneal tumors. When damaged, extension of the knee will be compromised.

While the obturator nerve lies in a more protected position along the lateral pelvic wall, it is important to consider that it is responsible for the adduction of the thigh. Compression to it may also manifest as paresthesias to the inner thigh (Howship–Romberg sign).

The psoas muscle arises from the transverse processes and bodies of T12 to L5 and inserts in the lesser trochanter of the femur, acting as a hip flexor and internal rotator. The psoas sheath circumferentially envelops the psoas muscle. When affected by infection, it may harbor abscesses that extend into the thigh, lateral to the femoral vessels. Worldwide, the most common etiology of psoas abscesses continues to be tuberculosis. In the United States, staphylococcal and *E. coli* infections are the most common causes.

Meralgia Paresthetica

MEROS (*thigh*) ALGOS (*pain*)

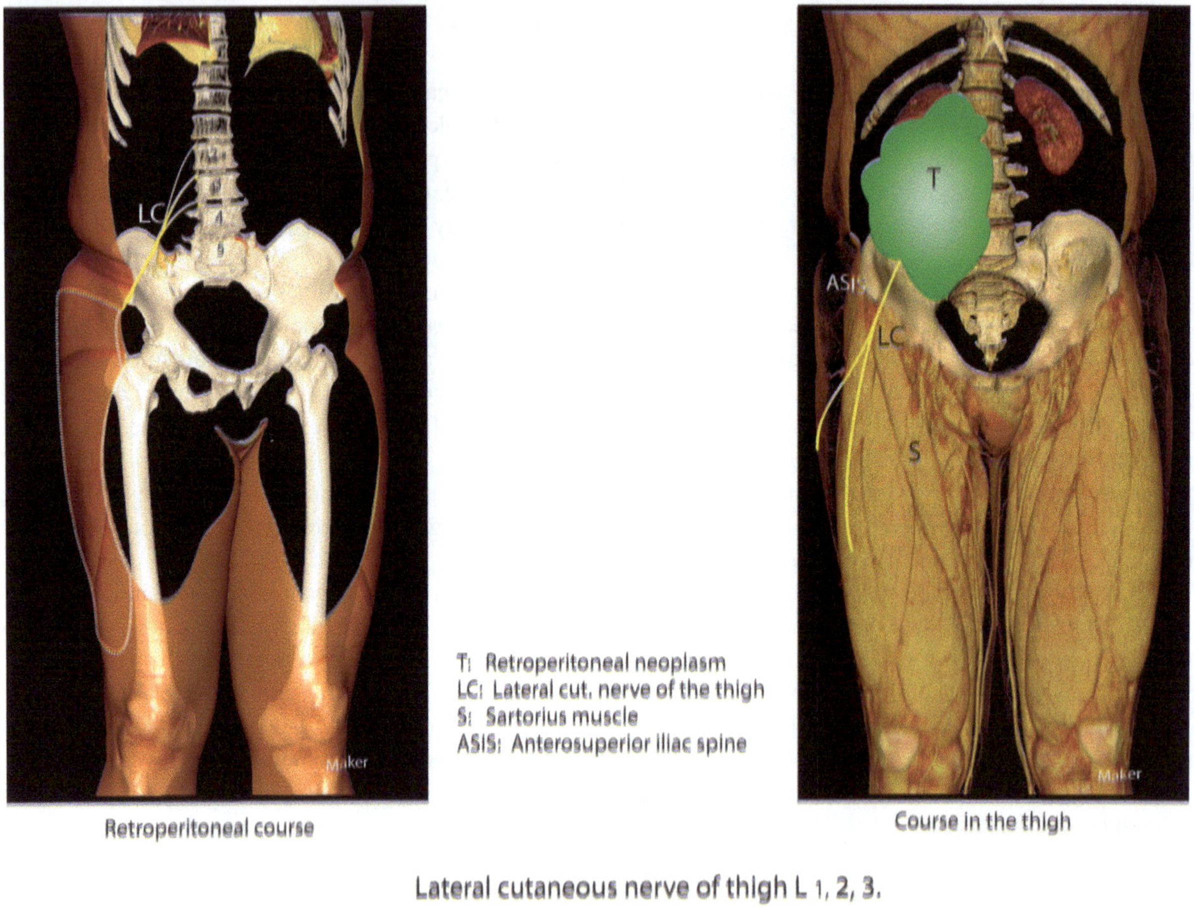

Fig. 10.1 Meralgia (thigh pain in Greek) paresthetica refers to the pain and paresthesia on the anterolateral aspect of the thigh as shown in the dotted area above. This condition is typically secondary to chronic injury to the lateral cutaneous nerve of the thigh near the anterior superior iliac spine. However, the presence of meralgia paresthetica should always raise suspicion for a retroperitoneal neoplasm as the lateral cutaneous nerve (L2, L3 with often contribution from L1) runs the entire length of the retroperitoneum. *T* retroperitoneum neoplasm, *LC* lateral cutaneous nerve of the thigh, *S* sartorius muscle, *ASIS* ant. sup. iliac spine

Answer

e

4. Select the *correct* statement.
   (a) Retroperitoneal sarcomas are a nonsurgical disease.
   (b) The Mattox maneuver includes the kocherization of the duodenum.
   (c) The Cattell maneuver is carried out from the left of the patient towards the right.
   (d) The spleen and pancreas are mobilized en bloc for retroperitoneal exposure to the suprarenal aorta.
   (e) The retroperitoneum can be fully exposed by a unilateral approach.

Comments Exposure of retroperitoneal structures is classically obtained by two maneuvers. The Cattell maneuver exposes the right retroperitoneum through a combination of mobilization of the right colon by incising the white line of Toldt and kocherization of the duodenum and pancreas (Fig. 10.2a–c).

The Mattox maneuver exposes the left retroperitoneum by mobilizing the left colon, spleen, stomach, and pancreatic tail. Neither of these maneuvers can give exposure to the entire retroperitoneum because dissection cannot be carried beyond the midline vascular structures. However, by combining them, a nearly complete access is obtained. Currently, it is possible to approach the retroperitoneum laparoscopically, either through the peritoneal cavity or through posterior and lateral approaches [3, 5] (Fig. 10.3).

While retroperitoneal sarcomas are most often painless, it is possible for them to cause symptoms through compression of retroperitoneal structures, including nerves and portions of the GI tract. Constitutional symptoms may also be present.

Retroperitoneal sarcomas rarely present with lymphatic spread. Hematogenous spread is more common, with the lung as the most often affected organ.

The treatment of retroperitoneal sarcomas is at this time essentially limited to surgery. While radiation therapy is valuable in extremity sarcomas, its application to the retroperitoneum is fraught with complications due to radiation toxicity to adjacent structures [8, 9] (Fig. 10.4).

a

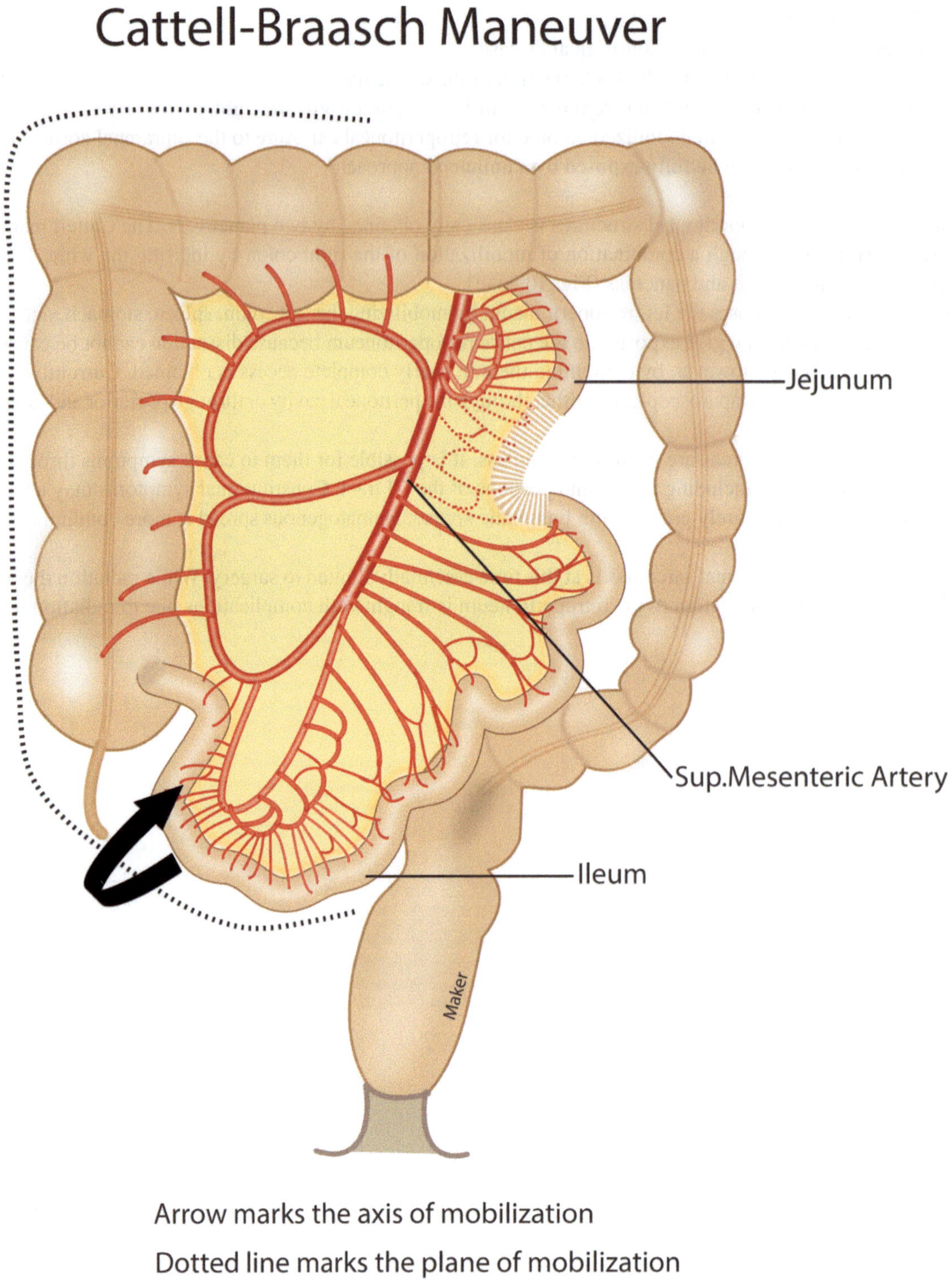

Fig. 10.2 (**a**) The goal of the Cattell–Braasch maneuver is to gain quick access to the right retroperitoneal space, including the inferior vena cava and the aorta. In the first step, an incision is made along the avascular *white line* (*Toldt line*), which is the embryological plane of fusion between the right colon and the retroperitoneum in the right paracolic gutter. This incision is extended along the lateral wall of the terminal ileum. The appropriate axis of mobilization is along the superior mesenteric artery, which is supplying the entire midgut with a plan to lift it anteriorly and fold it on itself towards the left upper quadrant of the abdomen

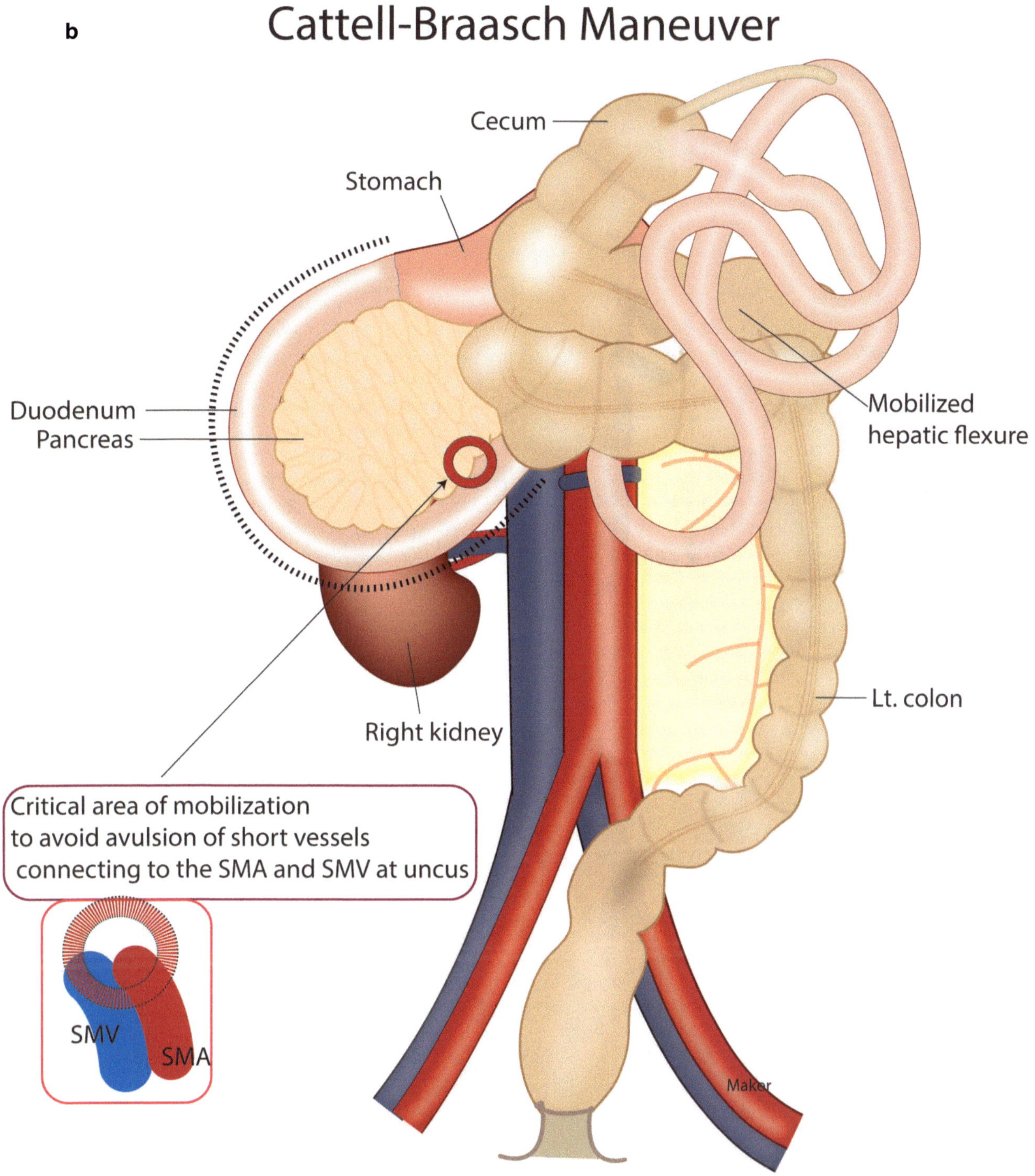

Fig. 10.2 (continued) (**b**) As the right colon, hepatic flexure, and small bowel are being mobilized to the left upper quadrant, one must be very cautious in the area of the uncus of the pancreas. Multiple arteries and veins to the rt. hemicolon as well as inferior pancreaticoduodenal vessels connect to the superior mesenteric vessels. Specifically, the superior mesenteric vein (SMV) is vulnerable in this exposure. Avulsion injuries from the superior mesenteric vein can cause brisk bleeding as it is a high-pressure vein. During this step, the duodenum is completely kocherized to gain additional exposure

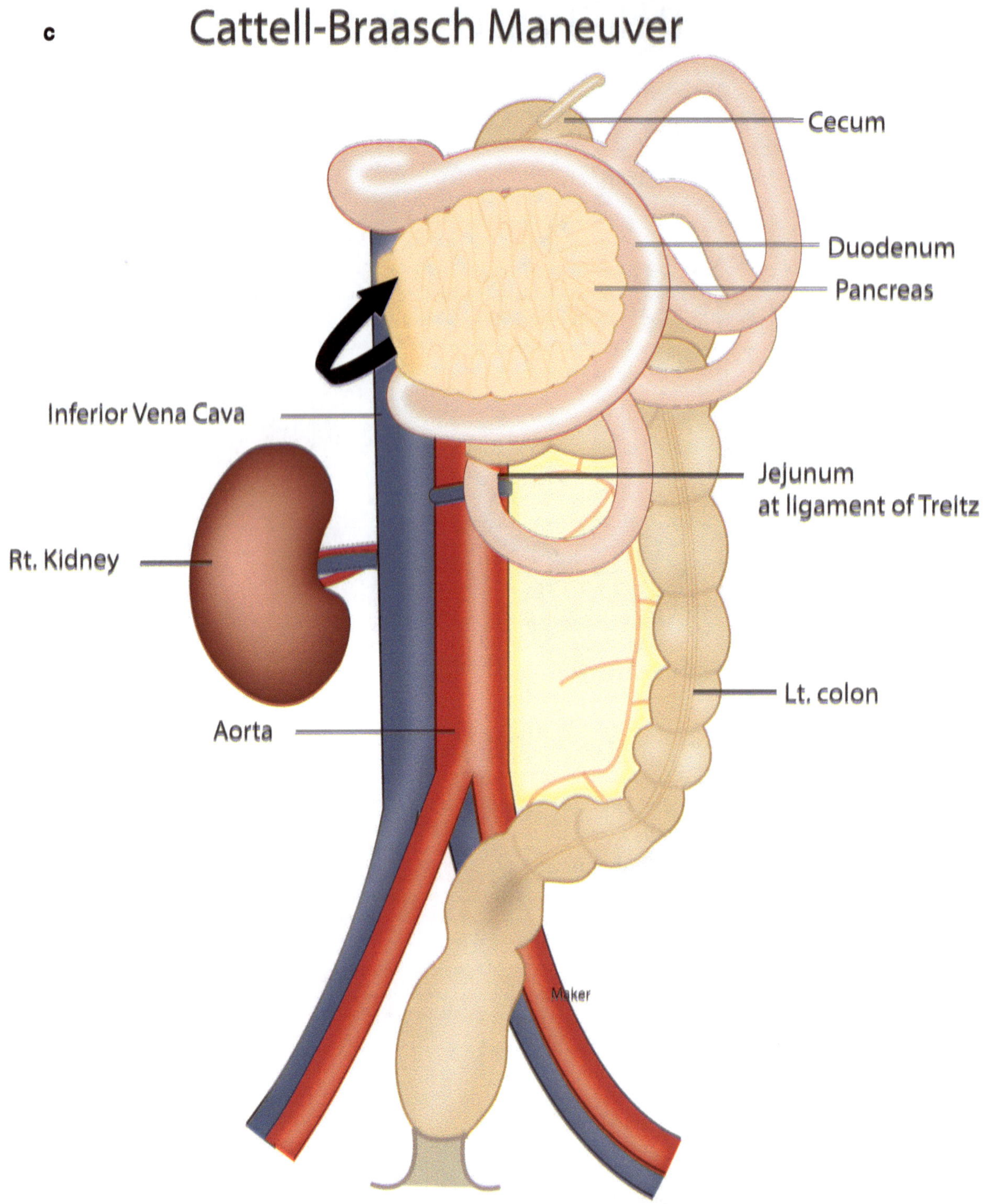

Fig. 10.2 (continued) (**c**) Mobilization of the duodenum and pancreas is carried past the inferior vena cava to the aorta. This is the last step in the Cattell–Braasch maneuver to complete the exposure of the retropancreatic inferior vena cava and aorta from the right side. This exposure is critical in traumatic injuries to this area as well as in the elective exposure of large adrenal, renal, and pancreatic neoplasms. The major limiting factor for adequate supracolic exposure in this area is the presence of the liver, especially when it is enlarged and/or firm and fibrotic. In the latter case, hepatic mobilization or an additional transthoracic exposure may be required

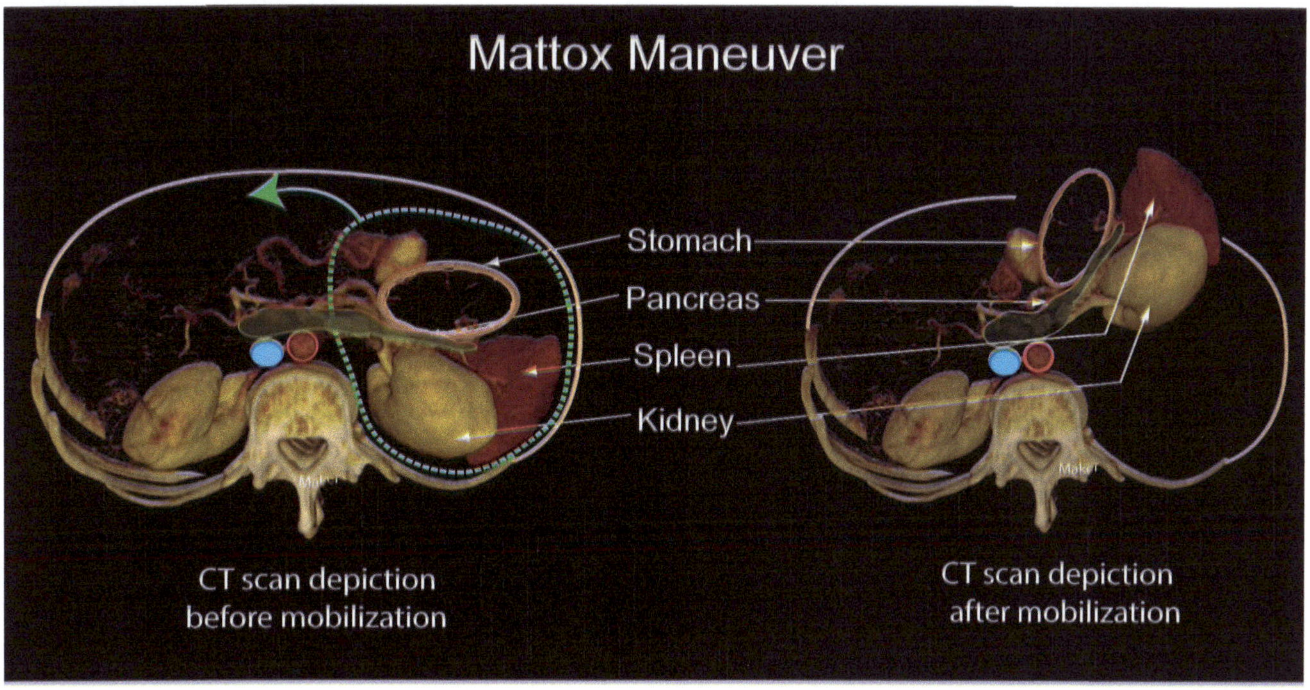

Fig. 10.3 The mattox maneuver results in an excellent exposure of the supracolic aorta and the left retroperitoneum by complete mobilization of the spleen and the distal pancreas along with the left colon and left kidney. The Cattell–Braasch maneuver, on the other hand, provides better exposure of the infracolic right retroperitoneum and inferior vena cava. Since the liver occupies the right supracolic compartment one will have to mobilize the right coronary and the falciform ligaments of the liver to gain access to the retrohepatic inferior vena cava

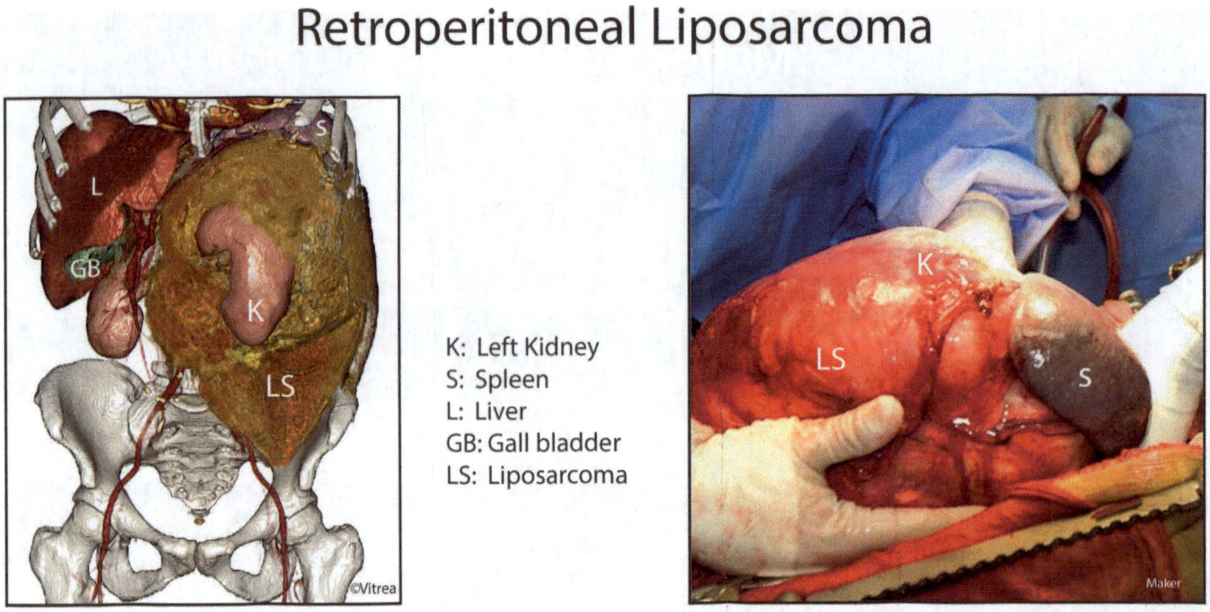

3D reconstruction of CT scan

Intraoperative view after mobilization of colon, small bowel and ligation of lumbar vessels feeding the tumor.

Fig. 10.4 This 60-year-old female presented with an enlarging mass in the left abdomen for over 2 years. CT scan was suggestive of a heterogenous retroperitoneal liposarcoma which had displaced the left kidney anteriorly, pushed the aorta to the right, and displaced the superior mesenteric artery anteriorly. Blood supply to the tumor was from the lumbar vessels. En bloc R0 resection was achieved using a combination of elements of the Cattell-Braasch and Mattox maneuvers to gain exposure of the retroperitoneum. The patient has no evidence of recurrence for over 4 years. *K* left kidney, *S* spleen, *L* liver, *GB* gallbladder, *LS* liposarcoma

Answer

d

5. Mark the *correct* answer.
   (a) IMA patency is preserved during endovascular infrarenal AAA stent grafting.
   (b) Massive upper GI bleeding secondary to aortoduodenal fistulas is initially treated with IV octreotide drip.
   (c) AAA development represents a failure of the aortic intima.
   (d) Bloody diarrhea after an AAA repair should prompt the suspicion of mesenteric ischemia.
   (e) AAA of 5.5 cm should be observed with yearly ultrasound studies.

Comments Aortic aneurysms are the expression of an inflammatory process affecting the media layer of the aorta. This inflammation leads to progressive weakening of the vessel wall, which expands under intraluminal pressure and increasing wall tension. As the aneurysm increases in size, so does the risk of rupture, crossing the risk–benefit threshold for repair at 5.5 cm. Other indications for repair are an increase of over 0.5 cm in 6 months and symptoms stemming from the aneurysm [10].

Abdominal aortic aneurysm repair, open or endovascular, routinely sacrifices the inferior mesenteric artery (which is often already occluded at the time of surgery), relying on collaterals from the superior mesenteric artery and hemorrhoidal arteries to supply the left colon. This is not feasible when such collaterals are disrupted, as in the case of a prior colon resection. In this setting, reimplantation of the IMA is needed. The IMA may also be a source of endoleak requiring embolization. When ischemia does occur, it often manifests itself as abdominal pain and bloody diarrhea. In this setting, colonoscopy is the best confirmatory test. Surgical resection of the affected bowel may be necessary [11, 12].

Aortoenteric fistulas are a rare but lethal complication of aortic aneurismal disease. They may present as recurrent gastrointestinal bleeding or as catastrophic hemorrhage. Treatment is surgical. Octreotide has no role in this setting [13].

Answer
d

6. Select the *correct* statement in relation to mesenteric ischemia.
   (a) The IMA is indispensable for adequate perfusion to the left colon.
   (b) The median arcuate ligament may compress the SMA causing symptoms of ischemia.
   (c) Embolic mesenteric ischemia is most likely to compromise the splenic flexure.
   (d) The layer of the intestinal wall most affected by ischemia is the mucosa.
   (e) Ischemia due to low-flow states most commonly compromises the cecum.

Comments Acute mesenteric ischemia may follow two etiologies: embolic and low flow. In the former, an embolus lodges itself in the mesenteric circulation, most often a proximal branch of the SMA, generating an area of ischemia in the distal small bowel and proximal colon. In the presence of compromised circulation, low-flow states may critically impair the perfusion of the watershed area between the SMA and IMA, corresponding to the splenic flexure. Through either mechanism, the layer of the intestine most affected is the mucosa, by virtue of having the most active metabolism, as well as being the furthest from the blood vessels. The median arcuate ligament of the diaphragm is not in relation to the SMA. However, it may compress the celiac trunk, causing gastric ischemia [14–16].

Answer
d

7. Select the *incorrect* statement.
   (a) As a general rule, the anastomotic networks between veins are richer than the ones between arteries.
   (b) The lumbar veins may be ligated.
   (c) The gonadal veins may be a source of pulmonary embolism in the presence of IVC filters.
   (d) Liver segments I and VIII may entrap the IVC in cirrhosis, contraindicating portacaval shunting.
   (e) Infrarenal ligation of the vena cava is contraindicated due to the lack of collaterals to carry the blood from the lower body to the heart.

Comments The lumbar veins are paired vessels that take origin from the sacral veins and ascend on either side of the spine, receiving the segmental tributaries at each vertebral level. They are continuous with the azygos vein on the right and the hemiazygos vein on the left. They are part of a rich network of collaterals to the vena cava and may be ligated. Although reserved for extreme circumstances, the vena cava may be ligated below the renal vessels [17]. Ligation above this level would lead to cessation of venous outflow from the kidneys, particularly if the gonadal veins are not patent [18].

Inferior vena cava filters are always placed below the renal vessels. They have been shown to reduce the risk of pulmonary embolism, but are ineffective at preventing embolic events arising from the gonadal vessels when placed in an infrarenal location [19].

The inferior vena cava is frequently dilated in the setting of hepatic cirrhosis. While this may be due to increased flow as well as increased right-sided heart pressures, constriction of the vena cava by the liver, the anomalous parenchyma may be present. The inferior vena cava may also be compressed by hepatic tumors [20].

Answer

e

8. Mark the *correct* statement about anastomotic networks in the abdomen.
   (a) The arc of Buhler communicates the celiac trunk and the superior mesenteric artery.
   (b) The arc of Riolan communicates the celiac trunk with the IMA.
   (c) The marginal artery of Drummond communicates the celiac trunk with the SMA.
   (d) Middle and inferior hemorrhoidal arteries arise from IMA
   (e) The SMA communicates with the internal iliac through the superior hemorrhoidal arteries.

Comments The arc of Buehler is an anastomosis between the celiac trunk and the superior mesenteric artery. Its presence is rather inconstant, being reported in only 4 % of mesenteric and celiac angiograms [21]. The arc of Riolan and the marginal artery of Drummond are both anastomotic pathways between the SMA and IMA. The arc of Riolan, also known as the meandering mesenteric artery, communicates the middle colic and the left colic artery. It is usually not detectable through angiography, and its presence signifies occlusion of either the SMA or IMA and, hence, should alert the surgeon of possible devascularization with its interruption [22]. The marginal artery of Drummond lies in close proximity to the colon and is more constantly found [14] (Figs. 10.5, 10.6, and 10.7).

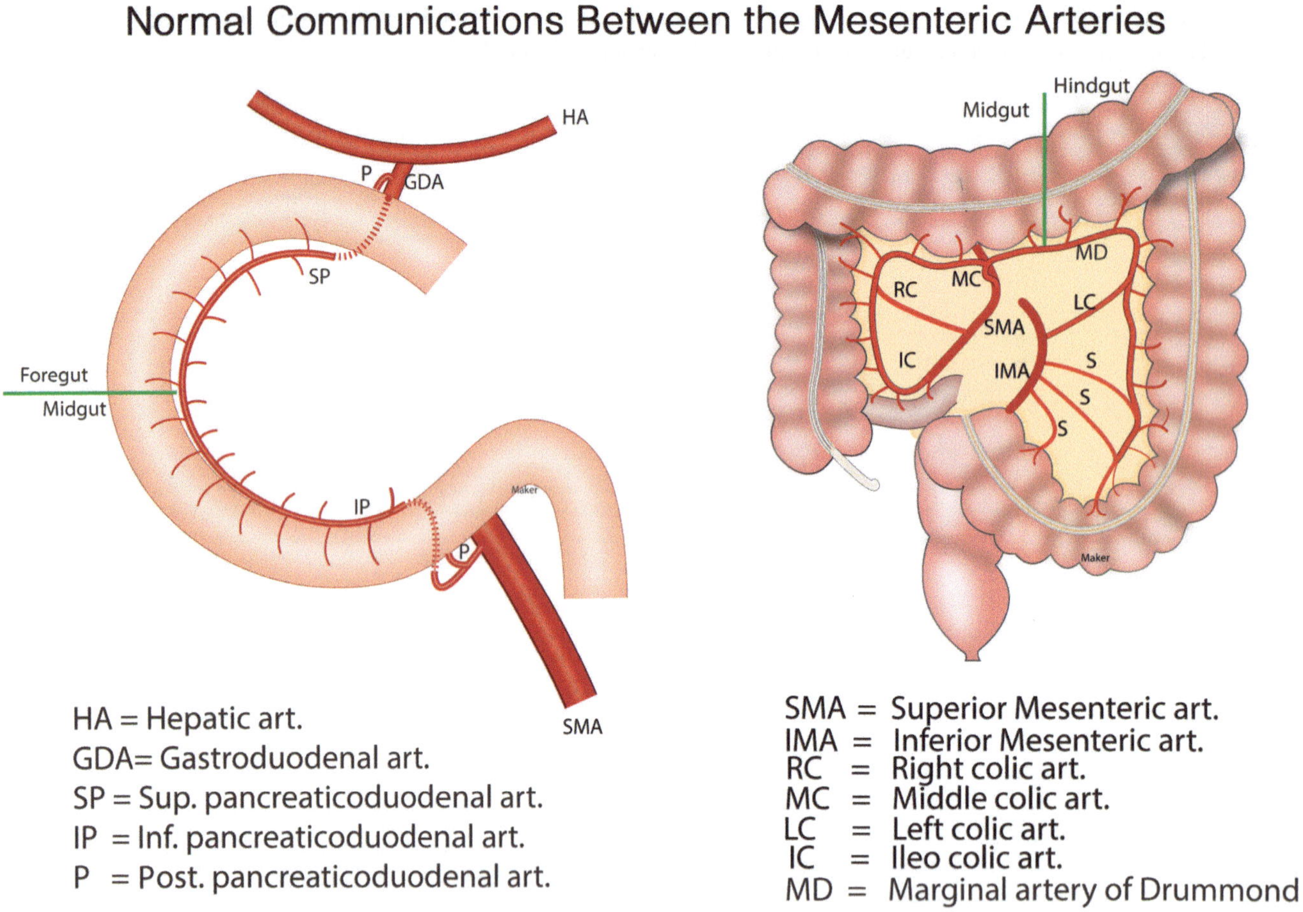

Fig. 10.5 Normal communication between mesenteric arteries. *HA* hepatic artery, *GDA* gastroduodenal artery, *SP* superior pancreaticoduodenal artery, *IP* inferior pancreaticoduodenal artery, *P* posterior pancreaticoduodenal artery, *SMA* superior mesenteric artery, *IMA* inferior mesenteric artery, *RC* right colic artery, *MC* middle colic artery, *LC* left colic artery, *IC* ileocolic artery, *MD* marginal artery of Drummond

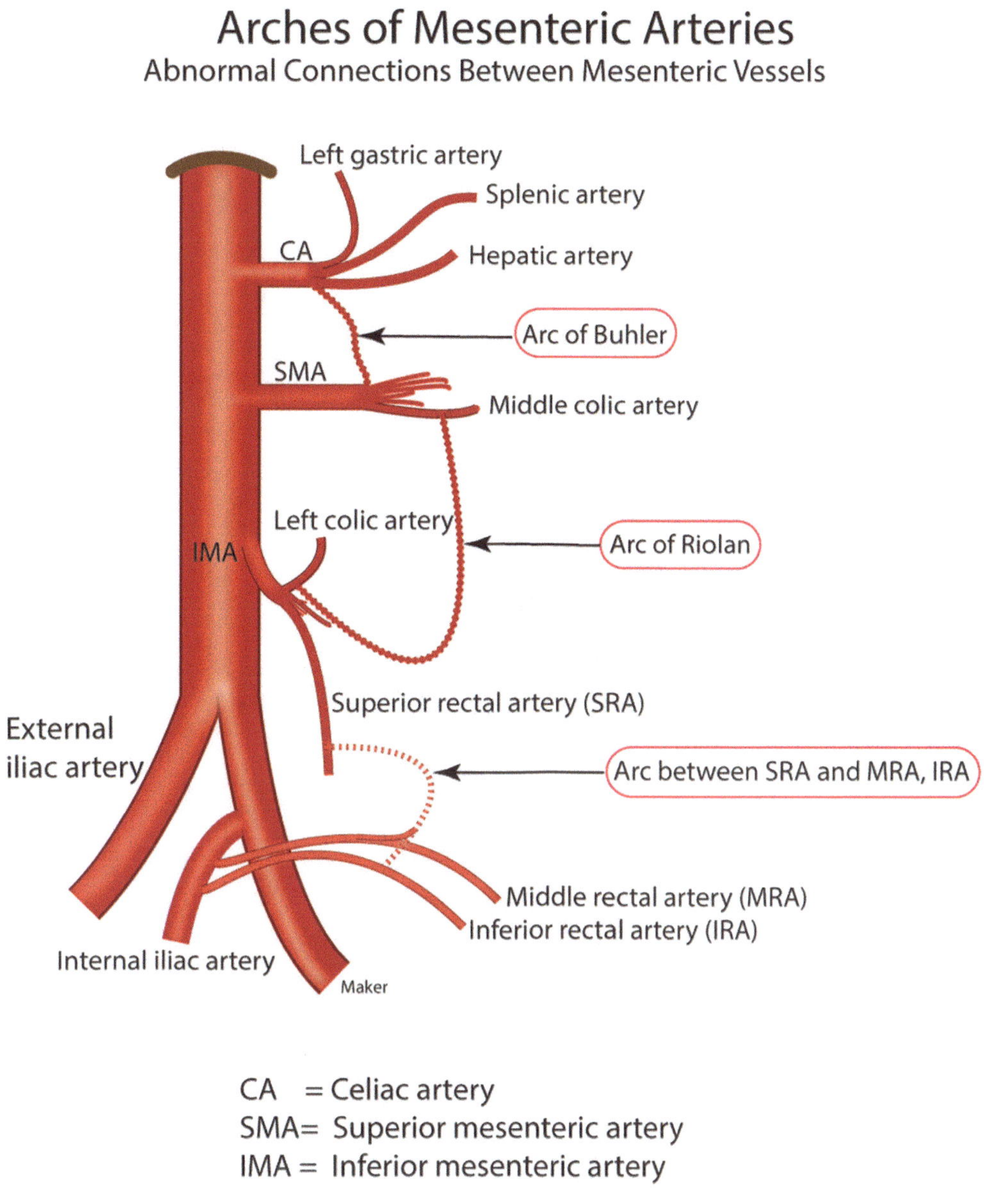

Fig. 10.6 Mesenteric vessels rarely communicate with each other by short bypasses called arches. Each of them may represent a unique set of problems in case of mesenteric ischemia and surgery in these areas. The arc of Buhler, when present, becomes an important collateral with retrograde flow in celiac artery stenosis. Arches between the superior rectal artery and the mid- and inferior rectal arteries produce unique challenges in colorectal ischemia in patients with aortoiliac disease. *CA* celiac artery, *SMA* superior mesenteric artery, *IMA* inferior mesenteric artery

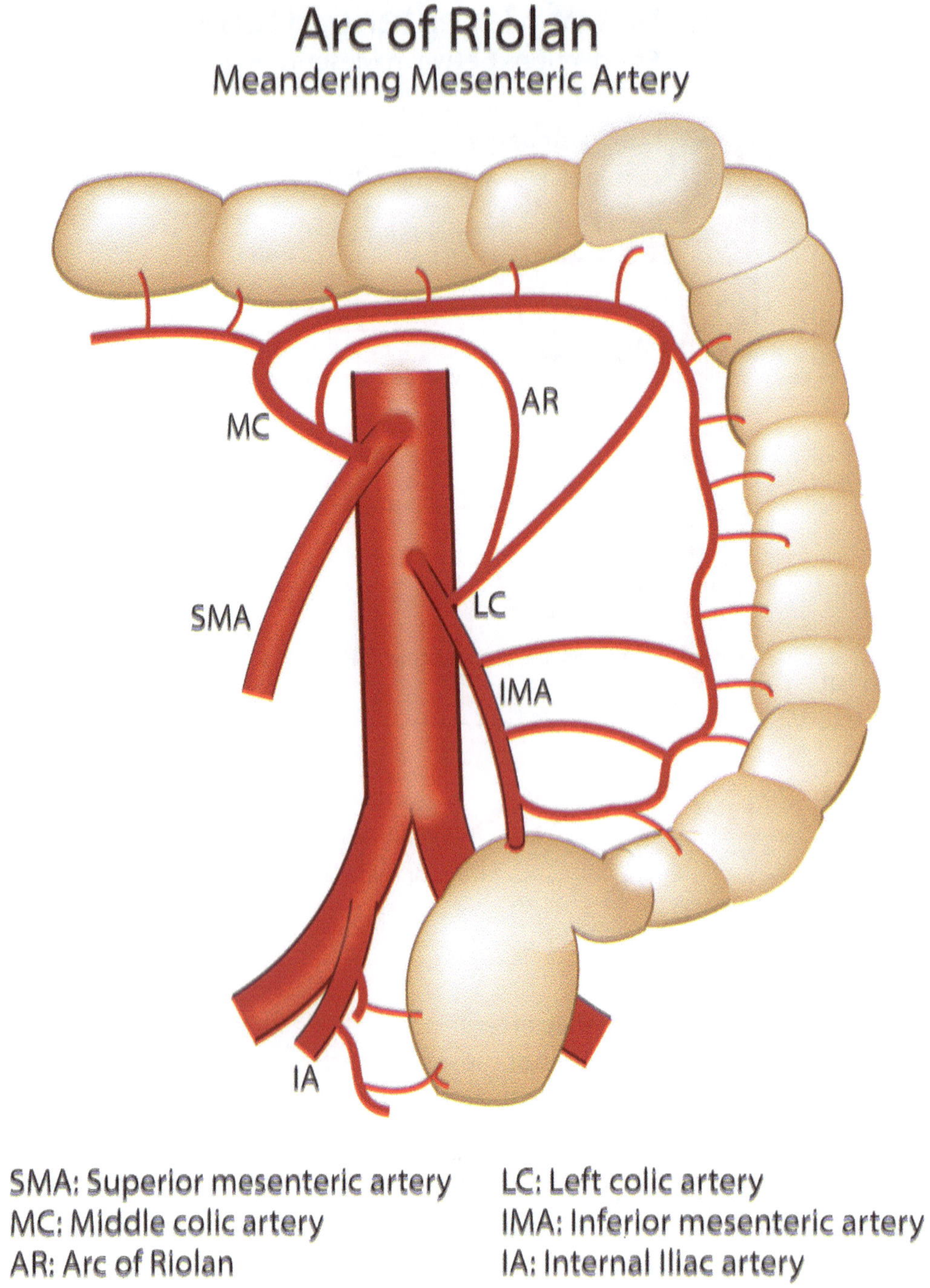

Fig. 10.7 The arc of Riolan is a short bypass, close to the base of the mesentery between the middle and the left colic artery. While it is rare and has many variations, it may produce challenges in understanding ischemic patterns in mesenteric thromboembolic disease and its treatment in each case. One of the common variations is a short arc between the proximal middle colic artery and a branch of left colic artery with or without a well-formed marginal artery of Drummond. *Note*: Jean Riolan, a French anatomist (1577–1657), made no mention of this arc in his writings but has been credited for his work on circulation. *SMA* superior mesenteric artery, *MC* middle colic artery, *AR* arc of Riolan, *LC* left colic artery, *IMA* inferior mesenteric artery, *IA* internal iliac artery

Answer

a

References

1. Hsieh CH, Wang YC, Yang HR, Chung PK, Jeng LB, Chen RJ. Extensive retroperitoneal and right thigh abscess in a patient with ruptured retrocecal appendicitis: an extremely fulminant form of a common disease. World J Gastroenterol. 2006;12(3):496–9.
2. Abulafi AM, Mee WM, Pardy BJ. Leaking abdominal aortic aneurysm presenting as an inguinal mass. Eur J Vasc Surg. 1991;5(6):695–6.
3. Nethercliffe J, Wood DN, Andrich DE, Greenwell TJ, Mundy AR. Retroperitoneal and transthoracic anatomy and surgical approaches. BJU Int. 2004;94(5):705–18.
4. Gupta R, Munoz JC, Garg P, Masri G, Nahman Jr NS, Lambiase LR. Mediastinal pancreatic pseudocyst – a case report and review of the literature. MedGenMed. 2007;9(2):8.
5. Lin PH, Chaikof EL. Embryology, anatomy, and surgical exposure of the great abdominal vessels. Surg Clin North Am. 2000;80(1):417–33, xiv.
6. Fargo MV, Konitzer LN. Meralgia paresthetica due to body armor wear in U.S. soldiers serving in Iraq: a case report and review of the literature. Mil Med. 2007;172(6):663–5.
7. Nouraei SA, Anand B, Spink G, O'Neill KS. A novel approach to the diagnosis and management of meralgia paresthetica. Neurosurgery. 2007;60(4):696–700.
8. Woodall CE, Scoggins CR. Retroperitoneal and visceral sarcomas: issues for the general surgeon. Am Surg. 2007;73(6):631–5.
9. Pisters PW, O'Sullivan B. Retroperitoneal sarcomas: combined modality treatment approaches. Curr Opin Oncol. 2002;14(4):400–5.
10. Lederle FA, Kane RL, MacDonald R, Wilt TJ. Systematic review: repair of unruptured abdominal aortic aneurysm. Ann Intern Med. 2007;146(10):735–41.
11. Pitton MB. Collateral vessels in endovascular aneurysm treatment. Abdom Imaging. 2004;29(4):514–7.
12. Brewster DC, Franklin DP, Cambria RP, Darling RC, Moncure AC, Lamuraglia GM, et al. Intestinal ischemia complicating abdominal aortic surgery. Surgery. 1991;109(4):447–54.
13. Heidemann J, Domagk D, Wessling J, Domschke W, Kucharzik TF. Recurrent obscure gastrointestinal bleeding caused by aorto-enteric fistula. Z Gastroenterol. 2006;44(9):981–4.
14. Lange JF, Komen N, Akkerman G, Nout E, Horstmanshoff H, Schlesinger F, et al. Riolan's arch: confusing, misnomer, and obsolete. A literature survey of the connection(s) between the superior and inferior mesenteric arteries. Am J Surg. 2007;193(6):742–8.
15. Ujiki M, Kibbe MR. Mesenteric ischemia. Perspect Vasc Surg Endovasc Ther. 2005;17(4):309–18.
16. Stoney RJ, Cunningham CG. Acute mesenteric ischemia. Surgery. 1993;114(3):489–90.
17. Jones VS, Shun A. Is the inferior vena cava dispensable? Pediatr Surg Int. 2007;23(9):885–8.
18. Blute ML, Boorjian SA, Leibovich BC, Lohse CM, Frank I, Karnes R. Results of inferior vena caval interruption by greenfield filter, ligation or resection during radical nephrectomy and tumor thrombectomy. J Urol. 2007;178(2):440–5.
19. Martin MJ, Salim A. Vena cava filters in surgery and trauma. Surg Clin North Am. 2007;87(5):1229–52.
20. Wachsberg RH, Levine CD, Maldjian PD, Simmons MZ. Dilatation of the inferior vena cava in patients with cirrhotic portal hypertension. Causes and imaging findings. Clin Imaging. 1998;22(1):48–53.
21. Saad WE, Davies MG, Sahler L, Lee D, Patel N, Kitanosono T, et al. Arc of buhler: incidence and diameter in asymptomatic individuals. Vasc Endovascular Surg. 2005;39(4):347–9.
22. Gourley EJ, Gering SA. The meandering mesenteric artery: a historic review and surgical implications. Dis Colon Rectum. 2005;48(5):996–1000.

Pharynx and Esophagus

11

1. Mark the *correct* statement regarding the embryogenesis of the pharynx.
   (a) The pharynx is derived from the branchial apparatus and foregut.
   (b) The pharyngeal pouches are mesodermal.
   (c) The pharyngeal clefts are endodermal.
   (d) The pharyngeal arches are ectodermal.
   (e) The pharyngeal floor is mesodermal.

Comments As explained in Chap. 1, the human branchial apparatus is formed by pharyngeal pouches (endoderm), arches (mesoderm), and clefts (ectoderm). The branchial apparatus, in continuity with the embryonic foregut form the adult pharynx. Contributions of these multiple structures are shown in Table 11.1 [1, 2].

Table 11.1 The human branchial apparatus is formed by pharyngeal pouches (endoderm), arches (mesoderm), and clefts (ectoderm). The branchial apparatus, in continuity with the embryonic foregut, forms the adult pharynx. Contributions of these multiple structures forming the adult pharynx

Embryologic origin	Adult structure
1st pharyngeal pouch	Eustachian tube
2nd pharyngeal pouch	Tonsillar fossa
3rd pharyngeal pouch	Pyriform sinus
4th pharyngeal pouch	Pyriform apex
5th pharyngeal pouch	Pharyngeal ventricle
6th pharyngeal pouch	Pharyngeal ventricle

Answer
a

V.K. Maker, E.D. Guzman-Arrieta, *Cognitive Pearls in General Surgery*,
DOI 10.1007/978-1-4939-1850-8_11, © Springer Science+Business Media New York 2015

2. Mark the *correct* statement regarding congenital pharyngeal anomalies.
   (a) Lingual thyroid glands are usually accompanied by mediastinal thyroid tissue.
   (b) The skin orifices of all pharyngeal fistulas are posterior to the sternocleidomastoid muscle.
   (c) The tract of second pharyngeal fistula crosses the carotid bifurcation.
   (d) The internal opening of the branchial cyst is at the base of the tongue.
   (e) Complete choanal atresia is asymptomatic at birth.

Comments The most common congenital anomalies of the neck are those derived from the thyroglossal duct (70 %), followed by anomalies of the branchial apparatus (30 %) [3, 4]. Thyroglossal duct cysts most often present as midline cervical masses located anywhere between the base of the tongue and the sternal notch. The tract most often goes through the body of the hyoid bone. While originally sterile, communication of the cyst with the pharynx through the foramen cecum and thyroglossal duct may predispose the cyst to infection. There is a small reported incidence of malignancy in this ectopic tissue (1 %), with papillary thyroid cancer being the most common type and a medullary carcinoma being embryologically impossible.

Thyroglossal duct cysts must be distinguished from the other two midline neck masses, which are dermoid cysts and the Delphian lymph node. This can be done on clinical grounds. Thyroglossal cysts move with swallowing but more importantly move superiorly with protrusion of the tongue. Dermoid cysts arise from the skin and hence move with the skin. The Delphian node is a lymph node draining the thyroid gland.

Considering that the thyroglossal duct does not communicate with the skin, it is thought that thyroglossal sinuses and fistula are not congenital, but rather represent secondary drainage of a cyst or abscess [5] (Fig. 11.1).

The presence of a lingual thyroid should raise a strong suspicion of the absence of additional thyroid tissue in the neck. Considering this, removal of lingual thyroid must be preceded by a thyroid scan. Lingual thyroid glands have no embryologic relation to mediastinal thyroid tissue. The former occur due to failure of descent of the thyroglossal duct that normally forms the medial thyroid anlagen. The latter is derived from anomalous decent of the lateral thyroid anlagen, derived from the fourth pharyngeal pouch.

Branchial anomalies may present as cysts, sinuses, or pharyngocutaneous fistulas (Table 11.2). The level at which these anomalies are located along the neck depends on their embryologic origin; however, all of them are anterior to the sternocleidomastoid muscle. The second arch is most commonly affected (95 % of cases). The definitive treatment of all branchial anomalies is complete excision [6, 7]. Choanal atresia results from the persistence of the nasobuccal membrane. When bilateral, infants present with apnea during quiet respiration, which is relieved during crying. This is due to the fact that neonates are nasal breathers during the first 6 weeks of life, but become mouth breathers while crying. In addition, those affected have copious nasal secretions. Treatment involves securing the airway through intubation followed by surgical repair or tracheostomy if repair is not possible. Choanal atresia is part of the CHARGE syndrome, composed of *c*oloboma, *h*eart defects, choanal *a*tresia, developmental *r*etardation, *g*enitourinary anomalies, and *e*ar abnormalities [8].

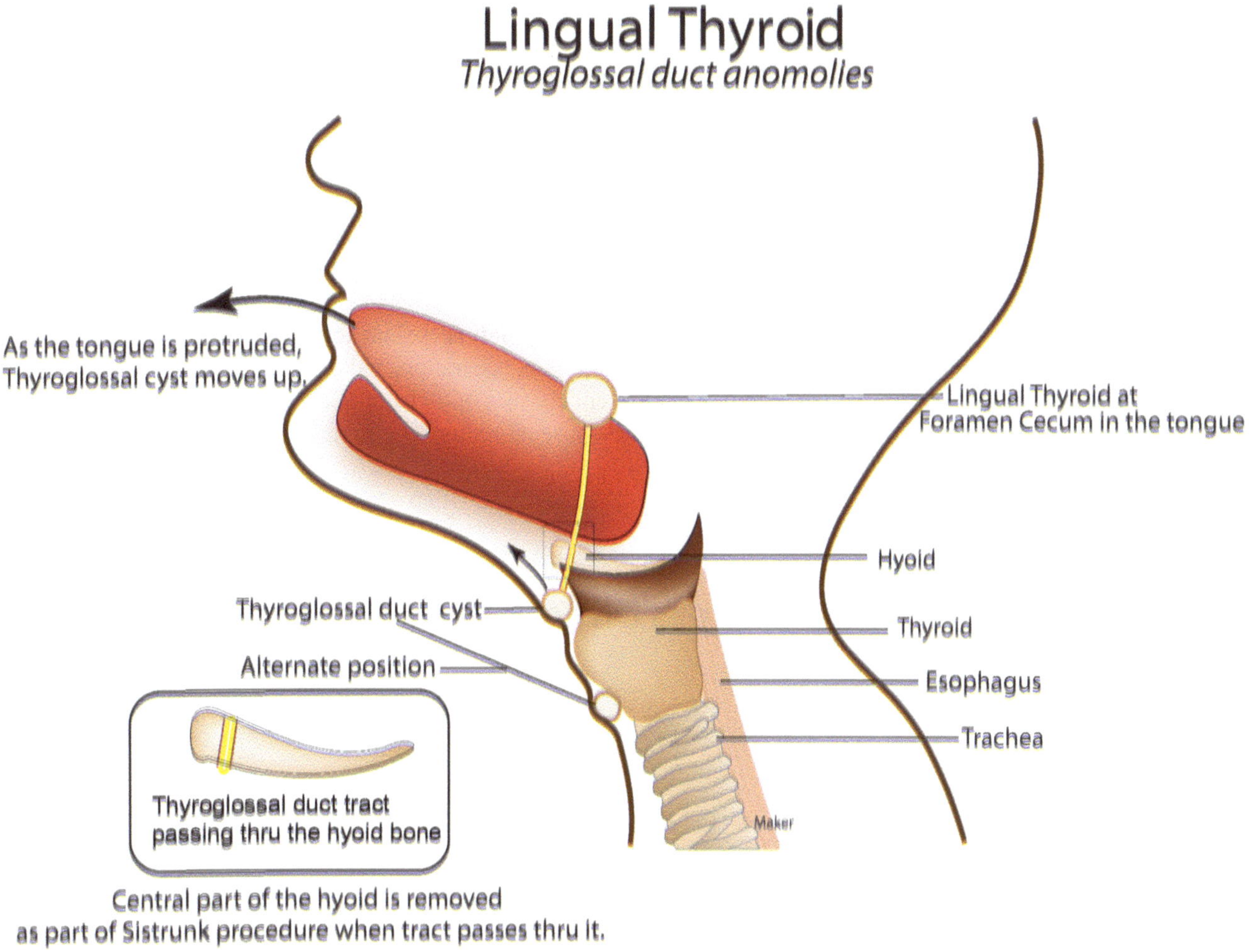

Fig. 11.1 A lingual thyroid is the most common site of an ectopic thyroid and represents non-descent of the thyroglossal duct from the foramen cecum at the base of the tongue. Most of the patients with a lingual thyroid do not have any other thyroid tissue. Unless causing dysphagia, dyspnea, or dysphonia, lingual thyroids are not excised

Table 11.2 Pharyngocutaneous fistulas course in relation to critical anatomic structures that may be injured during resection

Embryologic origin	External orifice	Internal orifice	Relations
First cleft	Between the external auditory canal and the angle of the mandible	External auditory canal or middle ear	Facial nerve and parotid gland
Second cleft	Lower anterior border of the sternocleidomastoid	Supratonsillar fossa	Carotid bifurcation and IX and XII cranial nerves
Third cleft	Lower anterior border of the sternocleidomastoid	Pyriform sinus	Internal carotid, hypoglossal, and glossopharyngeal nerves
Fourth cleft	Lower anterior border of the sternocleidomastoid	Pyriform apex or cervical esophagus	Right subclavian artery and aortic arch

Answer

c

3. Mark the *correct* statement regarding Zenker's diverticulum.
   (a) Zenker's diverticulum is most common on the right side.
   (b) Zenker's diverticulum occurs below the cricopharyngeus muscle.
   (c) Zenker's diverticulum is a true diverticulum.
   (d) Zenker's diverticulum is a traction diverticulum.
   (e) The key principle in the management of a Zenker's diverticulum is the cricopharyngeus myotomy.

Comments Zenker's diverticulum consists of a protrusion of pharyngoesophageal mucosa through Killian's triangle, a weak area above the superior esophageal sphincter (cricopharyngeus muscle). It is thought that Zenker's diverticulum arises due to the presence of a hypertonic cricopharyngeus resulting in increased pharyngeal swallowing pressures. This leads to the formation of a false (pulsion) diverticulum that most often lies in the left neck. Due to its lack of musculature, Zenker's diverticulum is unable to empty, collecting food particles causing reflux, aspiration, and severe halitosis [9, 10]. In view of the above-described pathophysiology, the key step in management consists of division of the cricopharyngeus muscle. The state of cricopharyngeus spasm has been attributed to gastroesophageal reflux. The initial test of choice to diagnose this condition is a barium esophagogram (Fig. 11.2).

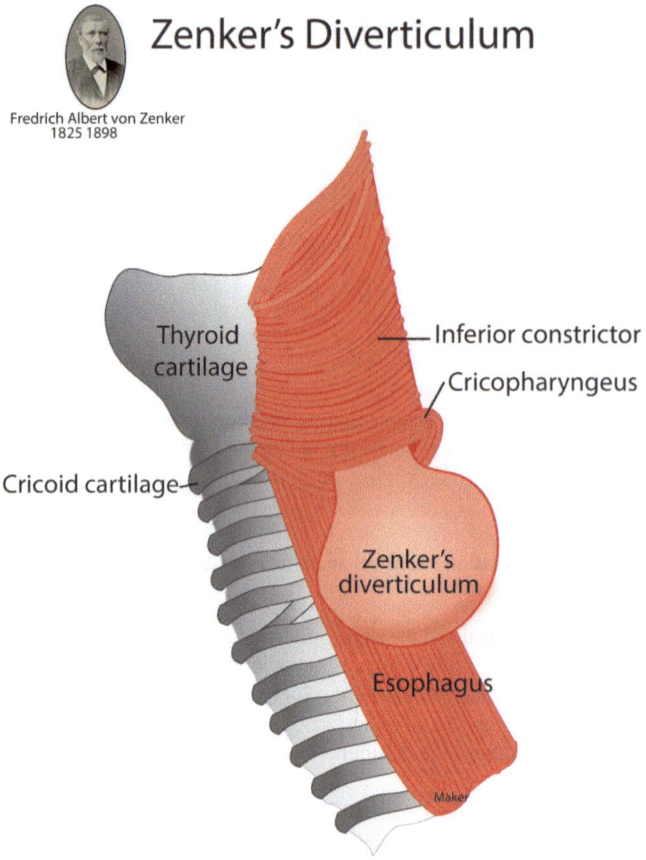

Fig. 11.2 Zenker's diverticulum is a false, i.e., mucosa-lined, diverticulum through the weak area in Killian's triangle formed between the inferior constrictor and cricopharyngeus muscles. It is a pulsion (pushed out) diverticulum secondary to the higher upper esophageal pressure

Answer
e

4. All of the following are correct *except*:
   (a) Enlarged adenoids in the adult may be due to neoplasia.
   (b) Juvenile nasopharyngeal angiofibromas should be biopsied.
   (c) Craniopharyngiomas arise from remnants of Rathke's pouch.
   (d) Upper aerodigestive tract and tonsil tumors may manifest as ear pain or enlarged cervical nodes.
   (e) Kursteiner cysts are pharyngeal pouch endoderm remnants attached to the parathyroid glands.

Comments Tonsil and adenoid enlargement are a common benign finding, especially in the pediatric population. However, occasionally occult malignancies (most often lymphoma and lymphosarcoma) may be present. While the prevalence of this finding is rare, special care should be taken when assessing older patients with tonsillar asymmetry and associated lymphadenopathy [11]. Ear pain in the absence of ear pathology may be due to tumor involvement of the Eustachian tubes. Similarly, the presence of enlarged upper cervical lymph nodes may be the consequence of metastatic spread of tonsillar carcinomas.

Juvenile nasopharyngeal angiofibromas are rare extremely vascular tumors seen almost exclusively in adolescent males. Their vascular nature preludes biopsy. While initially slow growing, they eventually invade the base of the skull and may cause significant bleeding. Traditionally, treatment has consisted of surgical resection following angiographic embolization [12].

Craniopharyngiomas are benign tumors arising from Rathke's pouch, the endodermal precursor to the anterior pituitary. While benign in nature, their treatment is difficult due to proximity with critical structures as well as their tendency to recur [13, 14].

Nasopharyngeal bursa or Thornwaldt's bursa is a notochord-derived recess in the posterior nasopharynx. Obstruction of its draining orifice may lead to cyst formation, resulting in nasal obstruction [15].

Kursteiner cysts are an anatomic variation of the parathyroid glands. They may be lined with differentiated parathyroid cells producing PTH.

Answer
b

5. Mark the *incorrect* statement.
   (a) Children with cleft palates suffer from chronic middle ear effusions due to improper opening of the Eustachian tubes.
   (b) Ipsilateral paralysis of the tongue is the most common neurological deficit after carotid endarterectomy.
   (c) The presence of laryngeal clicking suggests the existence of a retropharyngeal mass.
   (d) Advanced tumors of the base of the tongue require bilateral cervical lymphadenectomy.
   (e) Surgery for obstructive sleep apnea is based on the excision of redundant oropharyngeal tissue.

Comments Cleft palate results from the failed fusion of the maxillary prominences derived from the first pharyngeal arch and the middle nasal prominence. Difficulty in generation of negative intraoral pressures may lead to failure to thrive. The abnormal insertion of the tensor veli palatini (which acts as a sphincter to the pharyngeal opening of the Eustachian tube) predisposes to middle ear disease and conductive hearing loss [16].

Palatine tonsils are often inflamed due to self-limited viral and bacterial infections. However, these benign infections may progress to abscess formation, affecting the peritonsillar or parapharyngeal spaces, causing systemic septic symptoms as well as trismus [17].

Hypoglossal nerve injury is the most common nerve injury during carotid endarterectomy, and it is seen in approximately 2 % of cases, with higher rates being reported in the face of prior radiation or surgery. Interestingly, this condition constituted selection criteria for carotid stenting in the SAPPHIRE trial [18, 19]. Laryngeal clicking is a normal physical finding elicited by displacing the larynx laterally over the cervical spine. The loss of this finding has been associated to retrolaryngeal masses as well as to traumatic retrolaryngeal edema [20].

Treatment of cancers of the base of the tongue has shifted from radical resections to neoadjuvant chemoradiation coupled with organ-preserving surgery. The rich lymphatic drainage of the tongue determines that metastatic nodal involvement is often bilateral. This makes bilateral neck dissection necessary in patients with multiple nodal involvement [21].

The surgical treatment of obstructive sleep apnea is usually reserved for patients who have failed treatment with positive airway pressure. While excision of redundant oropharyngeal tissue (veloplasty and uvuloplasty) is an important treatment principle, other strategies include improving nasal airflow through septoplasty or turbinectomy and mobilizing the tongue anteriorly, either through genioglossus advancement or en bloc with the mandible through osseous distraction of the jaw [22].

Answer
c

6. Barrett's esophagus represents:
   (a) Metaplasia
   (b) Dysplasia
   (c) Anaplasia
   (d) Hypertrophy
   (e) Hyperplasia

Comments Barrett's esophagus represents an instance of metaplasia, in which a mature epithelium is replaced by another kind of mature epithelium due to environmental stresses. In the esophagus, the normal squamous epithelium is replaced by intestinal-like columnar epithelium. While the change in epithelial phenotype is reversible, it is a first step in the development of cancer. Dysplasia refers to a loss in the degree of cellular differentiation within a given tissue, leading to the replacement of fully differentiated cells by abnormal cells with altered microarchitecture. Anaplasia characterizes fully transformed cells and consists in the complete loss of cellular differentiation typical of cancer.

Hyperplasia and hypertrophy are both normal responses of tissues in order to cope with external stimuli. Both lead to an increase in tissue mass. Hyperplasia consists of an increase in the number of cells due to proliferation, whereas hypertrophy is characterized by the increase in the size of cells without an increase in number [23–25].

Answer

a

7. The esophagus is supplied by the following arteries *except*:
   (a) Inferior thyroid arteries
   (b) Tracheobronchial arteries
   (c) Splenic artery
   (d) Left gastric artery
   (e) Right gastric artery

Comments The esophagus receives its blood supply in a stepladder fashion from multiple, small segmental arteries shared with the surrounding organs. These branches contribute to the formation of a rich intramural capillary network, which allows mobilization and segmental resection of this organ. The cervical esophagus derives its blood supply mainly from the inferior thyroid arteries. The thoracic esophagus receives branches from the tracheobronchial arteries as well as multiple small branches arising directly from the descending aorta. Finally, the abdominal esophagus is supplied by branches of the inferior phrenic artery, the left gastric artery, and the splenic artery.

While vessels are of unimpressive caliber, the modest blood flow to the esophagus is sufficient to sustain its metabolic activity, dominated by peristalsis and minimal secretion of mucus. This blood supply, when preserved, is also sufficient to allow the healing of surgical anastomosis. The small caliber of these vessels allows the blunt mobilization during transhiatal esophagectomy [26] (Fig. 11.3).

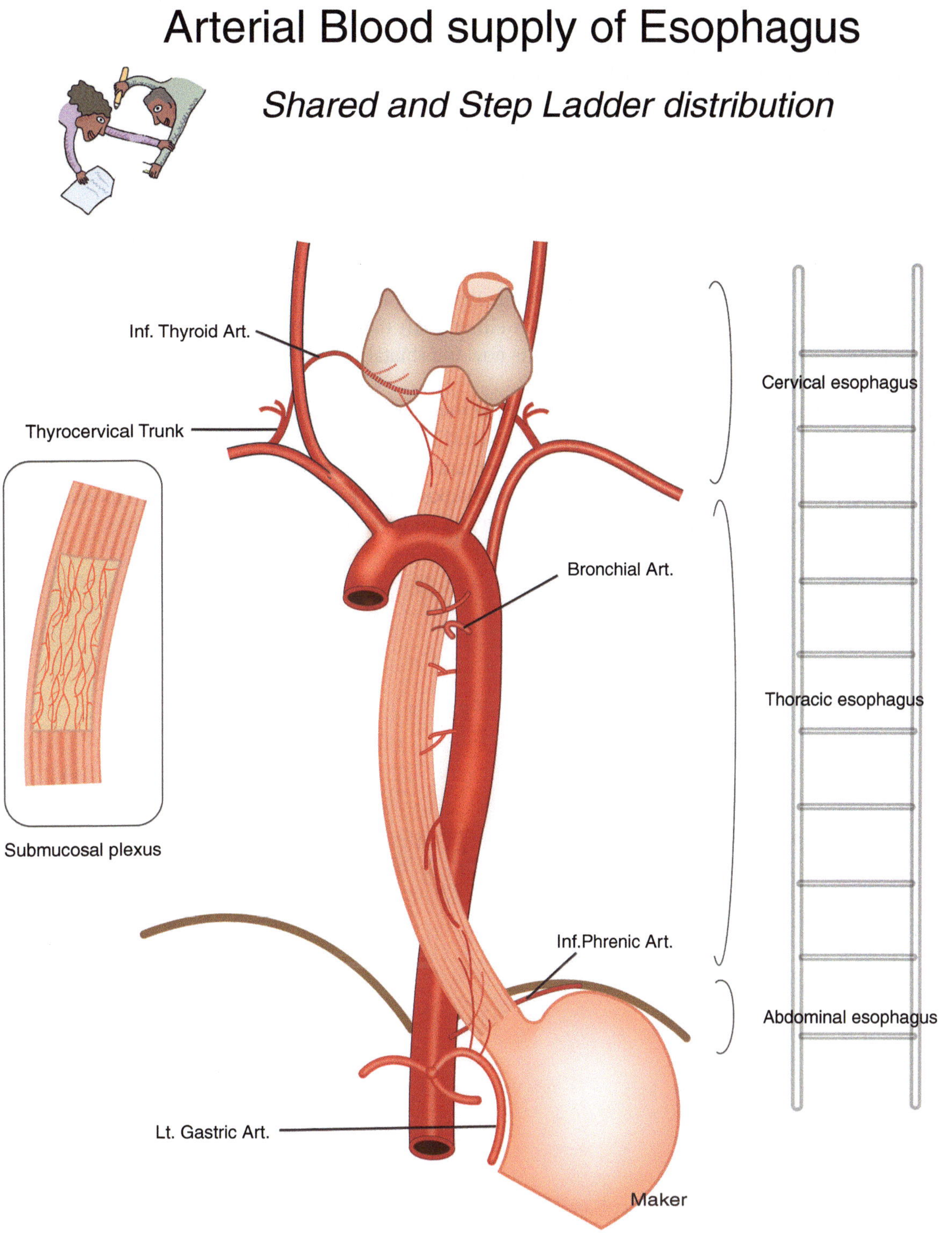

Fig. 11.3 Arterial blood supply to the esophagus is shared with other organs and comes in a stepladder fashion from the inferior thyroid artery in the neck; aortic, intercostal, tracheobronchial, and bronchoesophageal arteries in the chest; and left gastric and splenic arteries in the abdomen. In the esophageal submucosa, arterial blood supply to the esophagus forms a rich longitudinal anastomotic latticework. This cognitive pearl is helpful in dividing the esophagus at any level for anastomosis and even bluntly dissecting it in the intrathoracic space

Answer

e

8. Select the *correct* statement.
   (a) The cervical esophagus should be approached through a right cervical incision.
   (b) The mid-esophagus can be approached by left thoracotomy.
   (c) The lower third of the esophagus can be safely approached through a left thoracotomy.
   (d) A thoracic approach to the esophagus is associated with higher mortality.
   (e) Transthoracic esophagectomy relies mainly on blunt dissection.

Comments The different surgical approaches to the esophagus are based on its tortuous course. The esophagus arises in the midline at the level of the sixth cervical vertebra. From there, it takes a slightly leftward course towards the base of the neck. When it reaches T7, it angulates towards the right, only to return to the left in its lower third. As a consequence, the cervical esophagus is approached through a left neck incision, while the mid-thoracic esophagus is best reached through a right thoracotomy. The distal esophagus can be reached through either a left thoracotomy or through a transhiatal approach [26]. Another increasing popular approach to the esophagus is now transhiatal, where the entire esophagus is dissected up to the neck, with the anastomosis being created in the left neck.

The oncologic outcomes for transthoracic (Ivor Lewis) and transhiatal esophagectomy are comparable, although transthoracic esophagectomy exhibits a trend towards improved results. The Ivor Lewis approach consists of an initial laparotomy with assessment of the extent of infradiaphragmatic disease and complete mobilization of the stomach based on the left gastroepiploic artery and feeding jejunostomy, followed with repositioning of the patient for a right thoracotomy. The transhiatal approach to esophagectomy has been associated with less perioperative complications [27].

Answer
c

9. Mark the *true* statement regarding lower esophageal sphincter (LES) tone.
   (a) Decreased by gastrin and histamine
   (b) Increased by secretin and CCK
   (c) Decreased by progesterone
   (d) Increased by fatty meals, alcohol, and chocolate
   (e) Decreased by protein-rich meals

Comments See question 5.

Answer
c

10. Mark the *incorrect* statement.
    (a) The upper esophageal sphincter is tonically contracted.
    (b) The upper esophageal sphincter prevents aerophagia and reflux into the airway.
    (c) The pressure of the upper esophageal sphincter is much higher than that of the lower esophageal sphincter.
    (d) Esophageal perforations due to instrumentation usually occur at the level of the LES.
    (e) The esophagus has three constrictions determined by the cricopharyngeus muscle, the aorta along with the left main bronchus, and the LES.

Comments The esophagus has both an upper and a lower sphincter. The upper sphincter is in a state of constant contraction at a pressure of approximately 60 mmHg. It relaxes transiently to allow the passage of the food bolus and then contracts briefly to 90 mmHg, preventing reflux generated by esophageal peristalsis (which reaches 80 mmHg). In similar fashion, the lower esophageal sphincter acts as a barrier to gastroesophageal reflux. It has a lower resting pressure of approximately 30 mmHg. The cervical esophagus is the most common area of iatrogenic perforation.

The LES constitutes a functional entity rather than an anatomic, as there are no particular muscle fibers present to explain its function. It is identified as an area of elevated endoluminal pressure at the level of the esophageal hiatus, spanning 3–5 cm in length. The tone of the LES is modulated by multiple stimuli of neurologic, hormonal, and pharmacologic nature. In general, the parasympathetic system, also involved in swallowing, relaxes the LES, with the sympathetic system having an opposite effect. GI hormones that increase gastric acidity contract the LES, with the opposite being true of these that promote pancreatic secretion. Progesterone has a generalized effect in decreasing the tone of the smooth muscle, explaining in part the increased incidence of GERD and constipation during pregnancy [28–30].

The normal esophagus has no spontaneous peristalsis. Primary peristaltic wave starts after the act of swallowing. The glossopharyngeal nerve (IX) starts this voluntary reflex which is continued by the vagus nerve (X) in involuntary fashion.

Answer
d

11. All of the following are correct *except*:
    (a) Below the carina, the esophagus has only the smooth muscle.
    (b) The carina marks a watershed area for lymphatic flow. Above it lymph flows cephalad, below caudad.
    (c) Lymphatic vessels travel circumferentially in the esophagus, making circumferential tumor spread more likely than longitudinal extension.
    (d) The esophagus has two types of epithelium: stratified proximally and columnar distally.
    (e) The esophagus possesses a rich arterial and venous submucosal anastomotic network.

Comments As mentioned previously, the esophagus has a rich arterial anastomotic network. Arteries not only describe circular segmental anastomosis but also form multiple longitudinal collaterals. This pattern is also mimicked by the esophageal veins and lymphatics, allowing significant longitudinal tumor spread along the axis of this organ (Figs. 11.4 and 11.5).

The transition between the upper squamous epithelium and the lower columnar epithelium occurs in a progressive fashion in the vicinity of esophageal hiatus. The zone in which this transition is most noticeable is called the Z line. It is important to know that this line is not fixed in position and may migrate cephalad in the presence of gastroesophageal reflux [26].

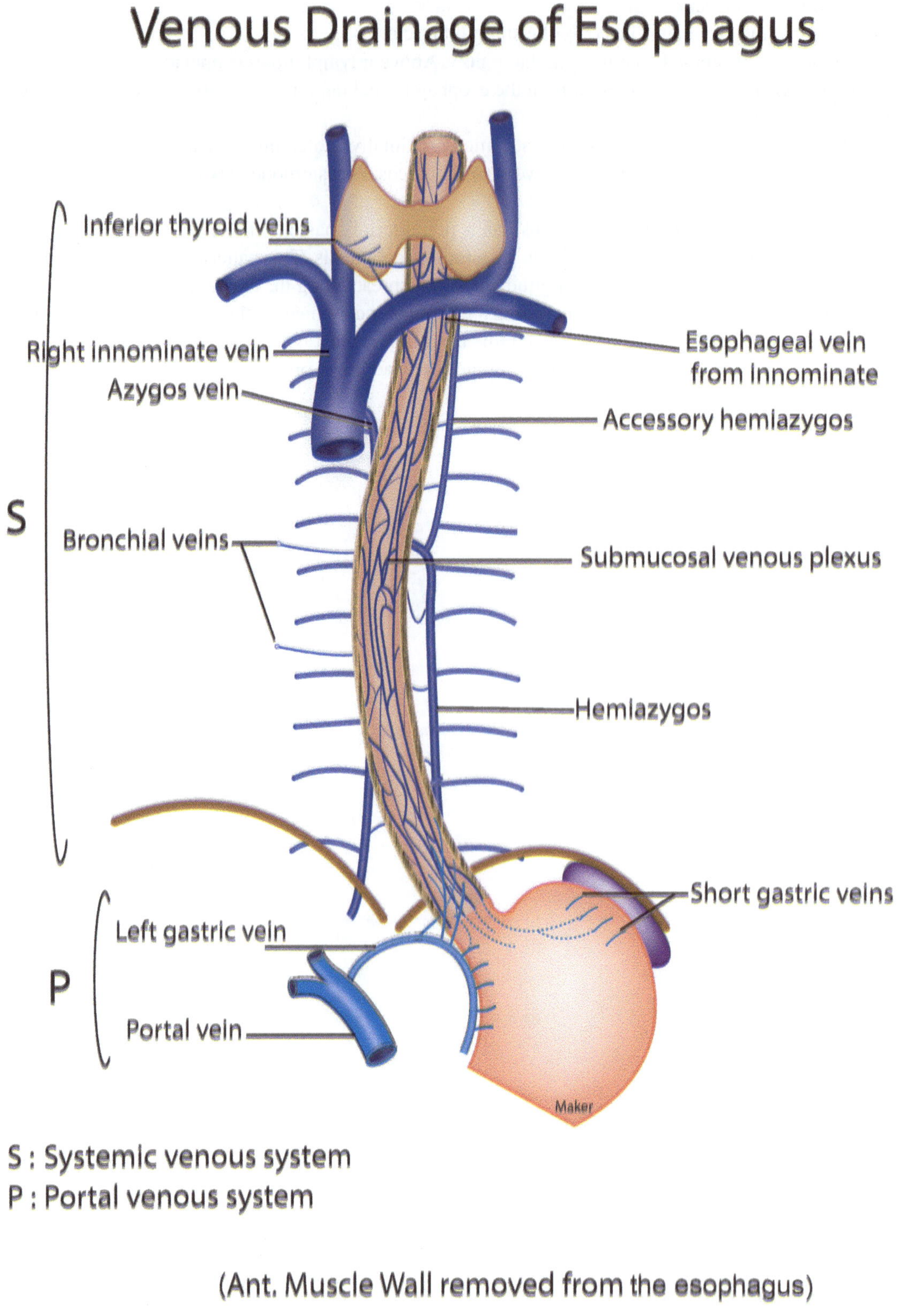

Fig. 11.4 Venous drainage of the esophagus is shared with other organs as well. It has an extensive submucosal longitudinal latticework of collateral veins just like the arterial supply of the esophagus. However, the distinct difference lies in the fact that the lower esophageal drainage is into a higher-pressure portal system as compared to the lower-pressure systemic veins of the cervical and thoracic esophagus. This cognitive pearl is clinically relevant in patients with portal hypertension

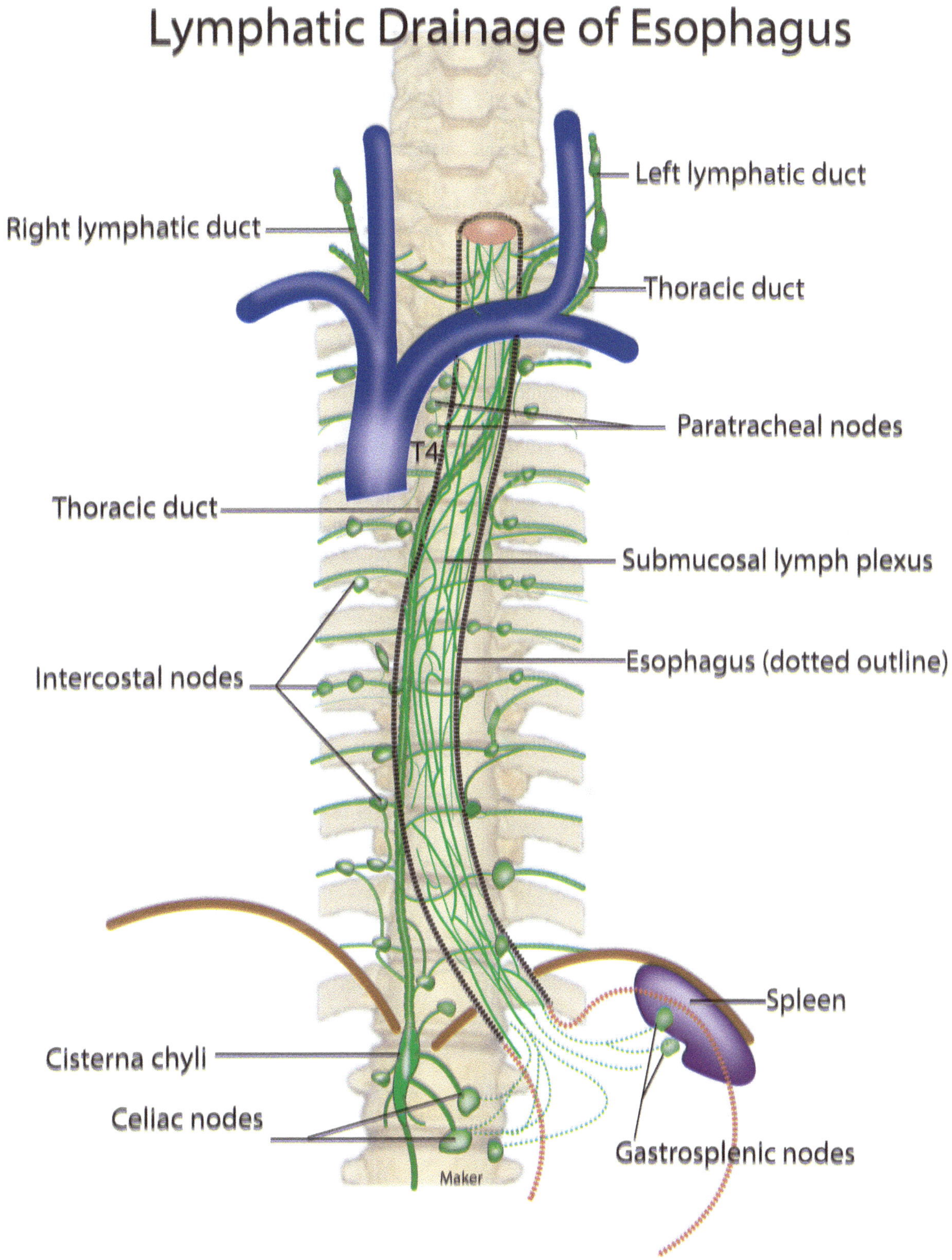

Fig. 11.5 The extensive submucosal longitudinal network of esophageal visceral lymphatics has no valves. Esophageal lymphatics may carry neoplastic cells of the esophagus for long distances in either direction, partly explaining the extraesophageal spread of cancers from the esophagus and the need for total esophagectomy for most esophageal cancers above the esophagogastric junction

Answer

c

12. Please select the *correct* statement regarding dysphagia.
    (a) Schatzki's ring is one of the most common causes of dysphagia.
    (b) Dysphagia can be seen in severe mitral stenosis.
    (c) Dysphagia lusoria is caused by bronchial compression of the esophagus.
    (d) Dysphagia is a sign of early esophageal carcinoma.
    (e) Plummer–Vinson syndrome associated with pernicious anemia.

Comments Schatzki's ring is synonymous with lower esophageal mucosal ring. It is a rare anomaly that is commonly asymptomatic. It occurs in association with hiatal hernias and GERD, which may play a role in its etiology. Treatment, in the form of dilatation, is reserved for symptomatic disease [31].

Severe mitral stenosis leading to massive left atrial enlargement can cause extrinsic compression of the esophagus, between the heart and vertebra. Hoarseness secondary to recurrent laryngeal nerve compression may be an associated finding [32].

Dysphagia lusoria is another uncommon cause of dysphagia secondary to a vascular ring, formed by an anomaly of the fourth aortic arch [33].

The esophagus is a relatively mobile organ in the mediastinum, having the protection of the lungs on either side. For carcinoma of the esophagus to produce dysphagia, it must invariably fix the esophagus in place to cause narrowing. Hence, by definition, when dysphagia is present in carcinoma of the esophagus, it is a locally advanced disease. It is ironic that the earliest symptom of esophageal carcinoma, i.e., dysphagia is indicative of advanced disease.

Plummer–Vinson syndrome comprised of the association of dysphagia secondary to an acquired upper esophageal web, iron-deficiency anemia, and glossitis. It most often presents in middle-aged women. The etiology of this syndrome is unclear. It has been associated with the development of squamous carcinoma of the esophagus [34].

Answer
b

13. All of the following are correct *except*:
    (a) Zenker's diverticulum is approached through a left neck incision.
    (b) Epiphrenic diverticula may arise at any level of the thoracic esophagus.
    (c) Epiphrenic diverticula are most often approached through a right posterolateral thoracotomy.
    (d) Resection of epiphrenic diverticula should be accompanied by esophagomyotomy.
    (e) Treatment of traction diverticula is largely nonoperative.

Comments Esophageal diverticula are somewhat infrequent acquired anomalies that occur most frequently in older adults. They can be divided by their mechanism into pulsion and traction diverticula or by the layers of their wall into true or false diverticula.

Both Zenker's and epiphrenic diverticula are caused by pulsion and are formed by the mucosa only, hence being classified as false. Pulsion occurs due to spasm of the underlying sphincter: the cricopharyngeus muscle or lower esophageal sphincter, respectively. It follows that myotomy will be the key surgical treatment principle. Both present most frequently on the left side. Even though they may occur at any level, epiphrenic diverticula are most frequent in the last 10 cm of the thoracic esophagus, making a left thoracotomy the approach of choice.

Traction diverticula involve all layers of the esophageal wall. They are most often located in the mid-esophagus, in the vicinity of the peritracheal lymph nodes. These nodes, when affected by fibrosis induced by granulomatous diseases (tuberculosis, histoplasmosis), retract and exert force on the esophageal wall. Most often they cause few symptoms, which improve with the treatment of the underlying disease. Less frequently, a significant inflammation may be present, leading to tracheoesophageal fistulization. In these cases, drainage and repair through thoracotomy are needed. Interposition flaps are recommended [35].

Answer
c

14. All of the following are correct *except*:
    (a) Negative intrathoracic pressure is a driving force for mediastinal contamination in esophageal perforation.
    (b) Boerhaave's syndrome is most often caused by foreign body or instrumental perforation of the distal esophagus.
    (c) Left-sided pleural effusions are a relatively late sign of esophageal perforation.
    (d) Spontaneous esophageal perforation is best approached through a seventh interspace left-sided thoracotomy.
    (e) A radiocontrast esophagogram is the confirmatory test of choice for esophageal perforation.

Comments Postemetic (barogenic) esophageal perforation was first described by Herman Boerhaave in 1724. His patient was a Dutch admiral who had ruptured esophagus after having a 3-day feast of food and alcohol [36].

It is caused by sudden increases in esophageal pressure due to retching with a closed upper esophageal sphincter. Rupture most often occurs in the left lateral aspect of the distal thoracic esophagus, which lies to the left of the midline. This determines the side for surgical approach.

The clinical diagnosis is based on Mackler's triad of vomiting, chest pain, and subcutaneous emphysema. However, atypical presentations may occur, and a high index of suspicion should be maintained, especially in the unwell patient. The initial diagnostic modality should be a Gastrografin swallow study, followed by thin barium if Gastrografin is nondiagnostic [37, 38].

Answer
d

15. All of the following are correct *except*:
    (a) Mallory–Weiss tears most often occur at the gastroesophageal junction.
    (b) Mallory–Weiss tears follow a longitudinal course along the distal esophagus and proximal cardia.
    (c) Mallory–Weiss tears extend along the lesser curve.
    (d) Mallory–Weiss tears are limited to the mucosa.
    (e) Mallory–Weiss tears are approached through a left-sided 7th space thoracotomy.

Comments Mallory–Weiss tears are disruptions of the mucosa of the distal esophagus and proximal stomach. They are secondary to forceful vomiting and retching, often times related to binge drinking. The mechanism is thought to involve propulsion and shearing of the stomach through the esophageal hiatus due to sudden increases in abdominal pressure. The presence of hiatal hernia is thought to be a predisposing factor and is found in up to 84 % of cases.

While most often the cause of self-limited bleeding, they may be responsible for the significant blood loss. Unlike esophageal varices, Mallory–Weiss tears create arterial bleeding. Diagnosis is established by endoscopy, during which the retroflexion maneuver is key. This modality may also be used therapeutically. Another alternative to control bleeding is angiographic embolization. If these approaches fail, the lacerated mucosa can be repaired through a high gastrostomy [39, 40].

Answer
e

References

1. Graham A. Development of the pharyngeal arches. Am J Med Genet A. 2003;119(3):251–6.
2. Graham A, Okabe M, Quinlan R. The role of the endoderm in the development and evolution of the pharyngeal arches. J Anat. 2005;207(5):479–87.
3. Todd NW. Common congenital anomalies of the neck. Embryology and surgical anatomy. Surg Clin N Am. 1993;73(4):599–610.
4. Waldhausen JH. Branchial cleft and arch anomalies in children. Semin Pediatr Surg. 2006;15(2):64–9.
5. Foley DS, Fallat ME. Thyroglossal duct and other congenital midline cervical anomalies. Semin Pediatr Surg. 2006;15(2):70–5.
6. Acierno SP, Waldhausen JH. Congenital cervical cysts, sinuses and fistulae. Otolaryngol Clin N Am. 2007;40(1):161–8.
7. Tracy Jr TF, Muratore CS. Management of common head and neck masses. Semin Pediatr Surg. 2007;16(1):3–13.
8. Rutter MJ. Evaluation and management of upper airway disorders in children. Semin Pediatr Surg. 2006;15(2):116–23.
9. Veenker EA, Andersen PE, Cohen JI. Cricopharyngeal spasm and Zenker's diverticulum. Head Neck. 2003;25(8):681–94.
10. Aly A, Devitt PG, Jamieson GG. Evolution of surgical treatment for pharyngeal pouch. Br J Surg. 2004;91(6):657–64.
11. Randall DA, Martin PJ, Thompson LD. Routine histologic examination is unnecessary for tonsillectomy or adenoidectomy. Laryngoscope. 2007;117(9):1600–4.
12. Enepekides DJ. Recent advances in the treatment of juvenile angiofibroma. Curr Opin Otolaryngol Head Neck Surg. 2004;12(6):495–9.
13. Garre ML, Cama A. Craniopharyngioma: modern concepts in pathogenesis and treatment. Curr Opin Pediatr. 2007;19(4):471–9.
14. Karavitaki N, Wass JA. Craniopharyngiomas. Endocrinol Metab Clin N Am. 2008;37(1):173–93.
15. Lin JH, Tai CF, Lee KW, Ho KY, Kuo WR, Wang LF. Huge Thornwaldt's cyst: a case report. Kaohsiung J Med Sci. 2006;22(10):524–8.
16. Arosarena OA. Cleft lip and palate. Otolaryngol Clin N Am. 2007;40(1):27–60, vi.
17. Tewfik TL, Al GM. Tonsillopharyngitis: clinical highlights. J Otolaryngol. 2005;34 Suppl 1:S45–9.
18. Cunningham EJ, Bond R, Mayberg MR, Warlow CP, Rothwell PM. Risk of persistent cranial nerve injury after carotid endarterectomy. J Neurosurg. 2004;101(3):445–8.
19. Yadav JS, Wholey MH, Kuntz RE, Fayad P, Katzen BT, Mishkel GJ, et al. Protected carotid-artery stenting versus endarterectomy in high-risk patients. N Engl J Med. 2004;351(15):1493–501.
20. Hansen SH. Laryngeal crepitus: an aid to diagnosis in non-fatal strangulation. Med Sci Law. 2001;41(4):284–6.
21. Han P, Hu K, Frank DK, Sessions RB, Harrison LB. Management of cancer of the base of tongue. Otolaryngol Clin N Am. 2005;38(1):75–85, viii.
22. Won CH, Li KK, Guilleminault C. Surgical treatment of obstructive sleep apnea: upper airway and maxillomandibular surgery. Proc Am Thorac Soc. 2008;5(2):193–9.
23. Guindi M, Riddell RH. Histology of Barrett's esophagus and dysplasia. Gastrointest Endosc Clin N Am. 2003;13(2):349–68, viii.
24. Hornick JL, Odze RD. Neoplastic precursor lesions in Barrett's esophagus. Gastroenterol Clin N Am. 2007;36(4):775–96, v.
25. Tang LH, Klimstra DS. Barrett's esophagus and adenocarcinoma of the gastroesophageal junction: a pathologic perspective. Surg Oncol Clin N Am. 2006;15(4):715–32.
26. Skandalakis JE, Ellis H. Embryologic and anatomic basis of esophageal surgery. Surg Clin N Am. 2000;80(1):85–155, x.
27. Pennathur A, Luketich JD. Resection for esophageal cancer: strategies for optimal management. Ann Thorac Surg. 2008;85(2):S751–6.
28. Hornby PJ, Abrahams TP. Central control of lower esophageal sphincter relaxation. Am J Med. 2000;108(Suppl 4a):90S–8.
29. Crookes PF. Physiology of reflux disease: role of the lower esophageal sphincter. Surg Endosc. 2006;20 Suppl 2:S462–6.
30. Gawrieh S, Shaker R. Peripheral mechanisms affecting the lower esophageal sphincter tone. Gastroenterol Clin N Am. 2002;31(4 Suppl):S21–33.
31. Jalil S, Castell DO. Schatzki's ring: a benign cause of dysphagia in adults. J Clin Gastroenterol. 2002;35(4):295–8.
32. Morgan AA, Mourant AJ. Left vocal cord paralysis and dysphagia in mitral valve disease. Br Heart J. 1980;43(4):470–3.
33. Levitt B, Richter JE. Dysphagia lusoria: a comprehensive review. Dis Esophagus. 2007;20(6):455–60.
34. Atmatzidis K, Papaziogas B, Pavlidis T, Mirelis C, Papaziogas T. Plummer-Vinson syndrome. Dis Esophagus. 2003;16(2):154–7.
35. Cassivi SD, Deschamps C, Nichols III FC, Allen MS, Pairolero PC. Diverticula of the esophagus. Surg Clin N Am. 2005;85(3):495–503, ix.
36. Adams BD, Sebastian BM, Carter J. Honoring the Admiral: Boerhaave-van Wassenaer's syndrome. Dis Esophagus. 2006;19(3):146–51.
37. Khan AZ, Strauss D, Mason RC. Boerhaave's syndrome: diagnosis and surgical management. Surgeon. 2007;5(1):39–44.
38. Vial CM, Whyte RI. Boerhaave's syndrome: diagnosis and treatment. Surg Clin N Am. 2005;85(3):515–24, ix.
39. Younes Z, Johnson DA. The spectrum of spontaneous and iatrogenic esophageal injury: perforations, Mallory-Weiss tears, and hematomas. J Clin Gastroenterol. 1999;29(4):306–17.
40. Morales P, Baum AE. Therapeutic alternatives for the Mallory-Weiss tear. Curr Treat Options Gastroenterol. 2003;6(1):75–83.

12 Stomach

1. Mark the *correct* statement regarding hypertrophic pyloric stenosis (HPS).
   (a) Symptoms most commonly appear before 2 weeks of age.
   (b) The palpation of a pyloric tumor (olive) has low specificity for the diagnosis of HPS.
   (c) The Ramstedt procedure consists of the division of the muscle fibers of the pylorus leaving the mucosa intact.
   (d) The Ramstedt procedure includes transverse closure of the longitudinal myotomy site.
   (e) Accidental mucosal perforation during a pyloromyotomy is treated with resection of the affected segment and anastomosis.

Comments Hypertrophic pyloric stenosis (HPS) is one of the most common surgical conditions in infancy, affecting 3 in 1,000 newborns. It is most common in white firstborn males. It presents between the 2nd and 12th week of life with postprandial non-bilious emesis. The etiology is unclear. Diagnosis can be made solely on clinical grounds, with the presence of a palpable "olive" having a high specificity. Ultrasound examination has at least 99 % sensitivity and specificity for this diagnosis. A pyloric channel measuring 15–20 mm, with a wall thickness of 3–5 mm and lack of relaxation are considered positive findings.

Treatment is the Ramstedt pyloromyotomy, a procedure in which the serosa and muscular layers are transected longitudinally, leaving the mucosa intact. In cases in which the mucosa is penetrated, it should be repaired. Current recommendations include closure of the original myotomy site, with creation of a new myotomy at a different site [1, 2].

Answer
c

V.K. Maker, E.D. Guzman-Arrieta, *Cognitive Pearls in General Surgery*,
DOI 10.1007/978-1-4939-1850-8_12,

2. Mark the *correct* statement regarding gastric anatomy.
   (a) The posterior part of the stomach is the anterior wall of the lesser sac.
   (b) The stomach has very limited mobility.
   (c) Gastric volvulus is one of the most common complications of gastric banding.
   (d) The lesser omentum may harbor replaced right hepatic arteries.
   (e) The gastrophrenic ligament contains the short gastric vessels.

Comments The stomach is a rather mobile organ, held in place at either end by the phrenoesophageal ligament proximally and the duodenum distally. This degree of motility allows it to rotate along its axis, creating a gastric volvulus. Gastric volvulus can be organoaxial (i.e., along the longitudinal axis or cascade volvulus along its horizontal axis). The most important predisposing factors are gastric distention and the shape of the stomach itself. Long, vertically oriented stomachs are prone to organoaxial volvulus, whereas broad horizontally oriented stomachs are predisposed to a cascade volvulus. Gastric volvulus has not been associated to gastric banding [3] (Fig. 12.1).

Due to its mobility, the stomach is often used to replace the esophagus in the chest. In order to mobilize the stomach, the short gastric vessels, the left gastric artery, the right gastric artery, and the left gastroepiploic artery are divided. In such cases, the right gastroepiploic artery may feed the entire stomach [4].

The stomach is attached to other abdominal organs through the derivatives of the ventral and dorsal mesogastria. The ventral mesogastrium forms the lesser omentum, which may harbor accessory or replaced left hepatic arteries arising from the left gastric artery. The dorsal mesentery forms the gastrosplenic ligament (which encases the short gastric vessels), the splenic capsule, and the splenophrenic ligament [5].

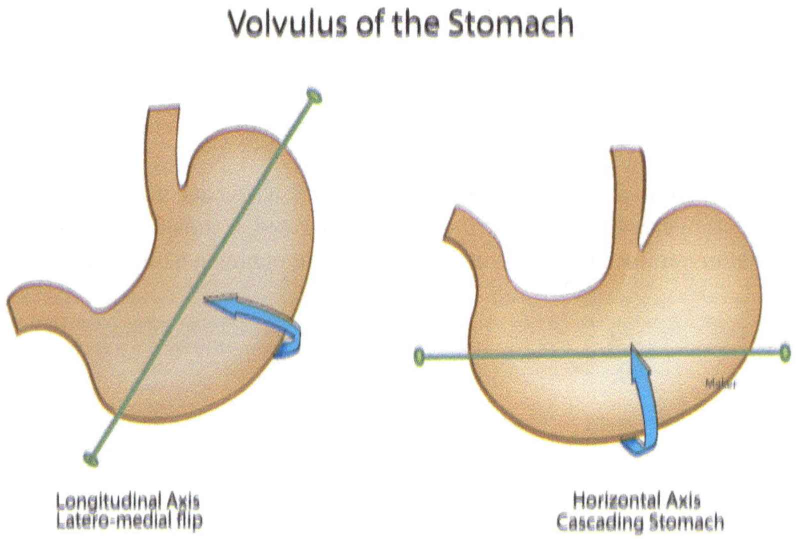

Fig. 12.1 By virtue of its bulky shape and fixed narrow ends, the stomach is prone to volvulus. This tendency increases when the stomach is herniated into the chest. In acute presentations, early diagnosis is critical for surgical treatment

Answer

a

3. All of the following are correct *except*:
   (a) The endocrine cells of the stomach are mainly located in the fundus and body.
   (b) G cells are located in the antrum.
   (c) D cells produce somatostatin.
   (d) Enterochromaffin-like cells produce histamine.
   (e) Intrinsic factor is produced by P cells (parietal cells).

Comments Gastric acid secretion is the sole function of the parietal cells. This is a finely regulated process, under the influence of neural, hormonal, and intraluminal stimuli. Parietal cells are located exclusively in the fundus and body of the stomach, which is the basis of limiting highly selective vagotomy to the branches of the nerve of Latarjet going to this portion of the stomach.

Located in the antrum, G cells, through gastrin production, are the most important positive regulators of acid secretion. They are stimulated by vagal efferents as well as by the presence of food in the gastric lumen. Gastrin reaches the oxyntic region of the stomach (fundus and body), where it stimulates the production of acid by parietal cells directly and indirectly, by inducing histamine release from enterochromaffin-like cells. The acidification of the gastric lumen stimulates somatostatin-producing D cells in the antrum, which inhibit G cells in a paracrine manner.

Interestingly D cells are also found in the oxyntic region of the stomach; however, in this location, they lack luminal receptors and do not respond to gastric acidification. Instead, they respond to the hormones released by duodenal acidification, namely, CCK, secretin, and gastric inhibitory peptide, and further downregulate gastric production.

M cells produce mucus. While they are located throughout the stomach, they are most abundant in the antrum. Chief cells share their location with parietal cells. They produce intrinsic factor, pepsin, and other digestive enzymes [6, 7] (Fig. 12.2).

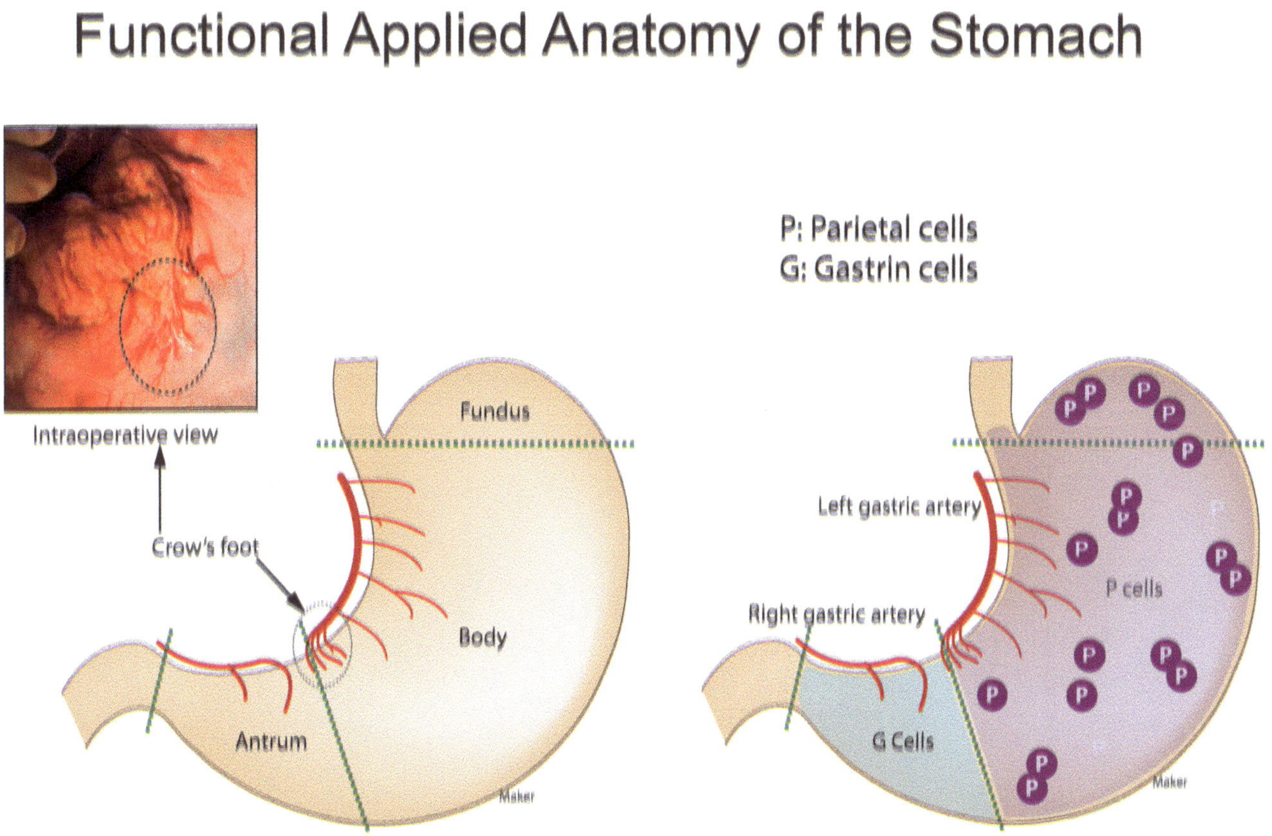

Fig. 12.2 The fundus and body of the stomach contain all the parietal cells which make hydrochloric acid, while the antrum contains all the G cells attributed to making gastrin. The left gastric artery finishes on the lesser curvature of the stomach in a "crow's-foot" distribution and marks the junction of the gastric fundus and body with the antrum and pylorus

Answer
a

4. Mark the *correct* statement in relation to celiac artery compression syndrome.
   (a) Celiac artery compression most commonly affects elderly individuals.
   (b) Celiac artery compression is always symptomatic.
   (c) In approximately 25 % of the population, the median arcuate ligament impinges on the celiac trunk.
   (d) Celiac trunk compression is best seen during expiration.
   (e) There are no routes of collateral circulation to compensate for decreases in flow across the celiac artery.

Comments Celiac artery compression syndrome, also known as median arcuate ligament syndrome, celiac band syndrome, or Dunbar's syndrome, mostly affects young and middle-aged women. The compression of the celiac trunk leads to intermittent gastric ischemia, causing symptoms of epigastric pain, mostly in the postprandial period, and is classically accompanied by an epigastric bruit and weight loss.

However, it has been suggested that while necessary, celiac compression may not be sufficient to produce this syndrome. As noted above, up to 25 % of the population has some degree of celiac trunk impingement, with symptomatic disease being much less common. It has been hypothesized that a disturbance in the rich collateral circulation of the stomach must also be present for symptoms to occur.

During deep inspiration, descent of the diaphragm and slight cephalad displacement of the aorta increase the degree of compression on the celiac trunk. This is best seen on lateral views through conventional angiography or CT scanning. Another key finding is the poststenotic dilatation of the celiac trunk and the formation of prominent collateral vessels.

Surgical repair has traditionally involved release of the median arcuate ligament with restoration of normal blood flow. However, considering the multiple etiologies of celiac artery compression, other procedures such as removal of enlarged lymph nodes or celiac ganglia may be needed. On occasions, the celiac trunk may be chronically scarred, making the creation of an aorto-celiac bypass necessary. More recently, laparoscopic release combined with celiac artery endovascular stenting has been proposed as an alternative. The fact that these interventions are sometimes ineffective highlights both the importance of ruling out other causes of abdominal pain and the complex pathophysiology of this entity [8–10].

Answer
c

5. Mark the *incorrect* statement regarding gastric nerve supply.
   (a) The hepatic nerve stems from the left vagus.
   (b) The right vagus innervates the distal pancreas and spleen.
   (c) The failure to divide the criminal nerve of Grassi leads to inadequate vagotomy.
   (d) The nerves of Latarjet give no branches to the antrum and pylorus.
   (e) The highly selective vagotomy must clear the nerve supply of the last 5–7 cm of esophagus.

Comments The left vagus nerve becomes anterior below the diaphragm and supplies all of the structures that develop in the ventral mesogastrium, i.e., the liver, biliary tree, and head of the pancreas. In a similar fashion, the right vagus, which becomes posterior, supplies the structures that arise in the dorsal mesogastrium (tail of the pancreas and spleen). In addition, the posterior vagus extends along the dorsal mesentery to the entire midgut. This explains why it is larger than the anterior vagus, and may even be comprised by two trunks.

The nerves of Latarjet arise from either vagus and run along the lesser curvature in the gastrohepatic ligament. They supply branches to the fundus and body of the stomach, ending in the pylorus. The nerves of Latarjet supply all the acid-secreting cells and control gastric emptying.

Highly selective vagotomy is also called parietal cell vagotomy. In principle, it divides all branches of the anterior and posterior nerves of Latarjet supplying the fundus and body of the stomach. In this surgery, it is important that the branches to all parietal cells be divided; hence, surgery must start 5 cm above the esophagogastric junction and finish just past the crow's-foot, in order to totally vagotomize the body and fundus of the stomach (Figs. 12.3 and 12.4).

One of the most often mentioned causes of incomplete vagotomy and ulcer recurrence is the failure to section the "criminal nerve of Grassi." This nerve is a branch of the posterior vagus, often arising above the diaphragm. When undivided, it may perpetuate gastric acid secretion. Vagal afferents supplying the oxyntic region of the stomach from the greater curvature have also been described [11].

Sympathetic innervation of the stomach arises from the T5 to T10. These fibers end in the celiac ganglia, where they synapse with ganglion cells that reach the stomach following the branches of the celiac artery. Afferent fibers follow the opposite route [12].

It must be remembered that incomplete vagotomy is not the only cause of ulcer recurrence after the surgical treatment of peptic ulcer disease. The possibilities of NSAID abuse, *H. pylori* infection, retained gastric antrum, gastrinoma, and hypercalcemia must also be considered [13].

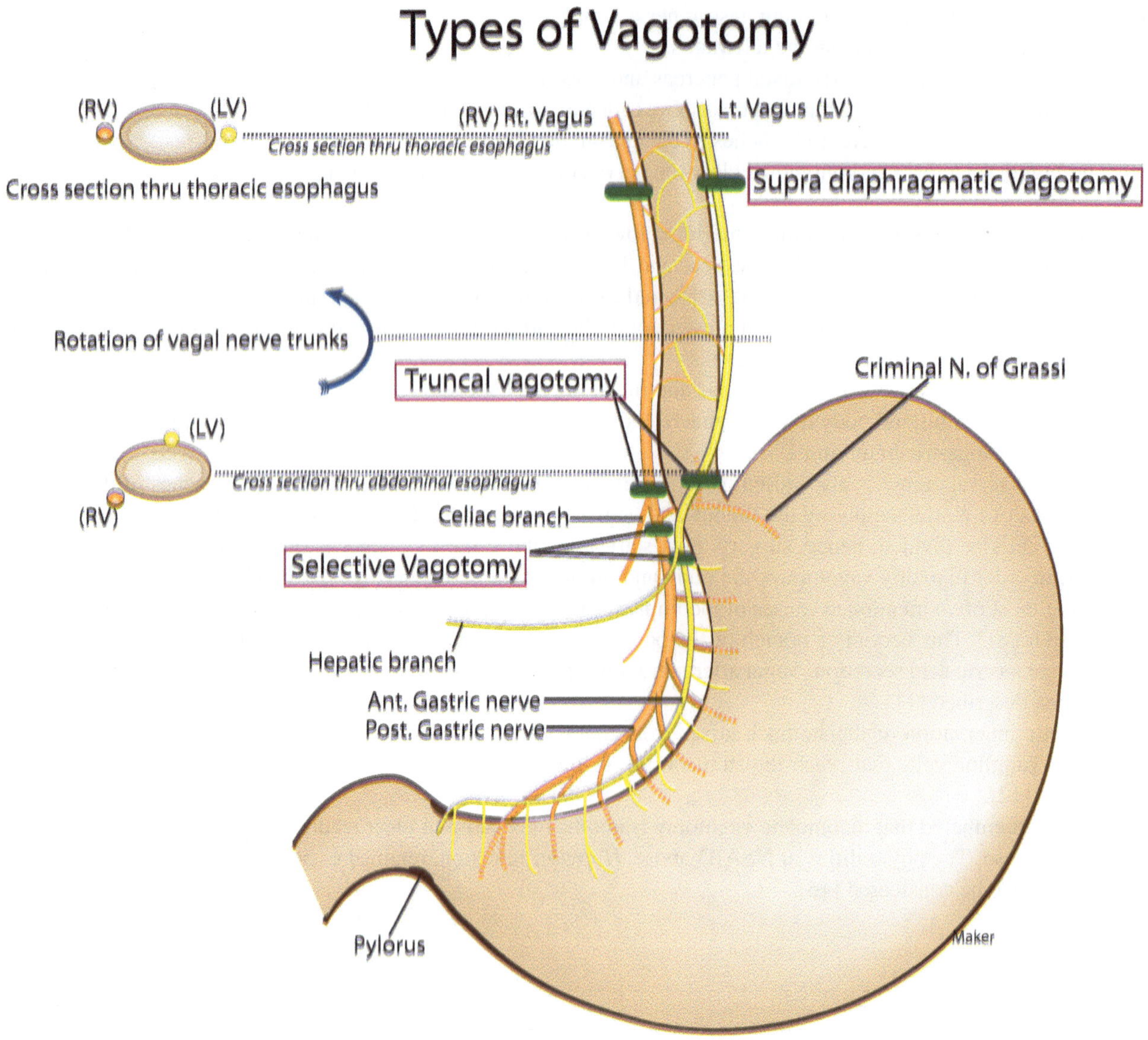

Fig. 12.3 Intra-abdominal truncal vagotomy is an effective operation for reducing acid output of the stomach but results in parasympathetic denervation of the entire foregut and midgut. Selective vagotomy limits parasympathetic denervation to the stomach by only dividing the anterior and posterior gastric nerves past the origin of the branches to other viscera. With this operation, there is a risk of missing vagal innervation to the acid-bearing parts of the fundus. Supradiaphragmatic or thoracic vagotomy is reserved for patients with resistant recurrent peptic ulcer where previous truncal vagotomy has failed and the intra-abdominal approach is no longer available secondary to a frozen abdomen or other causes

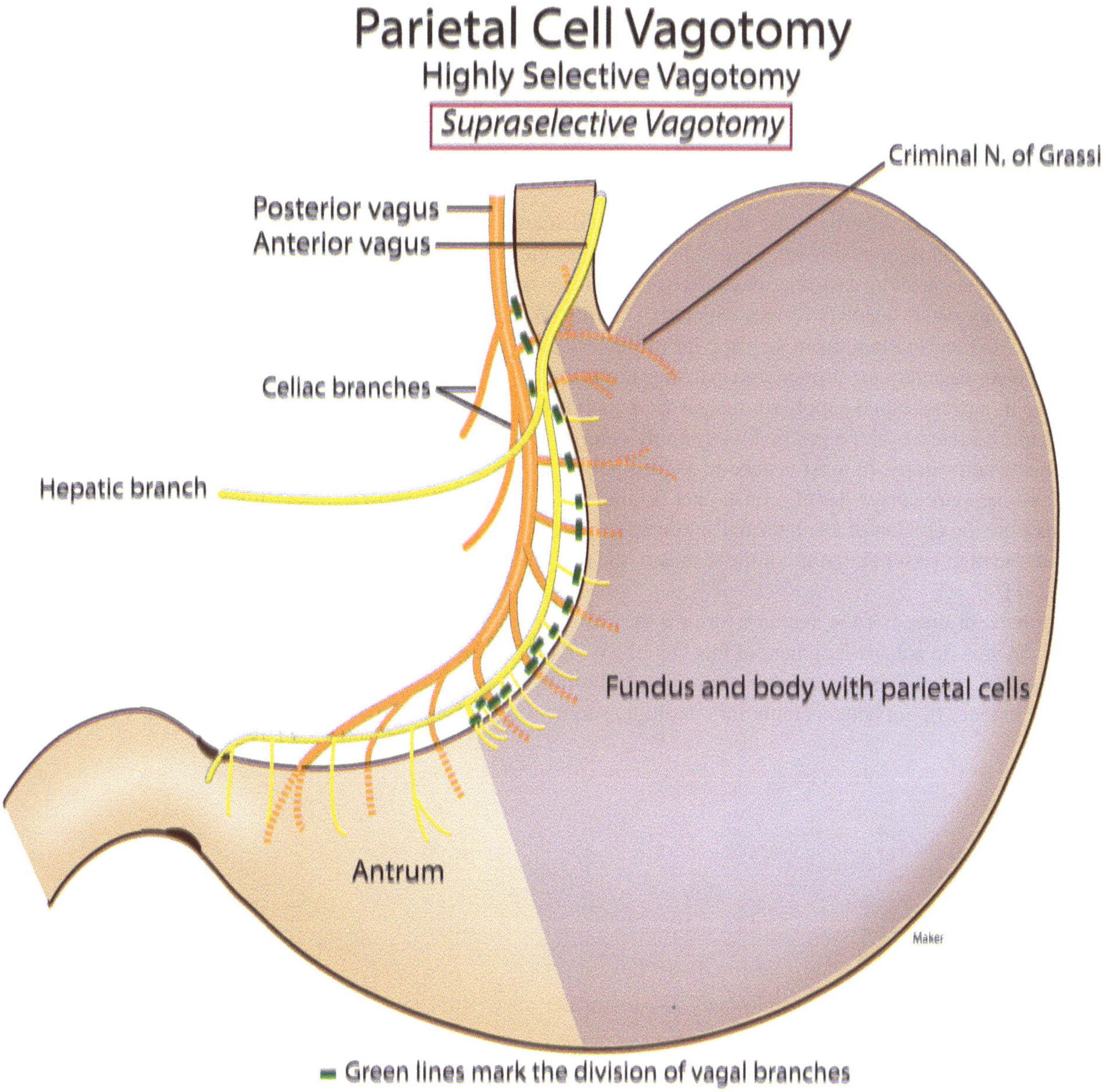

Fig. 12.4 Highly selective vagotomy (supraselective vagotomy) is performed by dividing all the parasympathetic nerves of the fundus and the cardia of the stomach. Anterior and posterior gastric nerves (nerves of Latarjet) are kept intact maintaining nerve supply to the antrum. All nerves entering the stomach from the distal 5 cm of esophagus up to the antrum are carefully divided including the nerve of Grassi. This procedure obviates the need for routine pyloroplasty as the motor function of the antrum is left intact. This procedure has the least post-vagotomy syndromes as complications

Answer
d

6. Mark the *true* statement.
   (a) Acute ligation of the left gastric artery will cause gastric infarction.
   (b) The lymphatic drainage of the stomach follows clear and mutually exclusive areas draining to distinct nodal basins.
   (c) Simple ligation of the gastroduodenal artery is sufficient to control a bleeding duodenal ulcer.
   (d) Extragastric arterial ligation will reliably control gastric bleeding sources.
   (e) The artery most responsible for the Dieulafoy ulcer (submucosal aneurysm) is the left gastric artery.

Comments The stomach is perhaps the segment of the GI tract with the richest blood supply. The lesser curve receives blood from the left and right gastric arteries, while the greater curve is supplied by the right and left gastroepiploic arteries, with contribution of the short gastric arteries derived from the splenic artery. These four arteries form an anastomotic network such that only one is needed to preserve gastric viability. While these arteries ultimately arise from the celiac trunk, the stomach may also receive blood from the superior mesenteric artery, via the inferior pancreaticoduodenal, which anastomoses to its superior counterpart, ultimately perfusing the right gastroepiploic artery. For example, the right gastroepiploic artery is the only arterial blood supply for the gastric pouch in esophagogastric reconstructions.

The multiple collaterals of the gastric blood supply determine that single ligation of a branch involved in a bleeding ulcer will not achieve hemostasis. In most instances, a three-point ligation is needed.

Dieulafoy ulcers are somewhat of a misnomer, in the sense that a classic peptic ulceration is not present. Rather, these lesions constitute the erosion of an abnormal submucosal arterial plexus. While these lesions where classically described as occurring on the high lesser curvature of the stomach, the term has been expanded to describe similar lesions in the GI tract as a whole [14].

The lymphatic drainage of the stomach forms a very complex network, which confers unpredictability to tumor spread from any given area. In acknowledgment of this fact, the lymphatic drainage of the stomach is not viewed as linear, traveling vascular branches; rather, it is conceived in concentric fashion, with nodal groups describing polygons of increasing diameter [15, 16]. The extent of lymphadenectomy for oncologic surgery coincides with this description [17, 18] (Fig. 12.5a–d).

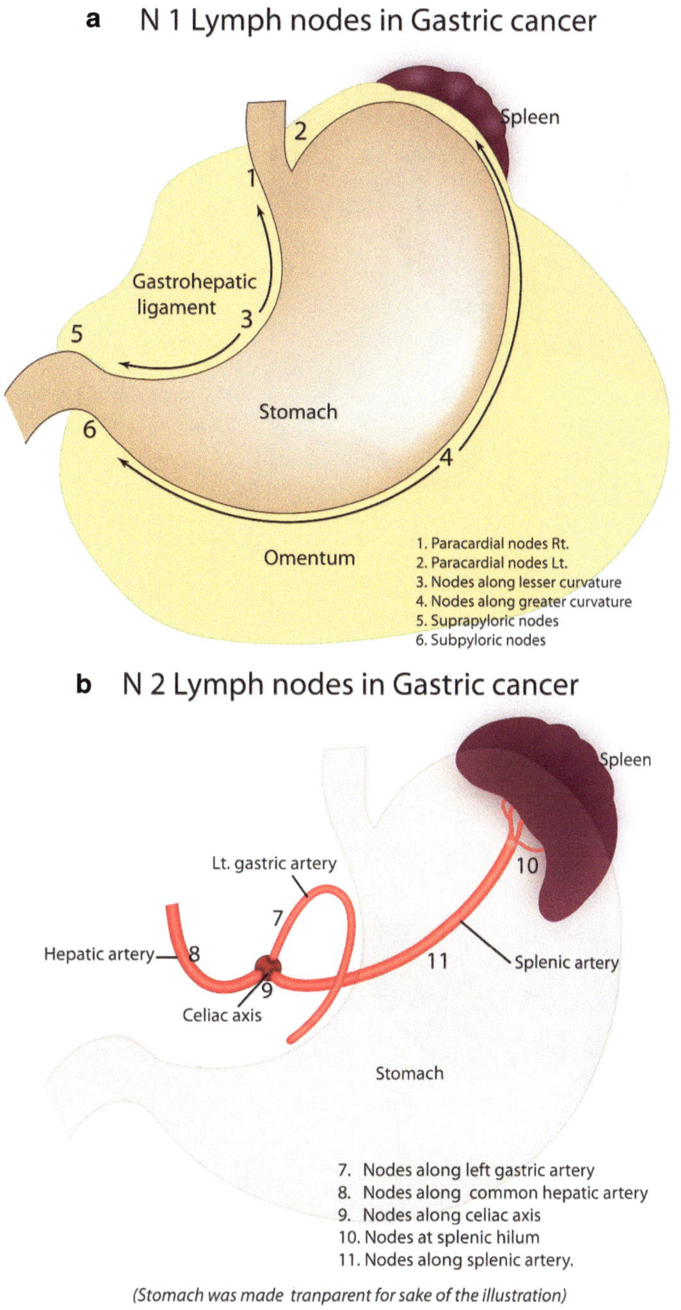

Fig. 12.5 (**a**) N1 lymph node stations are immediately perigastric. D1 gastric resection refers to the removal of the entire gastrohepatic ligament (lesser omentum) and the greater omentum, containing lymph node stations 1–6 as shown above en bloc with the gastrectomy specimen. (**b**) N2 lymph node stations are one step beyond the perigastric lymph nodes. They are located on the celiac axis and its branches, and include all the nodes on and around the celiac axis and extending along the splenic artery to the splenic hilum (stations 7–11). The present literature supports the extent of this resection in the West as D2. (**c**) N3 lymph node stations (12–14) are the posterior extension of the N2. In this dissection, all the posterior lymph nodes on the duodenal side of the gastric resection are removed starting from the hilum of liver superiorly to the root of the mesentery at L2 vertebra. This is considered a D3 resection. (**d**) N4 lymph node stations (15 and 16) are the most posterior and inferior extension of the lymphatic dissection. It includes nodes at the base of middle colic vein entering the superior mesenteric vein as well as periaortic nodes. This addition constitutes a D4 resection (with few modifications depending on the extent of cancer)

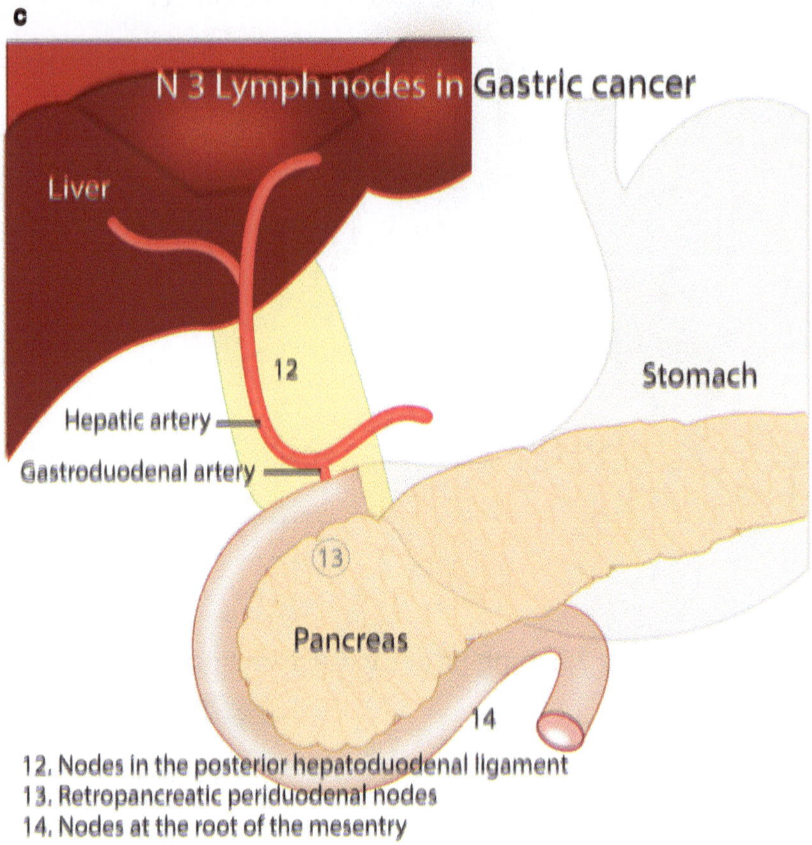

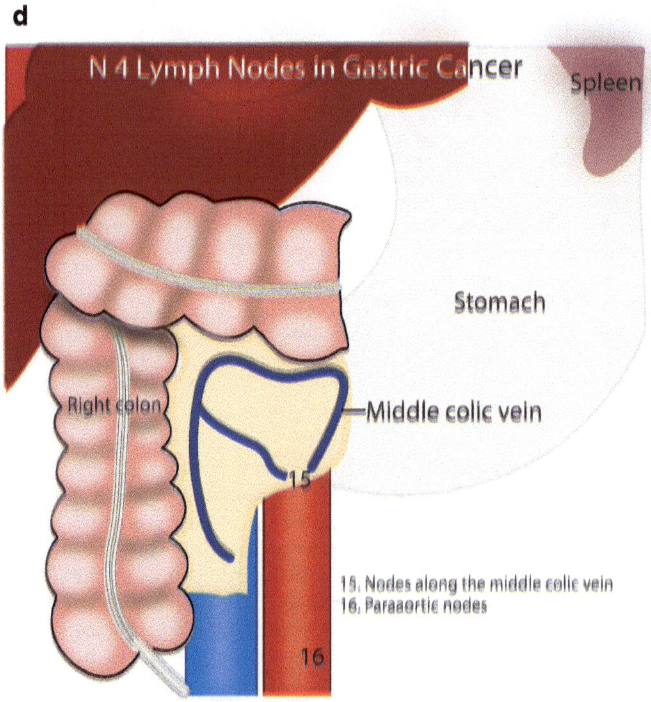

Fig. 12.5 (continued)

Answer
e

7. Mark the *correct* statement regarding gastric surgery complications.
   (a) Retained gastric antrum is typically seen after Billroth I reconstructions.
   (b) Afferent loop syndrome may lead to duodenal stump blowout.
   (c) The symptoms of early dumping are caused by fluctuations in blood sugar levels.
   (d) Efferent loop syndrome is characterized by bilious vomiting
   (e) Megaloblastic anemia after total gastrectomy is treated with oral B12 supplements.

Comments See question 8.

Answer
b

8. Mark the *correct* statement regarding gastric surgery complications.
   (a) Bacterial overgrowth occurs in the chronic afferent loop syndrome.
   (b) Reflux alkaline gastritis after a Billroth II reconstruction is always treated surgically.
   (c) Gastrojejunocolic fistulas occur after antecolic gastrojejunostomy.
   (d) Billroth I reconstructions are immune to dumping syndrome after vagotomy.
   (e) Interposition of retroperistaltic segments is used in the treatment of efferent loop syndrome.

Comments Retained gastric antrum is a complication of gastrectomy and Billroth II reconstruction. It occurs when a portion of the pylorus, containing gastrin-producing cells, is left in continuity with the defunctionalized duodenal limb. In this setting, the G cells in the stump are not exposed to the gastrin-induced decrease in pH, which causes a breakdown in the feedback system leading to hypergastrinemia, excessive acid production in the stomach remnant, and ulceration. In the case of retained gastric antrum, secretin administration will lower gastrin production, a feature that distinguishes it from gastrinoma. Treatment can be pharmacologic in the form of proton pump inhibitors, or surgical, with removal of the remainder of the antrum [19].

Efferent loop syndrome is a cause of abdominal pain and bilious vomiting, most often caused by obstruction of the efferent limb requiring surgical resolution. Afferent loop syndrome is another complication of Billroth II reconstructions, in which there is difficult emptying of the duodenal limb. The syndrome is characterized by postprandial upper abdominal pain and non-bilious vomiting, followed by large bilious emesis that produces relief. The causes include kinking, torsion, and obstruction of the afferent loop. Treatment consists of conversion to a Roux-en-Y anastomosis.

Marginal ulcers are seen at the gastrojejunal anastomosis. They can be on either side of the anastomosis, depending on whether the etiology is continued acid secretion (jejunal side) or bile reflux (gastric side). In either case, marginal ulcers can be a delayed cause of afferent and efferent loop syndromes, through scarring and stricture formation.

Chronically, a redundant afferent loop may also lead to bacterial overgrowth syndrome, characterized by weight loss, diarrhea, and megaloblastic anemia. However, a more frequent cause of megaloblastic anemia is the lack of intrinsic factor leading to vitamin B12 deficiency in total gastrectomy. In this case, the vitamin must replace parenterally, since oral supplements cannot be absorbed [20].

Dumping syndromes are caused by unregulated passage of food into the small bowel due to the absence of the pylorus. More precisely, the osmoregulatory function of the antrum and pylorus is lost. Dumping syndrome is a constellation of gastrointestinal and vasomotor symptoms, after consuming a high osmotic load, mainly in the form of simple carbohydrates.

Early dumping is thought to be a form of distributive shock, in which the passage of a high osmotic load into the small bowel produces acute volume depletion. Late dumping is explained by rebound hypoglycemia after rapid abortion of glucose into the bloodstream. While the above mechanisms appear to be important in explaining these two entities, it appears that gastrointestinal hormones also play an important and not fully understood role. Treatment involves dietary manipulations. If these result ineffectively, interposition of a retroperistaltic loop or a long isoperistaltic loop can be performed [21]. Another surgical alternative is the creation of "Henle's loop." This procedure consists of using a segment the efferent limb of a Billroth II reconstruction to construct a Billroth I reconstruction (Fig. 12.6).

Alkaline reflux gastritis and esophagitis are a consequence of the loss of the pyloric sphincter. This allows passage of bile into the stomach with concurrent destruction of the mucosal barrier. Clinical manifestations are dominated by postprandial burning epigastric pain. Endoscopy classically reveals bile staining of the stomach, esophagus, and in severe cases mouth and tongue. Medical treatment with cholestyramine yields moderate improvement of symptoms. The treatment of choice is diverting the biliary stream at least 20 cm away from the stomach through a gastrojejunostomy [22].

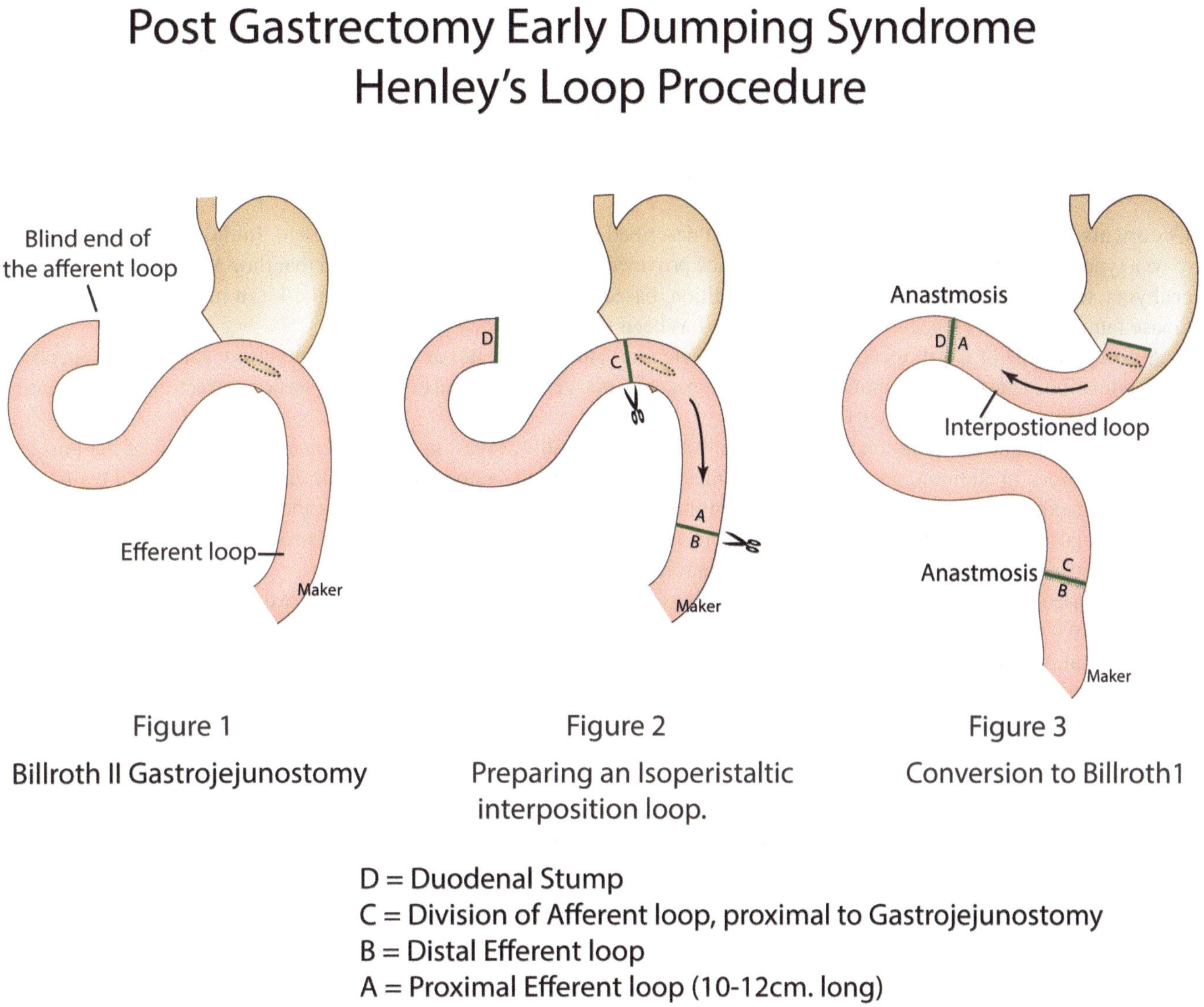

Fig. 12.6 Henle's loop procedure consists of interpositioning an isoperistaltic loop of the jejunum between the residual postgastrectomy stomach and the blind end of the duodenal afferent loop. In this procedure, a postgastrectomy Billroth II procedure is converted into a more physiologic Billroth I. *D* duodenal stump, *C* division of afferent loop, proximal to gastrojejunostomy, *B* distal efferent loop, *A* proximal efferent loop (10–12 cm long)

Answer

a

9. All of the following are correct *except*:
   (a) The interstitial cells of Cajal are responsible for generating spontaneous gastrointestinal motility.
   (b) The interstitial cells of Cajal give origin to GIST tumors.
   (c) The interstitial cells of Cajal are limited to the stomach.
   (d) The interstitial cells of Cajal express the c-kit receptor (CD117).
   (e) Gastrointestinal stromal tumors (GIST) are most common in the stomach.

Comments The interstitial cells of Cajal were first described in the stomach over a century ago. Initially, they were thought to be a type of primitive neuron. Currently, evidence provided chimeric models have shown that they arise from the gut mesenchyma, thus being endodermal in origin. In addition, based on their unique expression of c-kit (a member of the tyrosine kinase family), their presence in the entire GI tract has been well established [23].

A group of cells of Cajal, located in the high greater curvature of the stomach, play an important role in the generation and modulation of gastroenteric motility. They act as pacemakers, generating and organizing phasic contractions. Interestingly, this is the most common site of GIST.

The cells of Cajal also participate in the transmission of peristaltic waves, in a manner analogous to that of the Purkinje cells in the heart. In addition, they participate as mediators between the autonomic neurons and the myocytes. Finally, they have mechanoceptive properties that participate in the regulation of peristalsis. Supporting their role, the loss of interstitial cells of Cajal has been linked to multiple gastrointestinal motility disorders, such as gastroparesis, idiopathic intestinal pseudo-obstruction, achalasia, and chronic constipation [24–26].

Solely based on histologic criteria, most types of gastrointestinal mesenchymal tumors were difficult to distinguish. With the advent of c-kit staining, the distinction between GIST and leiomyosarcomas has become clear. The former arise from the cells of Cajal, whereas the latter are derived from smooth muscle cells. The overexpression of c-kit in GIST constitutes an effective therapeutic target which imatinib (Gleevec) attacks.

Reflecting the greater concentration of interstitial cells of Cajal in the stomach, 50–60 % of GIST occur in this organ, with 30–40 % arising in the small bowel, 5 % in the colon and rectum, and 5 % in the esophagus. Primary GIST outside the GI tract is rare.

Optimal treatment of GIST is based on complete en bloc surgical resection. Gleevec therapy is reserved for recurrent and residual disease, with a neoadjuvant role currently being explored. These tumors rarely metastasize. Their malignant potential is determined by size, location, mitotic rate, and degree of local invasiveness [27] (Fig. 12.7).

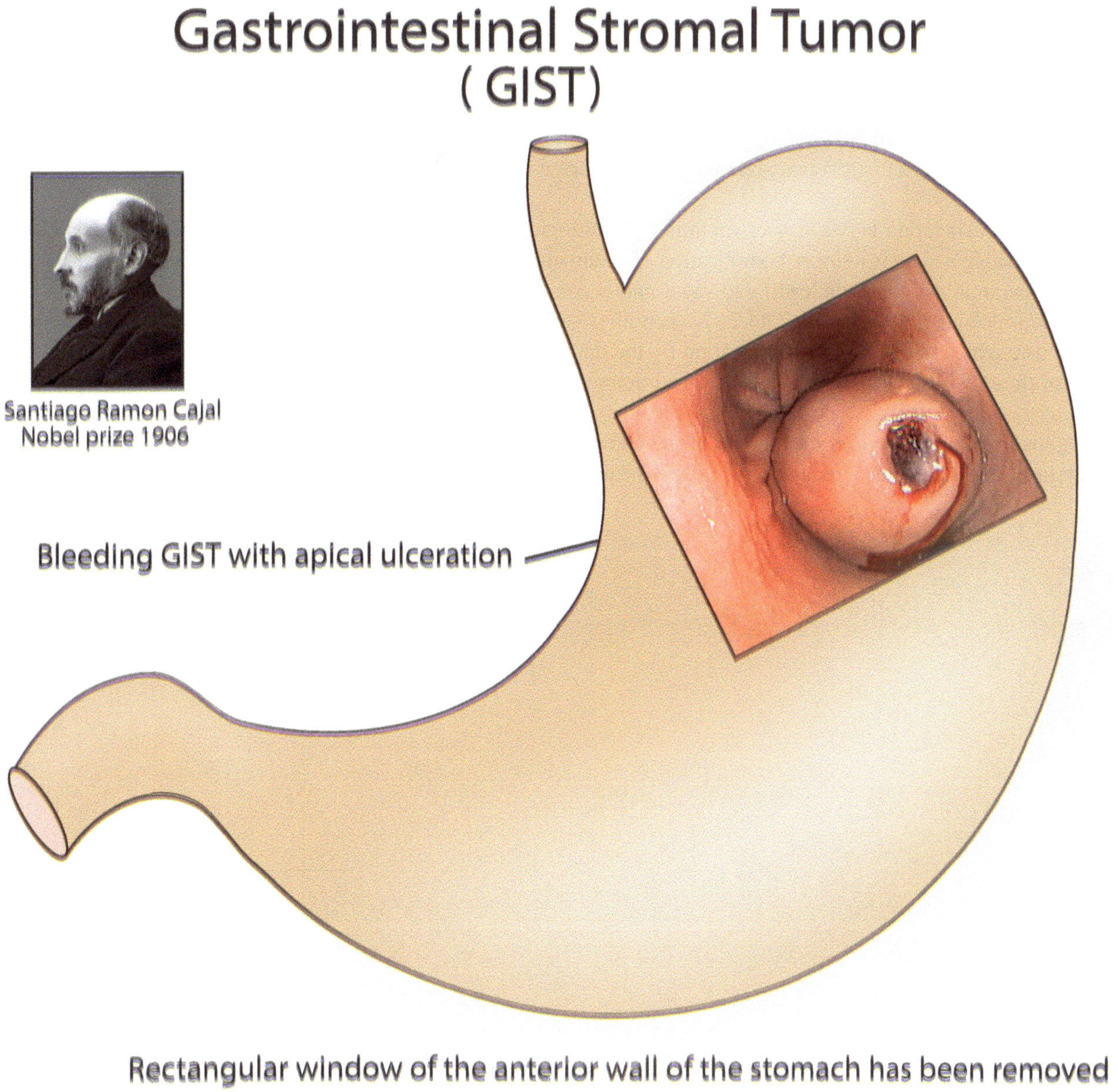

Fig. 12.7 Gastrointestinal stromal tumors arise from the submucosal interstitial cells of Cajal and develop into a submucosal neoplasm. In its classic presentation in the stomach, apical mucosa ulcerates with bleeding as the presenting symptom

Answer
c

10. All of the following are correct *except*:
    (a) NSAIDs increase the risk of peptic ulceration.
    (b) Cushing's ulcer is secondary to glucocorticoid administration.
    (c) Curling's ulcer is seen in patients with burns.
    (d) Critically injured patients should receive peptic ulcer prophylaxis.
    (e) The main complication of stress-related gastric mucosal disease is bleeding.

Comments The association between overwhelming physiologic stress and gastric ulceration and bleeding has been well established. Cushing's ulcer is a severe complication of traumatic brain injury. The mechanism of ulceration in thought to be related to intracranial hypertension leading to vagal nuclei compression and stimulation, generating excessive acid production and mucosal injury [28]. Curling's ulcer is seen after severe burns, in which hypovolemia leads to sloughing of the gastric mucosa, which is then prone to ulceration by the unopposed effect of gastric acid and pepsin [29]. Fortunately, the incidence of these two types of ulcers has decreased dramatically with the advent of gastric acid inhibition in the critically ill [30, 31].

Kissing ulcers are synchronous ulcerations of the anterior and posterior walls of the duodenum in the setting of gastric hypersecretion. They are considered more difficult to heal and more prone to complications than isolated ulcers [32, 33].

Answer

a

11. All of the following are correct *except*:
    (a) *H. pylori* requires urea to survive in acidic environments.
    (b) *H. pylori* attaches itself to the epithelium of the antrum and pylorus.
    (c) *H. pylori* gastritis is associated with gastric adenocarcinoma.
    (d) Gastric MALTomas can be cured through *H. pylori* eradication.
    (e) Gastric adenocarcinoma can be cured through *H. pylori* eradication.

Comments The gastric mucosal barrier covers all areas of the stomach. It is composed of a bicarbonate-rich mucus layer, the tightly joined epithelial cells, and the underlying blood vessels that remove acid and supply bicarbonate. When intact, this barrier allows the healthy stomach and duodenum to withstand exposure to acid, digestive enzymes, bacteria, and ingested irritants. The maintenance of this layer is modulated by multiple routes: intraluminal acid secretion, vagal stimuli, and prostaglandin production. Interestingly, the mucosal barrier is permeable to acid and pepsin secretion and yet does not allow their lateral diffusion. It is though that this property is due to the creation of temporary pores [34, 35].

H. pylori is unique in its ability to survive in the acidic environment of the stomach. To this end, it possesses multiple adaptations that allow it to resist or neutralize acidic environments. *H. pylori* inhabits the antrum and pylorus, where it burrows its way through the mucus with the use of flagella, attaching itself to the epithelium. The main acid-neutralizing defense of *H. pylori* is the presence of urease, which produces NH3 from urea, to buffer low pH. The detection of this enzyme or its activity is a useful test in the diagnosis of these bacteria [7].

The role of *H. pylori* as a carcinogen and ulcer-promoting agent has been extensively documented. Carcinogenesis is brought about by the combination of an indirect action through inflammation and a direct effect through gene modulation and mutation.

H. pylori-induced gastritis precedes the development of adenocarcinoma, with severe inflammation related to a higher likelihood of developing this malignancy. Although not fully clarified in its mechanism, the presence of inflammatory mediators has a cancer-promoting effect. *H. pylori* induces NF-kb activation in gastric epithelial cells, inhibiting apoptosis, enhancing cell growth, and promoting cell migration. It also induces dysregulation of DNA and RNA processing [36, 37].

Unfortunately, the eradication of *H. pylori* does not allow the regression of transformed cells. Paradoxically, the density of *H. pylori* colonization in the transformed mucosa is minimal when compared to that found in gastritis without dysplasia.

Perhaps the most convincing proof that *H. pylori* is involved in the pathogenesis of gastric MALT lymphoma lies in the fact that this tumor can be cured by eradication of the bacteria. It has been postulated that the inflammatory signals triggered by *H. pylori* promote the survival and proliferation of B cells, rendering them more prone to transformation.

Answer
e

12. All of the following are correct *except*:
    (a) Adenomatous gastric polyps are associated with gastric adenocarcinoma.
    (b) Hyperplastic gastric polyps may regress with *H. pylori* eradication.
    (c) Menetrier's disease is associated with exaggerated acid production.
    (d) Pernicious anemia is associated with chief and parietal cell destruction.
    (e) Antral cell hyperplasia may resolve with *H. pylori* eradication.

Comments There are three main types of gastric polyps. Fundic gland polyps are lesions with no malignant potential. They are associated in up to half of cases with familial adenomatous polyposis, and as such, may coexist with colon cancer.

Hyperplastic polyps are the most frequently found. They arise in the setting of chronic gastritis, often induced by *H. pylori*, and may regress with control of the infection. While they are not premalignant, they may harbor areas of dysplastic mucosa.

Adenomatous polyps, unlike the two prior types, are associated with gastric adenocarcinoma in as many as one fifth of cases. They may be removed endoscopically if pedunculated, smaller than 2 cm and with a clear base. It is important to know that removal of the polyp does not return the risk of cancer to baseline; on the contrary, synchronous carcinomas have been reported in up to 50 % of cases. This requires careful endoscopic initial evaluation and follow-up [38].

Menetrier's disease is a rare disorder of uncertain etiology, characterized by the development of very enlarged mucosal folds. These folds represent hyperplasia of the mucus-producing cells, with destruction of parietal and chief cells. Manifestations include protein loss from copious mucus production leading to hypoproteinemia, anemia, and hypochlorhydria. Abdominal pain, nausea, and vomiting are also present. This condition is associated with an increased risk of gastric cancer, treatment has traditionally been total gastrectomy, but EGFR antagonism may offer a molecular target [39].

Pernicious anemia is an antibody-mediated autoimmune disease, affecting the chief and parietal cells of the stomach, leading to achlorhydria and the lack of pepsinogen and acid production. It leads to chronic atrophic gastritis affecting the fundus and body of the stomach (type A, in contrast with type B gastritis involving the antrum as seen with *H. pylori*). This entity is significant because it is associated with a two- to fivefold increase in the risk of gastric cancer. Therapeutic efforts are limited to the administration of vitamin B12 [40].

In the 1970s, prior to the discovery of *H. pylori*, the association between an increased number of antral G cells, postprandial hypergastrinemia, and peptic ulcer disease was established. It was later found that the alkalinization of the antral milieu by *H. pylori* led to the said hyperplasia and that eradication of the bacteria led to its resolution. However, *H. pylori* is not present in all cases, and other causes must be explored [41].

Answer

a

References

1. Aspelund G, Langer JC. Current management of hypertrophic pyloric stenosis. Semin Pediatr Surg. 2007;16(1):27–33.
2. Naik-Mathuria B, Olutoye OO. Foregut abnormalities. Surg Clin N Am. 2006;86(2):261–84, viii.
3. Godshall D, Mossallam U, Rosenbaum R. Gastric volvulus: case report and review of the literature. J Emerg Med. 1999;17(5):837–40.
4. Soybel DI. Anatomy and physiology of the stomach. Surg Clin N Am. 2005;85(5):875–94, v.
5. Hiatt JR, Gabbay J, Busuttil RW. Surgical anatomy of the hepatic arteries in 1000 cases. Ann Surg. 1994;220(1):50–2.
6. Larsson LI. Developmental biology of gastrin and somatostatin cells in the antropyloric mucosa of the stomach. Microsc Res Tech. 2000;48(5):272–81.
7. Sachs G, Weeks DL, Melchers K, Scott DR. The gastric biology of Helicobacter pylori. Annu Rev Physiol. 2003;65:349–69.
8. Bech FR. Celiac artery compression syndromes. Surg Clin N Am. 1997;77(2):409–24.
9. Gloviczki P, Duncan AA. Treatment of celiac artery compression syndrome: does it really exist? Perspect Vasc Surg Endovasc Ther. 2007;19(3):259–63.
10. Loukas M, Pinyard J, Vaid S, Kinsella C, Tariq A, Tubbs RS. Clinical anatomy of celiac artery compression syndrome: a review. Clin Anat. 2007;20(6):612–7.
11. Donahue PE, Griffith C, Richter HM. A 50-year perspective upon selective gastric vagotomy. Am J Surg. 1996;172(1):9–12.
12. Skandalakis LJ, Donahue PE, Skandalakis JE. The vagus nerve and its vagaries. Surg Clin N Am. 1993;73(4):769–84.
13. Turnage RH, Sarosi G, Cryer B, Spechler S, Peterson W, Feldman M. Evaluation and management of patients with recurrent peptic ulcer disease after acid-reducing operations: a systematic review. J Gastrointest Surg. 2003;7(5):606–26.
14. Bech-Knudsen F, Toftgaard C. Exulceratio simplex dieulafoy. Surg Gynecol Obstet. 1993;176(2):139–43.
15. Kim HJ, Karpeh Jr MS, Brennan MF. Standardization of the extent of lymphadenectomy for gastric cancer: impact on survival. Adv Surg. 2001;35:203–23.
16. Meyer HJ, Jahne J. Lymph node dissection for gastric cancer. Semin Surg Oncol. 1999;17(2):117–24.
17. de Steur WO, Dikken JL, Hartgrink HH. Lymph node dissection in resectable advanced gastric cancer. Dig Surg. 2013;30(2):96–103.
18. Schmidt B, Chang KK, Maduekwe UN, Look-Hong N, Rattner DW, Lauwers GY, et al. D2 lymphadenectomy with surgical ex vivo dissection into node stations for gastric adenocarcinoma can be performed safely in Western patients and ensures optimal staging. Ann Surg Oncol. 2013;20(9):2991–9.
19. Katsinelos P, Zavos C, Paroutoglou G, Beltsis A, Kountouras J. Education and imaging. Gastrointestinal: retained gastric antrum. J Gastroenterol Hepatol. 2007;22(3):448.
20. Yilmaz S, Yekeler E, Dural C, Dursun M, Akyol Y, Acunas B. Afferent loop syndrome secondary to Billroth II gastrojejunostomy obstruction: multidetector computed tomography findings. Surgery. 2007;141(4):538–9.
21. Ukleja A. Dumping syndrome: pathophysiology and treatment. Nutr Clin Pract. 2005;20(5):517–25.
22. Scholmerich J. Postgastrectomy syndromes – diagnosis and treatment. Best Pract Res Clin Gastroenterol. 2004;18(5):917–33.
23. Sanders KM. Interstitial cells of Cajal at the clinical and scientific interface. J Physiol. 2006;576(Pt 3):683–7.
24. Ward SM, Sanders KM. Physiology and pathophysiology of the interstitial cell of Cajal: from bench to bedside. I. Functional development and plasticity of interstitial cells of Cajal networks. Am J Physiol Gastrointest Liver Physiol. 2001;281(3):G602–11.
25. Hirst GD, Edwards FR. Role of interstitial cells of Cajal in the control of gastric motility. J Pharmacol Sci. 2004;96(1):1–10.
26. Takaki M. Gut pacemaker cells: the interstitial cells of Cajal (ICC). J Smooth Muscle Res. 2003;39(5):137–61.
27. Katz SC, DeMatteo RP. Gastrointestinal stromal tumors and leiomyosarcomas. J Surg Oncol. 2008;97(4):350–9.
28. Alain BB, Wang YJ. Cushing's ulcer in traumatic brain injury. Chin J Traumatol. 2008;11(2):114–9.
29. Moran KT, O'Reilly T, Munster AM. A combined regimen for the prophylaxis of Curling's ulcer. Am Surg. 1987;53(10):575–6.
30. Marrone GC, Silen W. Pathogenesis, diagnosis and treatment of acute gastric mucosal lesions. Clin Gastroenterol. 1984;13(2):635–50.
31. Steinberg KP. Stress-related mucosal disease in the critically ill patient: risk factors and strategies to prevent stress-related bleeding in the intensive care unit. Crit Care Med. 2002;30(6 Suppl):S362–4.
32. Stabile BE, Hardy HJ, Passaro Jr E. 'Kissing' duodenal ulcers. Arch Surg. 1979;114(10):1153–6.
33. Pecora PG, Kaplan B. Corticosteroids and ulcers: is there an association? Ann Pharmacother. 1996;30(7–8):870–2.
34. Ham M, Kaunitz JD. Gastroduodenal defense. Curr Opin Gastroenterol. 2007;23(6):607–16.
35. Allen A, Flemstrom G. Gastroduodenal mucus bicarbonate barrier: protection against acid and pepsin. Am J Physiol Cell Physiol. 2005;288(1):C1–19.
36. Moss SF, Malfertheiner P. Helicobacter and gastric malignancies. Helicobacter. 2007;12 Suppl 1:23–30.
37. Chiba T, Marusawa H, Seno H, Watanabe N. Mechanism for gastric cancer development by Helicobacter pylori infection. J Gastroenterol Hepatol. 2008;23(8):1175–81.
38. Park DY, Lauwers GY. Gastric polyps: classification and management. Arch Pathol Lab Med. 2008;132(4):633–40.
39. Coffey RJ, Washington MK, Corless CL, Heinrich MC. Menetrier disease and gastrointestinal stromal tumors: hyperproliferative disorders of the stomach. J Clin Invest. 2007;117(1):70–80.
40. Toh BH, Alderuccio F. Pernicious anaemia. Autoimmunity. 2004;37(4):357–61.
41. Kwan CP, Tytgat GN. Antral G-cell hyperplasia: a vanishing disease? Eur J Gastroenterol Hepatol. 1995;7(11):1099–103.

13 Small Bowel

1. Select the *true* statement regarding the differences between the jejunum and ileum:
   (a) The ileum has more and larger lymphoid follicles.
   (b) The jejunum has thinner walls.
   (c) The root of the mesentery is attached from the right of the first lumbar vertebra to the left lower quadrant.
   (d) The ileum has a single line of arterial arcades with longer vasa recta.
   (e) The jejunum has three to five arcades with shorter vasa recta.

Comments The small bowel is the segment of the GI tract responsible for nutrient absorption. It receives its blood supply form the superior mesenteric artery, which distributes its branches along the mesentery. The small bowel mesentery originates to the left of L1–L2, at the level of the duodenojejunal junction. It travels diagonally towards the right sacroiliac joint, crossing anterior to the duodenum, pancreas, and great vessels.

There have been varied estimations of the length of the small bowel, with a 20–25 % elongation of the bowel reported in cadavers as compared to live subjects. Intraoperative measurements have shown an average length of 460 cm (15 ft), with a standard deviation of 78 cm (30 in.). No statistically significant differences in small bowel length on the basis of sex, height, age, and weight exist. Excluding the duodenum, the jejunum comprises approximately 30–40 % of the small bowel and the ileum 60–70 % [1].

Distinguishing the jejunum from the ileum may be difficult. Several criteria have been proposed, but none are completely reliable. It has been noted that the jejunum has thicker walls, a larger lumen, more prominent plicae circulares, and a single line of arterial arcades with longer vasa recta. All traits are related to the larger amount of nutrient it handles and its greater absorptive capacity. The jejunal mesenteric fat does not extend onto the bowel.

The ileum has more specialized absorptive functions, including the absorption of bile salts, fat-soluble vitamins, and vitamin B12. The ileum also possesses a greater concentration of lymphatic tissue (Peyer's patches), which are involved both in the maintenance of immune tolerance to gut antigens and nutrients and in the defense against pathogens. This abundance of lymphoid tissue explains the greater frequency of infectious bowel perforations in the terminal ileum, as well as the predilection of autoimmune disease and lymphomas for this segment of the GI tract [2].

Answer
a

V.K. Maker, E.D. Guzman-Arrieta, *Cognitive Pearls in General Surgery*,
DOI 10.1007/978-1-4939-1850-8_13,

2. Select the *incorrect* statement regarding the embryology of the small bowel:
   (a) The foregut and midgut meet just distal to the ampulla of Vater.
   (b) The axis of midgut rotation is the superior mesenteric artery.
   (c) Intestinal rotation occurs in a counterclockwise direction.
   (d) The first portion of the midgut to return to the abdomen is the cecum.
   (e) Intestinal malrotation leads to a shortened mesentery.

Comments Classically, the rotation of the small bowel has been described as occurring in three steps [3]:
Herniation into the yolk sac and 90° counterclockwise rotation
Reduction into the abdomen (jejunum first) and 180° counterclockwise rotation
Fixation with cecal descent

While herniation of the midgut has been explained by a disproportion in the size of the gut in comparison to the size of the abdomen, the driving force behind an en bloc midgut rotation has not been identified.

In complete malrotation there is less than 90° of rotation. The small bowel lies in the right abdomen, and the cecum is to the left, in the caudal portion of the abdomen. In incomplete malrotation there is near to 180° of rotation. Again, the small bowel lies in the right abdomen, with the cecum located cranially and to the left. In either case, the mesenteric attachment of the small bowel is narrow and prone to shortening. In addition, bands between the cecum and right body wall (Ladd's bands) cross in front of the duodenum, potentially compressing it [4]. Ladd's procedure addresses these defects as illustrated below (Fig. 13.1).

Embryologic studies in rat models suggest that there is no true midgut rotation; rather, the adult configuration of the midgut is the product of differential growth of segments of the small bowel. According to this model, the growth of the duodenojejunal region "pushes" the proximal jejunum behind the mesenteric vessels towards the left upper quadrant. The position of the cecum is attributed to the pattern of return of the bowel. Under this model, the anomalies termed "malrotation" are in reality a failure in the growth of the duodenojejunal junction that remains to the right of the midline [5].

What both models agree upon is that there is greater degree of growth in the segment proximal to the axis of the superior mesenteric artery than in the caudal part. This explains the proximity of Meckel's diverticulum to the ileocecal valve.

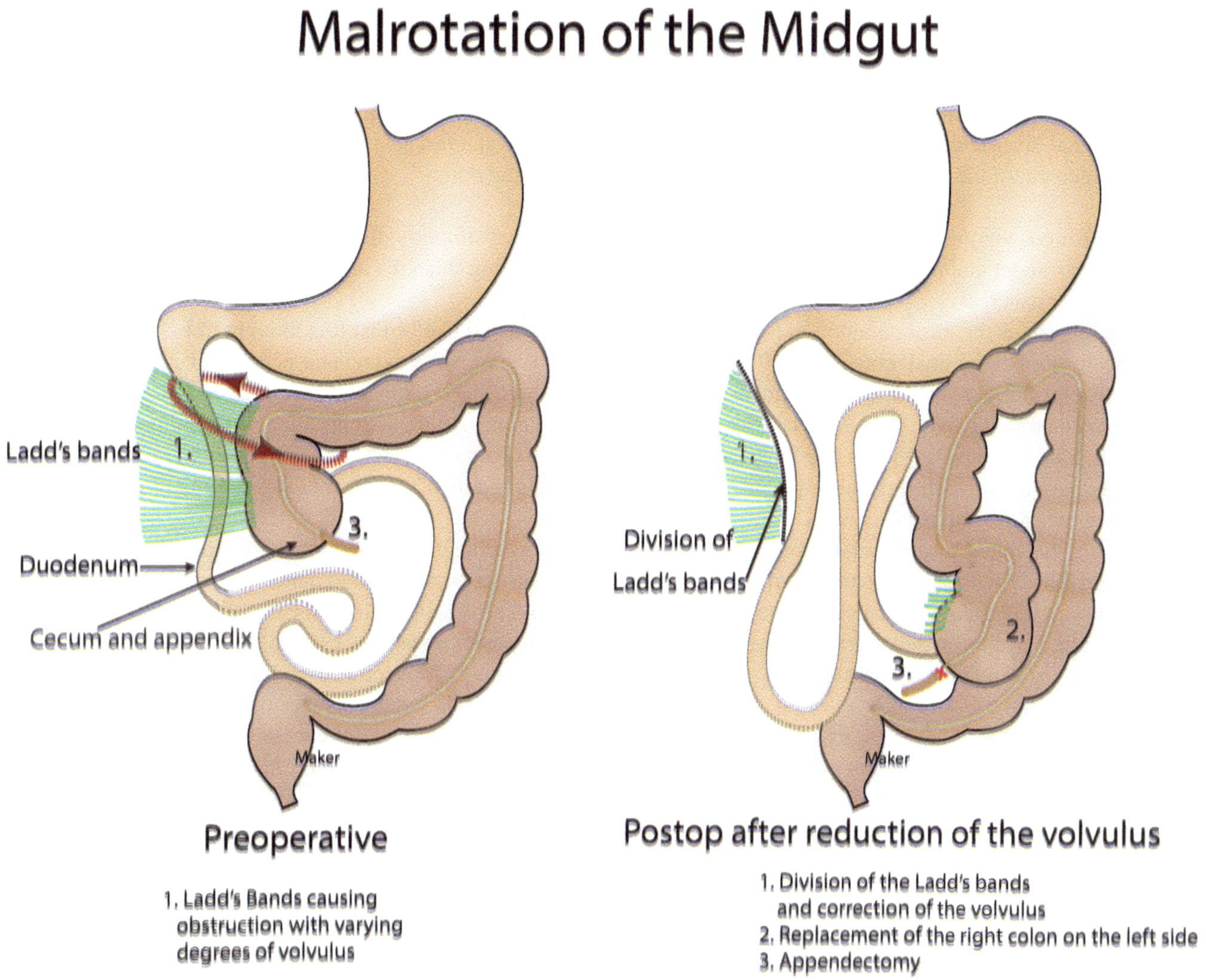

Fig. 13.1 Ladd's bands extend from the lateral abdominal wall to the cecum and cross over the duodenum. These bands form as part of the complex series of events during the rotation of the gut in the fetus. Midgut volvulus can be present in varying degrees from asymptomatic incomplete rotation to complete 360° midgut volvulus with impending vascular compromise if not recognized and treated emergently. The classic 3-step Ladd's procedure is illustrated

Answer
d

3. Select the *true* statement in relation to congenital pathology of the small bowel.
   (a) Duodenal atresia is accompanied by dilatation of the distal segment.
   (b) Intestinal atresia represents a failure of recanalization.
   (c) Duplicated intestinal segments are always located on the antimesenteric side of the normal intestine.
   (d) Duodenal diverticula are most commonly found opposite to the pancreas.
   (e) The segment of the small bowel most affected by diverticula is the ileum.

Comments Bilious vomiting in the neonatal period is suggestive of an obstruction distal to the ampulla of Vater, i.e., at the junction of the foregut and midgut. The three common anomalies affecting this area are duodenal atresia, midgut malrotation, and annular pancreas.

Duodenal atresia is the most common of the three, occurring in 1:10,000 live births. It is thought to be a result of failure in the recanalization of the small bowel at 8–10 weeks of gestation. It is commonly associated with annular pancreas, preduodenal portal vein, malrotation, biliary malformations, and esophageal atresia. The diagnosis is suggested by polyhydramnios and bile-stained amniotic fluid, reflecting the lack of passage into the more distal gastrointestinal tract. Although classically described in duodenal atresia, the double bubble sign can be seen in other forms of postampullary obstruction. Duodenal stenosis may have a more delayed and subtle presentation. Treatment consists of duodenoduodenostomy or resection of the duodenal web when present [6] (Fig. 13.2).

It is thought that intestinal atresia is the result of ischemia to the developing midgut. In fact, this condition has been experimentally reproduced by vascular ligation. Furthermore, intestinal atresia has been linked to maternal exposure to tobacco and other vasoconstricting agents. Patients with intestinal atresia present with obstruction during the first days of life. While failure to pass meconium is often quoted, atresias occurring later in fetal development may allow enough time for meconium to reach the bowel distal to the point of obstruction. Type 1 intestinal atresia (web) may be treated with web excision and stricturoplasty if needed. A search for further webs must be undertaken. Other types of atresia require re-anastomosis of the separated segments of the bowel. It is often necessary to resect segments of the bowel that have become excessively dilated [7].

Both the midgut and hindgut may give rise to duplicated segments of the intestine, being more common in the former, especially in the terminal ileum. They are typically located along the mesenteric border of the normal bowel, with which they have a shared blood supply. This feature dictates that they must be removed by segmental bowel resection and anastomosis. These structures have serosal, muscular, and mucosal layers. They often present by causing abdominal pain and obstruction or as an abdominal mass [8].

Duodenal diverticula are present in 5–22 % of the population. They are most often false diverticula located along the pancreatic border of the duodenum and may be in close proximity to the ampulla of Vater. While they are most often asymptomatic, they may give rise to inflammation, perforation, hemorrhage, and obstruction of the common bile duct and pancreatic duct [9].

Diverticula of the jejunum and ileum are much less frequent than those of the duodenum, affecting approximately 1 % of the population. 80 % are located in the jejunum, along the mesenteric border. Their incidence increases with age, a finding which is consistent with their occurrence through a pulsion mechanism generating false diverticula. Like duodenal diverticula, they are most often asymptomatic, but may give rise to inflammatory and hemorrhagic complications [10].

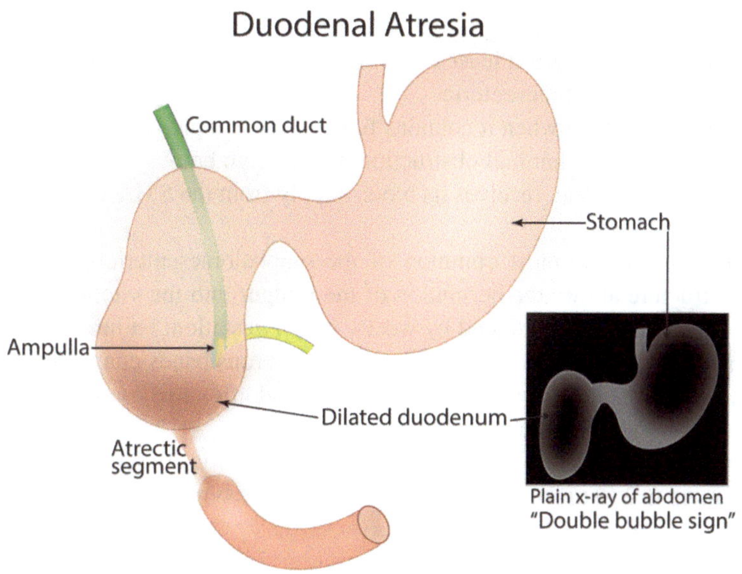

Fig. 13.2 In over 85 % of cases, the duodenum is atretic distal to the ampulla, thereby presenting with bilious emesis and without abdominal distention. Annular pancreas and midgut malrotation are in the differential diagnosis and must be ruled out

Answer
b

4. All of the following are correct *except*:
   (a) Meckel's diverticulum is usually found at least 2 ft away from the ileocecal valve.
   (b) Meckel's diverticulum is always antimesenteric.
   (c) Meckel's diverticulum may ulcerate when it contains functioning ectopic gastric mucosa.
   (d) Meckel's diverticulitis is caused by luminal obstruction by a foreign body.
   (e) Meckel's diverticulum, when present, receives its blood supply from the SMA.

Comments Meckel's diverticulum is the most common of the omphalomesenteric duct (vitelline duct) abnormalities. During embryonic life, this structure allows the herniation of the midgut into the vitelline sac and subsequent return. The omphalomesenteric duct usually becomes obliterated by weeks 8–9 of gestation. Failure in this process may lead to persistence of the omphalomesenteric duct, formation of sinuses, cysts, or fibrous bands connecting the ileum with the umbilicus and its most common anomaly, the Meckel's diverticulum [11, 12]. In addition to these anomalies, the urachus and umbilical veins may also give rise to pathology in this area (Fig. 13.3).

Meckel's diverticulum is a true diverticulum located over the antimesenteric border of the ileum, usually within 2 ft of the ileocecal valve. It is present in up to 2 % of the population. While mostly asymptomatic, they usually present within the first 2 years of life [13].

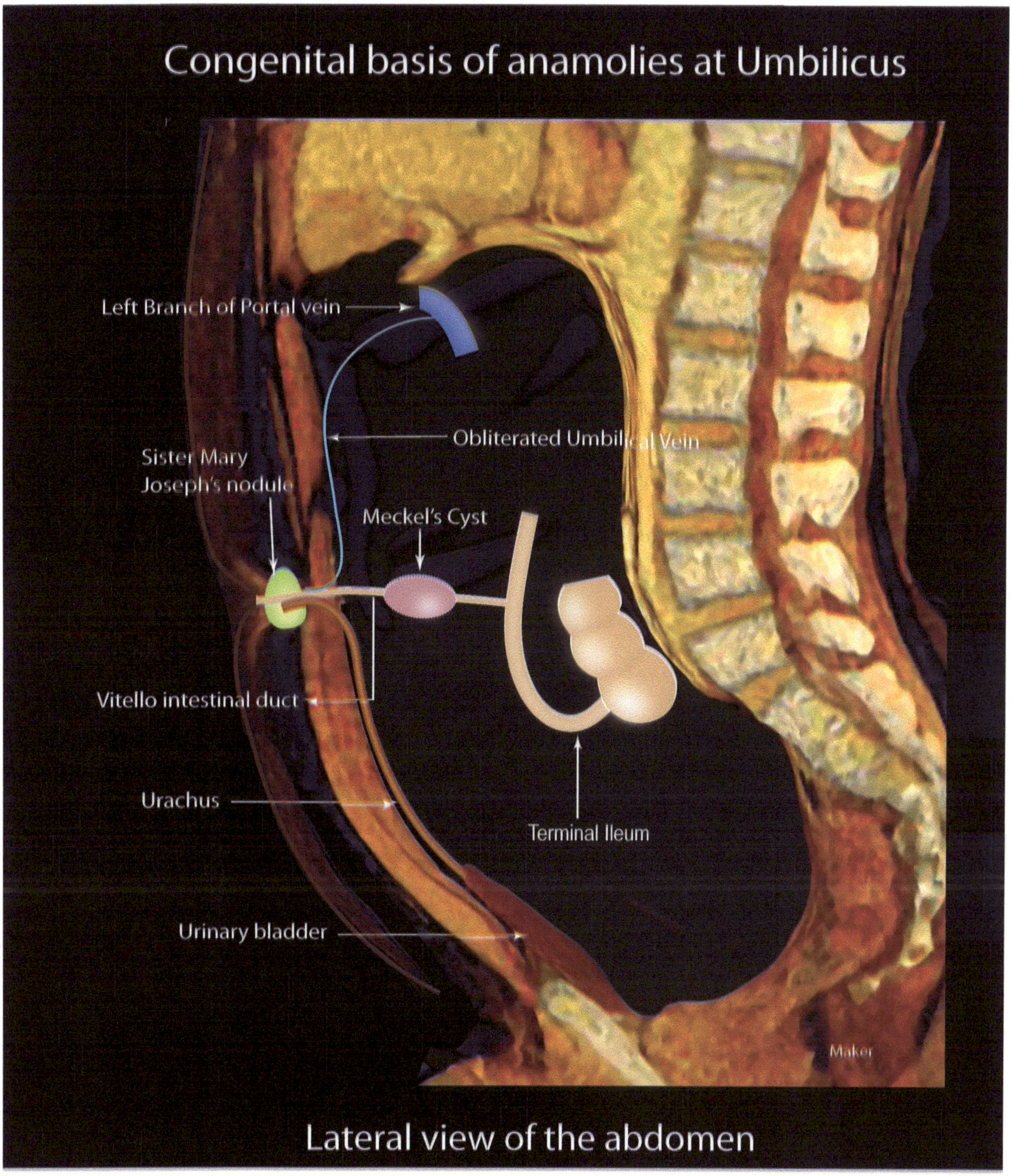

Fig. 13.3 Multiple clinical problems may manifest at the umbilicus based on the vestigial connections that existed between the mother and the fetus. The remnant of the vitellointestinal duct may present as an intestinal draining fistula, Meckel's cyst, Meckel's diverticulum, or even a tight band attaching the umbilicus to the intestine with its own set of problems. Remnants of the urachus may present as a urinary fistula or an urachal cyst. A patent umbilical vein likely forms secondary to portal hypertension and eventually developes into a caput medusa at the umbilicus. Sister Mary Joseph's nodule from a metastatic abdominal malignancy, and umbilical endometriosis, likely results from travel along the fetal pathway of peritoneal ligaments, veins, and lymphatics that drain towards the umbilicus

The most common presentation is obstruction, in which the diverticulum acts as a lead point for intussusception. When attached to the umbilicus, it may also serve as an axis for torsion.

Bleeding is the next most common complication, and it is caused by the presence of ectopic gastric mucosa leading to ulceration. In this setting, the ectopic mucosa and the diverticulum harboring it may be detected through a technetium-99m pertechnetate scan (Meckel's scan). Clinically, ectopic mucosa appears as a solid structure during the transillumination of the Meckel's diverticulum (Fig. 13.4).

Inflammation is clinically undistinguishable from acute appendicitis and is a finding of up to 1 % of appendectomies. A rare complication of a large Meckel's diverticulum is malabsorption and presence of multiple "Meckoliths."

Treatment of the complications of Meckel's diverticulum involves either wedge resection with transverse closure or segmental resection and anastomosis, depending upon the status of the adjacent bowel. The treatment of incidentally discovered Meckel's diverticula is controversial [14] (Fig. 13.5).

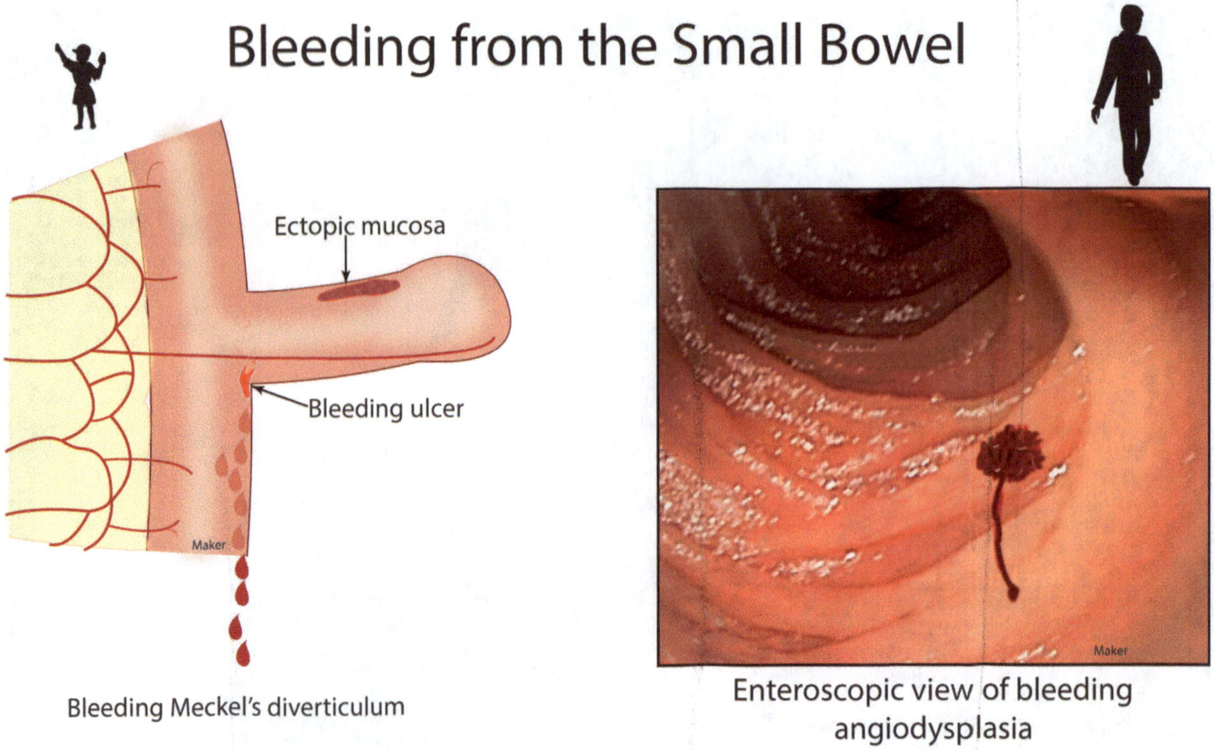

Fig. 13.4 The most common cause of lower GI bleeding in children is Meckel's diverticulum. Meckel's diverticulum contains ectopic mucosa over 60 % of the time. The most common ectopic mucosa is gastric, which may produce bleeding ulcers typically located at the junction with the small bowel. The vast majority of lesions causing GI bleeding can be seen with upper and lower endoscopy. Obscure GI bleeding in adults comes from small bowel angiodysplasia in 75 % of the patients

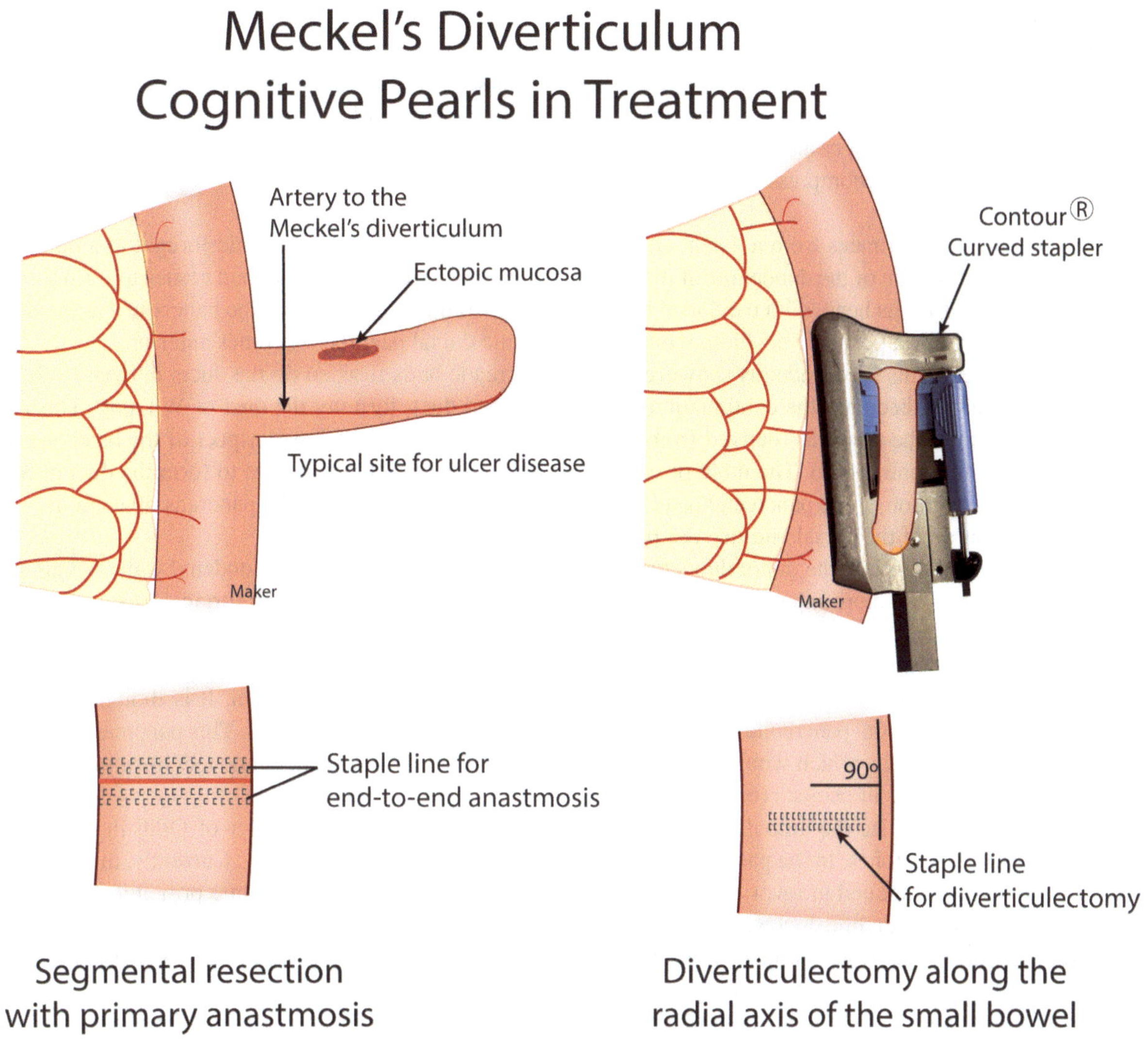

Fig. 13.5 A broad-based Meckel's diverticulum is treated with segmental resection of the ileum. A narrow-based diverticulum can be treated with diverticulectomy. The author's choice is to utilize the curved stapler fired at 90° from the longitudinal axis of the ileum to avoid narrowing of the lumen. A curved stapler helps with en bloc excision of the diverticulum with a cuff of the terminal ileum

Answer
a

5. All of the following are correct *except*:
   (a) The duct of Wirsung is derived from the ventral pancreatic bud.
   (b) The common bile duct may be accidentally sutured in the course of oversewing a bleeding duodenal ulcer.
   (c) A penetrating peptic ulcer can cause pancreatitis by eroding into the duct of Santorini.
   (d) An annular pancreas is best treated by division.
   (e) Papillotomy for biliary decompression is performed at an 11 o'clock position.

Comments The pancreas originates from a dorsal and ventral bud arising from the embryonic foregut at a point which is analogous to the second portion of the duodenum at the future sphincter of Oddi. The ventral bud comes to form the uncinate process and lower portion of the head, with the dorsal bud originating from the remainder of the pancreas. Paradoxically, the ventral bud comes to occupy a posterior position, while the embryonic dorsal pancreas becomes anterior.

Originally, each duct drains independently; however, as the pancreatic buds fuse, so do the ducts in over 70 % of cases. The duct of the ventral bud becomes the continuation of the dorsal bud duct, forming the duct of Wirsung. This duct then drains the body and tail of the pancreas (derived from the dorsal bud) as well as the lower aspect of the head and uncinate process (derived from the ventral bud). The more proximal part of the dorsal bud duct comes to form the duct of Santorini, which drains the upper portion of the pancreatic head. Failure of this ductal fusion leads to pancreas divisum, in which the duct of Santorini drains all of the dorsal bud-derived pancreatic tissue [15].

The duct of Santorini drains into the minor duodenal papilla, located in the anteromedial duodenal wall, 1–3 cm proximal to the major papilla. Being the more superficial of the two ducts, it may be injured during the surgical treatment of penetrating peptic ulcer disease.

Annular pancreas is the most common congenital pancreatic anomaly presenting in children. It constitutes a ring of normal pancreatic tissue encircling, and often constricting, the second portion of the duodenum. It is thought to represent a defect in the rotation of the ventral pancreatic bud as it rotates to the right to join the dorsal bud. This pancreatic tissue usually contains ductal structures within, which would be injured by division. In light of this, duodenoduodenostomy and duodenojejunostomy are the treatments of choice [16, 17].

It is often necessary to incise the ampulla of Vater and divide the fibers of the sphincter of Oddi in order to extract impacted common bile duct stones. In the past this was accomplished through a duodenotomy. Currently, this procedure has been almost completely abandoned in favor of an endoscopic approach. However, the anatomic principle of extending the line of incision into the common bile duct while protecting the pancreatic duct and associated sphincteric structures is applicable to both procedures. This is accomplished by incising the ampulla at an 11 o'clock position, which is the axis along which the common bile duct lays. In contrast, the pancreatic duct is located between the 3 and 5 o'clock position. It is thought that injury to the pancreatic duct can predispose to acute pancreatitis by making biliary reflux into the pancreas more likely [18] (Fig. 13.6).

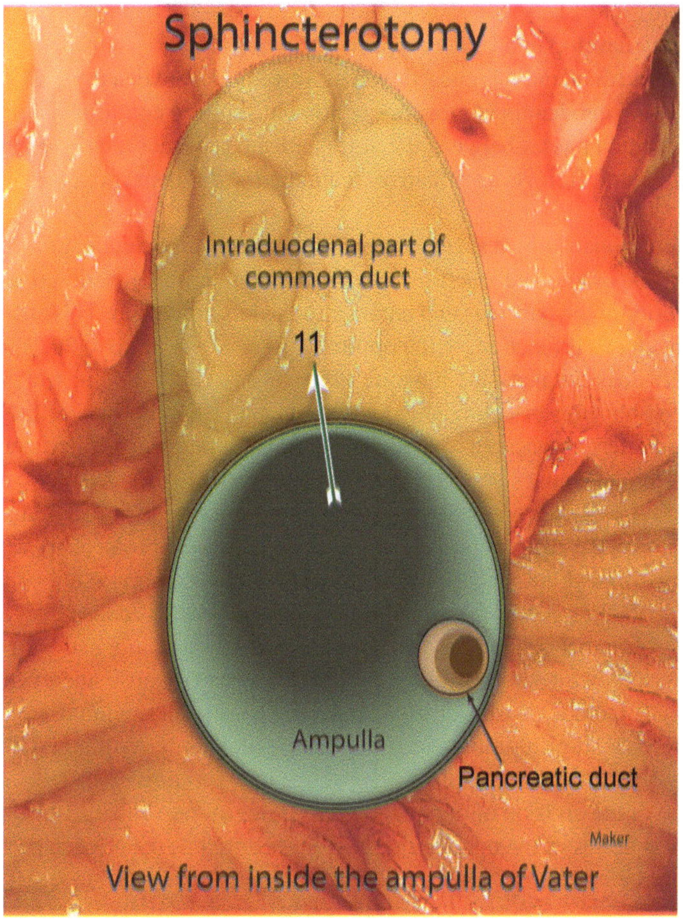

Fig. 13.6 Sphincterotomy is a relatively common procedure where the sphincter of Oddi is safely divided at close to the 11 o'clock position, which is along the direction of the intraduodenal common duct. Injury to the pancreatic duct can thereby be avoided during this procedure

Answer
d

6. Select the *incorrect* statement.
   (a) Quadriplegic patients may develop duodenal compression syndrome.
   (b) Vascular compression of the duodenum is caused by a narrow angle between the aorta and superior mesenteric artery.
   (c) Vascular compression of the duodenum is most frequently an acquired condition.
   (d) The first part of the duodenum passes between the aorta and superior mesenteric artery.
   (e) Transection of the ligament of Treitz is an effective treatment for duodenal compression syndrome.

Comments The ligament of Treitz, also known as the suspensory muscle of the duodenum, is a band of fibromuscular tissue arising from the left crus of the diaphragm and inserting into the duodenojejunal junction. It is fixed to the celiac trunk in its middle portion. It courses posterior to the pancreas and anterior to the left renal vein. This structure is often very tenuous and does not appear to serve any mechanical function, to the point that its absence in up to 20 % of the population is asymptomatic [19]. The ligament of Treitz does *not* mark the junction of the foregut and midgut, which actually occurs in the second portion of the duodenum at the sphincter of Oddi. This location is also the point where the superior pancreaticoduodenal (foregut–celiac trunk) meets the inferior pancreaticoduodenal (midgut–superior mesenteric artery).

The third portion of the duodenum courses between the aorta and the superior mesenteric artery, which normally forms a 40 to 60° angle that allows passage without compression. Narrowing of this angle may be caused by wasting of the inframesenteric fat pad (due to weight loss and quadriplegia), decrease in the degree of thoracic spine kyphosis, and downward traction on the mesentery or retroperitoneal masses. In these settings, vascular compression of the duodenum may arise. This entity has been classically described in young females undergoing scoliosis correction surgery with perioperative weight loss. Manifestations include postprandial abdominal pain, nausea, bilious vomiting, and weight loss [20] (Fig. 13.7).

CT angiography is useful in the diagnosis and ruling out the presence of aortic aneurysms or masses that may present similarly. Conservative treatment includes nasogastric decompression and nasojejunal feeding in attempts to restore the inframesenteric fat pad. The optimal surgical treatment is duodenojejunostomy. While gastrojejunostomy is also feasible, it may not alleviate the duodenal obstruction and result in persistence of symptoms.

Strong's procedure consisted of the division of the ligament of Treitz (of no value as an isolated treatment) and downward mobilization of the 3rd and 4th portions of the duodenum. This procedure has the advantage of not violating the integrity of the bowel but has been shown to be ineffective in up to 25 % of cases [21].

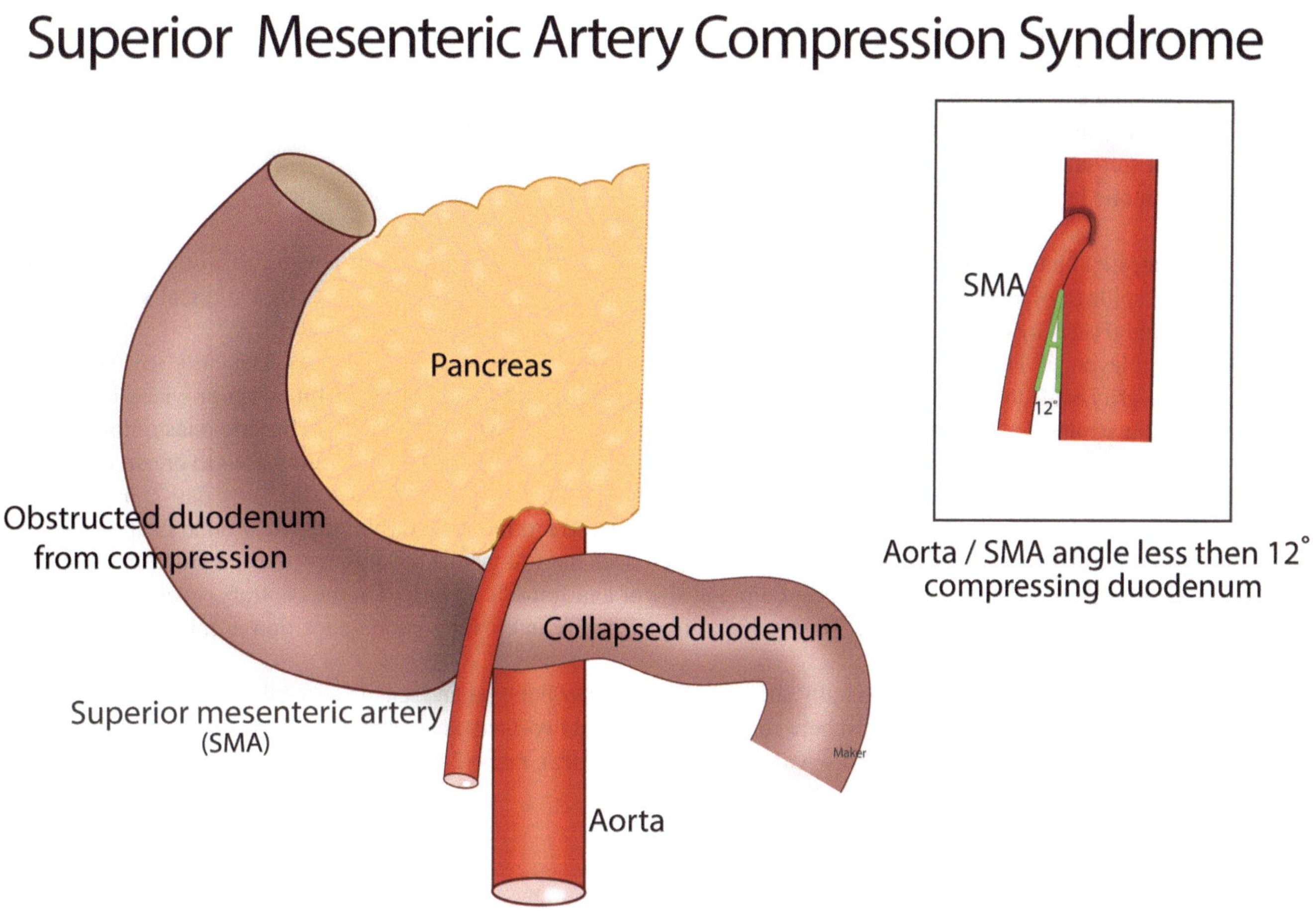

Fig. 13.7 The superior mesenteric artery courses distally from its origin, creating a tight space at its apex through which runs the third portion of the duodenum and the left renal vein. When this critical space gets tighter, the proximal duodenum becomes obstructed from extrinsic compression causing superior mesenteric artery syndrome

Answer

d

7. All of the following are correct *except*:
   (a) Stapled anastomoses are eversion-type anastomoses as compared to inversion anastomosis in the hand-sewn method.
   (b) The bursting strength of inversion anastomosis is higher than that of eversion anastomosis.
   (c) The antimesenteric side of the intestine has the poorest blood supply.
   (d) Lack of serosal coverage is associated with higher leak rates.
   (e) Anastomotic hematomas are an important cause of tissue ischemia and anastomotic failure.

Comments Intestinal anastomosis must appose two segments of the GI tract in a manner leading to wound healing while preventing the spillage of enteric contents. These functions are often accomplished by sutures and surgical staples. While devices that hold tissues by compression alone have been developed, their use is not widespread [22].

The different layers of the intestinal wall serve different roles in the healing of an anastomosis. The early reestablishment of mucosal integrity seals the anastomosis and acts as a barrier to intestinal bacteria. The submucosa provides mechanical strength to the anastomosis. The apposition of the serosal layer minimizes the rate of leakage. Enteric anastomosis has the lowest bursting strength (50 %) 2–3 days after being created, point at which the staples or sutures used to create the anastomosis play their most crucial role. Thereafter, bursting pressure increases, reaching almost a 100 % by day 7. Interestingly, neither glucocorticoids nor radiation therapy appears to play an important role in disturbing enteric wound healing.

While blood supply is crucial for adequate wound healing, it does not follow that the antimesenteric border of the bowel – which has the poorest blood supply – is the most common site of anastomotic leakage. On the contrary, in end-to-end anastomosis, it is the mesenteric side that fails. This is due to the difficulty in creating good apposition at this level, especially when the mesentery is bulky [23].

Stapled anastomosis has been experimentally shown to have greater bursting and tensile strength than sutured anastomosis. No significant differences appear to exist between single layer and two-layer anastomosis. All three types of anastomosis (stapled, single layer, and double layer hand sewn) have comparable leak rates [24].

Answer
d

8. All of the following regarding short bowel syndrome are true *except*:
   (a) Patients with less than 120 cm of the remaining small bowel develop symptoms of short gut syndrome.
   (b) Patients with less than 60 cm of the small bowel and no ileocecal valve become dependent on total parenteral nutrition.
   (c) Ileal resection is better tolerated than jejunal resection.
   (d) Retroperistaltic small bowel interpositions delay small bowel emptying.
   (e) Preservation of the ileocecal valve with 45 cm of the ileum may prevent parenteral nutrition dependency in short bowel syndrome.

Comments Short bowel syndrome is the result of massive bowel resections most often performed for the treatment of mesenteric infarction (adults) and small bowel volvulus or necrotizing enterocolitis (children). Advances in the treatment of Crohn's disease have made it a less frequent etiology.

The abnormalities in the absorption of water and macronutrients and fat-soluble vitamins (A, D, E, and K) are most dependent on the extent of bowel resected, while particular micronutrient deficiencies are determined by the area of the bowel that is resected.

The bowel has considerable functional reserve capacity, which allows the resection of up to 50 % of the small bowel. Resections of 50–70 % may lead to transient malabsorption which can be resolved by intestinal adaptation. Interestingly, in this setting the colon acquires the capacity to absorb short-chain fatty acids. However, resections greater than 70 % or those that leave less than 100–120 cm of the small bowel determine the development of short gut syndrome. Loss of bowel is better tolerated if the ileocecal valve is preserved.

The duodenum and terminal ileum have specific absorptive properties that cannot be replaced by other segments of the bowel. The duodenum is responsible for the absorption of calcium, magnesium, iron, and folic acid. The terminal ileum absorbs vitamin B12 and bile salts. Vitamins B1, B2, B6, and C are absorbed by the entire small bowel.

After massive small bowel resection, the exposure to nutrients is necessary to induce adaptation. Anatomic adaptation achieves an increase of the small bowel absorptive area by increases in length and diameter of the remaining bowel, as well as by hyperplasia of the mucosa. Physiologic adaptation includes a decrease in peristalsis and an increase in the absorptive capacity for some nutrients at a cellular level. The ileocecal region not only delays small bowel emptying but also induces adaptation of the remainder of the bowel through the release of trophic factors [25].

Surgical interventions have been reserved for patients in whom nonoperative treatments have failed and should be performed after small bowel adaptation has been maximized. Approaches include bowel lengthening, interposition of an antiperistaltic segment of the bowel, and creation of artificial valves to delay intestinal transit. Whenever possible, reincorporation of the colon by takedown of ileostomies and jejunostomies should be performed. Small bowel transplantation by itself or combined with liver transplantation has the potential to cure short gut syndrome and the hepatic complications of long-term TPN and is becoming a more frequently used alternative [2, 26].

Answer

c

9. All of the following are correct regarding mesenteric ischemia *except*:
   (a) The superior mesenteric artery is the most common site of visceral embolism.
   (b) The ileum has better collateral circulation than the jejunum.
   (c) Thrombotic occlusion is associated with preexisting atherosclerosis.
   (d) The splenic flexure is the area of the bowel with the least circulation.
   (e) SMA embolism primarily compromises the right colon.

Comments The superior mesenteric artery arises at the level of L1, approximately 1 cm below the origin of the celiac trunk. Its branches are the inferior pancreaticoduodenal, middle colic, right colic, 4–6 jejunal branches, 9–13 ileal branches, and the ileocolic artery, which is a terminal artery. The greater number of branches to the ileum, together with the more developed anastomotic arcades, renders this portion of the small bowel more tolerant of ischemic insults.

Splanchnic blood flow varies widely in relation to digestion. At rest flow is approximately 300 ml/min, exhibiting a waveform typical of a high-resistance outflow bed. During digestion, flow quadruples and becomes antegrade throughout the cardiac cycle. This variation is the physiologic basis for the manifestations of chronic mesenteric ischemia.

Acute mesenteric ischemia is usually the result of embolism (50 %), thrombosis (25 %), and nonocclusive mesenteric ischemia (25 %). Mesenteric vein thrombosis is a rare cause.

SMA emboli usually arise from the heart. The majority lodge distal to the origin of the middle colic artery, where the artery starts to taper after giving rise to this large vessel. In contrast, SMA thrombi occur at the origin of the vessel, flush with the aorta, and are associated with atherosclerotic disease in this area.

Nonocclusive mesenteric ischemia is the product of low flow. Causes include cardiogenic shock, sepsis, and pressor-induced vasospasm. The areas most affected are those with the least collateral circulation, namely, the splenic flexure, the distal sigmoid, and proximal rectum. This form of mesenteric ischemia is becoming more frequent as the population of critically ill patients rises. Interestingly, mesenteric ischemia may be worsened in these patients by enteral feeding and may result in necrosis and perforation [27, 28] (Fig. 13.8).

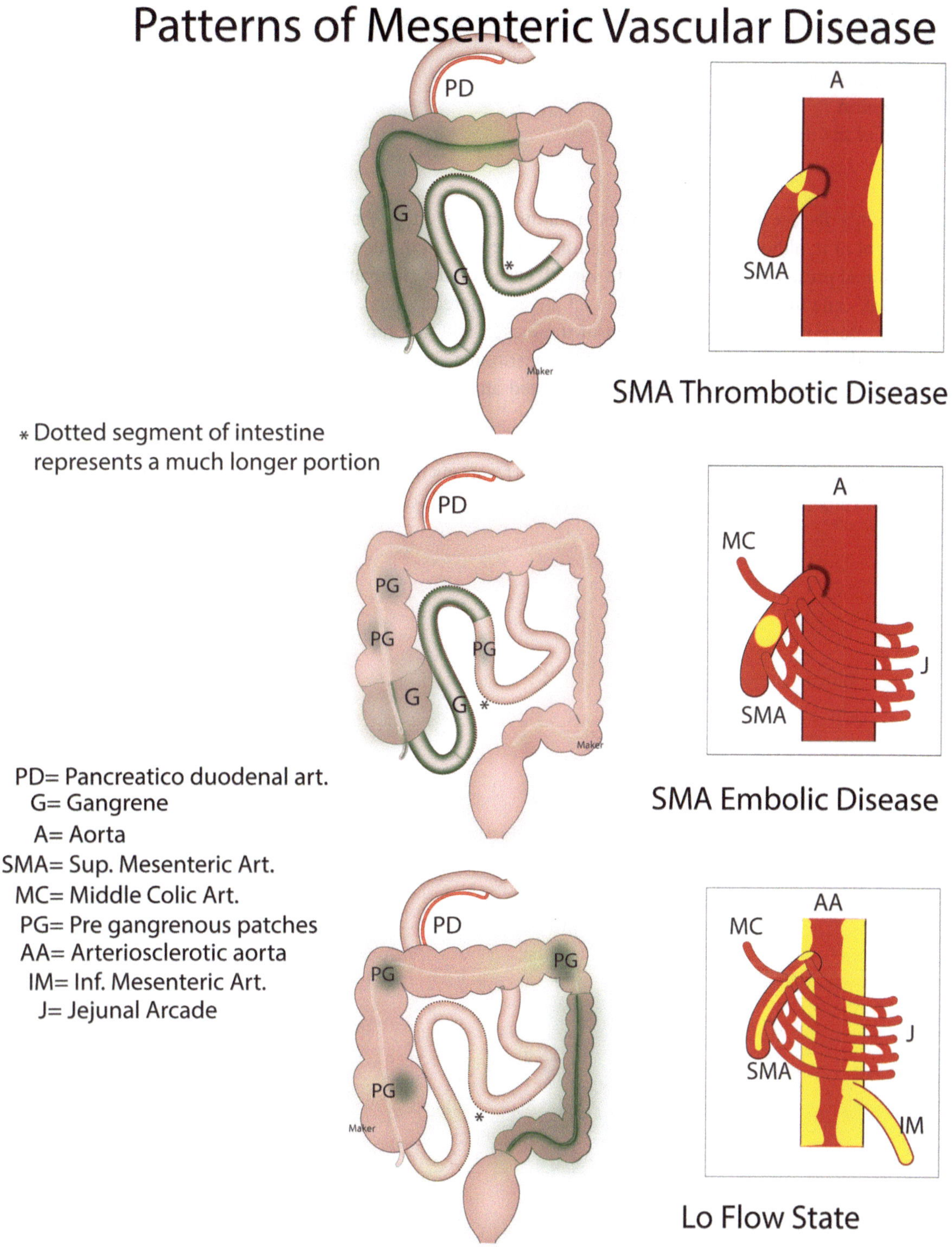

Fig. 13.8 Superior mesenteric artery thrombotic disease typically affects the origin of the artery from the aorta, and hence, the entire midgut is at risk of ischemic gangrene. Collaterals from pancreaticoduodenal arterial arcades often result in sparing of the very proximal jejunum. Embolic disease, on the other hand, often spares the jejunum and right colon as the embolus obstructs distal to the origin of the middle colic artery, where the diameter of the artery is smaller. In low-flow states, while the entire GI tract is at risk, the predominant ischemic changes are in the distal colon along the distribution of the inferior mesenteric artery. There is anorectal sparing because of its systemic blood supply and collaterals from the other branches of the iliac arteries. *PD* pancreaticoduodenal artery, *G* gangrene, *A* aorta, *SMA* superior mesenteric artery, *MC* middle colic artery, *PG* pregangrenous patches, *AA* arteriosclerotic aorta, *IM* inferior mesenteric artery, *J* jejunal arcade

Answer
e

10. All of the following are intraoperative findings in Crohn's disease *except*:
    (a) Creeping fat
    (b) Interloop abscesses
    (c) Fistulization
    (d) Sparing of the ileocecal valve
    (e) Stricture

Comments Crohn's disease is a granulomatous inflammatory condition that affects the full thickness of the GI tract and can affect any segment of it, although it is most commonly described in the distal small bowel and colon.

While the clinical presentation may be quite varied, based on the stage and severity of the disease, as well as the segment affected, there are some intraoperative findings that are considered typical.

Among these, creeping fat or encroachment of the mesenteric fat onto the intestinal wall is pathognomonic. It has been hypothesized that this hypertrophy of fat tissue may constitute a counterregulatory mechanism to the inflammatory process. It has been shown that these adipocytes produce elevated amounts of adiponectin, which has anti-inflammatory properties [29].

Given that Crohn's disease affects the entire intestinal wall, perforation is a possibility. When contained, abscesses may form between loops of the bowel. Alternatively, these perforations may exteriorize creating fistulas.

As the disease runs its course, inflammation subsides and a fibrotic reaction takes place, generating strictures [30, 31] (Fig. 13.9a, b).

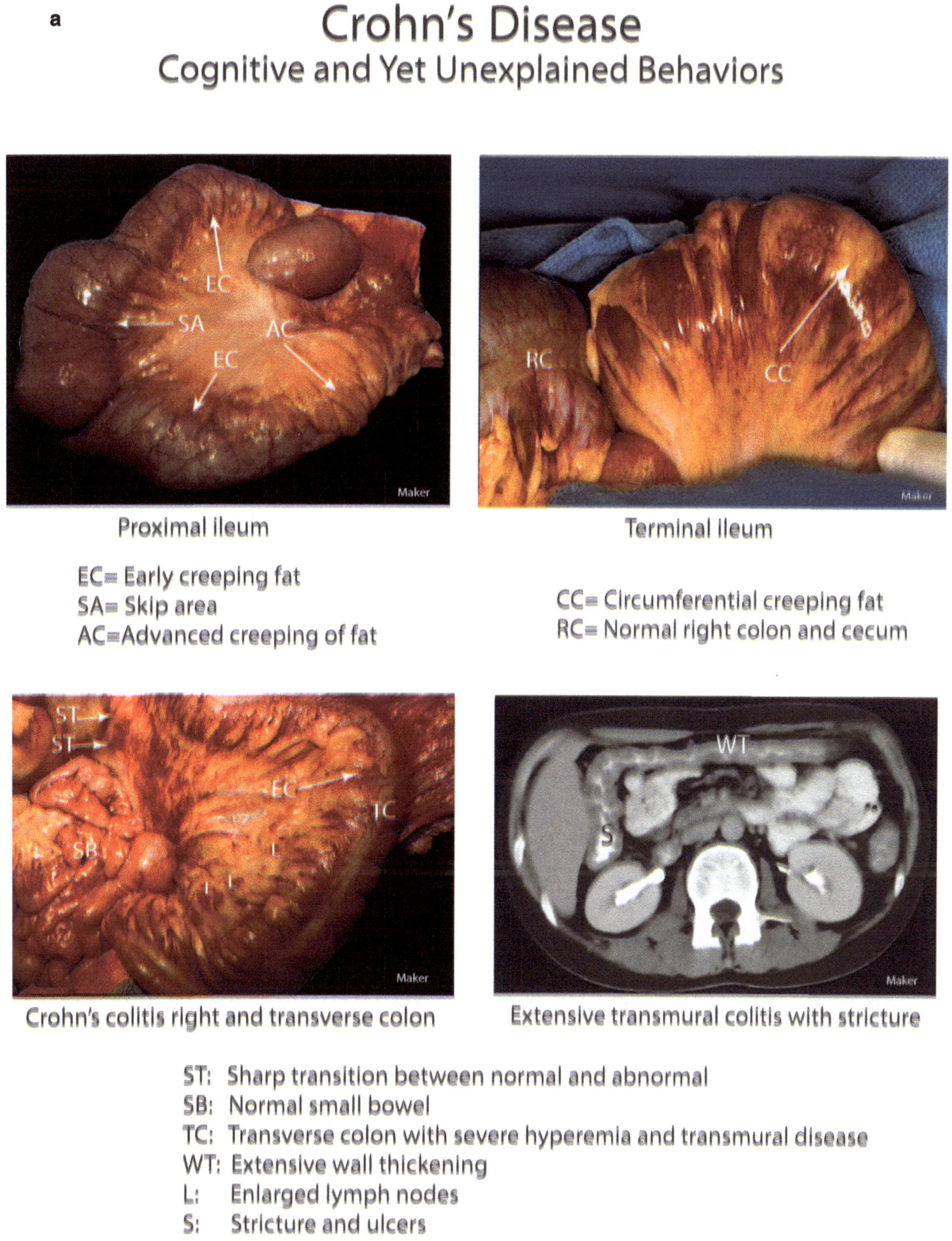

Fig. 13.9 (**a**) Crohn's disease is known for predictable behaviors, and yet some of its behaviors have defied common cognition, e.g., skip areas and sharp transition points even in a chronic setting of the disease. Illustrations above show creeping fat of different degrees corresponding to the severity of the trans-serosal disease, hyperemia, lymphadenopathy, and extensive narrowing of the right and transverse colon on CT scan. *ST* sharp transition between normal and abnormal, *SB* normal small bowel, *TC* transverse colon with severe hyperemia and transmural disease, *WT* extensive wall thickening, *L* enlarged lymph nodes, *S* stricture and ulcers. (**b**) Normal small bowel mesentery is a sandwich of the two layers of the visceral peritoneum containing blood vessels, lymphatics, lymphoid tissue and macrophages in the packing of fat. Two layers of the visceral peritoneum of the mesentry continue as the serosa of the small bowel and provide an excellent pathway for mesenteric fat to creep on to the bowel. Creeping fat may well be a physiological process of sealing the trans-serosal injury of Crohn's disease with an immunocompetent tissue wrap

b

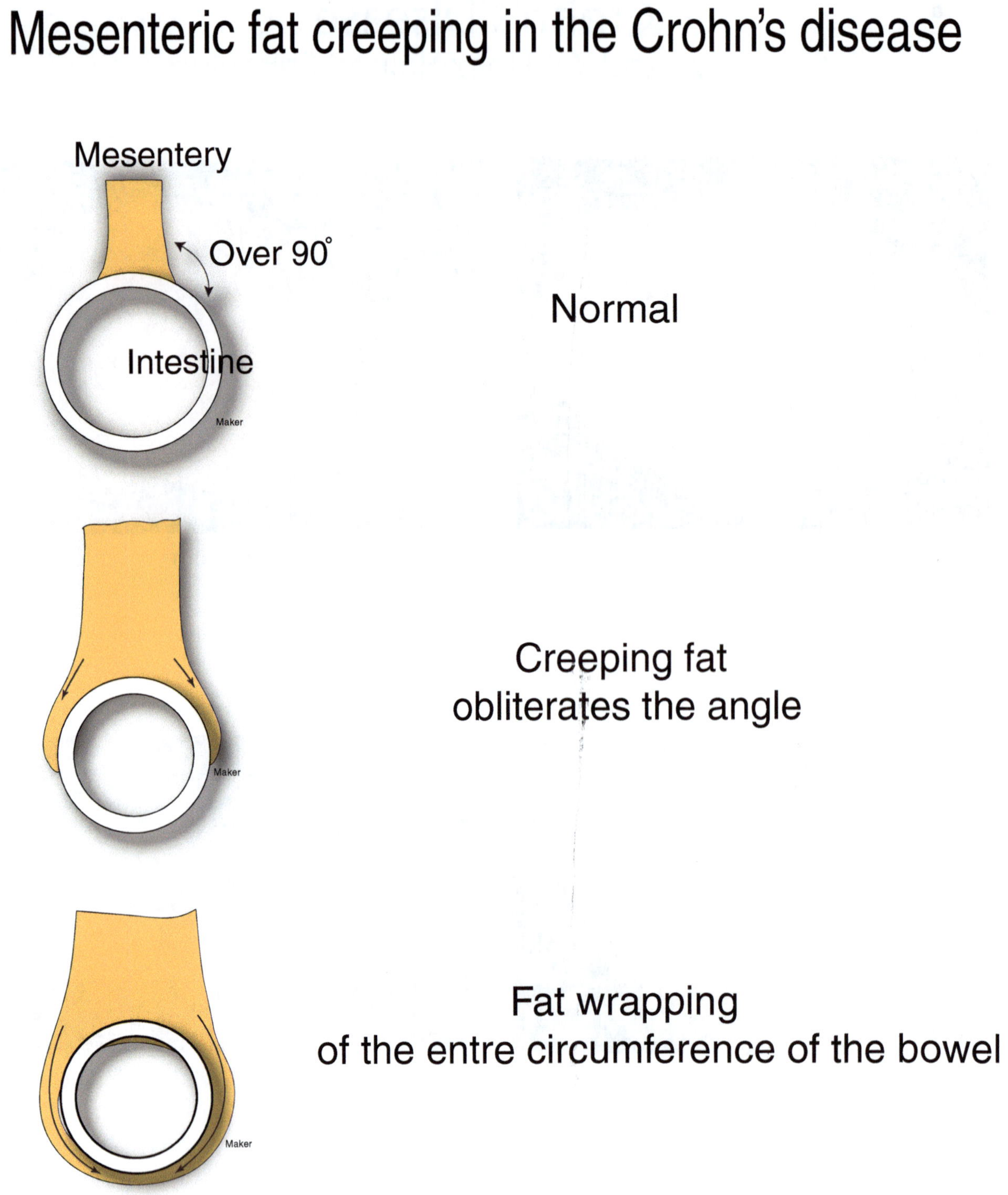

Fig. 13.9 (continued)

Answer
d

References

1. Hosseinpour M, Behdad A. Evaluation of small bowel measurement in alive patients. Surg Radiol Anat. 2008;30:653–5.
2. Misiakos EP, Macheras A, Kapetanakis T, Liakakos T. Short bowel syndrome: current medical and surgical trends. J Clin Gastroenterol. 2007;41(1):5–18.
3. Kluth D, Jaeschke-Melli S, Fiegel H. The embryology of gut rotation. Semin Pediatr Surg. 2003;12(4):275–9.
4. Millar AJ, Rode H, Cywes S. Malrotation and volvulus in infancy and childhood. Semin Pediatr Surg. 2003;12(4):229–36.
5. Kluth D, Kaestner M, Tibboel D, Lambrecht W. Rotation of the gut: fact or fantasy? J Pediatr Surg. 1995;30(3):448–53.
6. Naik-Mathuria B, Olutoye OO. Foregut abnormalities. Surg Clin North Am. 2006;86(2):261–84, viii.
7. Gosche JR, Vick L, Boulanger SC, Islam S. Midgut abnormalities. Surg Clin North Am. 2006;86(2):285–99, viii.
8. Jancelewicz T, Simko J, Lee H. Obstructing ileal duplication cyst infected with Salmonella in a 2-year-old boy: a case report and review of the literature. J Pediatr Surg. 2007;42(5):E19–21.
9. Martinez-Cecilia D, Arjona-Sanchez A, Gomez-Alvarez M, Torres-Tordera E, Luque-Molina A, Valenti-Azcarate V, et al. Conservative management of perforated duodenal diverticulum: a case report and review of the literature. World J Gastroenterol. 2008;14(12):1949–51.
10. Kassahun WT, Fangmann J, Harms J, Bartels M, Hauss J. Complicated small-bowel diverticulosis: a case report and review of the literature. World J Gastroenterol. 2007;13(15):2240–2.
11. Moore TC. Omphalomesenteric duct malformations. Semin Pediatr Surg. 1996;5(2):116–23.
12. Snyder CL. Current management of umbilical abnormalities and related anomalies. Semin Pediatr Surg. 2007;16(1):41–9.
13. Yahchouchy EK, Marano AF, Etienne JC, Fingerhut AL. Meckel's diverticulum. J Am Coll Surg. 2001;192(5):658–62.
14. Zani A, Eaton S, Rees CM, Pierro A. Incidentally detected Meckel diverticulum: to resect or not to resect? Ann Surg. 2008;247(2):276–81.
15. Androulakis J, Colborn GL, Skandalakis PN, Skandalakis LJ, Skandalakis JE. Embryologic and anatomic basis of duodenal surgery. Surg Clin North Am. 2000;80(1):171–99.
16. Maker V, Gerzenshtein J, Lerner T. Annular pancreas in the adult: two case reports and review of more than a century of literature. Am Surg. 2003;69(5):404–10.
17. Paraskevas G, Papaziogas B, Lazaridis C, Gigis P, Papaziogas T. Annular pancreas in adults: embryological development, morphology and clinical significance. Surg Radiol Anat. 2001;23(6):437–42.
18. Leung JW, Leung FW. Papillotomy performance scoring scale – a pilot validation study focused on the cut axis. Aliment Pharmacol Ther. 2006;24(2):307–12.
19. Kim SK, Cho CD, Wojtowycz AR. The ligament of Treitz (the suspensory ligament of the duodenum): anatomic and radiographic correlation. Abdom Imaging. 2008;33(4):395–7.
20. Welsch T, Buchler MW, Kienle P. Recalling superior mesenteric artery syndrome. Dig Surg. 2007;24(3):149–56.
21. Merrett ND, Wilson RB, Cosman P, Biankin AV. Superior mesenteric artery syndrome: diagnosis and treatment strategies. J Gastrointest Surg. 2008;13:287–92.
22. Kaidar-Person O, Rosenthal RJ, Wexner SD, Szomstein S, Person B. Compression anastomosis: history and clinical considerations. Am J Surg. 2008;195(6):818–26.
23. Thompson SK, Chang EY, Jobe BA. Clinical review: healing in gastrointestinal anastomoses, part I. Microsurgery. 2006;26(3):131–6.
24. Enestvedt CK, Thompson SK, Chang EY, Jobe BA. Clinical review: healing in gastrointestinal anastomoses, part II. Microsurgery. 2006;26(3):137–43.
25. Drozdowski L, Thomson AB. Intestinal mucosal adaptation. World J Gastroenterol. 2006;12(29):4614–27.
26. Keller J, Panter H, Layer P. Management of the short bowel syndrome after extensive small bowel resection. Best Pract Res Clin Gastroenterol. 2004;18(5):977–92.
27. McKinsey JF, Gewertz BL. Acute mesenteric ischemia. Surg Clin North Am. 1997;77(2):307–18.
28. Rosenblum JD, Boyle CM, Schwartz LB. The mesenteric circulation. Anat Physiol Surg Clin N Am. 1997;77(2):289–306.
29. Yamamoto K, Kiyohara T, Murayama Y, Kihara S, Okamoto Y, Funahashi T, et al. Production of adiponectin, an anti-inflammatory protein, in mesenteric adipose tissue in Crohn's disease. Gut. 2005;54(6):789–96.
30. Bandzar S, Gupta S, Platt MO. Crohn's disease: a review of treatment options and current research. Cell Immunol. 2013;286(1–2):45–52.
31. Buchner AM, Blonski W, Lichtenstein GR. Update on the management of Crohn's disease. Curr Gastroenterol Rep. 2011;13(5):465–74.

14 Appendix

1. Right hemicolectomy is indicated in the following cases *except*
   (a) Carcinoid tumors greater than 2 cm or with extension into the mesoappendix
   (b) Adenocarcinoma of the appendix
   (c) Cystic masses involving the base of the appendix
   (d) Symptomatic duplication of the cecum
   (e) Twisted appendix epiploica

Comments Appendectomy is one of the most commonly performed emergency operations. On occasion, the surgeon is faced with unexpected findings mimicking the presentation of appendicitis, which require specific treatments. Tumors are found in approximately 0.1 % of appendectomies. Carcinoid tumors are the most frequent type, followed by adenocarcinoma of the appendix and by benign tumors. It is important to point out that all tumors of the appendix may be accompanied by synchronous disease, making a full exploration of the abdomen imperative [1].

Carcinoid tumors are neuroendocrine neoplasms derived from the Kulchitsky cells, present in the epithelium of the GI tract. These cells participate in the regulation of enteric motility, secretion, and permeability through the production of serotonin and other mediators. The appendix is the most common site of carcinoid tumors in the GI tract, followed by the small intestine and rectum. The incidence of appendiceal carcinoid tumors in appendectomy specimens is as high as 1 in 200. Currently, most appendiceal carcinoid tumors are found during surgery for acute appendicitis. Carcinoid syndrome is a late presentation of disease, associated with hepatic and pulmonary involvement. The degree of invasiveness correlates well with the size of the tumor. Tumors smaller than two centimeters, with no involvement of the appendiceal base, are best treated by appendectomy with complete mesoappendiceal excision. Larger tumors or those involving the base or the mesoappendix require a right hemicolectomy. Carcinoid tumors have high association with adenocarcinoma of the GI tract [2–6].

Primary adenocarcinomas of the appendix are rare neoplasms constituting only 0.5 % of all GI malignancies. They are often unrecognized at the time of surgery and identified during the pathologic analysis of the specimen. The ideal treatment consists of right hemicolectomy. Appendectomy alone may result in increased mortality and reoperation for a completion hemicolectomy is appropriate, especially in cases that are poorly differentiated, invade the mucosa, or have nodal involvement [7–9].

V.K. Maker, E.D. Guzman-Arrieta, *Cognitive Pearls in General Surgery*,
DOI 10.1007/978-1-4939-1850-8_14, © Springer Science+Business Media New York 2015

Appendiceal mucoceles are associated with benign and malignant processes (mucinous cystoadenocarcinoma). Proper management is imperative, due to the risk of development of pseudomyxoma peritonei. In the past, right hemicolectomy was advocated for all appendiceal mucoceles, but currently this operation is reserved for tumors confirmed by frozen section that are involving the base of the appendix and local nodes. In all cases encountered laparoscopically, conversion to an open procedure is recommended to reduce the risk of tumor seeding and subsequent development of pseudomyxoma peritonei [10].

Cystic duplication of the cecum is a congenital malformation usually identified during childhood, typically presenting as an abdominal mass associated with intussusception, obstruction, or bleeding. These masses are found in the mesenteric side of the bowel, with which they intimately share their blood supply, making segmental en bloc resection necessary [11, 12].

Torsion of appendices epiploica (epiploic appendagitis) may mimic acute appendicitis. Resection of the infarcted appendix epiploica is indicated. High-resolution CT scanners help make this diagnosis in a vast majority of patients. Performing a simultaneous appendectomy is controversial [13].

Answer

e

2. All of the following are correct *except*:
   (a) The appendicular artery is an end artery.
   (b) During pregnancy, the appendix is displaced cephalad and to the right.
   (c) Appendiceal position affects the risk for acute appendicitis.
   (d) The best landmark for locating the appendix is the convergence of the three taenia coli.
   (e) The appendicular artery is a branch of the ileocolic artery.

Comments The main blood supply of the appendix comes from the appendicular artery, which is the end branch of the superior mesenteric artery. The appendicular artery represents the distal extension of the ileocolic artery. This artery courses within the mesoappendix giving multiple perpendicular branches to the appendix. The appendix may receive additional blood supply from small branches derived from the cecal artery [14].

During pregnancy, the uterus displaces the cecum laterally and superiorly. During early pregnancy, patients with appendicitis may complain of right lower quadrant pain, but later on appendicitis may present as right upper quadrant or right flank pain [15].

The appendiceal tip may be located in any position in relation to the cecum; however, the base of the appendix can be reliably found at the confluence of the taenia coli, which is the preferred landmark for its localization. The location of the appendix has not been shown to increase the risk for appendicitis. However, it may change the clinical presentation of acute appendicitis and in some cases result in delayed diagnosis and increased morbidity (Fig. 14.1).

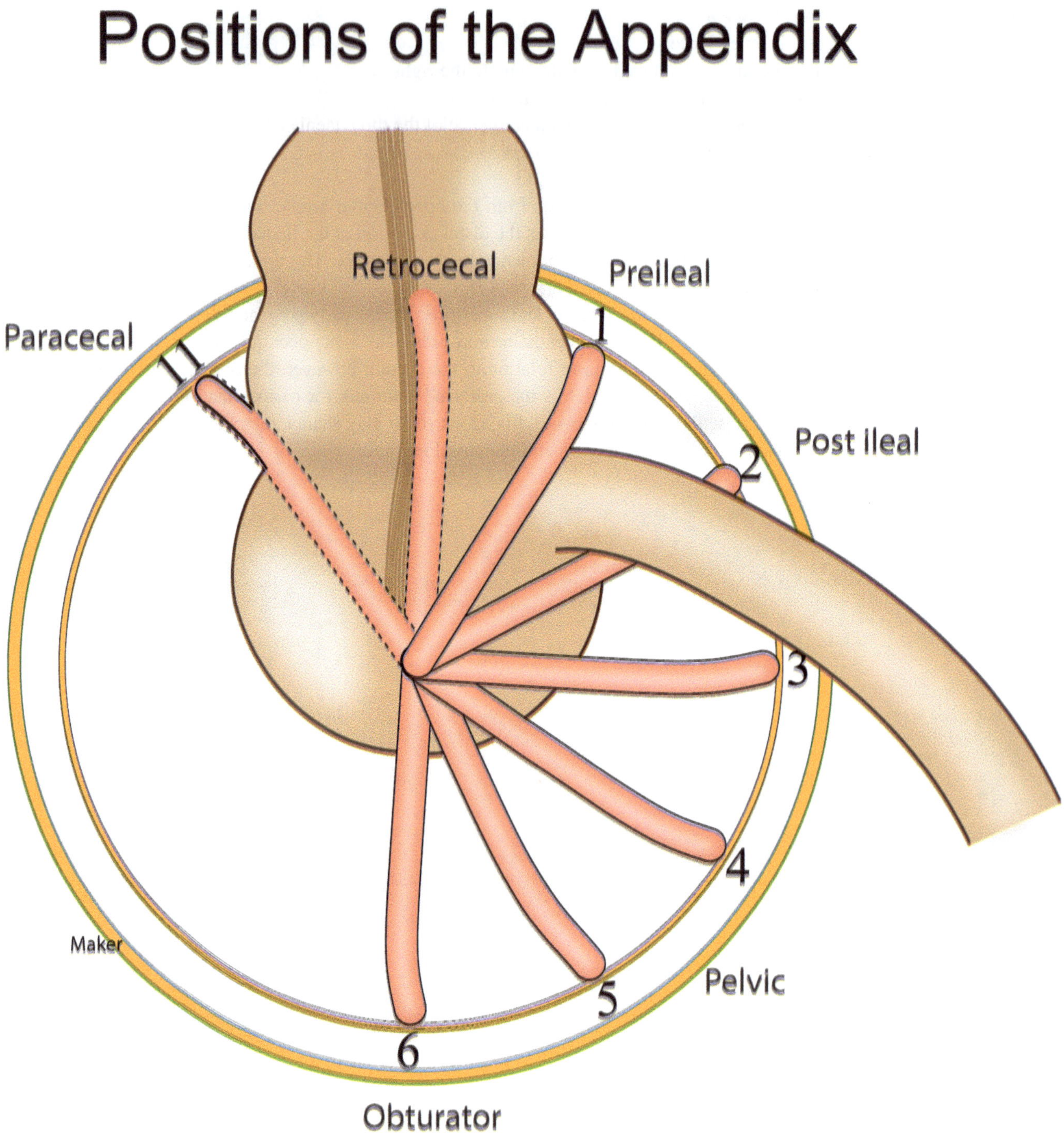

Fig. 14.1 Depending on the location of the appendix on the clock, appendicitis will present with unique findings in addition to the classic presentation. Pre-ileal and post-ileal positions can present with diarrhea, especially in children. Three o'clock position of the appendicitis may lie on the ureter or genitofemoral nerve and can present with symptoms mimicking ureteric colic. Depending on the length of the appendix and location, 4, 5, and 6 o'clock appendicitis could present diagnostic challenges mimicking pelvic inflammatory disease, urinary tract infection, or diverticulitis. In this location, there can also be a positive obturator sign. In paracecal and retrocecal positions, classic Mcburney's point tenderness may be missing and findings may well relate to flank pain with a positive psoas sign

Answer

c

3. Mark the *correct* statement in relation to the signs and symptoms of acute appendicitis:
   (a) The psoas and obturator sign usually coexist in the same patient.
   (b) Perforated appendicitis is accompanied by pneumoperitoneum.
   (c) Acute appendicitis in patients with intestinal malrotation presents with lower abdominal pain.
   (d) Appendicitis may occur in an inguinal hernia.
   (e) Vomiting typically precedes pain in adult acute appendicitis.

Comments The psoas and obturator signs are mutually exclusive. Both are caused by irritation of the adjacent muscle due to contact with the inflamed appendix. This manifests as pain during stretching. The psoas sign is typical of retrocecal appendicitis, whereas the obturator sign is present when the appendix is located in the anterior pelvis.

As a general rule, perforation of hollow abdominal organs leads to pneumoperitoneum; however, appendiceal perforation is an exception to this rule. Appendices perforate distal to the point of obstruction, which impedes the passage of gas from the cecum to the peritoneal cavity. Furthermore, the capacity of the normal appendix is only 0.2–0.5 ml, a volume too small to produce pneumoperitoneum. Rarely, pneumoperitoneum may be present if the perforation happens at the base of the appendix, allowing direct leakage from the cecum (Fig. 14.2).

Pain in appendicitis classically follows an orderly progression of symptoms. There is at first vague periumbilical pain that progresses into more localized somatic pain as inflammation ensues (Fig. 14.3).

Complete malrotation of the bowel is characterized by the presence of the cecum in the upper abdomen, usually to the left of the midline. After the surgical correction of intestinal malrotation, the cecum is placed in the left lower quadrant. In view of the anomalous position the appendix occupies after the correction of intestinal malrotation, prophylactic appendectomy is a part of the Ladd's procedure with the intent to avoid future atypical presentations of appendicitis.

Vomiting in inflammatory surgical pathology of the bowel usually follows the onset of pain. The contrary is true in gastroenteritis [16].

The first appendectomy was performed by Amyand in 1735 on a boy presenting with an inflamed appendix in a right inguinal hernia. Furthermore, the appendix was found to be perforated by a previously swallowed pin. Hernias containing the vermiform appendix are now named Amyand hernia [17, 18].

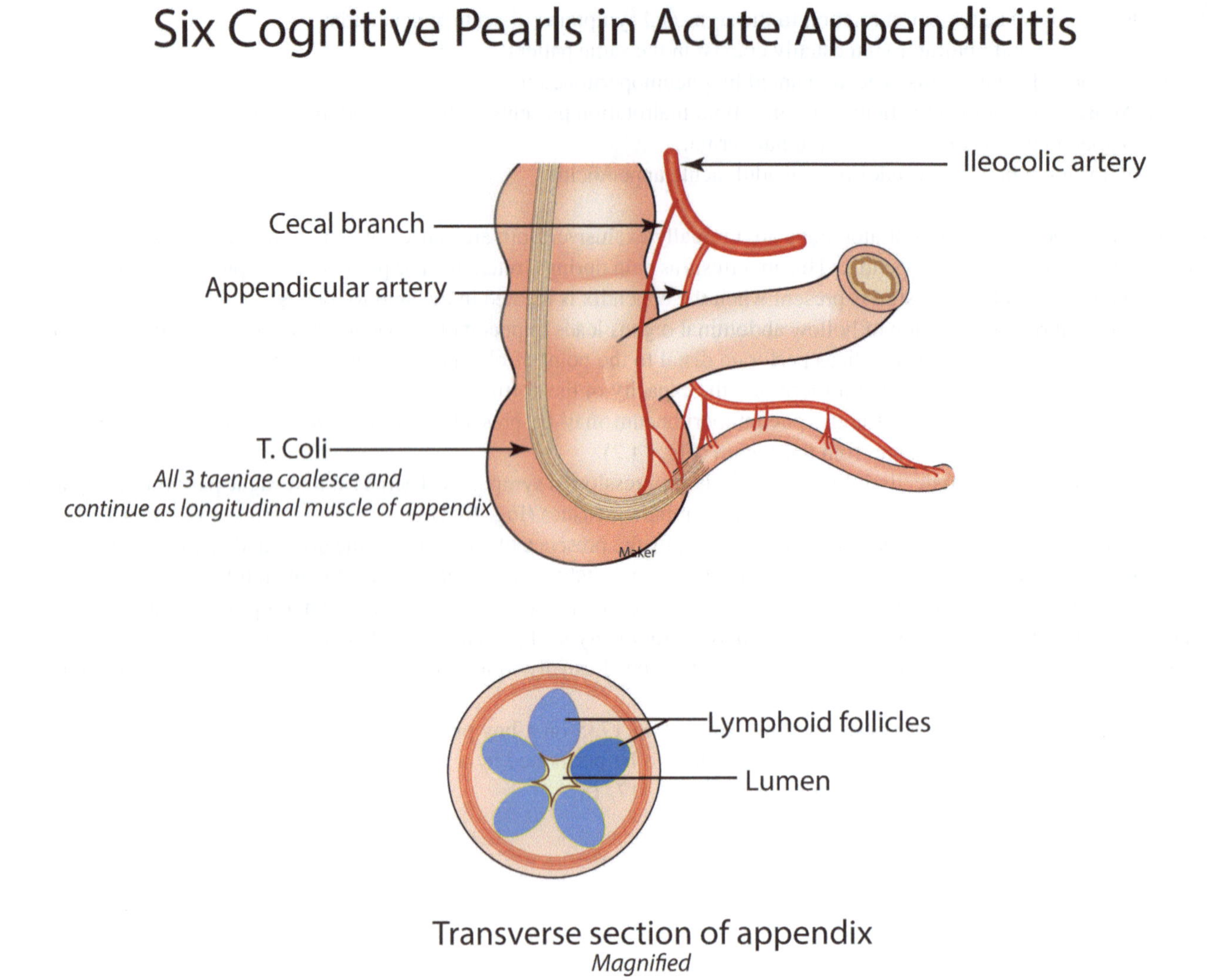

Fig. 14.2 *1* Obstruction of the proximal lumen of the appendix must happen to develop appendicitis. *2* Obstruction of the lumen of the appendix is a closed loop obstruction. *3* The luminal volume capacity of the normal appendix is 0.1 ml. *4* Lymphoid tissue makes up the bulk of the submucosa, except in the elderly. *5* 0.5 ml of the mucous in the appendix will well exceed lymphatic and venous filling pressure of the appendicular wall. As a result of obstruction of the appendiceal orifice, intraluminal pressure of the appendix may reach 60 cm. of water with as little as 0.5 ml of mucous. *6* Even though the base of the appendix has collateral blood supply, the appendicular artery is an end artery

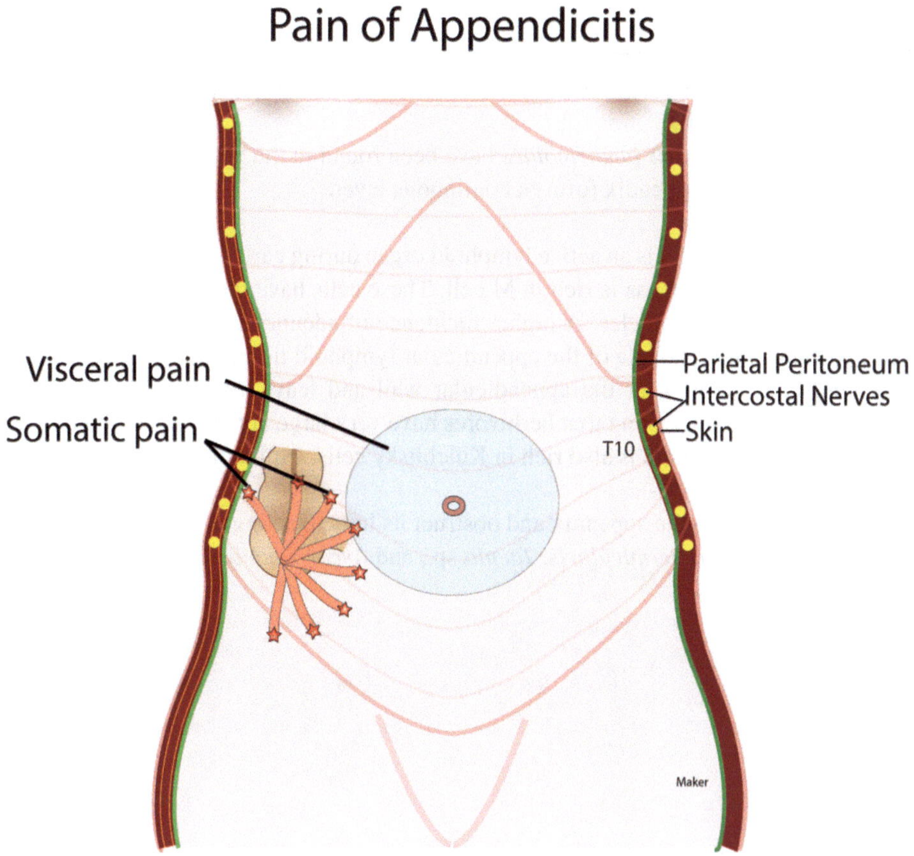

Fig. 14.3 Distention of the obstructed appendix produces the initial vague periumbilical visceral pain that is mediated through the visceral nerves. As the disease progresses, the inflamed serosa of the appendix touches the parietal peritoneum initiating the localized somatic pain, mediated through spinal nerves. Somatic pain is localized in the area of contact between appendicitis and the parietal peritoneum depending on its anatomical position

Answer

d

4. All of the following are correct *except*:
   (a) The appendiceal mucosa is poor in M cells.
   (b) The lymphatic tissue in the appendix gradually decreases in size after puberty.
   (c) The appendix has Kulchitsky cells.
   (d) *Enterobius vermicularis* and *Ascaris lumbricoides* have been found in the appendix.
   (e) The longitudinal muscle of the appendix forms a continuous layer.

Comments Like the thymus, the appendix is an active lymphoid organ during early life, which declines in function with age. In line with this role, the appendiceal mucosa is rich in M cell. These cells have the function of transporting antigens from the lumen to the submucosal lymphoid follicles. A higher incidence of adenocarcinoma of the colon has been reported in patients with previous appendectomy. The role of the appendicular lymphoid tissue in this association is debated [19].

Lymphoid follicles constitute the bulk of the appendicular wall and leave a narrow lumen that is likely to become obstructed causing appendicitis. It is interesting that herbivores have very large appendices with large lumens and extremely low incidence of appendicitis. The appendix is also rich in Kulchitsky cells, explaining the frequency of carcinoid tumors in this organ.

Intestinal parasites may migrate into the appendix and obstruct its lumen, acting as a fecalith. The literature reports cases of appendicitis secondary to *Enterobius vermicularis*, *Taenia* sp., and *Ascaris lumbricoides* [20, 21].

Answer

a

5. Incidental appendectomy is performed in the following cases *except*:
   (a) Midgut volvulus
   (b) Meckel's diverticulitis
   (c) Cholecystectomy
   (d) Laparotomy done for Crohn's ileitis
   (e) Chronic right lower quadrant pain of unknown etiology

Comments Incidental appendectomy is performed less liberally than in the past. Although this is usually a safe procedure, attention should be paid to assess the risk of developing future appendicitis in balance with the potential use of the appendix for future reconstructive surgery of the biliary system and urinary tract. In addition, the association between appendectomy and increased incidence of colorectal cancer should be considered.

As mentioned before, appendectomy is indicated during the correction of a midgut volvulus associated with malrotation, due to the anomalous position of the appendix at the end of the operation.

Appendectomy during surgery for Meckel's diverticulitis is usually accepted, especially considering that the surgical scars may confuse the diagnosis of acute appendicitis. However, the incidental removal of a Meckel's diverticulum during appendectomy is not routinely advised.

The appendix may be removed to simplify the differential diagnosis in patients expected to have multiple episodes of right lower quadrant pain, such as those with Crohn's disease. Incidental appendectomy is performed provided the appendiceal base is intact.

Finally, other groups that may benefit from incidental appendectomy include patients with an appendicolith, patients with exceedingly high reoperative risk, patients expected to have major adhesions, and handicapped patient unable to provide a good history or expected to present atypically (e.g., spinal cord injury) [22, 23].

Answer

c

6. All of the following are correct *except:*
   (a) The appendix has a broad base in the neonate.
   (b) Acute appendicitis is rare under the age of 2.
   (c) Diffuse peritonitis following acute appendicitis is more common in the pediatric population.
   (d) Acute appendicitis may present with diarrhea.
   (e) The appendix is atrophic in children and develops with puberty.

Comments Acute appendicitis is the most common surgical pathology in the pediatric population; however, it is rare before the age of 2 because the appendix has a relatively broad base and short length, making obstruction less likely. During childhood the appendix develops proportions similar to those of the adult and is more prone to obstruction due to the abundant lymphoid tissue that may reactively enlarge.

Diffuse peritonitis is more common in the pediatric population due to delayed diagnosis, as well as a decreased capacity to contain intra-abdominal infections due to lack of development of the omentum. Pediatric appendicitis may mimic gastroenteritis more closely than adult appendicitis, with diarrhea being a common symptom [24].

Answer

e

References

1. Connor SJ, Hanna GB, Frizelle FA. Appendiceal tumors: retrospective clinicopathologic analysis of appendiceal tumors from 7,970 appendectomies. Dis Colon Rectum. 1998;41(1):75–80.
2. Tchana-Sato V, Detry O, Polus M, Thiry A, Detroz B, Maweja S, et al. Carcinoid tumor of the appendix: a consecutive series from 1237 appendectomies. World J Gastroenterol. 2006;12(41):6699–701.
3. Goede AC, Caplin ME, Winslet MC. Carcinoid tumour of the appendix. Br J Surg. 2003;90(11):1317–22.
4. Modlin IM, Tang LH. The gastric enterochromaffin-like cell: an enigmatic cellular link. Gastroenterology. 1996;111(3):783–810.
5. Kulke MH, Mayer RJ. Carcinoid tumors. N Engl J Med. 1999;340(11):858–68.
6. Moertel CG, Dockerty MB, Judd ES. Carcinoid tumors of the vermiform appendix. Cancer. 1968;21(2):270–8.
7. Manigrasso A, Candioli S, Pironi D, La TV, Panarese A, Romani AM, et al. Adenocarcinoma of the appendix. A case report and review of the literature. G Chir. 2007;28(3):73–81.
8. Ozakyol AH, Saricam T, Kabukcuoglu S, Caga T, Erenoglu E. Primary appendiceal adenocarcinoma. Am J Clin Oncol. 1999;22(5):458–9.
9. Hata K, Tanaka N, Nomura Y, Wada I, Nagawa H. Early appendiceal adenocarcinoma. A review of the literature with special reference to optimal surgical procedures. J Gastroenterol. 2002;37(3):210–4.
10. Dhage-Ivatury S, Sugarbaker PH. Update on the surgical approach to mucocele of the appendix. J Am Coll Surg. 2006;202(4):680–4.
11. Choong CK, Robertson RW, Beasley SW, Frizelle FA. Congenital caecal cystic duplication presenting with caecal volvulus in an elderly woman. Int J Colorectal Dis. 1997;12(4):256–8.
12. Oudshoorn JH, Heij HA. Intestinal obstruction caused by duplication of the caecum. Eur J Pediatr. 1996;155(4):338–40.
13. Jain S, Connell R, Kefford D. Torsion of an appendix epiploica: a rare cause of acute abdominal pain. J Obstet Gynaecol. 2002;22(5):564–5.
14. Ouattara D, Kipre YZ, Broalet E, Seri FG, Angate HY, Bi N'Guessan GG, et al. Classification of the terminal arterial vascularization of the appendix with a view to its use in reconstructive microsurgery. Surg Radiol Anat. 2007;29(8):635–41.
15. Tracey M, Fletcher HS. Appendicitis in pregnancy. Am Surg. 2000;66(6):555–9.
16. Cartwright SL, Knudson MP. Evaluation of acute abdominal pain in adults. Am Fam Physician. 2008;77(7):971–8.
17. Milanchi S, Allins AD. Amyand's hernia: history, imaging, and management. Hernia. 2008;12(3):321–2.
18. Hutchinson R. Amyand's hernia. J R Soc Med. 1993;86(2):104–5.
19. Corr SC, Gahan CC, Hill C. M-cells: origin, morphology and role in mucosal immunity and microbial pathogenesis. FEMS Immunol Med Microbiol. 2008;52(1):2–12.
20. da Silva DF, da Silva RJ, da Silva MG, Sartorelli AC, Rodrigues MA. Parasitic infection of the appendix as a cause of acute appendicitis. Parasitol Res. 2007;102(1):99–102.
21. Walshe T, Kavanagh DO, Bennani F, Eustace PW. The escaped worm. J Am Coll Surg. 2006;203(4):579.
22. Wolff BG. Current status of incidental surgery. Dis Colon Rectum. 1995;38(4):435–41.
23. Lynch CB, Sinha P, Jalloh S. Incidental appendectomy during gynecological surgery. Int J Gynaecol Obstet. 1997;59(3):261–2.
24. Morrow SE, Newman KD. Current management of appendicitis. Semin Pediatr Surg. 2007;16(1):34–40.

Large Intestine and Anorectum

15

1. Select the *true* statement.
   (a) Auerbach's plexus is located in the submucosa.
   (b) Meissner's plexus is located in the muscularis propria.
   (c) Absence of parasympathetic ganglia causes a segment of the bowel to be contracted and unable to conduct peristalsis.
   (d) Aganglionosis is the sole cause of megacolon.
   (e) In Hirschsprung's disease, the dilated colon lacks ganglion cells.

Comments The enteric nervous system is composed of a large population of diverse neural crest-derived cells forming complex plexuses within the bowel wall. While this network is subject to higher neurological and endocrine signals, it is also capable of functioning independently in regulating motility, secretion, and blood flow in the GI tract.

The midgut and hindgut are under the influence of the autonomic nervous system. The vagus nerve and the sacral plexus provide parasympathetic innervation and, in general, promote secretion, absorption, and peristalsis. In opposition, the sympathetic fibers derived from the thoracic and lumbar spinal cord inhibit peristalsis, increase the tone of the sphincters, and decrease secretion and absorption [1].

The foregut and midgut are colonized in craniocaudal fashion by neural crest cells originating in the vagal nuclei, whereas the hindgut is colonized from the sacral neural crest at a slightly later stage in development. These cells appear to migrate following chemotactic signals in the form of glial cell-derived neurotrophic factor (GDNF), which binds the product of the RET proto-oncogene. Interestingly, RET mutations are the chief genetic defect associated with Hirschsprung's disease. These mutations explain the association of Hirschsprung's disease and MEN2A syndrome [2–4].

Auerbach's plexus is located between the circular and longitudinal muscular layers, while Meissner's plexus resides in the submucosa. Additionally, a distinct population of glial cells located in the outer submucosa forms Schabadasch's plexus. While the function of these plexus was thought to be related to their location (i.e., Auerbach's for motility and Meissner's for mucosal secretion), it appears that both are highly interconnected and participate jointly in the regulation of all bowel functions, while coordinating afferent signals from the autonomic nervous system [5, 6].

Hirschsprung's disease is characterized by an absence of ganglion cells (involving both Meissner's and Auerbach's plexuses) in the affected segment of the colon. As a result, the affected segment is unable to relax creating a functional obstruction. Aganglionosis most often affects the distal hindgut; however, the absence of ganglion cells has been demonstrated in the proximal colon and small bowel. While the bowel proximal to the zone of aganglionosis is histologically normal, it often suffers passive dilatation secondary to a distal functional obstruction. Differential diagnoses include constipation, meconium ileus, meconium plug, small left colon syndrome, and intestinal neuronal dysplasia, making biopsy necessary to confirm the diagnosis [7, 8].

In the United States, Chagas disease is seen as a cause of megacolon with increasing frequency in relation to immigrants from endemic areas (Brazil, Argentina, Peru, and Bolivia). This disease is caused by *Trypanosoma cruzi*, an intracellular parasite with affinity for cells of the autonomic nervous system. This protozoan causes "mega" syndromes affecting the heart, esophagus, small bowel, and colon.

Answer
c

V.K. Maker, E.D. Guzman-Arrieta, *Cognitive Pearls in General Surgery*,
DOI 10.1007/978-1-4939-1850-8_15, © Springer Science+Business Media New York 2015

2. The lymph nodes draining the colon are classified into the following groups *except*:
   (a) Epiploic – Along the greater omentum
   (b) Epicolic – On the colonic wall, beneath the serosa
   (c) Paracolic – Along the marginal artery of Drummond
   (d) Intermediate – Along the colonic branches of the superior and inferior mesenteric arteries
   (e) Pre-/para-aortic – At the root of the superior and inferior mesenteric arteries

Comments Interest in the anatomy of colonic lymphatics has increased due to the well-established association between the number of lymph nodes obtained in a colon cancer resection and survival. It has been well established that adequate colon resections should contain 12 or more lymph nodes. It is possible that greater lymph node retrieval may result in survival improvements [9]. In addition, there is currently interest in the role of sentinel node mapping in the treatment of colon cancer, although its practical application has not been fully defined [10, 11]. Colon lymphatics are categorized in a four-tier system including epicolic, paracolic, intermediate, and pre-/para-aortic nodes. While these node levels form a concentric pattern, lymphatic drainage is not necessarily radial towards the preaortic nodes. On the contrary, lymph may flow cephalad or caudal along a given level, generating anomalous drainage patterns [12] (Fig. 15.1).

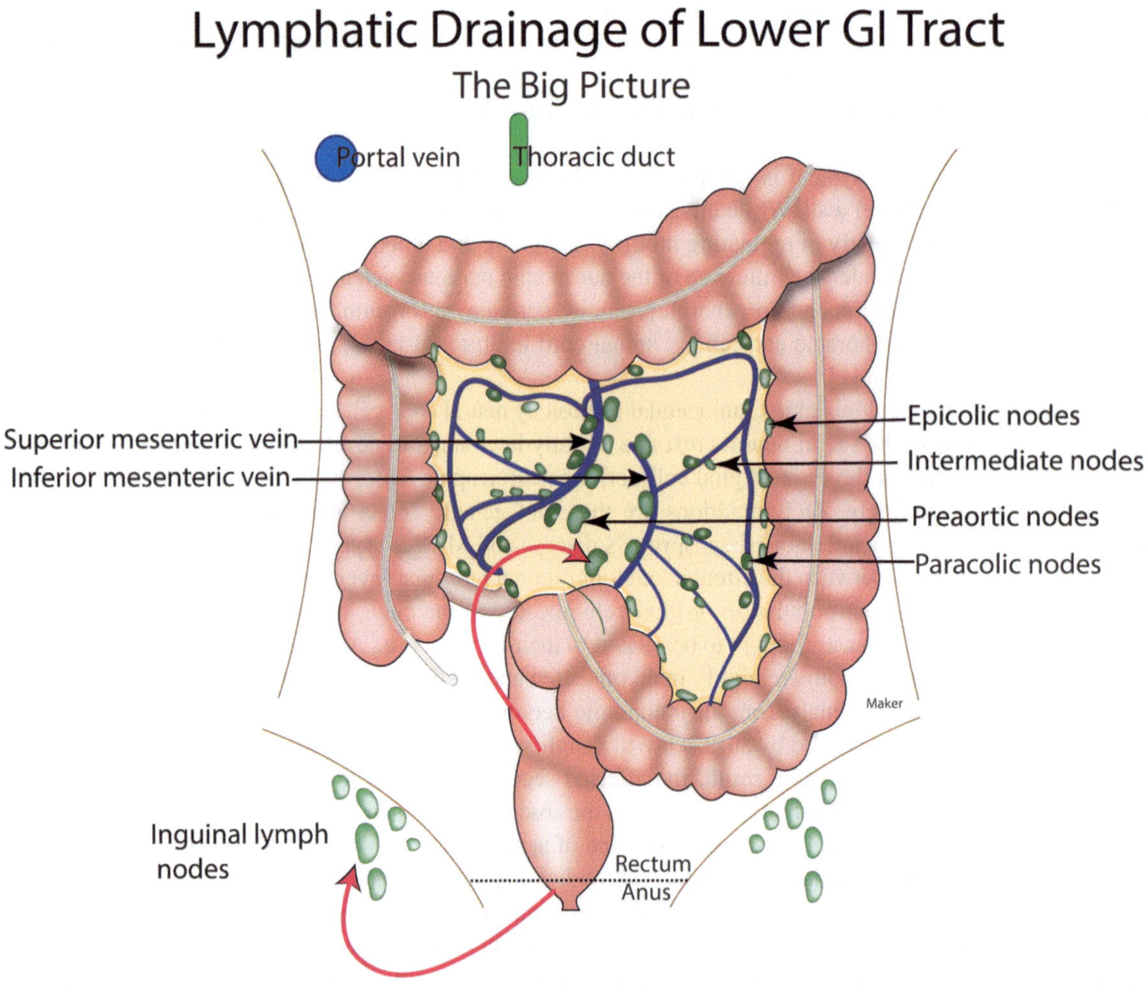

Fig. 15.1 Lymphatic drainage of the colon parallels the superior and inferior mesenteric vein tributaries through pericolonic and intermediate nodes to the preaortic lymph nodes. Lymphatic drainage of the rectum follows through the mesorectal nodes to the preaortic nodes. Ectodermal anus and anal canal neoplasms as well as very low rectal neoplasms may spread to the inguinal and mesorectal lymph nodes, similar to the dual portal and systemic venous drainage of this area. Eventually all lymphatics will reach the thoracic duct via its intestinal or lumbar trunks and veins to the hepatic portal system via mesenteric veins

Answer

a

3. All of the following are correct *except*:
   (a) The marginal artery of Drummond communicates the ileocolic, right colic, middle colic, left colic, and sigmoid arteries.
   (b) The arc of Riolan is an inconstant vessel communicating the IMA and SMA along the distal transverse mesocolon.
   (c) The critical point of Sudeck marks the place where the superior rectal artery can be ligated without devascularizing a long rectosigmoid stump.
   (d) The right mesocolon is less vascular than the left, hence the preference for the former when executing retrocolic gastrojejunostomies.
   (e) Each epiploic appendage has its own blood supply and its torsion will produce infarction.

Comments Please see question 4.

Answer

d

4. All of the following are correct *except*:
   (a) A watershed area for vascular, lymphatic, and neural supply exists at the junction of the middle and distal thirds of the transverse colon.
   (b) The upper rectum drains into the inferior mesenteric nodes.
   (c) Anastomosis between the superior and middle and inferior rectal veins constitutes a site for portosystemic shunting responsible for secondary hemorrhoids.
   (d) Testicular cancers drain into the inguinal lymph nodes.
   (e) The distal anal canal drains into the inguinal lymph nodes.

Comments The three main mesenteric vessels (celiac trunk, superior mesenteric artery (SMA), and inferior mesenteric artery (IMA)) are connected by ample anastomotic networks. These networks allow communication between branches as well as between the mesenteric and systemic circulations. Their capacity to accommodate blood flow is illustrated by the fact that the lower extremities may be perfused through branches of the inferior mesenteric artery in aortoiliac occlusive disease.

In the colon, the main anastomotic network is formed by the marginal artery of Drummond, which lies in proximity to the colon and gives rise to the vasa recta. This vessel communicates the branches of the SMA and IMA. The arc of Riolan (also known as meandering mesenteric artery) is a less constant anastomosis between the middle colic and the left colic artery. It lies closer to the root of the mesentery than the marginal artery of Drummond. Enlargement of these vessels reflects the presence of collateral flow due to vascular occlusion. Absence of this anastomosis may occur in up to 50 % of cases, creating a watershed at the splenic flexure. Due to its vulnerability to ischemia induced by colonic resections, this area has been named the "Griffiths' critical point" [13–15]. The left mesocolon has less collaterals than the right; as such, it is the preferred side for tunneling retrocolic anastomosis.

The critical point of Sudeck was described at the beginning of the twentieth century in an effort to promote the viability of the rectosigmoid stump in left colic resections. At the time, it was thought necessary to preserve the most distal arcade of the rectosigmoid vessels by ligating the superior rectal artery proximal to it. However, intramural collaterals of the rectosigmoid can preserve a stump extending up to 8–10 cm from the peritoneal reflection, making the critical point of Sudeck an item of historical interest [16, 17].

Epiploic appendages are fat-filled sacs of visceral peritoneum supplied by terminal vessels independent of the colonic wall circulation. This determines that appendagitis will not result in colonic perforation. They number approximately 100 in the normal individual and are most abundant in the sigmoid colon (57 %) and cecum (26 %) [18].

The blood supply and lymphatic drainage of the anorectum reflect its origin from two distinct embryologic entities, namely, the distal hindgut (endoderm) and the anal pit (ectoderm). As such, blood supply to the proximal anorectum is provided by the superior rectal artery, which is the terminal branch of the inferior mesenteric artery. This artery extends distally to the dentate line, which marks the endoderm–ectoderm junction. Lymphatic drainage for this segment is directed towards the mesenteric nodes. The middle sacral artery arises from the posterior wall of the distal aorta and provides blood to the posterior wall of the rectum and upper anal canal.

In contrast, blood supply to the anorectum distal to the dentate line is provided by the paired middle and inferior rectal arteries, both branches of the internal iliac (pudendal) arteries. Lymphatic drainage of this area is towards the inguinal nodes, constituting an exception where lymphatic drainage does not follow the blood vessels. Like anal cancers, vaginal, scrotal, and perineal malignancies drain into the inguinal lymph nodes. On the other hand, testicular cancers, like ovarian cancers, drain to the preaortic nodes. Of note, the rectal arteries and veins also receive the name "hemorrhoidal" [19] (Fig. 15.2).

The rich communications between the rectal vessels, both arterial and venous, allow the presence of functional shunts, important in decompressing portal hypertension and providing collateral arterial supply to the distal GI tract and lower extremities [20, 21].

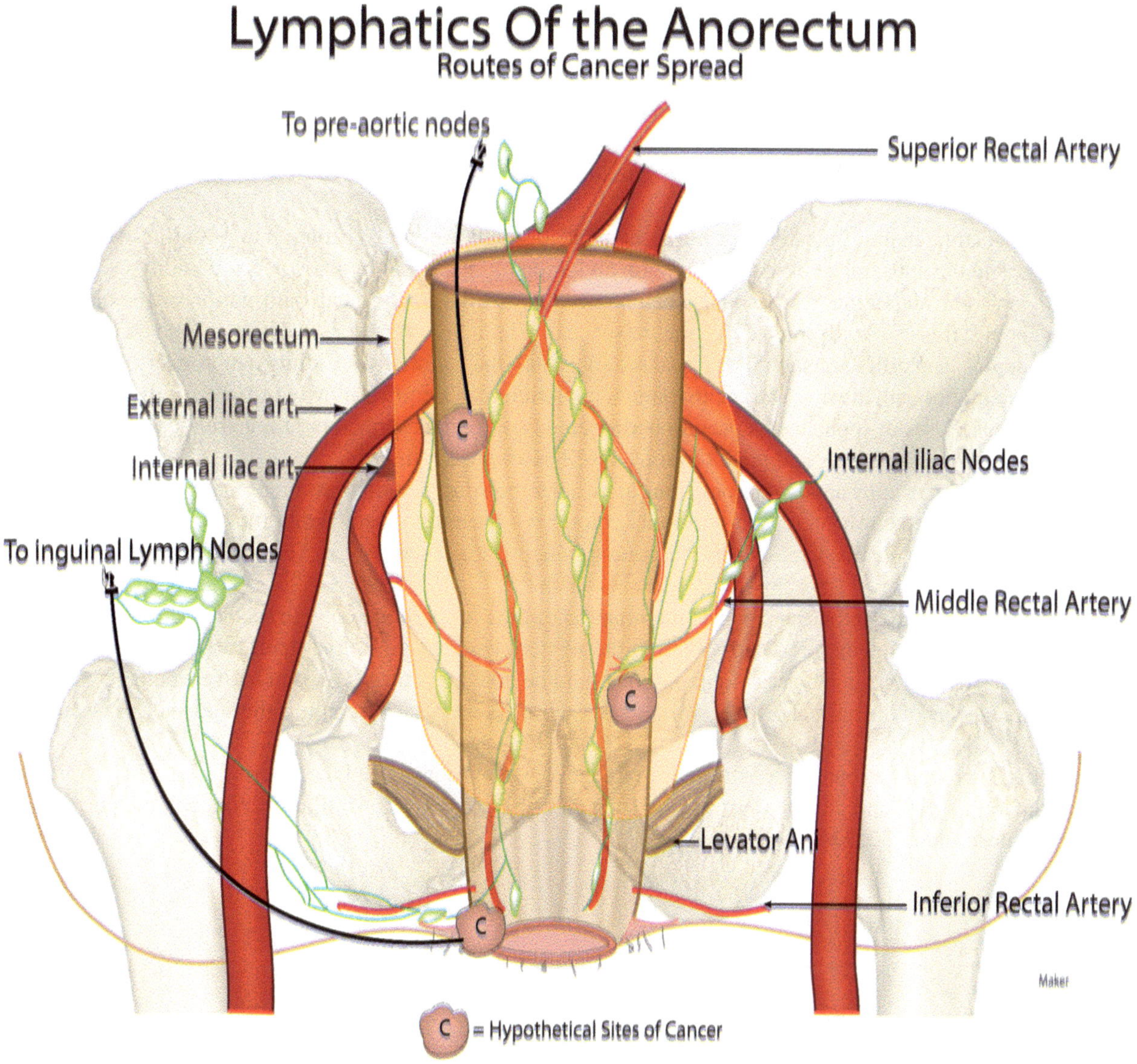

Fig. 15.2 The anorectal area has dual lymphatic and venous drainage. The rectum largely drains into the preaortic nodes after going through the mesorectum, while the anal canal and an overlapping junctional zone may additionally drain into inguinal lymph nodes along the middle and inferior rectal veins. To properly harvest these nodes, an en bloc total mesorectal excision is the standard of care for resectable tumors of the rectum which have infiltrated past the mucosa

Answer
d

5. All the following are correct *except*:
   (a) Interposition of the bowel between the liver and diaphragm may be confused with pneumoperitoneum.
   (b) Pneumoperitoneum may be asymptomatic.
   (c) The ascending or descending colon may interpose in retrorenal position.
   (d) Posterior perforations of the colon remain confined to the retroperitoneum.
   (e) Pneumoscrotum after colonoscopy suggests perforation.

Comments The hepatic flexure of the colon or other segments of the bowel may become interposed between the liver and the diaphragm, giving the appearance of free air on plain abdominal films, a finding known as Chilaiditi's sign. This can be accompanied by episodic abdominal pain and has been named Chilaiditi's syndrome. Confirmation of the diagnosis can be made by CT scanning. It is important to note that the presence of Chilaiditi's sign does not rule out the coexistence of other abdominal pathologies, and diligence should be exercised in finding the cause of coexisting symptoms [22–24].

Pneumoperitoneum does not always warrant abdominal exploration or signify hollow viscus perforation, especially in an asymptomatic patient. Cases of spontaneous pneumoperitoneum have been described in female runners, pneumatosis intestinalis, and extension from the thorax and mediastinum as well as after cunnilingus.

The colon may come to occupy anomalous positions in the abdomen due to alterations in normal bowel rotation. Instances of retrogastric, retrosplenic, retrohepatic, and retrorenal colon have been described. While these conditions are most often asymptomatic, they should be considered when interpreting imaging studies as well as before embarking on interventional procedures [25–27].

Posterior perforations of the colon can create contamination of the retroperitoneum with secondary infection of the structures therein. The most common cause of perforation in the western hemisphere is diverticulitis. Often, this condition presents with contained perforations in the pericolonic fat. It should be noted that these are pseudodiverticula, as their wall does not contain all three layers of the normal colonic wall. Rather, these are mucosal herniations through sites of perforator blood vessel entry (Fig. 15.3).

The psoas muscle provides a route of spontaneous drainage towards the groin and the anterior thigh [28, 29]. Drainage of purulent material to the spine and gluteal area has also been described [30, 31]. In similar fashion, colonic perforations may manifest as pneumoscrotum [32, 33].

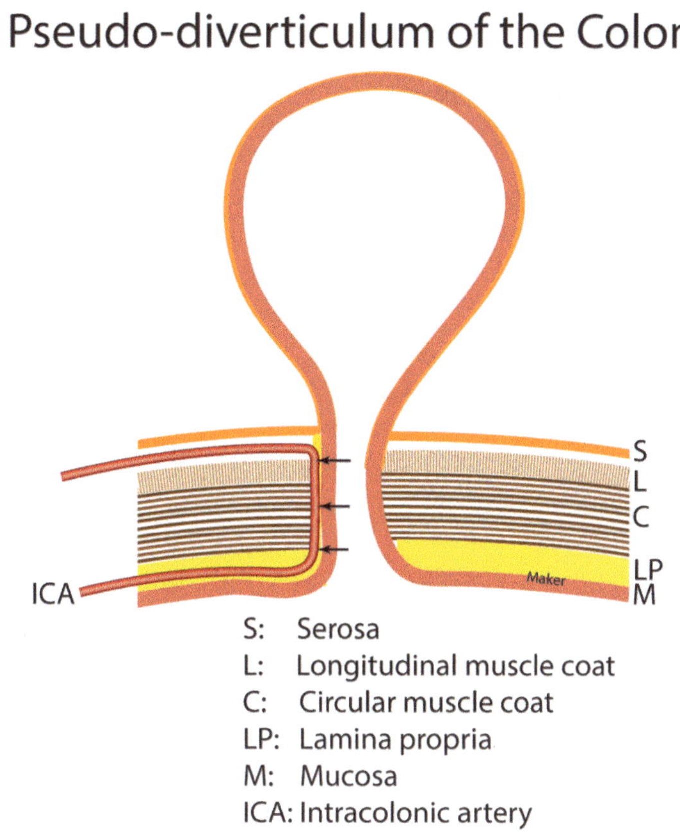

Fig. 15.3 Classic diverticular disease of the colon actually represents pseudodiverticula as they do not own a muscle coat and hence are unable to contract or empty themselves. The neck of each diverticulum has an intracolonic artery sharing the same defect through which the mucosal diverticulum protrudes out. This is the same artery which when eroded in diverticular disease causes hemorrhage and, in cases of diverticulitis, undergoes thrombosis contributing to micro-perforation and resultant abscess formation. *S* serosa, *L* longitudinal muscle coat, *C* circular muscle coat, *LP* lamina propria, *M* mucosa, *ICA* intracolonic artery

Answer

d

6. The following are landmarks for the junction of the sigmoid colon and rectum *except*:
   (a) 3rd sacral vertebra
   (b) Level at which the sigmoid mesentery disappears
   (c) Sacral promontory
   (d) Level at which the taenia coli coalesce
   (e) Level at which the superior rectal artery divides

Comments Please see question 7.

Answer
c

7. Select the *true* statement regarding the anal canal above and below the dentate line.
   (a) Below the dentate line, the anal canal has simple columnar epithelium.
   (b) The most common form of cancer above the dentate line is squamous cell carcinoma.
   (c) The most sensitive part of the anal canal lies above the dentate line.
   (d) The most common cancer below the dentate line is treated with the Nigro protocol.
   (e) Circumferential stapled hemorrhoidopexy is an ectodermal operation.

Comments Like with the gastroesophageal junction, multiple and sometimes conflicting landmarks have been cited to describe the limits of the rectum. The junction of the sigmoid colon and rectum is best defined by the coalescence of the taenia coli into a continuous longitudinal muscle layer. This distinction is very important in the setting of colonic diverticulosis, which by definition does not cross over to the rectum. The level of this transition, as well as the level of the peritoneal reflection, is subject to individual variations. There tends to be a concordance between the disappearance of the sigmoid mesentery, the uppermost valve of Huston, and the upper border of the third sacral vertebra as useful landmarks between the sigmoid colon and rectum.

Distally, the dentate line and the uppermost aspect of the anal sphincter complex have been cited as separating the rectum from the anal canal. This distinction becomes less important when the anorectum is considered as a functional unit. However, the sphincter complex and its function must be considered when contemplating the different options for surgical excision.

On the other hand, the dentate line is useful when considering the type of epithelium and malignancies derived thereof. The epithelium above the dentate line is derived from the hindgut endoderm and is columnar. Below the dentate line, it is derived from the ectoderm and is squamous. In between the two, there is a transition zone, whose behavior more closely resembles that of the endoderm. Functionally, it is thought that the transition zone serves an important role in sensing the nature of the rectal contents.

In concordance with the above division, the sensory nerve supply above the dentate line is autonomic and allows essentially pain-free procedures at this level (internal hemorrhoid banding and stapled hemorrhoidopexy). In contrast, the epithelium below the dentate line has a rich somatic nerve supply, making it very sensitive and explaining the symptoms originated by pathology in this area [34, 35] (Fig. 15.4).

The most common cancer of the anal canal is squamous cell cancer. Unlike anal adenocarcinoma, which requires surgical excision, squamous cell carcinomas are primarily treated with radiation and chemotherapy (Nigro protocol), with surgery reserved for treatment failures and recurrences. Current recommendations advocate the use of mitomycin combined with 5-FU and 5,000 Rads. Bowen's disease is anal squamous carcinoma in situ. It does not require treatment using the Nigro protocol; rather, it is treated with topical 5-FU and close follow-up.

Melanoma of the anal canal is a rare tumor. Its treatment is based on the principles guiding the management of cutaneous melanoma, that is, wide excision and sentinel node mapping and excision [36].

Cognitive Anatomy of the Anorectum

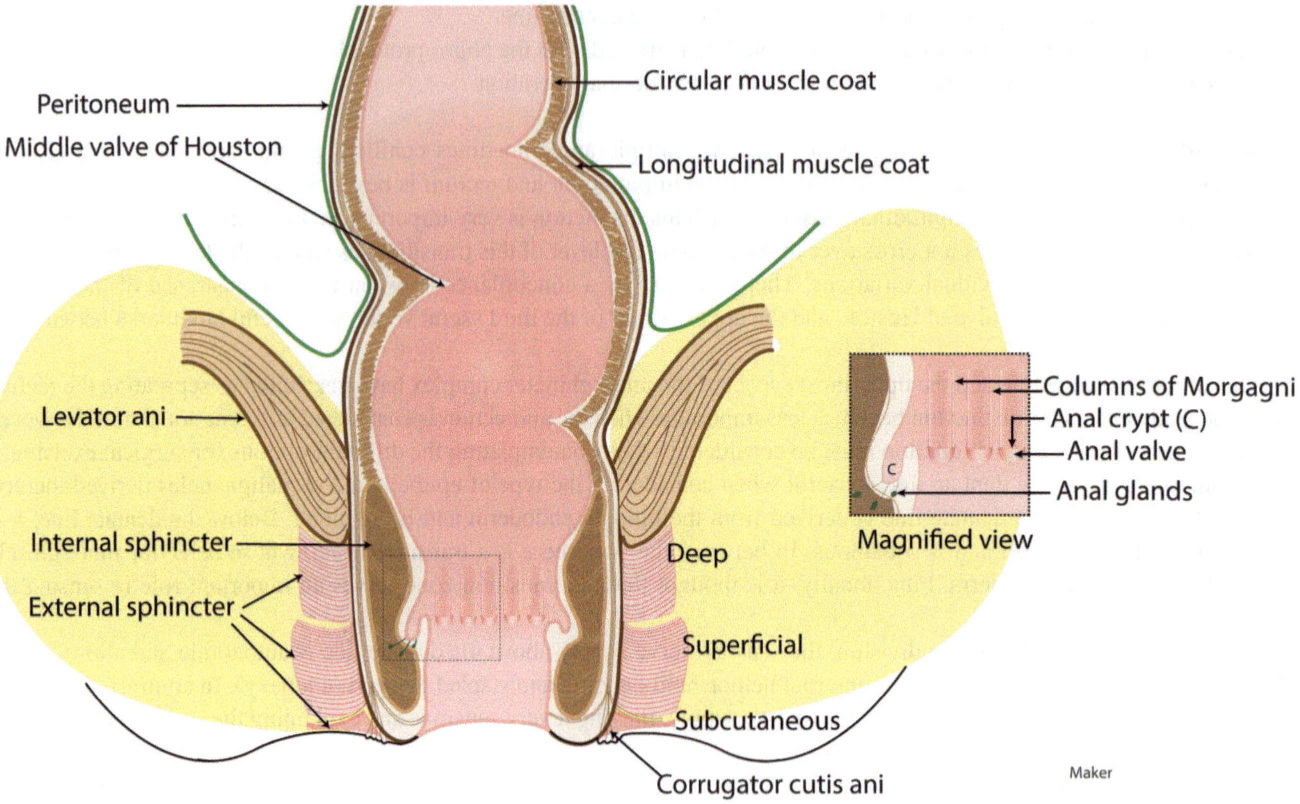

Fig. 15.4 The anorectal junction is marked by the *dentate line*, which represents a series of pockets called crypts. Each pocket is suspended at the bottom of two mucosal pleats named the columns of Morgagni. Inside the crypts are the openings of the anal glands, which secrete mucous to help lubricate the anus as the sphincter relaxes during a bowel movement. The corrugator cutis ani muscle is the insertion of the longitudinal muscle coat and, as the name implies, is responsible for corrugation of the immediate perianal skin

Answer
d

8. Match the following tumor locations with the most appropriate operation

(a) Cancer of the cecum	1. Left hemicolectomy
(b) Cancer of the mid transverse colon	2. Low anterior resection
(c) Cancer of the proximal rectum	3. Right hemicolectomy
(d) Cancer of the descending colon	4. Extended right hemicolectomy
(e) Cancer of the distal rectum	5. Abdominal perineal resection

Comments The surgical treatment of colorectal cancer (open or laparoscopic) is based on the vascular pedicles to different sections of the colon and the associated lymphatic drainage basins. While at least 2 cm distal margin of resection must be considered, they rarely become determinants of the extent of resection. Colon cancer tends to have more proximal than distal spread, determining recommendations of 5–7 cm proximal margins. Surgery of the rectum and anus must take into account the involvement of the sphincter complex.

Right hemicolectomies resect the segment supplied by the ileocolic and right colic artery, while left hemicolectomies involve the territory of the left colic artery. Either resection may be, respectively, "extended" to the territory supplied by the right or left branch of the middle colic artery. The sigmoid colon may be resected independently.

Resections of the rectum must consider the distance between the tumor and the sphincter complex. Again, at least a 2 cm margin must be achieved, determining that if such margin is obtainable, a low anterior sphincter preserving resection should be performed. In contrast, if this margin does not exist, and more so if the sphincter complex is involved, an abdominoperineal approach must be taken [37–39] (Fig. 15.5a, b).

Reconstruction of intestinal transit after colon resection is often carried out via creation of stapled anastomosis. As mentioned in prior chapters, these anastomoses offer wide patency, satisfactory bursting strength and convenience. There are several technical principles to take into consideration. These are illustrated below, as they apply to ileocolic anastomosis (Fig. 15.6).

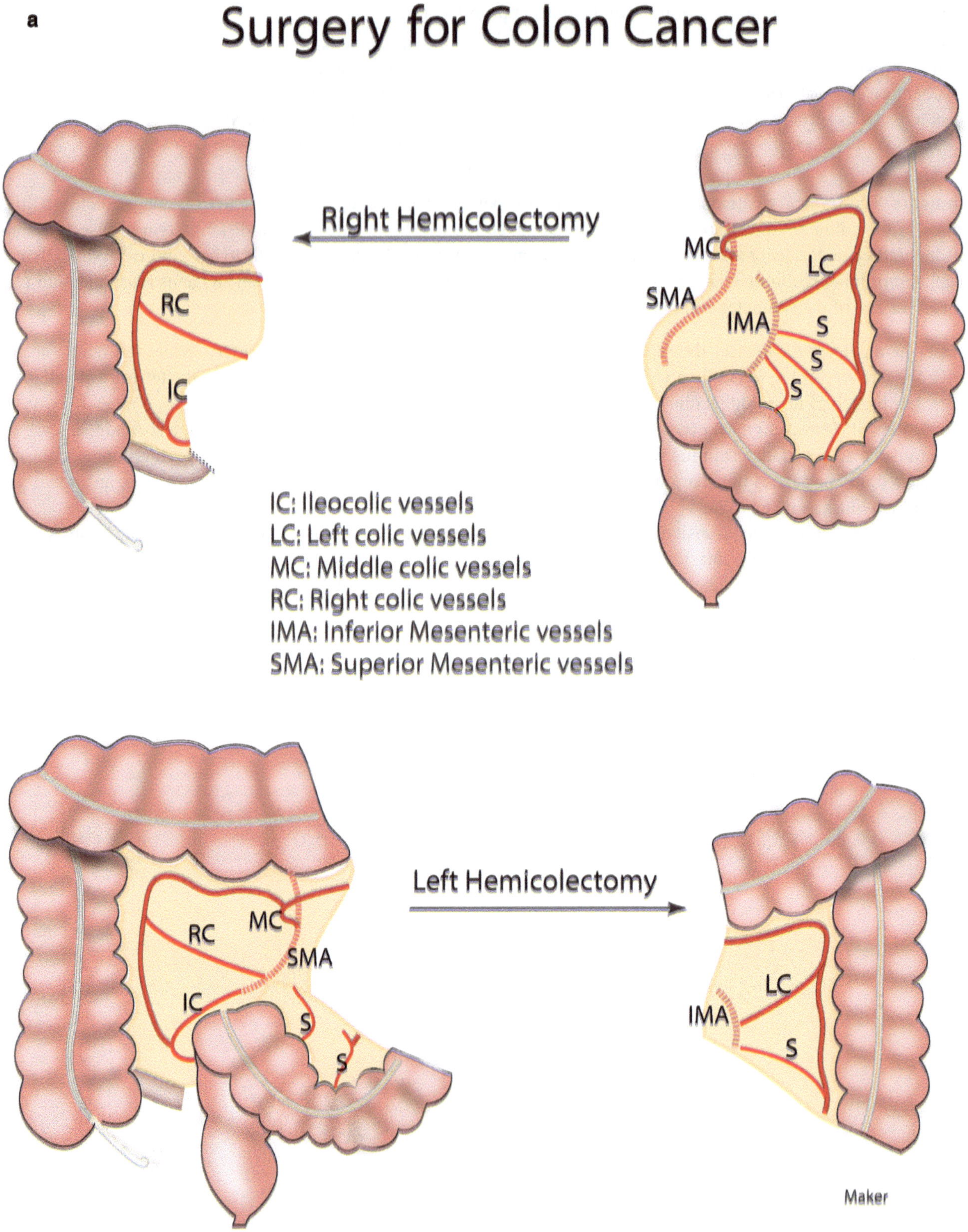

Fig. 15.5 (**a**) Surgery for cancer of the right colon consists of removing the right colon en bloc with its lymph node drainage basin along the ileocolic and right colic bundles, and ending to the right of midcolic vessels. Similarly, left hemicolectomy is for cancers of the left colon removing lymph node drainage basins from left of the midcolic vessels and including the left colic and first branches of the sigmoid vessels. Cancer of the transverse colon between the two flexures may require extended right or left hemicolectomy including midcolic lymph node basins. *IC* ileocolic vessels, *LC* left colic vessels, *MC* middle colic vessels, *RC* right colic vessels, *IMA* inferior mesenteric vessels, *SMA* superior mesenteric vessels. (**b**) Low anterior resection refers to the removal of the rectosigmoid through an anterior abdominal approach as compared to the abdominoperineal resection where an additional perineal approach is added to remove the perianal skin, anorectal canal, and ischio-anal fossa contents of fat and lymph nodes. En bloc resection of the mesorectal pad of fat and lymph nodes is part of both procedures. *SMA* superior mesenteric vessels, *IMA* inferior mesenteric vessels, *RC* right colic vessels, *MC* middle colic vessels, *LC* left colic vessels, *IC* ileocolic vessels, *RA* anorectum with ischiorectal tissues, *MR* mesorectum

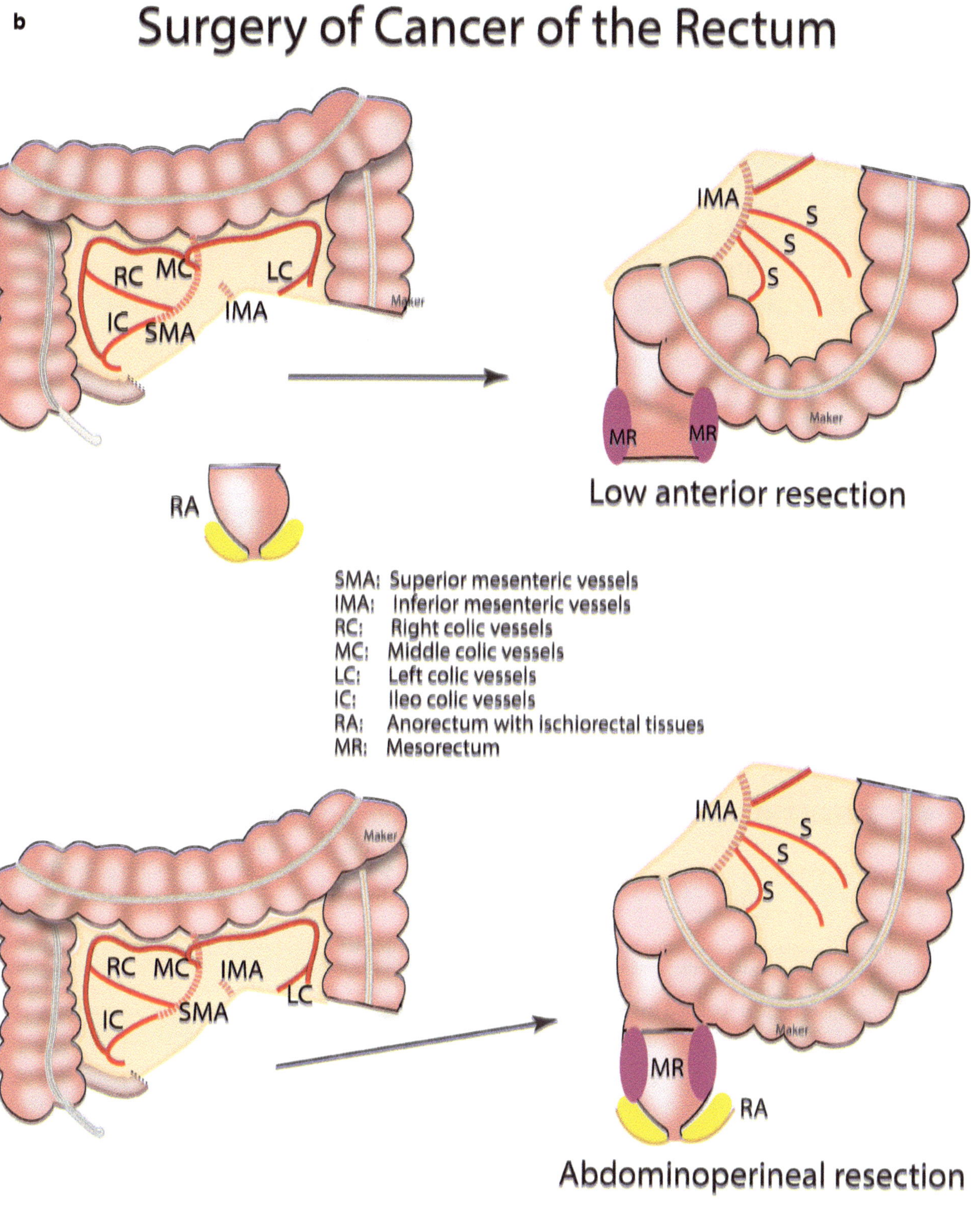

Fig. 15.5 (continued)

Cognitive Principles of a Stapled Anastomotic Technique

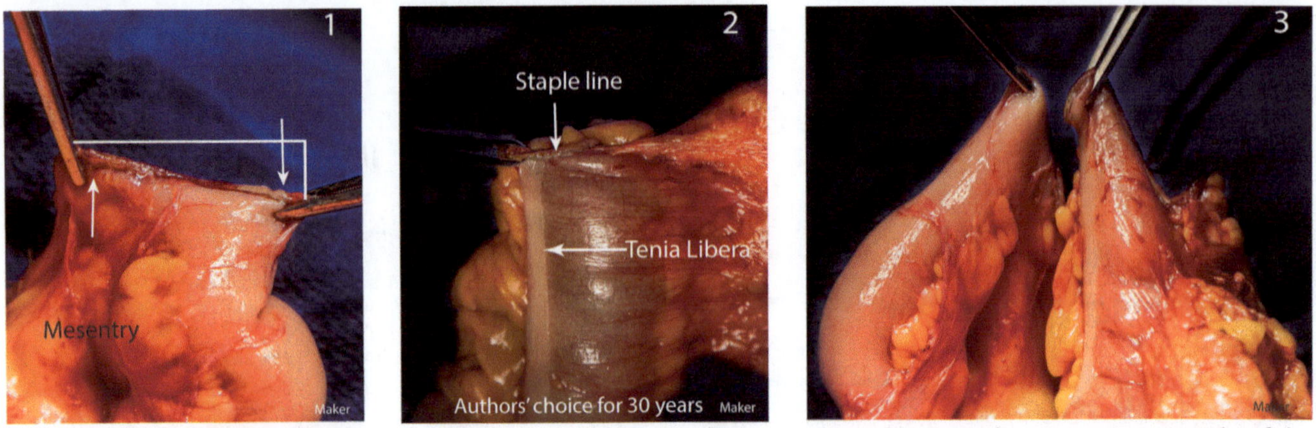

1. Bowel is divided obliquely so that the antimesenteric side is lower to maximize its blood flow.

2. Colon is turned in a way that Tinea libera is on the free end of the staple line.

3. Tinea libera and antimesenteric side of the small bowel are brought together in preparation for anastomosis.

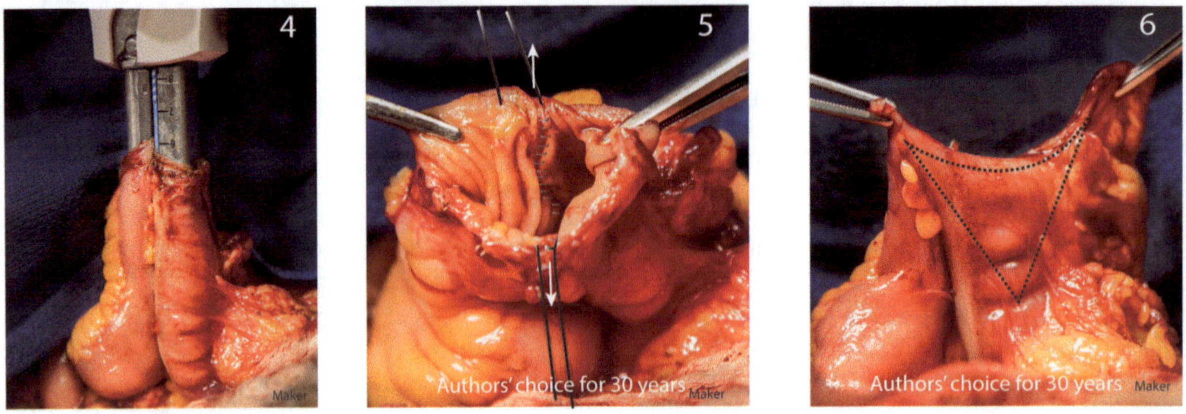

4. Small rectangular openings are made at the staple lines to snuggly fit GIA limbs.

5. Two ends of anastomotic staple lines are pulled in opposite directions to set up for a triangular closure.

6. Final staple line is constructed so as to form a triangle effectively separating all three staple lines.

Fig. 15.6 While the example shown is an ileotransverse colon anastomosis, the principles apply to most stapled GI anastomoses. The bowel is divided obliquely to angle lower on the antimesenteric side (Step 1). After the GIA stapling instrument is fired, the resultant two anastomotic staple lines are separated (Step 5) to form a triangle with the apex of the staple line clearly visible in the bowel for inspection of integrity and control of bleeders at the staple line. The final staple line is completed, typically with a TA stapler creating a triangular anastomotic opening (Step 6)

Answer

a, 3; b, 4; c, 2; d, 1; e, 5

9. The following are correct in relation to abdominoperineal resection (APR) *except*:
   (a) Waldeyer's fascia should be preserved during APR to prevent bleeding from the presacral vein plexus.
   (b) Denonvilliers' fascia separates the prostate from the rectum and constitutes the anterior plane of abdominal dissection during an APR.
   (c) APR includes the resection of the inguinal lymph nodes.
   (d) An APR results in a transient neurogenic bladder.
   (e) Mesorectal excision addresses radial margins.

Comments Abdominoperineal resection aims for the en bloc resection of the rectum, anus, sphincter complex, mesorectum, and ischio-anal fat tissue.

The anterior limit of the abdominal resection is Denonvilliers' fascia, which separates the prostate and bladder from the rectum in the male and the vagina and rectum in the female. Posteriorly, Waldeyer's fascia constitutes the limit of resection. Beneath this fascia lies the presacral venous plexus. Laterally, the resection extends to the pelvic sidewalls, preserving the endopelvic fascia. Dissection along these planes is carried caudally as low as possible and constitutes the total mesorectal excision.

The perineal portion of this operation involves creating a perianal incision extending from the center of the perineum to the coccyx and from one ischial tuberosity to another.

Lymphatic excision is carried out along the superior hemorrhoidal vascular pedicle. Even though the distal anorectum drains to the inguinal nodes, they are not normally removed during an abdominoperineal resection [40–44].

Answer
c

10. All of the following are true *except*:
    (a) The mesorectum separates the rectum from the presacral fascia and lateral pelvic walls.
    (b) Total mesorectal excision occurs through a relatively bloodless field.
    (c) Mesorectal excision markedly reduces the incidence of subsequent local recurrence of rectal cancer.
    (d) The distal edge of the mesorectum finishes into a tonguelike projection at which point the rectum has the smallest diameter.
    (e) Mesorectal resection taper in towards the distal rectum.

Comments Even though the rectum lacks a true mesentery, the term mesorectum has been coined to refer to the 2–3 cm thick circumferential envelope of fibrous and fatty tissue surrounding the rectum. This envelope is in turn surrounded by the visceral layer of the pelvic fascia and extends to the level of the rectal sphincter complex. Dissection is carried through the relatively bloodless plane between the visceral and parietal pelvic fascia.

The recognition of the mesorectum and its complete excision in the treatment of rectal cancer has yielded great survival benefits by improving control of the circumferential radial margins of rectal resections.

Successful total mesorectal excision is carried out from the presacral fascia to Denonvilliers' fascia along the pelvic sidewalls. Distally, the mesorectum should be transected at a right angle, avoiding "coning in" into the distal rectum. The specimen thus produced consists of the rectum covered by a smooth bilobed mass of fibrous and fatty tissue [45–47] (Fig. 15.7).

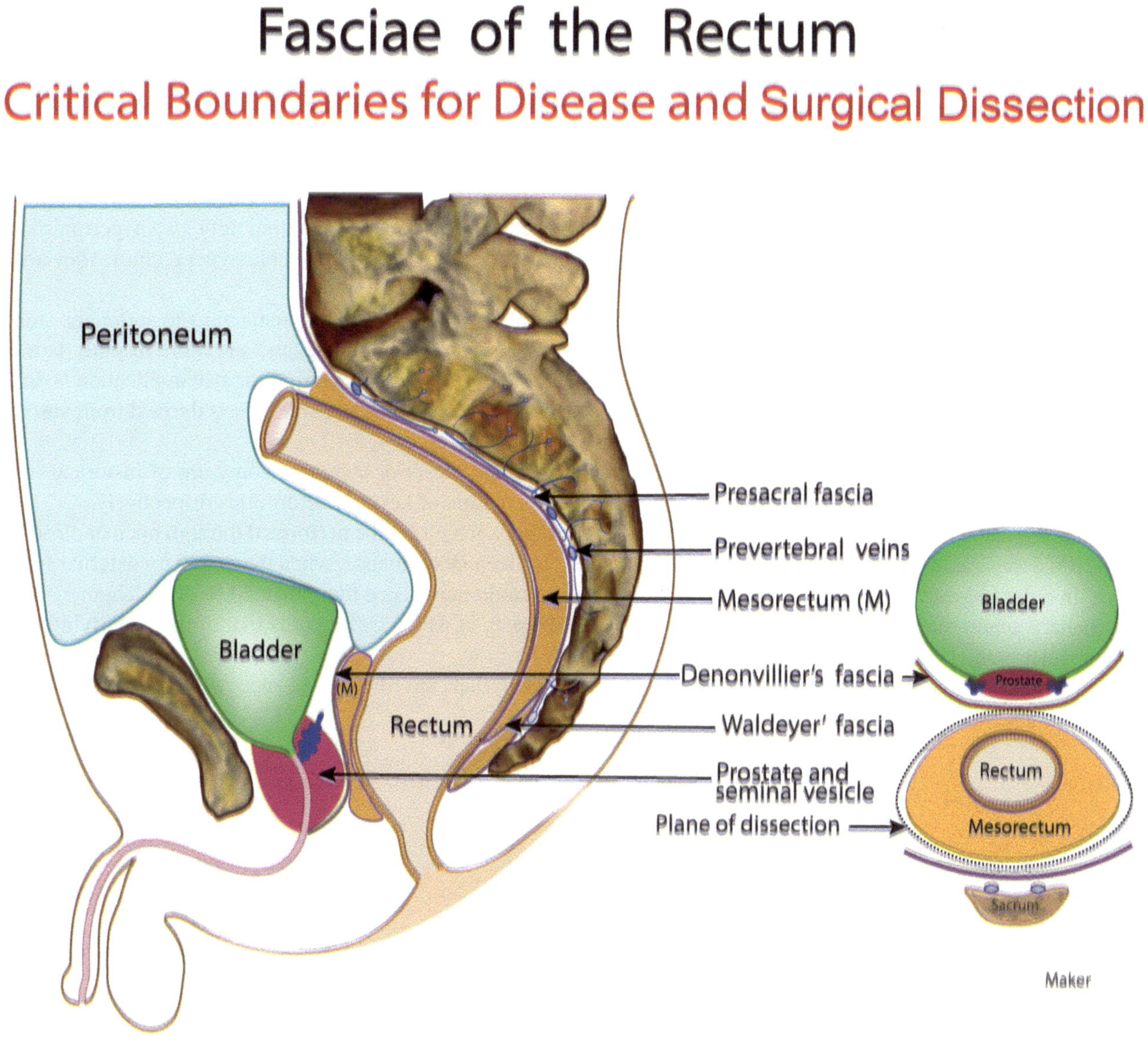

Maker

Fig. 15.7 The infraperitoneal rectum is well demarcated with strong fascial layers which help localize spread of infection and cancer. These layers are excellent surgical planes of division for the surgeon. Denonvilliers' fascia anteriorly separates the prostate, seminal vesicles, and their rich periprostatic venous plexus from the rectum. Presacral and Waldeyer's fasciae posteriorly create an excellent plane of division of the mesorectum from the sacrum and presacral veins

Answer
e

11. All of the following are correct *except*:
    (a) Posterior midline sphincterotomy results in a keyhole deformity.
    (b) Lateral internal sphincterotomy ideally should involve the entire internal sphincter.
    (c) Lateral internal sphincterotomy can be performed through closed or open techniques.
    (d) The initial treatment for anal fissure is stool softeners and nitroglycerine ointment.
    (e) The internal sphincter is responsible for maintaining continence during REM sleep.

Comments Primary anal fissures are tears in the anoderm that result from passage of hard stool through a hypertonic sphincter complex. They are a source of intense anorectal pain with defecation as well as bright red blood per rectum. They are most often located in the posterior midline.

The treatment of anal fissures involves both medical and surgical options. Medical treatment aims to soften the stool and relax the hypertonic internal anal sphincter via the use of nitrates, calcium channel blockers, and more recently botulinum toxin. When these treatments fail, surgery is indicated. Of note, the nitroglycerin preparation for anal application is different from the transdermal preparation used for the treatment of angina. However, both share side effects derived from vasodilatation such as headache.

Surgical therapies disrupt the internal sphincter. Digital stretch and posterior sphincterotomy are of historical interest. They have been abandoned due to a high rate of incontinence and creation of keyhole deformities respectively.

Current surgical therapy consists of lateral internal sphincterotomy, which can be performed through open or closed techniques with comparable results. This procedure may also result in sleep incontinence, when the voluntary external sphincter relaxes. In order to avoid incontinence, division of the sphincter should not exceed more than 50 % of its length.

Secondary anal fissures may occur in inflammatory bowel disease, in which treatment is that of the underlying disease, with sphincterotomy being contraindicated.

In cases where sphincterotomy is not feasible, rectal advancement flaps have been used successfully [48, 49].

Answer
b

12. All of the following are correct *except*:
    (a) Internal hemorrhoid bundles are 3, 7, and 11 o'clock in the prone jackknife position.
    (b) The valves of Houston help with fecal continence.
    (c) The anal crypts lie between the columns of Morgagni.
    (d) The anal valves are the remnant of the embryologic membrane separating the hindgut from the proctodeum.
    (e) The columns of Morgagni result from the junction of the wide hindgut with the narrower proctodeum.

Comments Hemorrhoids are venous cushions located beneath the epithelium of the anal canal. They are usually located in three groups: right anterior, right posterior, and left lateral, corresponding to 1, 5, and 9 o'clock in the jackknife position. Based on their epithelial lining and relation to the dentate line, they are classified into internal and external. Internal hemorrhoids are lined by mucosa and have very little sensitivity, whereas external hemorrhoids are covered by squamous epithelium and have great sensitivity. Hemorrhoids may occur primarily or secondarily to portal hypertension, ascites, and venous hypertension of any etiology [50].

The transverse folds of the rectum, also known as valves of Houston, are mucosal folds with varying degrees of muscular support. While their number has classically been quoted as three, they can be more numerous or totally absent. Their function is not completely understood. It has been proposed that they retard fecal passage, that they aid in continence, and that they induce a spiral motion upon passing stool. The middle valve of Houston is found approximately 8 cm from the anal verge and coincides with the rectal peritoneal reflection [51].

The embryologic junction of the distal hindgut and the proctodeum leaves several anatomic remnants. The best know of which is the dentate line, representing the epithelial junction between endoderm and mesoderm. It is thought that the anal valves, located between the columns of Morgagni represent the cloacal membrane. In turn, the columns of Morgagni may represent the plication of the distal hindgut as it meets with the proctodeum, which has a smaller caliber.

The columns of Morgagni join in their distal aspect, forming the anal crypts. These crypts are small mucosal pockets containing the opening of the anal glands. Anal glands typically secrete mucus, which collects in the crypts and supplies mucosal lubrication at the time of defecation [52].

Answer
a

13. All of the following are correct *except*:
    (a) Perianal hidradenitis suppurativa represents multiple anal fistulas.
    (b) Multiple perianal fistulous tracts are suggestive of Crohn's disease.
    (c) Perianal fistulas posterior to the transverse perianal plane stem from the posterior midline crypt.
    (d) Anterior perianal fistulas have radial tracts.
    (e) Hidradenitis suppurativa represents inflammatory disease of the apocrine glands.

Comments Hidradenitis suppurativa, also known as Verneuil's disease, consists of the chronic infection of apocrine glands leading to scarring, fibrosis, and sinus tract formation. It may arise in any region where these glands are located, namely, the axillae, nipples, inframammary folds, perineum, and buttocks. Treatment is difficult, and antibiotics alone are often unsuccessful. Surgical treatment involves incision and drainage, as well as various degrees of excision of the affected skin [53–55].

Anal fistulas track from the skin opening to an anal crypt. In the absence of malignancy or Crohn's disease, they follow Goodsall's rule. This rule states that fistulas anterior to the rectum follow a straight radial path to the closes crypt. In contrast, fistulas posterior to the rectum follow a curved path to the posterior midline crypt.

In the presence of Crohn's disease, fistulas tend to be multiple and follow unpredictable tracts. In this setting, traditional fistulotomy is often nonconductive to healing. Controlling disease activity systemically and achieving sphincter preservation are of paramount importance [56].

Answer

a

14. All of the following are correct *except*:
   (a) Human papillomavirus infection affects mucosal epithelia throughout the body.
   (b) Anal condylomata acuminata exhibit exophytic growth.
   (c) Buschke–Lowenstein tumors have both exophytic and endophytic growth.
   (d) Anal squamous cell carcinoma is characterized by invasion into adjacent tissues.
   (e) Perianal Paget's disease is associated with visceral malignancies in 50 % of cases.

Comments Human papillomaviruses (HPVs) are a group of double-stranded DNA viruses that infect keratinocytes of the skin, anogenital tract, mouth, larynx, and esophagus. During the 1970s, their association with epithelial neoplasms in these areas was demonstrated and viral DNA was found in the mutated cells. While there are over 30 types of HPV, types 6 and 11 are associated with 90 % of the benign lesions, while types 16 and 18 are found in 70 % of the malignant lesions. The strategy of viral replication seems to be associated with the malignant potential of different strains. Low-risk HPV types replicate in episomes, while high-risk HPV incorporates its genome into the host cell DNA, triggering malignant transformation [57].

Anal condylomata acuminata are soft cauliflower-like skin lesions induced by HPV. These lesions do not extend beyond the epidermal basal layer. While atypical mitotic cells may be found at this level, there is overall an orderly maturation of keratinocytes. When caused by HPV 6 and 11, these lesions may have a tendency to recur after excision, but rarely progress to carcinoma.

Buschke–Lowenstein tumors, also known as giant condylomas or verrucous carcinomas, are exophytic papillomatous tumors of the perianal and genital area, also associated with HPV infection [16, 18]. These lesions tend to burrow into adjacent tissues (endophytic growth), such as the ischio-anal fossa and perianal tissues. They are also associated with sinuses and fistulas. However, there is no demonstrable microscopic infiltration, and cells are more or less differentiated [58].

Bowen's disease or squamous cell carcinoma in situ is most often seen in the face, hands, and trunk, with the perianal region being an uncommon site. Lesions are often scaly plaques. Microscopically, basal cell atypia with an intact basal membrane are defining traits. These lesions have been linked to HPV 16. Treatment is carried out by excision.

Invasive squamous cell carcinoma represents the full oncogenic effects of HPV infection. These lesions may be flat, ulcerated, or papillomatous on physical exam. Microscopically, they all share the cellular atypia and frank invasion of underlying tissues.

Occasionally, anal or perianal tissues removed for pathologies such as fistulas or hemorrhoids are found to have serendipitous condylomas with varying grades of dysplasia or even squamous cell carcinoma. Completely excised low-grade lesions require no further treatment. However, high-grade lesions merit further workup, surveillance, and even re-excision, especially in patients with immunosuppression and other factors that may make them more prone to progression.

Anal and perianal Paget's disease arises from the apocrine sweat glands located in this area. These lesions are often eczematous and pruritic, although they may present as perianal masses in later stages. While distinct from squamous cell carcinoma in terms of their cell of origin (apocrine sweat gland vs. squamous epithelium) and etiology (HPV is not associated with Paget's disease), these lesions may be difficult to distinguish. Of note, Paget's disease coexists with synchronous visceral malignancies in up to 50 % of cases. Association with cancer of the anus, rectum, colon, stomach, and prostate has been reported. Resection is considered curative [59].

Anorectal melanomas represent 1 % of all melanomas and are often mistaken for benign lesions, with diagnostic delay and the associated poor prognosis being very common. Initially, treatment involved radical surgery in the form of abdominoperineal resection and inguinal lymph node dissection. However, currently, wide excision with sphincter preservation is the favored strategy [60].

Answer
a

15. All of the following are correct *except*:
    (a) Anal abscesses and fistulas originate in the intersphincteric space.
    (b) Anal fistulas occur after 30 % of anal abscesses.
    (c) Ischiorectal abscesses may extend contralaterally anterior to the rectum.
    (d) Sphincter preservation is a key goal in the treatment of anal abscesses and fistulas.
    (e) Obliteration of the internal opening is a necessary step in the treatment of anal fistulas.

Comments Anorectal abscesses and fistulas are thought to have a common origin in the infection of the glands of the anal crypts of Morgagni. These glands are located in the intersphincteric space, which would predict that abscesses should be predominantly located in this space; however, this is seldom the case. Other etiologies such as Crohn's disease, anal fissures, and trauma have also been defined.

Classification systems based on the cryptoglandular theory of abscess formation have been developed. According to this system, the infection originates as an intersphincteric abscesses. From here, the infection may track cephalad, forming supralevator abscesses or caudally giving rise to perianal abscesses. Lateral extension through the external sphincter produces ischiorectal abscesses, which may extend contralaterally behind the rectum thus forming horseshoe abscesses.

The importance of this classification lies in that it increases awareness of the potential routes of spread for infection, facilitating the planning of an optimal strategy for complete abscess drainage [61] (Fig. 15.8).

In analogous fashion, fistulas may follow a caudal course between the sphincters, in which case they are considered intersphincteric fistulas. Suprasphincteric fistulas are similar to supralevator abscesses and drain to the perineum thought the levator muscles. Transphincteric fistulas follow the same pattern of extension of ischiorectal abscesses. Extrasphincteric fistulas do not originate in the anal glands.

Treatment principles of fistulas included clearly defining the anatomy, drainage of associated abscesses, eradication of the fistulous tract, and preservation of continence. Perhaps the most important step consists of eliminating the internal orifice [62].

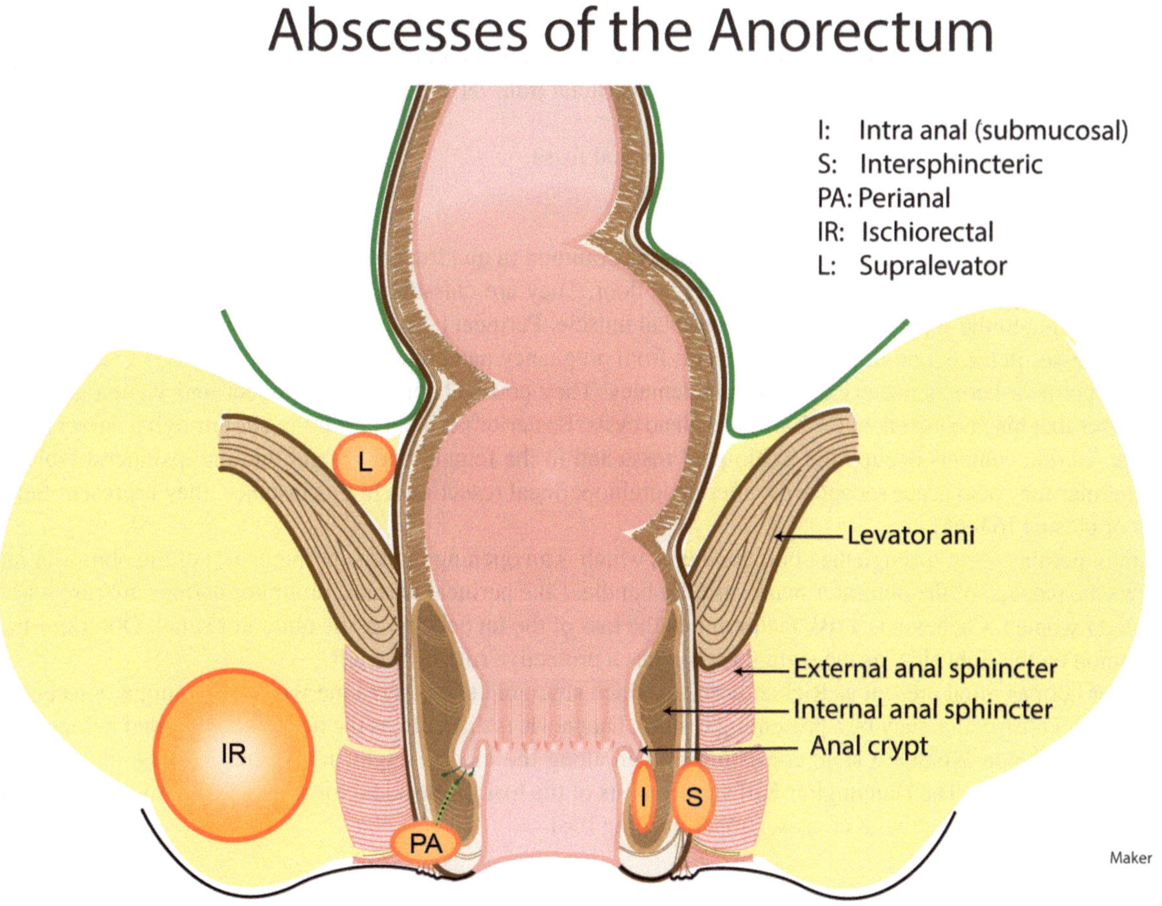

Fig. 15.8 Most abscesses of the anorectum start in the crypt glandular complex and track in spaces as shown above. Abscesses from idiopathic inflammatory bowel disease may track directly from the disease segment, and treatment always includes treating the primary disease. The majority of anorectal fistulas also originate from the crypt glandular complex, which becomes the internal opening of the fistula. *I* intra-anal (submucosal), *S* intersphincteric, *PA* perianal, *IR* ischiorectal, *L* supralevator

Answer

c

16. All of the following are correct *except*:
    (a) Perineal hernias consist of the protrusion of a viscus through the floor of the pelvis.
    (b) Perineal hernias always occur anterior to the superficial transverse perineal muscle.
    (c) Perineal hernias are always located laterally.
    (d) In the male, perineal hernias occupy the ischio-anal fossa.
    (e) The adductor muscles conceal obturator hernias.

Comments Perineal hernias are very rare in humans, but common in quadrupeds. They consist of the protrusion of a hernia sac containing abdominal contents through the pelvic floor. They are classified into anterior and posterior, based on their location in relation to the superficial transverse perineal muscle. Perineal hernias are more frequent in elderly females (5:1) due to weaknesses in the pelvic floor that may result from pregnancy and childbirth.

Anterior perineal hernias occur exclusively in females. They course lateral to the bladder and vagina and manifest as vulvar masses that may be mistaken for Bartholin gland cysts. Posterior perineal hernias occur through a defect in the levator ani muscle. Hernia contents occupy the ischio-anal fossa and in the female may extend into the ipsilateral labia. Posterior perineal hernias may also occur secondarily, after abdominoperineal resections. In this instance, they represent failure of the pelvic floor closure [63–65].

Obturator hernias occur through the obturator canal, which is an opening in the superior aspect of the obturator membrane that allows the passage of the obturator neurovascular bundle. Like perineal hernias, obturator hernias are rare and typically affect elderly women. Cachexia is a risk factor due to the loss of the fat occupying the obturator canal. Obturator hernias are most common on the right side, as the sigmoid colon has a protective role on the left.

Obturator hernias often present as Richter hernias, which strangulate and perforate without causing a bowel obstruction. However, bowel obstruction may be a presenting feature. Diagnosis is difficult, as the hernia is concealed below the adductor muscles. The Howship–Romberg sign, consisting of pain along the medial thigh (in the course of the obturator nerve), is present in 50 % of cases. The Hannington-Kiff sign consists of the loss of the adductor reflex. Diagnosis of obturator hernias is most frequently established with cross-sectional imaging [66].

Answer
b

References

1. Timmermans JP, Hens J, Adriaensen D. Outer submucous plexus: an intrinsic nerve network involved in both secretory and motility processes in the intestine of large mammals and humans. Anat Rec. 2001;262:71–8.
2. Burns AJ. Migration of neural crest-derived enteric nervous system precursor cells to and within the gastrointestinal tract. Int J Dev Biol. 2005;49:143–50.
3. Martucciello G. Hirschsprung's disease, one of the most difficult diagnoses in pediatric surgery: a review of the problems from clinical practice to the bench. Eur J Pediatr Surg. 2008;18:140–9.
4. Moore SW, Zaahl MG. Multiple endocrine neoplasia syndromes, children, Hirschsprung's disease and RET. Pediatr Surg Int. 2008;24:521–30.
5. Scheuermann DW, Stach W. Fluorescence microscopic study of the architecture and structure of an adrenergic network in the plexus myentericus (Auerbach), plexus submucosus externus (Schabadasch) and plexus submucosus internus (Meissner) of the porcine small intestine. Acta Anat (Basel). 1984;119:49–59.
6. Furness JB. The enteric nervous system: normal functions and enteric neuropathies. Neurogastroenterol Motil. 2008;20 Suppl 1:32–8.
7. Lau ST, Caty MG. Hindgut abnormalities. Surg Clin N Am. 2006;86:301–16, viii.
8. Knowles CH. New horizons in the pathogenesis of gastrointestinal neuromuscular disease. J Pediatr Gastroenterol Nutr. 2007;45 Suppl 2:S97–102.
9. Tornroos A, Garvin S, Olsson H. The number of identified lymph node metastases increases continuously with increased total lymph node recovery in pT3 colon cancer. Acta Oncol. 2009;48:1152–6.
10. Thomas KA, Lechner J, Shen P, Waters GS, Geisinger KR, Levine EA. Use of sentinel node mapping for cancer of the colon: "to map or not to map". Am Surg. 2006;72:606–11; discussion 11–2.
11. Stojadinovic A, Allen PJ, Protic M, et al. Colon sentinel lymph node mapping: practical surgical applications. J Am Coll Surg. 2005;201:297–313.
12. Govindarajan A, Baxter NN. Lymph node evaluation in early-stage colon cancer. Clin Colorectal Cancer. 2008;7:240–6.
13. Fisher Jr DF, Fry WJ. Collateral mesenteric circulation. Surg Gynecol Obstet. 1987;164:487–92.
14. Rosenblum JD, Boyle CM, Schwartz LB. The mesenteric circulation. Anatomy and physiology. Surg Clin N Am. 1997;77:289–306.
15. Gourley EJ, Gering SA. The meandering mesenteric artery: a historic review and surgical implications. Dis Colon Rectum. 2005;48:996–1000.
16. Goligher JC. The adequacy of the marginal blood-supply to the left colon after high ligation of the inferior mesenteric artery during excision of the rectum. Br J Surg. 1954;41:351–3.
17. Bertelli L, Lorenzini L, Bertelli E. The arterial vascularization of the large intestine. Anatomical and radiological study. Surg Radiol Anat. 1996;18 Suppl 1:A1–6, S1-59.
18. Hiller N, Berelowitz D, Hadas-Halpern I. Primary epiploic appendagitis: clinical and radiological manifestations. Isr Med Assoc J. 2000;2:896–8.
19. Sakorafas GH, Zouros E, Peros G. Applied vascular anatomy of the colon and rectum: clinical implications for the surgical oncologist. Surg Oncol. 2006;15:243–55.
20. Khaira HS, Silverman SH, Obeid ML. Critical lower limb ischaemia following excision of the rectum. Cardiovasc Surg. 1998;6:424–6.
21. Sivanesan S, Tam W. Images of interest. Hepatobiliary and pancreatic: colonic manifestations of portal hypertension. J Gastroenterol Hepatol. 2005;20:1124.
22. Glatter RD, April RS, Miskovitz P, Neistadt LD. Severe recurrent abdominal pain: an anatomical variant of Chilaiditi's syndrome. Med Gen Med. 2007;9:67.
23. Lo BM. Radiographic look-alikes: distinguishing between pneumoperitoneum and pseudopneumoperitoneum. J Emerg Med. 2010;38:36–9.
24. Saber AA, Boros MJ. Chilaiditi's syndrome: what should every surgeon know? Am Surg. 2005;71:261–3.
25. Unal B, Kara S, Aktas A, Bilgili Y. Anatomic variations of the colon detected on abdominal CT scans. Tani Girisim Radyol. 2004;10:304–8.
26. Prassopoulos P, Gourtsoyiannis N, Cavouras D, Pantelidis N. Interposition of the colon between the kidney and the psoas muscle: a normal anatomic variation studied by CT. Abdom Imaging. 1994;19:446–8.
27. Pinto A, Brunese L, Noviello D, Catalano O. Colonic interposition between kidney and psoas muscle: anatomical variation studied with CT. Radiol Med. 1997;94:58–60.
28. Lee KN, Lee HL, Yoon JH, et al. A case of mucinous adenocarcinoma of the colon presenting with psoas abscess. Korean J Gastroenterol. 2008;52:120–3.
29. Debes JD, Lopez-Morra H, Dickstein G. A psoas abscess caused by Pseudomonas aeruginosa due to diverticular perforation. Am J Gastroenterol. 2006;101:2168.
30. Hopton B, Barron D, Ambrose S, Millner P. The flatulent spine: lumbar spinal infection secondary to colonic diverticular abscess: a case report and review of the literature. J Spinal Disord Tech. 2008;21:527–30.
31. Sinha DD, Sharma C, Gupta V, Chaturvedi V, Sharma V. Post-traumatic retroperitoneal colonic injury presenting as gluteal abscess. Indian J Gastroenterol. 2004;23:151–2.
32. Yang B, Jiang SX, Fan ZL. Pneumoscrotum induced by spontaneous colon perforation: a case report and review of the literature. Zhonghua Nan Ke Xue. 2007;13:744–5.
33. Fu KI, Sano Y, Kato S, et al. Pneumoscrotum: a rare manifestation of perforation associated with therapeutic colonoscopy. World J Gastroenterol. 2005;11:5061–3.
34. Zbar AP, Guo M, Pescatori M. Anorectal morphology and function: analysis of the Shafik legacy. Tech Coloproctol. 2008;12:191–200.
35. Skandalakis JE. Comment on surgical anatomy. Arch Surg. 2000;135:1115.
36. Gervasoni Jr JE, Wanebo HJ. Cancers of the anal canal and anal margin. Cancer Invest. 2003;21:452–64.
37. Sternberg A. Carcinoma of the colon: margins of resection. J Surg Oncol. 2008;98:603–6.
38. Soop M, Nelson H. Is laparoscopic resection appropriate for colorectal adenocarcinoma? Adv Surg. 2008;42:205–17.
39. Ruo L, Guillem JG. Surgical management of primary colorectal cancer. Surg Oncol. 1998;7:153–63.
40. Radcliffe A. Can the results of anorectal (abdominoperineal) resection be improved: are circumferential resection margins too often positive? Color Dis. 2006;8:160–7.

41. Lange MM, Rutten HJ, van de Velde CJ. One hundred years of curative surgery for rectal cancer: 1908–2008. Eur J Surg Oncol. 2009;35:456–63.
42. Lindsey I, Guy RJ, Warren BF, Mortensen NJ. Anatomy of Denonvilliers' fascia and pelvic nerves, impotence, and implications for the colorectal surgeon. Br J Surg. 2000;87:1288–99.
43. Lindsey I, Warren BF, Mortensen NJ. Denonvilliers' fascia lies anterior to the fascia propria and rectal dissection plane in total mesorectal excision. Dis Colon Rectum. 2005;48:37–42.
44. Chessin DB, Guillem JG. Abdominoperineal resection for rectal cancer: historic perspective and current issues. Surg Oncol Clin N Am. 2005;14:569–86, vii.
45. Enker WE, Thaler HT, Cranor ML, Polyak T. Total mesorectal excision in the operative treatment of carcinoma of the rectum. J Am Coll Surg. 1995;181:335–46.
46. Enker WE. Total mesorectal excision–the new golden standard of surgery for rectal cancer. Ann Med. 1997;29:127–33.
47. Parfitt JR, Driman DK. The total mesorectal excision specimen for rectal cancer: a review of its pathological assessment. J Clin Pathol. 2007;60:849–55.
48. Bhardwaj R, Parker MC. Modern perspectives in the treatment of chronic anal fissures. Ann R Coll Surg Engl. 2007;89:472–8.
49. Nelson R. Operative procedures for fissure in ano. Cochrane Database Syst Rev. 2005;(11):CD002199.
50. Acheson AG, Scholefield JH. Management of haemorrhoids. BMJ. 2008;336:380–3.
51. Shafik A, Doss S, Ali YA, Shafik AA. Transverse folds of rectum: anatomic study and clinical implications. Clin Anat. 2001;14:196–203.
52. Fenger C. The anal transitional zone. Acta Pathol Microbiol Immunol Scand Suppl. 1987;289:1–42.
53. Balik E, Eren T, Bulut T, Buyukuncu Y, Bugra D, Yamaner S. Surgical approach to extensive hidradenitis suppurativa in the perineal/perianal and gluteal regions. World J Surg. 2009;33:481–7.
54. Mitchell KM, Beck DE. Hidradenitis suppurativa. Surg Clin N Am. 2002;82:1187–97.
55. Rubin RJ, Chinn BT. Perianal hidradenitis suppurativa. Surg Clin N Am. 1994;74:1317–25.
56. Singh B, Mc CMNJ, Jewell DP, George B. Perianal Crohn's disease. Br J Surg. 2004;91:801–14.
57. Monk BJ, Tewari KS. The spectrum and clinical sequelae of human papillomavirus infection. Gynecol Oncol. 2007;107:S6–13.
58. Levy A, Lebbe C. Buschke-Lowenstein tumour: diagnosis and treatment. Ann Urol (Paris). 2006;40:175–8.
59. Longacre TA, Kong CS, Welton ML. Diagnostic problems in anal pathology. Adv Anat Pathol. 2008;15:263–78.
60. Billingsley KG, Stern LE, Lowy AM, Kahlenberg MS, Thomas Jr CR. Uncommon anal neoplasms. Surg Oncol Clin N Am. 2004;13:375–88.
61. Rickard MJ. Anal abscesses and fistulas. ANZ J Surg. 2005;75:64–72.
62. Nelson R. Anorectal abscess fistula: what do we know? Surg Clin N Am. 2002;82:1139–51, v–vi.
63. Baleato Gonzalez S, Vilanova JC, Lopez Carreira L, Gracia-Figueiras R, Pazos Gonzalez G, Ortiz-Teran L. Perineal hernia. Emerg Radiol. 2009;16:395–8.
64. Gomez Portilla A, Cendoya I, Uzquiza E, et al. Giant perineal hernia: laparoscopic mesh repair complemented by a perineal cutaneous approach. Hernia. 2010;14:199–201.
65. Rayhanabad J, Sassani P, Abbas MA. Laparoscopic repair of perineal hernia. JSLS. 2009;13:237–41.
66. Salameh JR. Primary and unusual abdominal wall hernias. Surg Clin N Am. 2008;88:45–60, vii.

16 Liver

1. All of the following are correct *except*:
   (a) The postsinusoidal liver and the heart share a common origin in the hepatocardiac mesoderm.
   (b) The liver mesenchyme originates from the transverse septum.
   (c) Hepatocytes and biliary structures are derived from the foregut endoderm.
   (d) Placental blood flows through the portal system before reaching the systemic circulation.
   (e) The liver harbors hematopoietic stem cells in fetal life.

Comments Liver development is a complex process involving multiple interactions between the endoderm and the mesoderm. The hepatic bud derived from the foregut endoderm gives rise to hepatoblasts that will later differentiate into hepatocytes and cholangiocytes (bile duct cells). The mesoderm provides the structural framework, blood vessels, and hematopoietic elements [1].

Cells from the liver bud migrate and intermingle with the cells and connective tissue of the mesenchyme, which provides a scaffold for the nascent hepatocytes, bile ducts, and sinusoids. Concurrently, the developing liver accommodates hematopoietic stem cells, which participate in fetal hematopoiesis and later disappear. The extrahepatic ducts share a common developmental pathway with the pancreatic ducts. The mechanism through which the intra- and extrahepatic ducts anastomose remains to be elucidated [2].

Within the liver, the elements of the portal triad (portal vein, hepatic artery, and bile duct) travel together within a fibrous sheath, which is an invagination of Glisson's capsule. This anatomical relationship forms the basis of the modern intraglissonian approach to liver resections. The embryological development of this pattern is not well understood.

Fetal circulation presents two main shunts that are absent in the adult. These shunts reflect the substitution of pulmonary and hepatic function by the placenta. The ductus venosus allows nutrient-rich blood returning from the placenta to bypass the liver and reach the systemic circulation by communicating the left branch of the portal vein with the inferior vena cava. In the adult, the obliterated ductus venosus becomes an important landmark to dissect the left hepatic vein. The second fetal shunt is the ductus arteriosus. It connects the pulmonary artery with the aorta, allowing the majority of the oxygen-rich blood from the right heart to bypass the non-ventilated lungs of the fetus to reach the systemic circulation [3, 4].

Answer
d

V.K. Maker, E.D. Guzman-Arrieta, *Cognitive Pearls in General Surgery*,
DOI 10.1007/978-1-4939-1850-8_16, © Springer Science+Business Media New York 2015

2. All of the following are correct *except*:
   (a) Riedel's lobe is a mass of liver tissue extending downwards from the right lobe.
   (b) Riedel's lobe is a normal anatomic variant.
   (c) Riedel's lobe may present as a palpable right upper quadrant mass.
   (d) Riedel's lobe may harbor primary or metastatic disease of the liver.
   (e) Riedel's is considered as a separate additional segment.

Comments Riedel's lobe was first described in 1888. It is a tonguelike projection of the right lobe of the liver that may present as a palpable right upper quadrant mass. It is present in approximately 3 % of the population as a normal anatomic variant. It is not an independent liver segment; instead, it shares its portal triad elements with the adjoining liver. Riedel's lobe may harbor benign and malignant tumors and may be susceptible to torsion requiring surgical intervention [5–7] (Fig. 16.1).

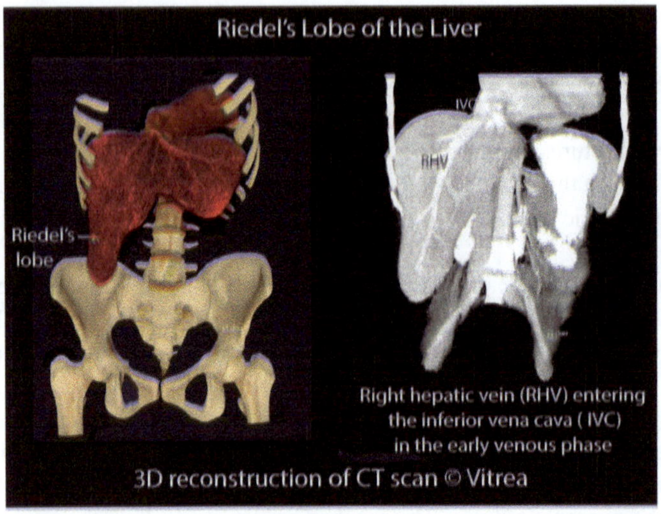

Fig. 16.1 3D reconstruction of CT scan © Vitrea. Riedel's lobe is a normal, albeit uncommon, variant of the right lobe of the liver and is neither an additional lobe nor an extra segment

Answer
e

3. All of the following are correct *except*:
   (a) Cantlie's line divides the liver into right and left lobes.
   (b) The falciform ligament divides the left lobe of the liver into lateral and medial sectors.
   (c) Lobar anatomy is based on the hepatic venous system.
   (d) Segmental anatomy is based on the branching of the portal triad.
   (e) The caudate lobe forms part of the left lobe of the liver.

Comments The liver is divided into eight functional segments based on the branching pattern of the portal triad (portal vein, hepatic artery, and bile duct), in conjunction with planes established by the hepatic veins. While there is some correlation with superficial anatomical landmarks, the said divisions are not dependent on them.

The first functional division of the liver dates to 1888, when Rex showed that the falciform ligament was not a true landmark for the right and left lobe of the liver. Instead, he proposed that the liver was divided into two equal-sized lobes by a plane drawn from the left border of the gallbladder to the inferior vena cava. In 1897 Cantlie confirmed this finding, and the line marking this division bears his name.

In the 1950s, Couinaud, Healy, Schroy, Goldsmith, and Woodburne proposed further division of the liver into segments defined by the branching of the portal triad. In 1982 Bismuth integrated these systems into the classification we use today, which is echoed by the Brisbane Terminology of Hepatic Anatomy and Resection published in the year 2000.

In this system, the liver is progressively divided into lobes, sectors (or sections), and segments, with the caudate lobe being an independent segment based on its supply by both the right and left portal triad and its direct venous drainage into the vena cava (Fig. 16.2).

As illustrated below, the middle hepatic vein, which courses along Cantlie's line, divides the liver into two lobes of similar mass. Each lobe is further divided by the right and left hepatic veins into sectors. On the left, there are a lateral and a medial sector. On the right side, there are anterior and posterior sectors. Finally, the transverse fissure, which is an imaginary line drawn along the right and left portal branches, divides the liver into superior and inferior segments [8–10] (Fig. 16.3).

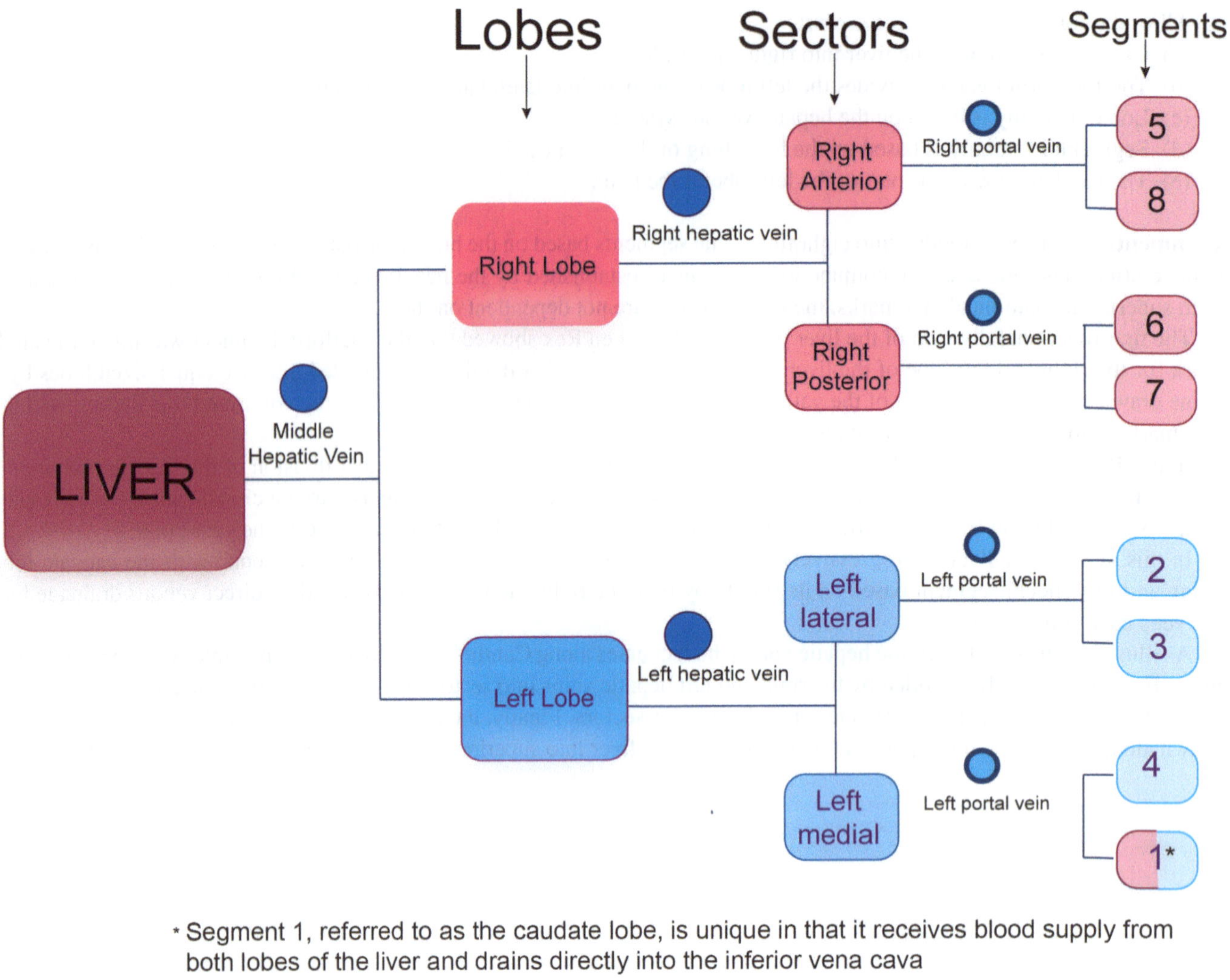

Fig. 16.2 The liver is elegantly and functionally divided into eight segments. Each segment is fed by its own bundle wrapped in the glissonian sheath consisting of the branches of the portal vein, hepatic artery, and the bile duct. The middle hepatic vein marks the division of liver into the right and left lobes. Right lobe has an anterior and a posterior sector in relation to the right hepatic vein and each sector in turn has two liver segments. The left lobe of the liver has a lateral sector with segments 2 and 3, while the medial sector has segments 4 and 1. Segment 1, also called the caudate lobe, is unique that it gets portal blood supply from both lobes and drains directly into the inferior vena cava

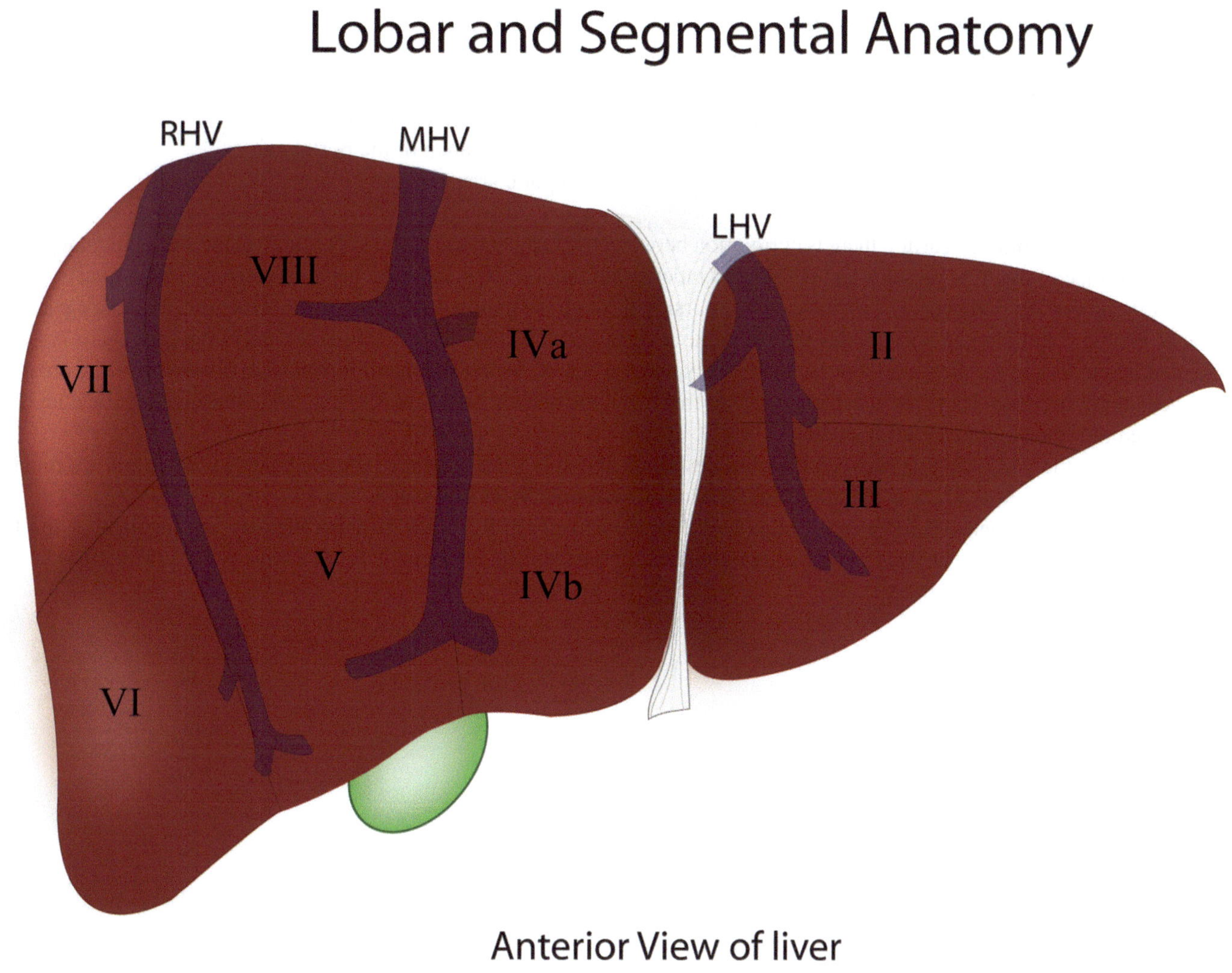

Fig. 16.3 Hepatic veins mark the division of liver into sectors, while the segmental anatomy depends on the portal vein inflow. All of the eight liver segments are represented in the anterior view of the liver except segment 1. Segments 5–8 are in the *right* lobe of the liver while segments 1–4 in the *left* lobe. Segment 1 is often referred to as the caudate lobe. According to location, it belongs to the left lobe of the liver but gets varying degrees of portal venous supply from both lobes and drains directly into inferior vena cava. It is best seen in the inferior view of the liver and has the most variations. *RHV* right hepatic vein, *MHV* middle hepatic vein, *LHV* left hepatic vein

Answer

e

4. All of the following are correct *except*:
   (a) Segment 4 (quadrate lobe) lays anterior to the porta hepatis.
   (b) Segment 1 (caudate lobe) lays posterior to the porta hepatis.
   (c) Cantlie's line is drawn from the left of the gallbladder fossa to the inferior vena cava.
   (d) The umbilical vein runs through the falciform ligament to the left branch of the portal vein.
   (e) The ligamentum venosum connects the portal vein to the hepatic artery.

Comments As mentioned earlier, there is correlation between liver segmentation and superficial anatomical landmarks. The visceral surface of the liver presents an "H"-shaped indentation that outlines the porta hepatis (gateway to the liver).

To the right of the porta hepatis, we have a line coursing through the gallbladder fossa towards the inferior vena cava. This line is named Cantlie's line and divides the liver into a right and left lobe. To the left of the porta hepatis, there is a line formed by the fissure for the round ligament anteriorly and the fissure for the ligamentum venosum posteriorly. The crossbar between these two lines is the porta hepatis itself. At this level, the hepatic artery, portal vein, and common hepatic duct have bifurcated into their right and left branches.

Anterior to the porta hepatis, between the lines described above lies the quadrate lobe (segment IV). Behind, we find the caudate lobe (segment I). Of note, the gallbladder belongs anatomically to segment 5.

The ligamentum venosum represents obliterated ductus venosus. In the adult, it helps identify the junction of the left hepatic vein to the vena cava. This anatomical landmark is helpful during left hepatic lobectomies [9, 10] (Fig. 16.4).

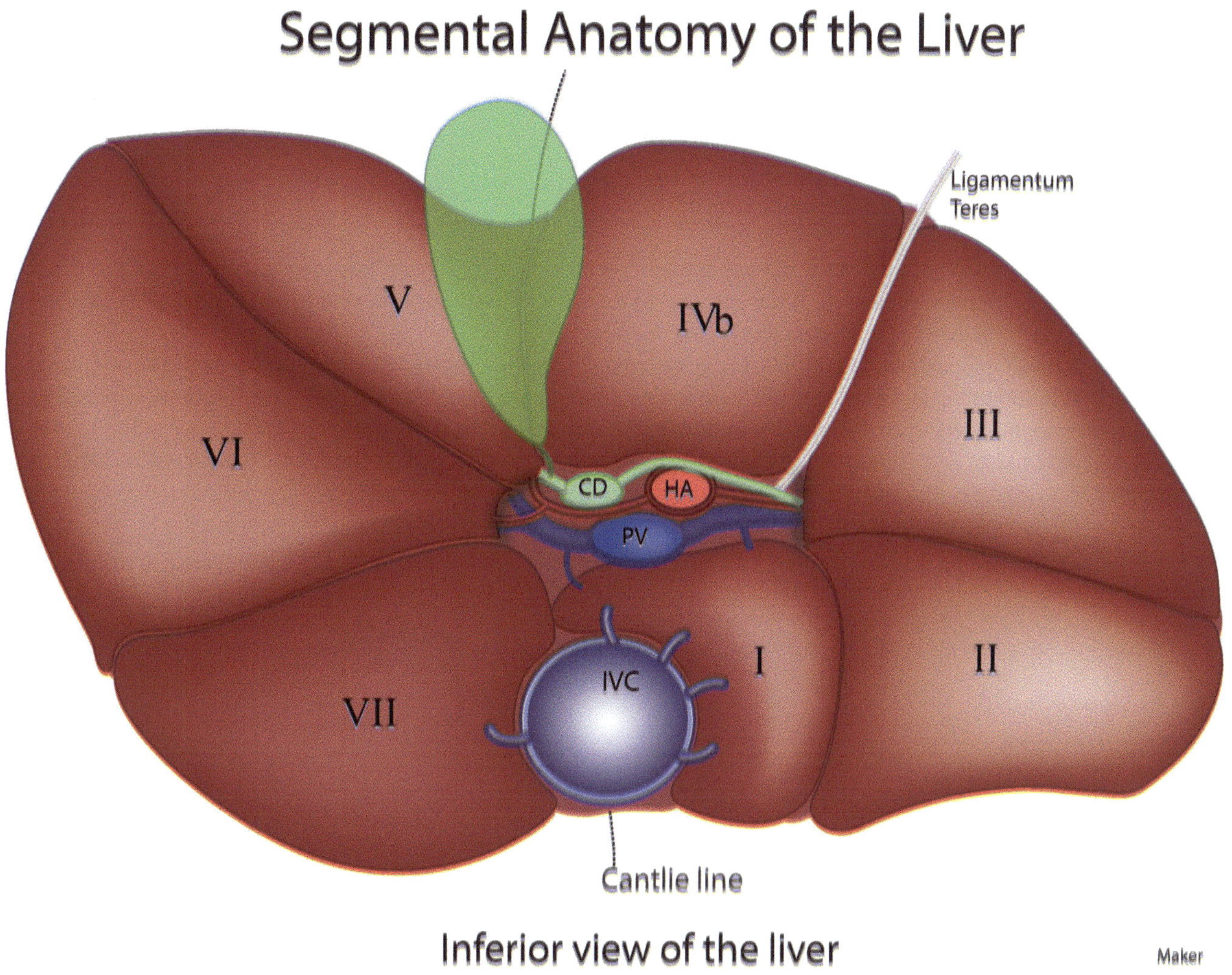

Fig. 16.4 Inferior view of the liver shows all of the segments of the liver except segments 8 and 4a which represent the dome of the liver. Cantlie's line is an imaginary plane between the gallbladder fossa and the inferior vena cava in both inferior and anterior views and represents the division of liver into the right and left lobes. This line follows the middle hepatic vein in the intraparenchymal liver. Gallbladder anatomically belongs to segment 5 and its fossa often abuts segment 4b. The caudate lobe of the liver often has a caudate process, which crosses over to the right lobe, and a caval ligament that runs posterior to the IVC attaching to segment VII. *CD* common duct, *HA* hepatic artery, *PV* portal vein, *IVC* inferior vena cava

Answer
e

5. All of the following are correct *except*:
   (a) The caudate lobe receives portal structures from both the right and left main branches.
   (b) The caudate process of the caudate lobe extends to and may make contact with segment 7 thus surrounding the inferior vena cava.
   (c) The caudate lobe is hypotrophic in Budd–Chiari syndrome.
   (d) The caudate lobe drains directly into the vena cava.
   (e) The caudate lobe is posterior to the porta hepatis.

Comments The caudate lobe of the liver is unique in that it receives branches from both the right and left portal triads and drains directly into the inferior vena cava. It lies anterior to the cava. The caudate process of the caudate lobe, connecting segments I to VII, may encircle the vena cava to varying degrees.

The venous drainage of caudate lobe of the liver is not affected by thrombosis of the hepatic veins in Budd–Chiari syndrome (hepatic vein thrombosis). Given that this lobe drains directly into the vena cava, its venous outflow is preserved. In fact, this lobe is noticeably enlarged, as it comes to replace the function of the remaining liver tissue.

Resection of the caudate lobe is practiced with increasing frequency and safety. It is commonly incorporated in right hepatectomies [9–11].

Answer

c

6. Select the incorrect association:
   (a) Extended right hepatic lobectomy: Segments IV, V, VI, VII, and VIII (trisegmentectomy)
   (b) Left hepatic lobectomy: Segments I II, III, and IV
   (c) Left lateral lobectomy: Segments II and III
   (d) Extended left lobectomy: Segments I, II, III, IV, VI, and VII
   e) Radical cholecystectomy: Segments IVB and V

Comments Liver resections have become progressively safer over the past 50 years, due in great part to the recognition of liver segments and anatomic resections. Reasons supporting the use of anatomic resections over nonanatomic wedge resections include superior oncologic outcomes, preservation of functional liver parenchyma, reduction of blood loss, and greater chance of achieving an en bloc resection without specimen fracture (Fig. 16.5).

In general, hepatic lobectomy refers to the excision of all the liver parenchyma to either side of Cantlie's line (with or without segment I for the left). Resections extended to include segments V and VIII with the left lobe or segment IV with the right lobe are termed "trisegmentectomy."

Other possible resections not named in the above table include right anterior sector resection (V and VIII), right posterior sector resection (VI and VII), left medial resection (IV), and caudate lobectomy (I). Like segment I, all liver segments can be excised individually [8].

A liver resection of particular clinical relevance is that of segments IVB and V, in the context of treatment of gallbladder cancer (Fig. 16.6).

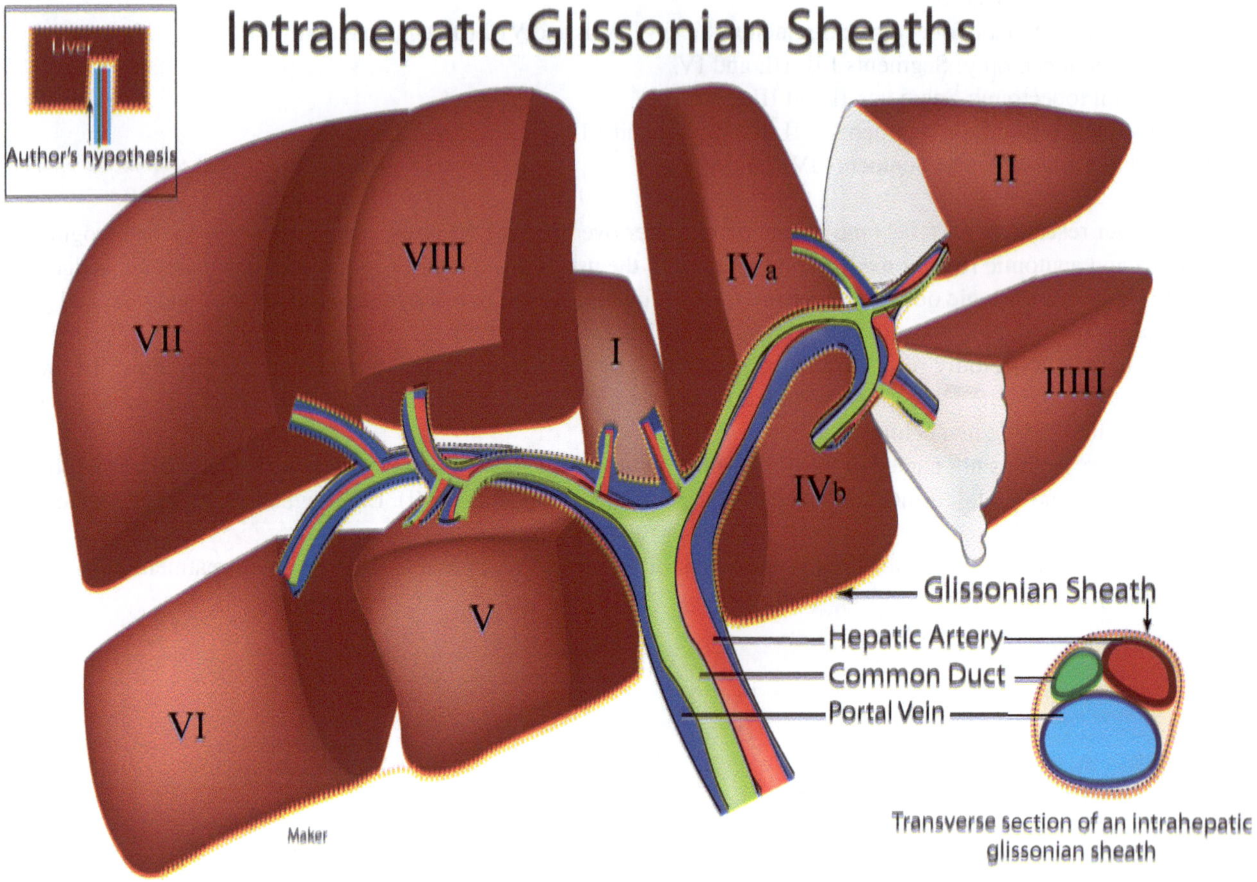

Fig. 16.5 Glisson's capsule of the liver encapsulates all of the three structures of the portal triad. It is possible that embryologically this portal trinity appears to have become invaginated into the liver surrounded by a sheath of Glisson's capsule into each lobe, sector, and segment. Irrespective of the hypothetical etiology, an intrahepatic approach to segmental liver surgery is made possible and requires identification and ligation of a single pedicle that contains all three structures of the portal triad within the glissonian sheath

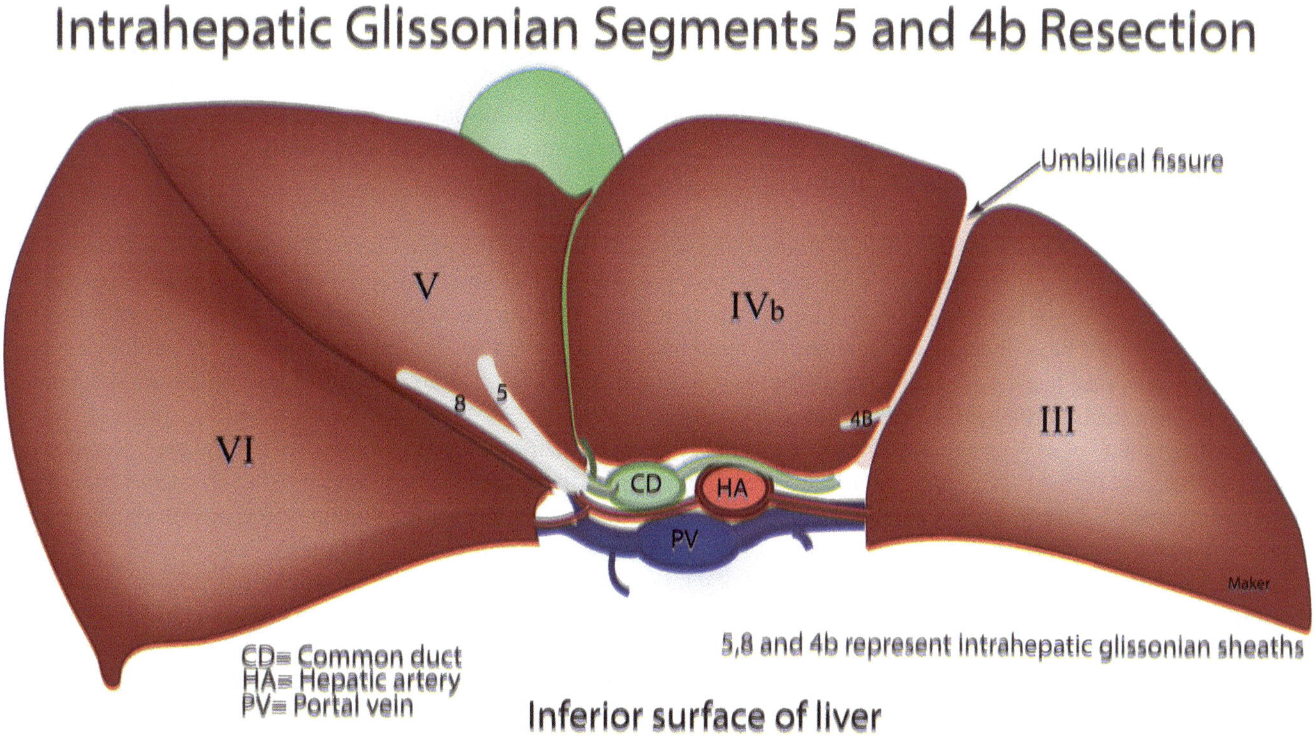

Fig. 16.6 To achieve R0 resection for early gallbladder cancer, one of the preferred treatments is cholecystectomy with en bloc segment 5 and 4b resection along with portal lymphadenectomy. Segments 5 and 4b pedicles can be safely accessed through an intrahepatic glissonian approach. The glissonian sheath for the segment 5 comes of the right anterior sectoral pedicle, while the segment 4b pedicle is supplied within the glissonian sheath coming through the umbilical fissure. *CD* common duct, *HA* hepatic artery, *PV* portal glissonian vein

Answer

d

7. All of the following are correct *except*:
   (a) Twenty-five percent of liver blood flow comes from the hepatic artery and 75 % from the portal vein.
   (b) The portal vein should never be ligated.
   (c) Central veins drain into the hepatic venous system forming the postsinusoidal network.
   (d) There are functional intrahepatic anastomoses between the right and left hepatic arteries.
   (e) The hepatic veins drain into the inferior vena cava.

Comments The liver has a dual blood supply through the hepatic artery and the portal vein. The portal vein provides 75 % of the blood volume to the liver; however, since the gut has used part of the oxygen content in this blood, it only provides for 50 % of the oxygen needs. However, portal blood is rich in nutrients coming from the bowel. The hepatic artery brings the remaining 25 % of the blood volume and supplies the other half of the oxygen needs. The terminal branches of the porta and hepatic artery reach the hepatic sinusoids, where they mix as blood flows towards the central vein. Multiple central veins will then join to form the branches of the hepatic veins (Fig. 16.7).

There is a gradient of oxygen and nutrient concentration as blood flows from the portal triad to the central vein. Hepatocytes closest to the triad (zone 1) have more nutrients available, whereas those close to the central vein have less (zone 3). In between lies zone 2. This gradient explains why hypoperfusion to the liver is most damaging to the centrolobular hepatocytes, while toxic substances are more damaging to those in the periphery (Fig. 16.8).

The microcirculation of the liver is unique in that blood inflow to the liver from the portal vein and hepatic arteries enters the sinusoids, which are of low pressure and slow flow, allowing hepatocytes to come into contact with the blood in order to fulfill their metabolic role. Sinusoids drain into the central veins continuing on the hepatic veins, forming the outflow of the liver. Waste products of the liver do not enter the venous circulation; rather, they are excreted through the bile ducts into the GI tract (Fig. 16.9).

Injury to the portal vein is best treated by repair. However, in circumstances where it is not possible or practical to repair the portal vein, ligation may be undertaken, provided there is flow through the hepatic artery and that there are collaterals to accommodate splanchnic venous return. When both the hepatic artery and portal vein are injured, preference should be given to the repair of the portal vein. It is also possible to ligate or embolize the hepatic artery [12].

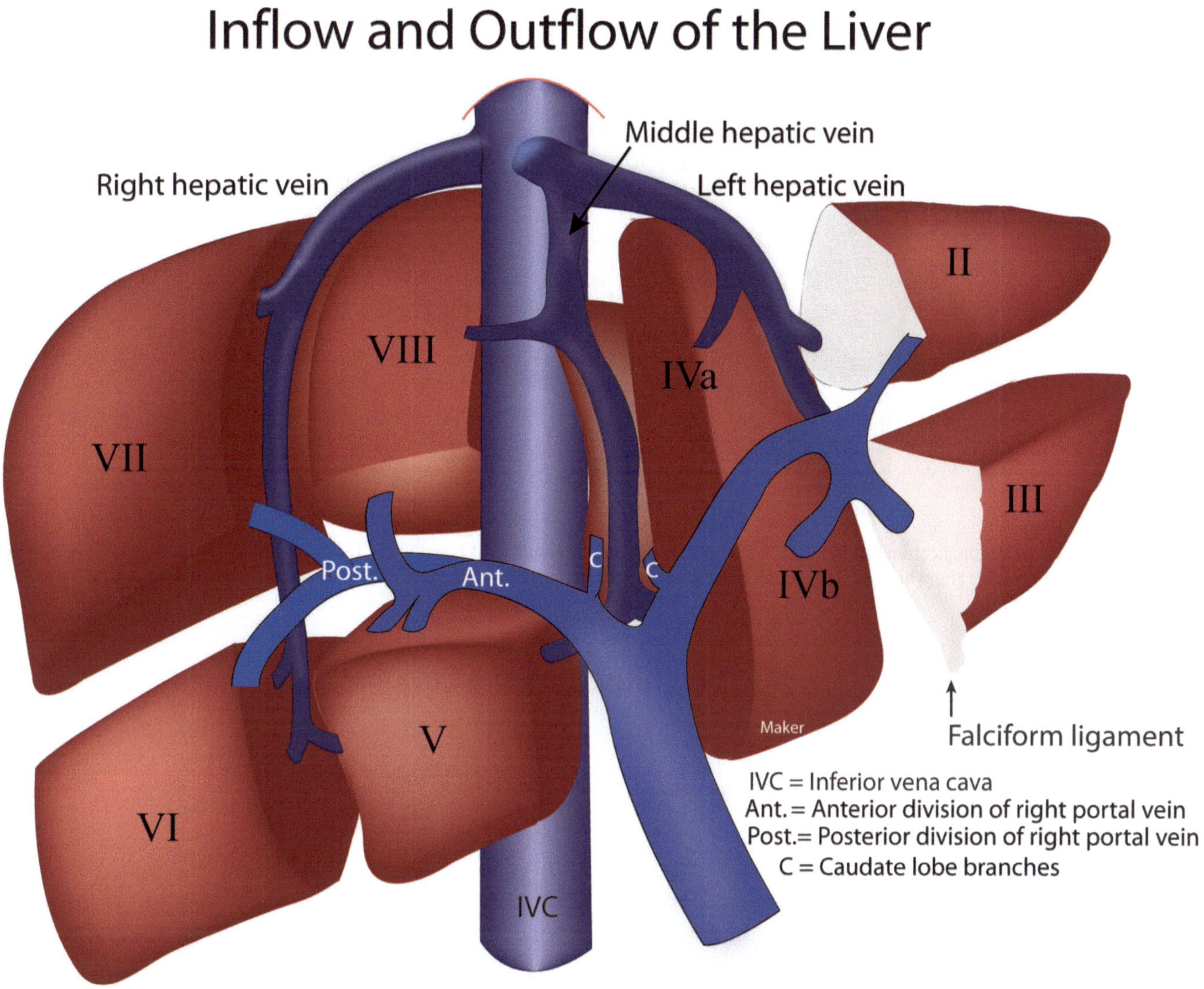

Fig. 16.7 The liver receives all the end products of digestion from the GI tract via the portal vein, and after complex processing returns them to the systemic circulation via the hepatic veins into the inferior vena cava. Each segment of the liver is individually supplied by a portal vein and in turn outflow is through one of the three major hepatic veins. The caudate lobe is not well seen in this diagram straddling posteriorly and to the left of cava. *IVC* inferior vena cava, *Ant* anterior division of right portal vein, *Post* posterior division of right portal vein, *C* caudate lobe branches

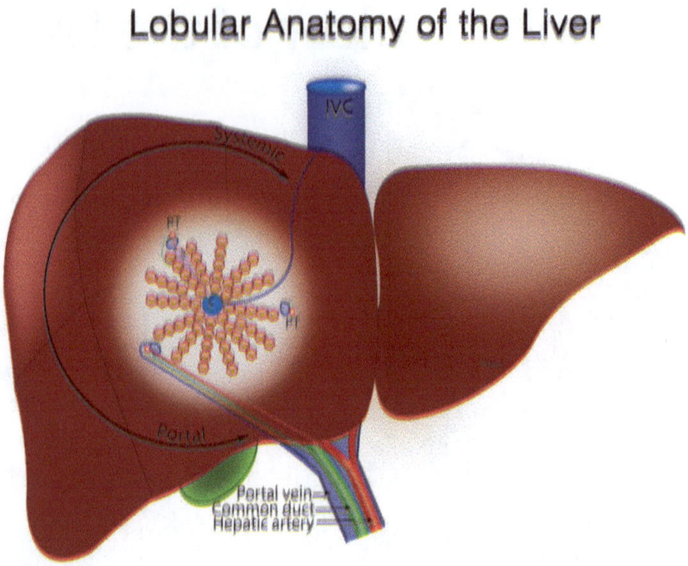

Fig. 16.8 Functional histological unit of the liver is a lobule, consisting of columns of hepatocytes fed by portal triads located at its periphery. Each lobule has a central vein, which drains through hepatic veins into the inferior vena cava. *PT* portal triad, *S* sinusoid, *C* central vein, *IVC* inferior vena cava

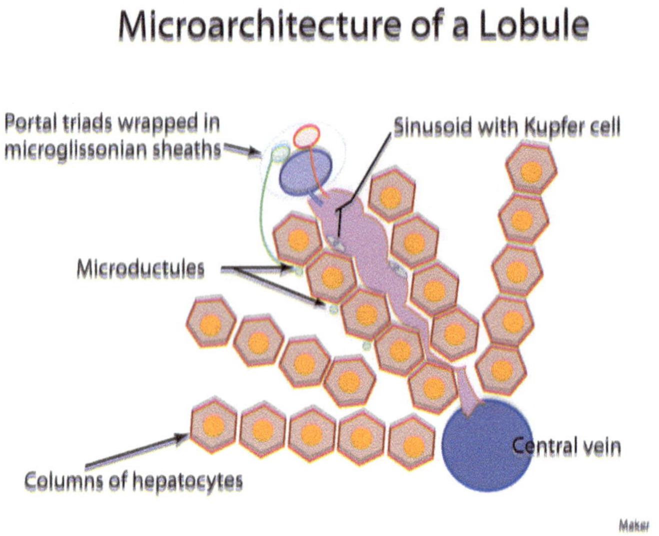

Fig. 16.9 In its most basic functional anatomy, hepatocytes pick up nutrients and oxygen from a sinusoidal ocean formed by a portal venous and hepatic artery capillary. Complex proteins and other manufactured products are sent through the central veins into the systemic circulation, while the waste is excreted in the biliary microductules that empty into the duodenum

Answer

b

8. All of the following are correct *except*:
   (a) Proximal splenorenal shunts have higher incidence of encephalopathy than distal splenorenal shunts.
   (b) Distal splenorenal shunts effectively decompress esophageal varices.
   (c) Transjugular intrahepatic portosystemic shunts (TIPS) are now the standard of care for chronic variceal bleeding.
   (d) Side-to-side portacaval shunts are the most effective operation for decreasing portal hypertension but carry the highest incidence of encephalopathy.
   (e) Mesocaval shunts are contraindicated in liver transplant candidates.

Comments From an anatomical standpoint, portal hypertension can be classified as right sided or left sided. The former is caused by liver cirrhosis and elevates the pressure of all the portal system, leading to esophageal varices. The latter is caused by occlusion and the portal vein, generating splenomegaly and a redirection of splenic venous return via the short gastric vessels, which may become varicose (Fig. 16.10).

The advent of endoscopic interventions and transjugular intrahepatic portosystemic shunts (TIPS) for the control of acute bleeding from esophageal varices, together with the increasing use of liver transplantation has limited the frequency with which surgical portosystemic shunts are created. Nonetheless, these procedures may still play a role in selected patients.

Surgical portosystemic shunts are classified into nonselective and selective. The first group includes end-to-side portacaval shunts, side-to-side portacaval shunts, large-diameter interposition shunts, proximal splenorenal shunts, and mesocaval shunts. In general these shunts decrease the incidence of variceal bleeding but cause worsened liver function and encephalopathy, with no net survival advantage. Liver function deteriorates because nonselective shunts allow the passage of blood coming from the gut directly into the systemic circulation. This blood is rich in ammonia and other toxic substances that are normally cleared by the liver and are responsible for hepatic encephalopathy.

Side-to-side shunts are superior to end-to-side shunts because they relieve sinusoidal and splanchnic hypertension, significantly reducing ascites formation. As a group, these operations are only indicated in the control of hemorrhage after nonoperative therapy has failed.

Selective portacaval shunts mainly decompress the esophageal varices. They are the left gastric to cava shunt (rarely used) and the distal splenorenal shunt, also known as Warren shunt. This operation diverts blood from the esophagus to the spleen via the short gastrics and from there into the renal vein. While in principle this operation preserves antegrade portal flow, in reality collaterals develop making the shunt nonselective with time. This seems to occur in spite of ligation of the left gastric vein as well as disconnection of the splenic vein and its pancreatic tributaries. In addition, this operation increases ascites formation. From a practical standpoint, Warren shunts offer no definitive long-term advantage over nonselective shunts in regard to the development of hepatic encephalopathy.

TIPS behave like side-to-side portosystemic shunts and carry similar rates of encephalopathy. Outcomes have been noted to be worse in patients with elevated MELD scores (>25). However, the ability to calibrate the diameter of the shunt based on portal pressure limits this complication. The main advantage of TIPS over conventional surgery lies in its minimally invasive nature and the lack of interference with future hepatic transplant surgery. The main disadvantage is the risk for stenosis and occlusion as well as the need for ongoing monitoring. The incidence of these complications has been reduced with the use of covered stents.

The traditional view has been that TIPS nor surgical shunting should be performed with the intent of preventing bleeding from asymptomatic esophageal varices. In this setting, these procedures may paradoxically decrease survival due to decline in liver function and encephalopathy. For these patients, endoscopic therapies are the best option [13, 14].

However, as procedural outcomes have improved for TIPS, there is a growing recognition that this procedure may have a role as a preventive intervention, in addition to its established utility as a salvage option for refractory bleeding (Fig. 16.11).

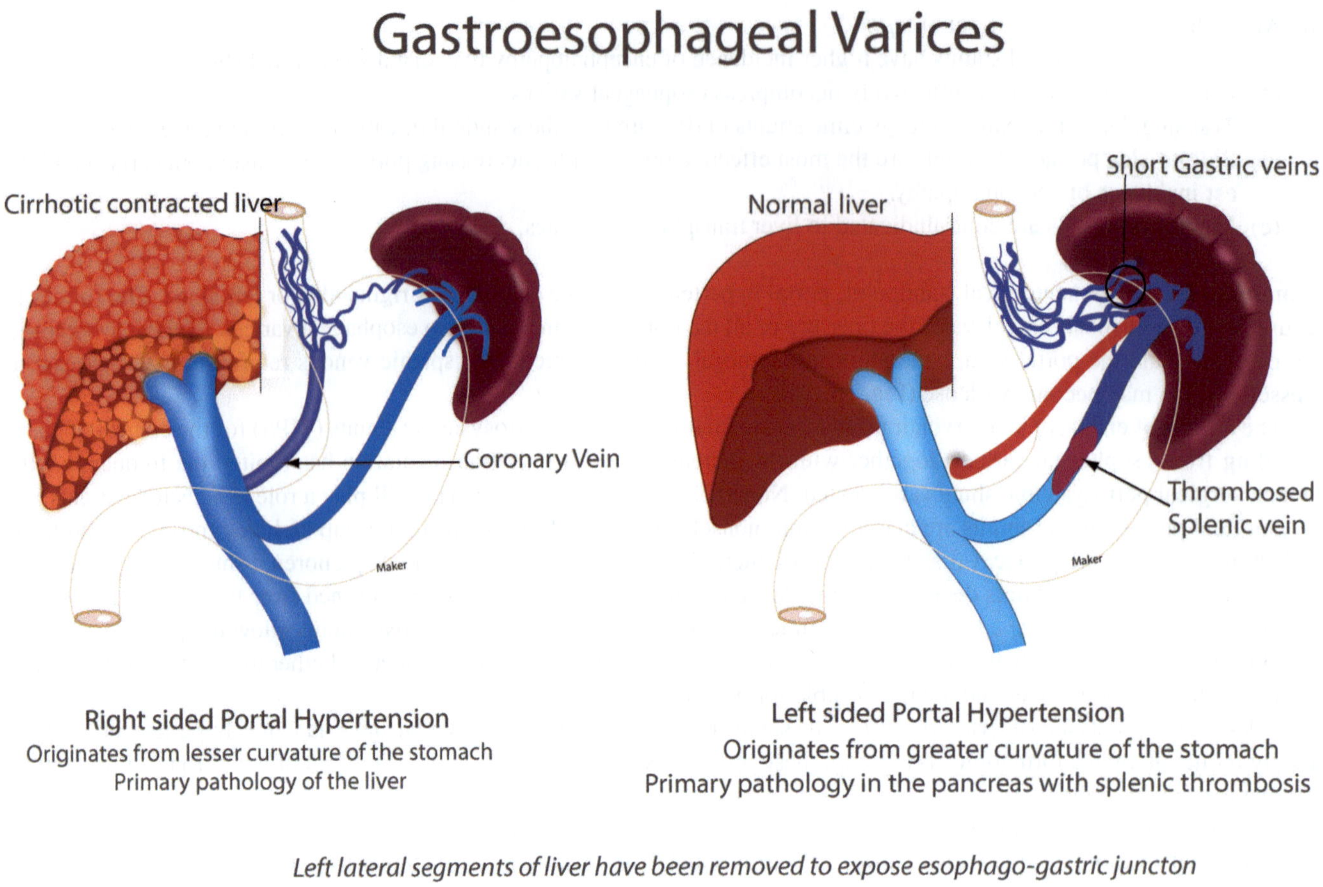

Fig. 16.10 Cirrhotic liver disease causes portal hypertension eventually resulting in gastroesophageal varices. The major contributor is the left coronary vein that originates at lesser curvature of the stomach. In splenic vein thrombosis, usually secondary to the chronic pancreatitis, portal hypertension starts on the left side, with short gastric veins on the greater curvature backing up into the systemic, esophageal azygos veins

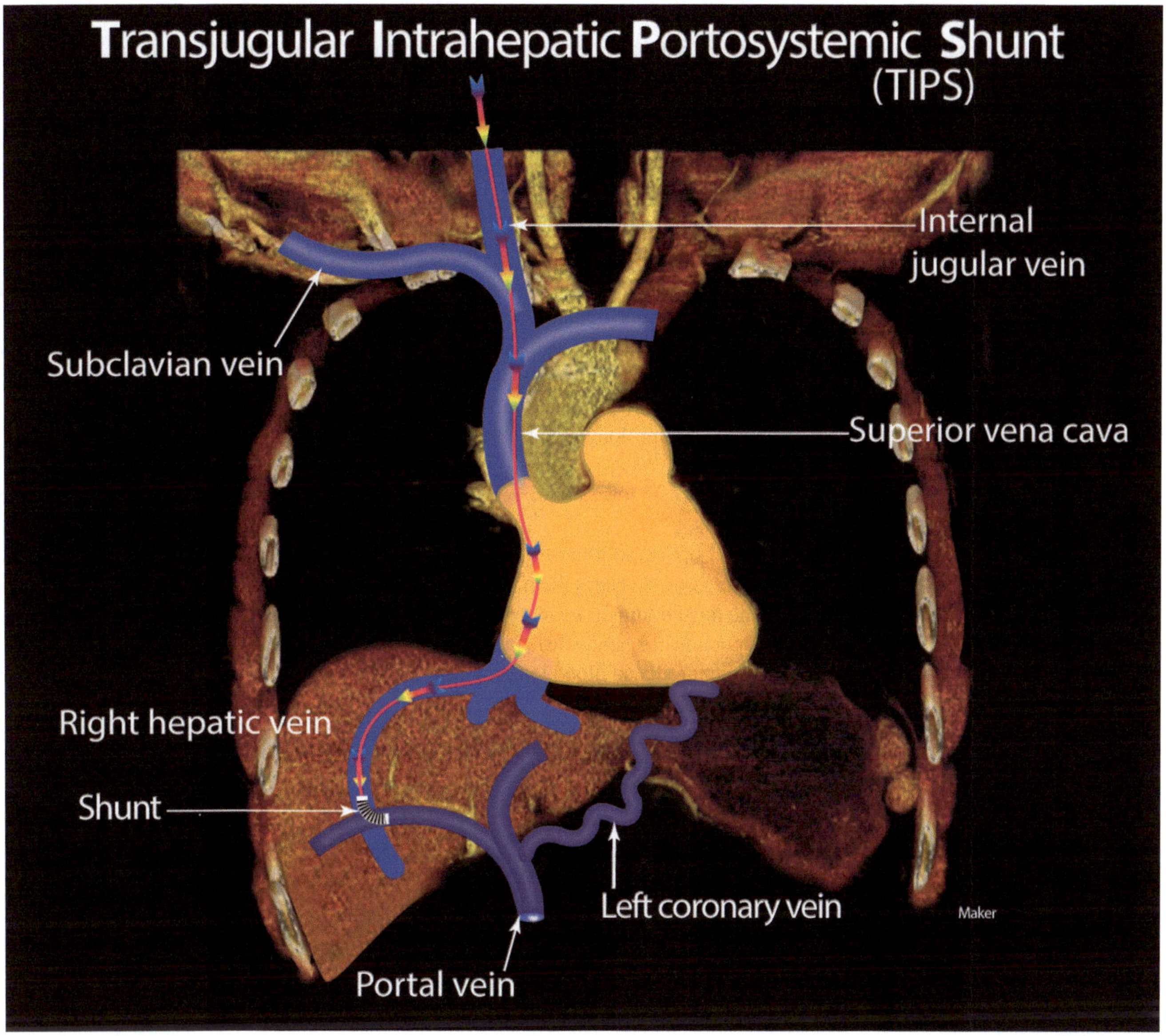

Fig. 16.11 Deployment of a covered intrahepatic stent between the hepatic and portal venous system is employed for the treatment of portal hypertension and is a viable alternative in selected cases with low MELD scores. These shunts are inserted through the internal jugular vein to the liver, and deployed through a hepatic vein to an adjoining portal venous tributary

Answer
e

9. All of the following are correct *except*:
   (a) The Pringle maneuver is the temporary extrahepatic occlusion of the structures of the portal triad in the hepatoduodenal ligament.
   (b) Limiting transfusions during liver surgery improves survival.
   (c) Liver resections should be performed under low central venous pressure.
   (d) Hepatic bleeding not controlled by the Pringle maneuver is likely to have the hepatic veins or inferior vena cava as a source.
   (e) Atrio-caval shunting is the treatment of choice for retrohepatic cava injuries.

Comments The Pringle maneuver consists of the temporary occlusion of the elements of the portal triad at the level of Winslow's hiatus. The main concept behind this technique is that the liver tolerates ischemia better than hemorrhage. It has been shown that the continuous clamping of the portal triad can be withstood for up to 90 min; shorter times are usually recommended. In practice, intermittent clamping of the portal triad is preferred. This is done using 15–20 min of clamping with 5 min brakes. Intermittent clamping has been shown to yield similar reductions in blood loss as continuous clamping, with the added benefit that total clamped time may be prolonged to as long as 120 min, allowing the completion of challenging resections or other procedures [15].

Evidence now exists supporting the maintenance of low central venous pressure during liver resections. This approach decreases blood loss and the need for transfusions.

The liver is one of the most common injured organs in blunt trauma. The elements of the portal triad are enveloped by invaginations of Glisson's capsule. This investing layer renders them more resistant to shear forces that otherwise disrupt the branches of the hepatic vein, making them the most common source of hepatic hemorrhage after blunt trauma. Fortunately, the low pressure of the hepatic veins allows spontaneous hemostasis in the majority of cases. This pattern of injury limits the usefulness of the Pringle maneuver, in that while it reduced blood inflow to the liver, it does not directly address the bleeding from the outflow veins [16].

Retrohepatic cava injuries carry a high mortality. While in the past primary repair was advocated, more current literature focuses on not disrupting, but rather reinforcing the tamponade that exists around the injury [17] (Fig. 16.12).

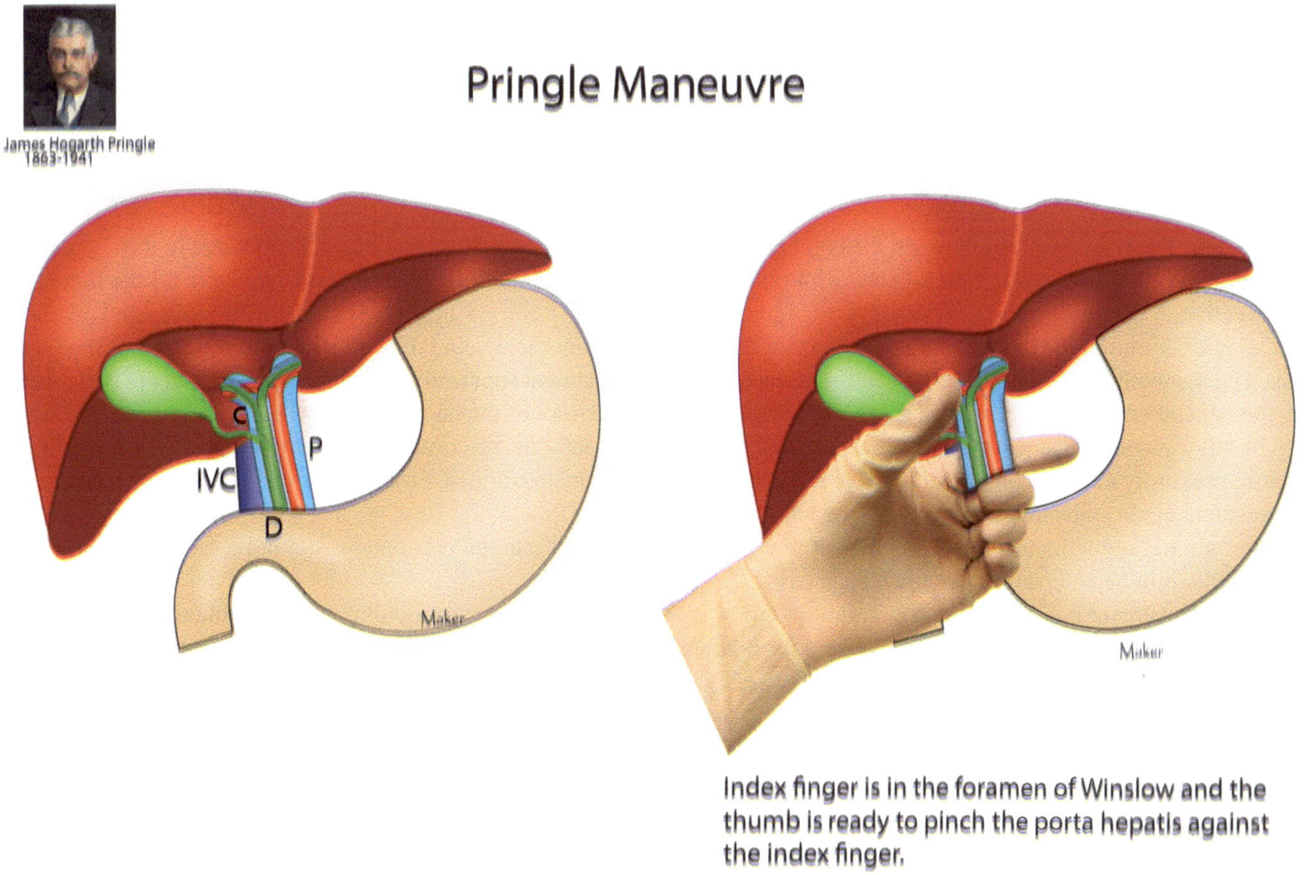

Fig. 16.12 Pringle maneuver for reducing bleeding in the liver surgery has stood the test of time for over a century. The medial free edge of the hepatoduodenal ligament contains the portal vein, hepatic artery, and the common duct. By inserting one's index finger through the foramen of Winslow and compressing the portal triad between the thumb and index finger, all of the inflow to the liver can be occluded with the rare exception of an anomalous hepatic artery coursing outside the pinched area. This occlusion can alternatively be performed with a nontraumatic instrument or touniquet. *C* caudate lobe of the liver, *P* portal vein, hepatic artery, and common duct, *D* duodenum, *IVC* inferior vena cava

Answer

e

10. All of the following are correct *except*:
    (a) The falciform ligament represents the ventral mesogastrium.
    (b) Brisk bleeding during the mobilization of the left triangular ligament comes from musculophrenic vessels.
    (c) The gastrohepatic ligament is avascular and can be divided with impunity.
    (d) The right triangular ligament connects the right lobe of the liver to the parietal peritoneum.
    (e) The retrocaval ligament bridges the right and left lobes posteriorly.

Comments The liver develops between the two layers of the ventral mesogastrium and hence is attached in the right upper quadrant with ligaments on its four aspects, with only a small bare area superiorly and posteriorly, where all the ligaments join together.

The inferior end of the falciform ligament carries the obliterated umbilical vein on its way to the left branch of the portal vein. The ligament itself is avascular; however, as one dissects the ligament superiorly and posteriorly, it splits in two revealing the hepatic veins. This constitutes an excellent landmark for exposure of the hepatic outflow.

The left triangular ligament connects the entire left lobe to the diaphragm and contains musculophrenic vessels, which run in close proximity to the diaphragm. Division of this ligament should be performed close to the liver. Towards its medial end, the ligament again splits into two exposing the left and middle hepatic veins.

The right triangular ligament anchors the entire right lobe to the right parietal peritoneum and in its most superior aspect leads to the right hepatic vein and suprahepatic cava.

The gastrohepatic ligament is indeed very thin and avascular, except at its right border, where it contains the three elements of the porta hepatis, also forming the anterior boundary of the foramen of Winslow. This becomes an important landmark for the Pringle maneuver.

The retrocaval ligament bridges the right and left lobes behind the cava. It may be absent or may contain a tongue of liver parenchyma. Multiple veins from the right lobe enter the inferior vena cava directly in addition to the right and middle hepatic veins at this level [9].

Answer

e

References

1. Kaestner KH. The making of the liver: developmental competence in foregut endoderm and induction of the hepatogenic program. Cell Cycle. 2005;4:1146–8.
2. Lemaigre F, Zaret KS. Liver development update: new embryo models, cell lineage control, and morphogenesis. Curr Opin Genet Dev. 2004;14:582–90.
3. Kessler J, Rasmussen S, Kiserud T. The fetal portal vein: normal blood flow development during the second half of human pregnancy. Ultrasound Obstet Gynecol. 2007;30:52–60.
4. Zaret KS. Liver specification and early morphogenesis. Mech Dev. 2000;92:83–8.
5. Kudo M. Riedel's lobe of the liver and its clinical implication. Intern Med. 2000;39:87–8.
6. Yano K, Ohtsubo M, Mizota T, et al. Riedel's lobe of the liver evaluated by multiple imaging modalities. Intern Med. 2000;39:136–8.
7. Zamfir R, Brasoveanu V, Boros M, Herlea V, Popescu I. Hepatocellular carcinoma in Riedel's lobe. Chir (Bucur). 2008;103:121–3.
8. Liau KH, Blumgart LH, DeMatteo RP. Segment-oriented approach to liver resection. Surg Clin N Am. 2004;84:543–61.
9. Skandalakis JE, Skandalakis LJ, Skandalakis PN, Mirilas P. Hepatic surgical anatomy. Surg Clin N Am. 2004;84:413–35, viii.
10. Abdalla EK, Vauthey JN, Couinaud C. The caudate lobe of the liver: implications of embryology and anatomy for surgery. Surg Oncol Clin N Am. 2002;11:835–48.
11. Chaib E, Ribeiro Jr MA, Silva Fde S, Saad WA, Cecconello I. Caudate lobectomy: tumor location, topographic classification, and technique using right- and left-sided approaches to the liver. Am J Surg. 2008;196:245–51.
12. Buckman RF, Pathak AS, Badellino MM, Bradley KM. Portal vein injuries. Surg Clin N Am. 2001;81:1449–62.
13. Rikkers LF, Sorrell WT, Jin G. Which portosystemic shunt is best? Gastroenterol Clin N Am. 1992;21:179–96.
14. Wolff M, Hirner A. Current state of portosystemic shunt surgery. Langenbeck's Arch Surg. 2003;388:141–9.
15. Smyrniotis V, Farantos C, Kostopanagiotou G, Arkadopoulos N. Vascular control during hepatectomy: review of methods and results. World J Surg. 2005;29:1384–96.
16. Abdalla EK, Noun R, Belghiti J. Hepatic vascular occlusion: which technique? Surg Clin N Am. 2004;84:563–85.
17. Lee SK, Carrillo EH. Advances and changes in the management of liver injuries. Am Surg. 2007;73:201–6.

17 Extrahepatic Biliary Tract and Gallbladder

1. All of the following are correct *except*:
   (a) The caterpillar cystic arteries are multiple branches supplying the gallbladder from an aberrant right hepatic artery.
   (b) Accessory hepatic arteries should always be preserved as they often are the only blood supply to a part of the liver.
   (c) The most common variation of the hepatic arterial supply is a replaced right hepatic artery arising from the superior mesenteric artery (SMA).
   (d) The cystic artery may cross posterior to the common bile duct.
   (e) Ligation of the common hepatic artery results in fulminant hepatic necrosis.

Comments The proper hepatic artery most commonly arises from the common hepatic artery (a branch of the celiac trunk) after the takeoff of the gastroduodenal artery. It then courses towards the liver and branches into the right and left hepatic arteries and subsequent segmental branches.

Anatomical variations in this vascular tree are common as the biliary tree originates at the junction of foregut and midgut (i.e., middle of the second portion of the duodenum at the ampulla of Vater). While the primary artery of the foregut is the celiac artery, the SMA supplies the entire midgut with the two communicating at the origin of the biliary tree.

The above-described classic anatomy is present in 75 % of cases. In 10 % of cases, the right hepatic artery arises from the SMA, in which case it courses towards the liver to the right of the bile duct coming behind the pancreas. This course puts the artery at risk both during biliary and pancreatic surgery [1] (Fig. 17.1).

Also in 10 % of cases, the left hepatic artery arises from the left gastric artery, reaching the liver through the gastrohepatic ligament (lesser omentum). In 3 % of cases, both the right and left hepatic arteries have an anomalous origin. In 2 % of cases, the common hepatic artery originates from the SMA.

Anomalous hepatic arteries may be accessory or replaced. Like the name implies, accessory arteries coexist with anatomically normal branches and may be sacrificed. On the other hand, replaced arteries are the only supply to a given area of liver parenchyma and should be preserved. In practice, all anomalous liver arteries must be considered replaced rather than accessory.

The cystic artery is classically described as a branch of the right hepatic artery, reaching the gallbladder deep to the lymph node of Lund in Calot's triangle. However, as is the case with all biliary vascular anatomy, anatomical variations are present. One of such variations is the caterpillar cystic artery, reported in 4–16 % of cases. In this setting, a right hepatic with a premature division, or arising from the SMA courses anomalously close to the cystic duct, often giving multiple small branches to the cystic duct and gallbladder. This anatomy may predispose to injury to the right hepatic artery as it can be confused with the cystic artery [2] (Fig. 17.2).

While the cystic artery normally reaches the gallbladder coursing anterior to the common bile duct, it may also be found posterior to it, case in which it originates from the left hepatic artery. Venous drainage of the gallbladder occurs directly into the liver, while lymphatic flow is directed towards the lymph node of Lund (also known as Calot's node) and from there to the superior pancreaticoduodenal nodes.

Although counterintuitive, ligation of the larger common hepatic artery is well tolerated, as opposed to ligation of the hepatic proper. This is because the more proximal ligation allows collateral blood flow from the SMA to reach the liver via the pancreaticoduodenal arcades, reconstituting the gastroduodenal artery to form the hepatic artery proper [3].

V.K. Maker, E.D. Guzman-Arrieta, *Cognitive Pearls in General Surgery*,
DOI 10.1007/978-1-4939-1850-8_17, © Springer Science+Business Media New York 2015

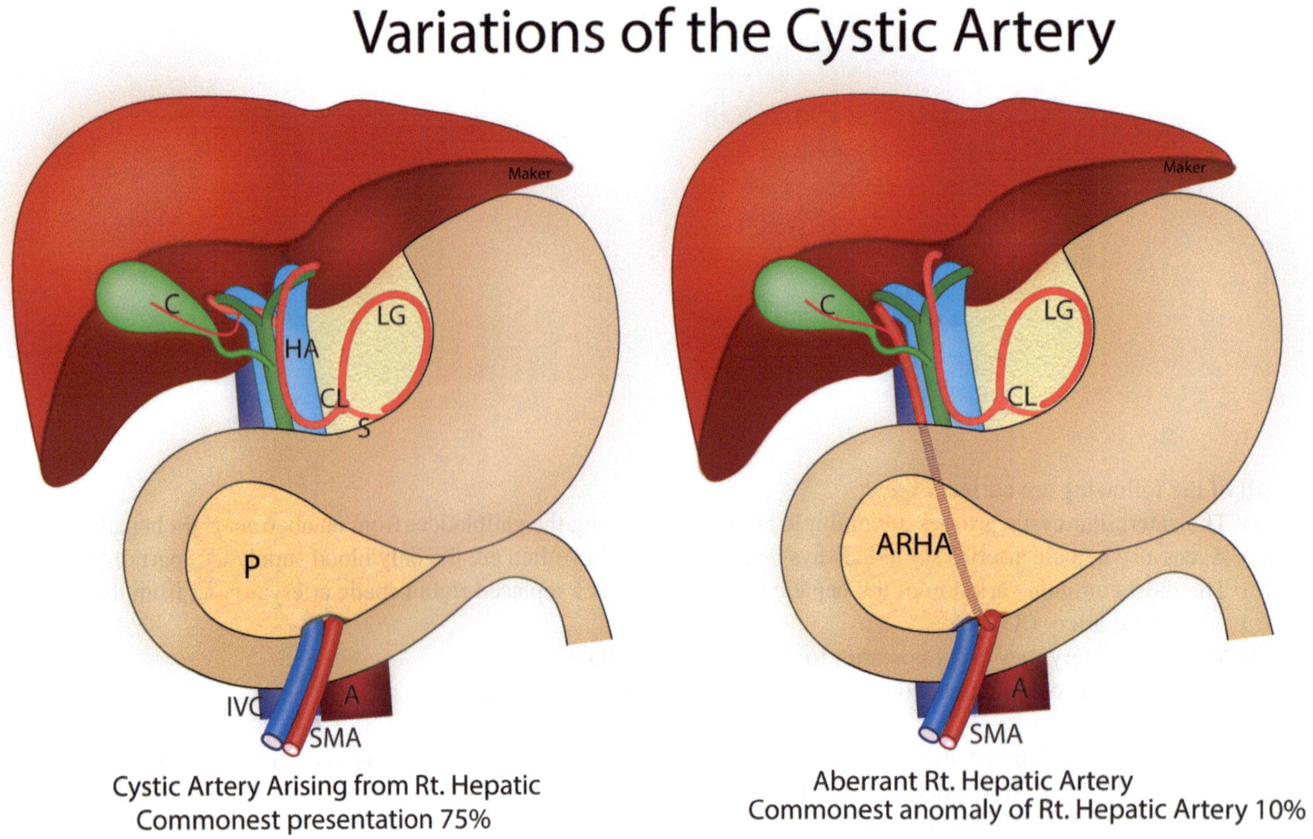

Fig. 17.1 Variations in biliary anatomy are the rule, and a few of them can lead to major errors in the biliary surgery. The gallbladder anatomically belongs to the right lobe of the liver, and hence, the cystic artery commonly arises from the right hepatic artery. In 10 % of population, the right hepatic artery takes origin from the superior mesenteric artery, runs posterior to the pancreas, and lies to the right in the porta hepatis where it gives off the cystic artery, making the right hepatic artery prone to injury in this location. *HA* hepatic artery, *S* splenic artery, *P* pancreas, *A* aorta, *IVC* inferior vena cava, *C* cystic artery, *LG* left gastric artery, *CL* celiac trunk, *SMA* superior mesenteric artery and vein, *ARHA* aberrant right hepatic artery

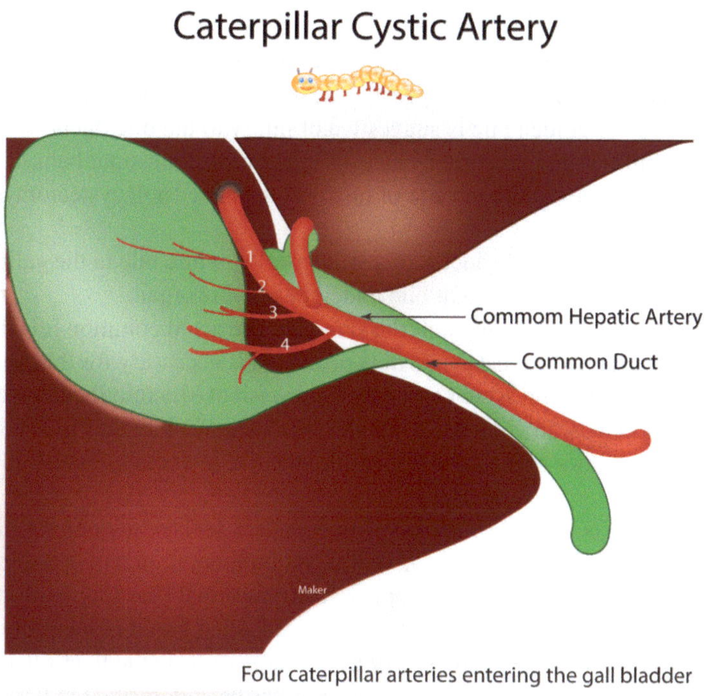

Fig. 17.2 There are multiple variations in the arterial blood supply to the gallbladder. Depicted here are the "caterpillar" cystic arteries. In this case, there are four cystic arteries arising from the common hepatic and the right hepatic artery. Also depicted is the abnormal course of the right hepatic artery running close to the gallbladder fossa and entering the liver outside the porta hepatis

Answer
e

2. All of the following are correct *except*:
   (a) White bile in the biliary tree is consistent with cystic duct obstruction.
   (b) The postoperative drainage of green bile is suggestive of injury to the duodenum.
   (c) The postoperative drainage of golden bile is suggestive of injury to the bile ducts.
   (d) Blood in the bile (hemobilia) is an uncommon cause of upper gastrointestinal hemorrhage.
   (e) The common bile duct is the most common site of bile leakage after cholecystectomy.

Comments Normally, bile in the common bile duct is of a golden color, while bile in the gallbladder is of a dark green color, reflecting the iso-osmotic concentration process that bile undergoes in this organ.

The presence of "white bile" (which is actually colorless) in the obstructed common bile duct is often a source of puzzlement. Experimental studies have established that cystic duct occlusion is necessary for this finding to be present. It is thought that in this setting, the rise in biliary duct pressure causes the backwash of bile into the liver, as bile is replaced by the secretions of the biliary duct mucous glands. In contrast, when the cystic duct is patent, black bile is found. In this setting, it is postulated that the absorptive capabilities of the gallbladder limit the rise in ductal pressure allowing antegrade bile flow with subsequent concentration [4, 5].

In similar fashion, long-standing occlusion of the cystic duct causes replacement of the bile contained therein by mucus secretion. This condition often occurs in the absence of significant inflammation and is termed "hydrops."

Periodic right upper quadrant pain, associated with upper gastrointestinal bleeding in absence of a primary gastrointestinal source, is caused by hemobilia. This condition is often diagnosed when blood is seen coming out of the ampulla of Vater on upper endoscopy and/or an abnormal CT scan demonstrating a large mass in the liver filled with liquid material. The most common cause of this condition is trauma to the liver; however, it has been described in hepatic malignancies [6].

Bile leakage occurs in 0.5–3 % of laparoscopic cholecystectomies. The most common source of leakage is the common bile duct, followed by the accessory ducts of Luschka and common bile duct injuries [7]. Bile draining directly from the biliary tree is usually golden in color. As bile mixes with gastric and pancreatic secretions in the intestine, it takes on a darker green color, as typically seen in duodenal leaks.

Answer
e

3. All of the following are correct *except*:
   (a) Duplicate gallbladders may share a common cystic duct or drain independently into the bile duct.
   (b) Gallbladders with a Phrygian cap deformity have increased incidence of perforation.
   (c) The gallbladder may be found under the left lobe of the liver.
   (d) A gallbladder may be totally intrahepatic.
   (e) Mirizzi's syndrome represents extraluminal obstruction of the common bile duct from a gallstone in Hartmann's pouch.

Comments Duplication of the gallbladder is present on 0.02–0.03 % of the population. The embryologic origin lies in the duplication of the cystic primordium during the 5th–6th week of gestation. While this anomaly is most often diagnosed incidentally at the time of surgery or through various imaging modalities, it may be a source of biliary disease, even after a history of cholecystectomy [8].

Left-sided gallbladders have a prevalence of 0.1–0.7 %. They are located to the left of the falciform ligament, under the left lobe of the liver. Left-sided gallbladders may represent an anomalous rotation of a normal gallbladder primordium, case in which the cystic duct enters the right side of the hepatic duct after making a sharp hairpin turn. Conversely, they may arise from an anomalous left-sided primordium, situation in which the cystic duct follows a straight course in the left side of the hepatic duct. While most left-sided gallbladders are asymptomatic, they may also be a source of biliary symptoms in the apparent absence of a gallbladder [9, 10].

Phrygian cap deformity of the gallbladder is the most common congenital anomaly of the biliary tract. It consists of a folding of the gallbladder in a shape similar to Santa Claus's hat. While many consider it to be an innocuous anatomical variation, their presence may be associated with biliary stasis and cholelithiasis [11].

Mirizzi's syndrome is an infrequent cause of obstructive jaundice. It is caused by extrinsic compression of the common bile duct by a stone impacted in Hartmann's pouch or cystic duct. Its occurrence is predisposed by the existence of a long cystic duct or Hartmann's pouch running parallel to the common hepatic duct, with which they share a common wall. There are times in which the cystic duct and common hepatic duct are wrapped by a fibrous sheath. Compression of the common bile duct may result in decubitus fistulization with significant disruption of the biliary structures. Treatment of this condition is challenging. Dissection of Calot's triangle is made difficult due to chronic inflammation. Attempts at total cholecystectomy are likely to result in large defects in the common hepatic duct or common bile duct. In order to avoid this, partial cholecystectomy, and stone removal with or without T tube drainage, has been advocated. Unfortunately this approach has met with a high incidence of biliary strictures. Mirizzi's syndrome has been associated with an elevated incidence of cholangiocarcinoma. With this in mind, total excision with choledocoduodenostomy or choledocojejunostomy has been performed. This procedure can be very challenging, as the common bile duct is often not dilated. Endoscopic decompression via stenting should be reserved for patients who are not surgical candidates [12] (Fig. 17.3).

Different degrees of incorporation of the gallbladder into the liver parenchyma are a common finding. However, true intrahepatic gallbladders are rare. By definition they are entirely enveloped by Glisson's capsule. They are associated with an increased incidence of cholelithiasis. Due their location, excision is challenging [13].

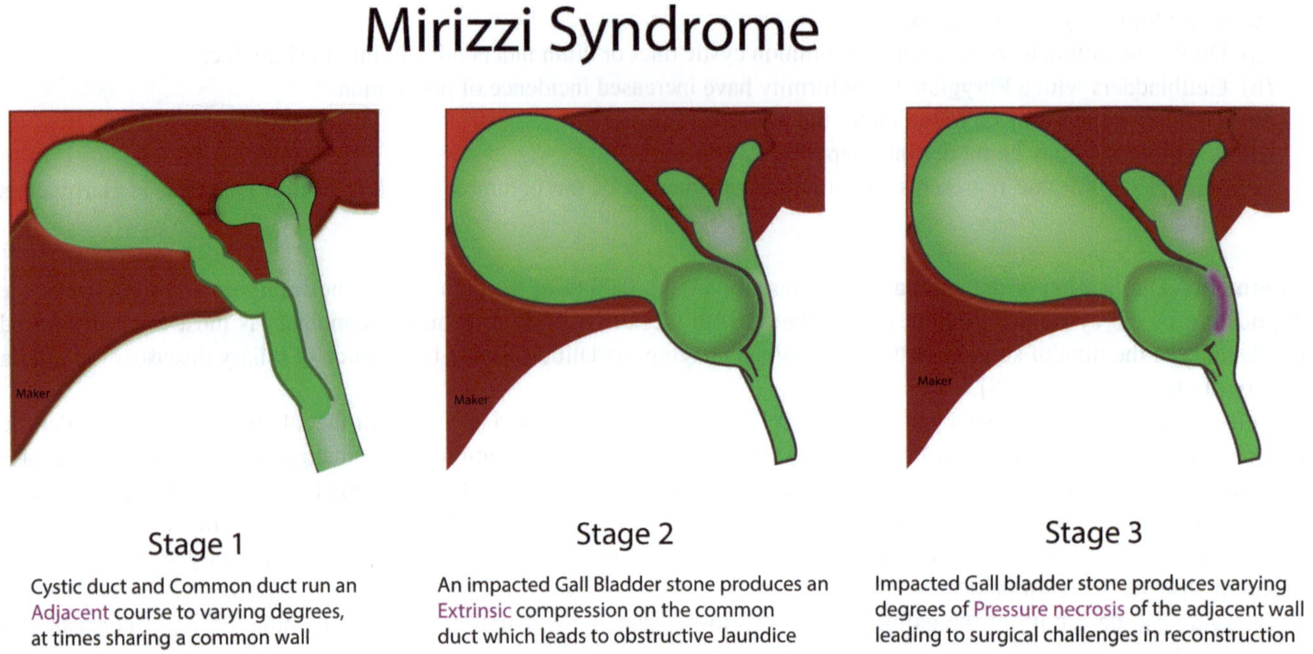

Fig. 17.3 Mirizzi's syndrome

Answer

b

4. All of the following are correct *except*:
   (a) The most common form of choledochal cyst is a single fusiform extrahepatic dilatation.
   (b) Caroli's disease consists of multiple intrahepatic dilatations.
   (c) Choledochal cysts are pseudocysts secondary to gallstone pancreatitis.
   (d) Choledochal cysts should be resected due to the high likelihood of cholangiocarcinoma.
   (e) Choledochal cysts are associated with repeated episodes of cholangitis.

Comments Choledochal cysts are congenital dilatations of the bile ducts that span single fusiform dilatations of the common bile duct to multiple intra and extrahepatic cyst formation. Pancreatobiliary maljunction is the key anatomic defect predisposing to cyst formation. It is defined as extramural junction of the pancreatic and biliary duct, devoid of the normal sphincter mechanism. The length of the common pancreaticobiliary channel has been reported to be approximately 5 mm, whereas it often measures in excess of 15 mm in patients with choledochal cysts.

This anomaly would allow the passage of pancreatic juices (phospholipase A-2, amylase, and lipase) into the biliary tree, leading to weakening of the duct wall and subsequent cystic degeneration. Experimental proof of this hypothesis has been established. Dogs in which the pancreatic juices are diverted into the biliary tree via the gallbladder develop choledochal cysts. Furthermore, both in experimental models and humans, exposure of the biliary epithelium to pancreatic juices leads to adenomatous metaplasia and malignant degeneration, making early resection imperative. The incidence of cholangiocarcinoma associated with choledochal cysts increases with age. It is 2 % in patients diagnosed in their 20s and as high as 43 % in those in their 60s. Overall, the incidence is 16 % [14].

Choledochal cysts have been classified as follows: (Fig. 17.4).

The Todani classification of choledochal cysts implies that all the types are brought about by the same pathophysiologic process as discussed above. However, this view has been challenged. It has been proposed that only types I and IV are secondary to reflux of pancreatic enzymes. Type II cysts are viewed as variations of gallbladder duplication, while type III (choledochoceles) are considered variations of duodenal duplication cysts, a view that is supported by their type of epithelial lining. Finally, Caroli's disease would result from a ductal plate malformation, associated with genetic defects and with polycystic disease of the kidney. Furthermore, types II, III, and V are commonly *not* associated with pancreaticobiliary maljunction [15].

While the classical presentation of choledochal cyst is that of a female infant of Asian background with jaundice, pain, and an abdominal mass, choledochal cysts are being diagnosed with increased frequency in adults of both sexes and diverse ethnicity.

Treatment of choledochal cysts involves excision of the cysts, cholecystectomy, and hepatico-enteric reconstruction. Given that epithelial changes may exceed the margins of cystic degeneration, resection often involves the segment spanning the very proximal common hepatic duct to the common bile duct just above the pancreas. Focal intrahepatic cystic degeneration requires liver resection, while diffuse involvement warrants transplant [16–19].

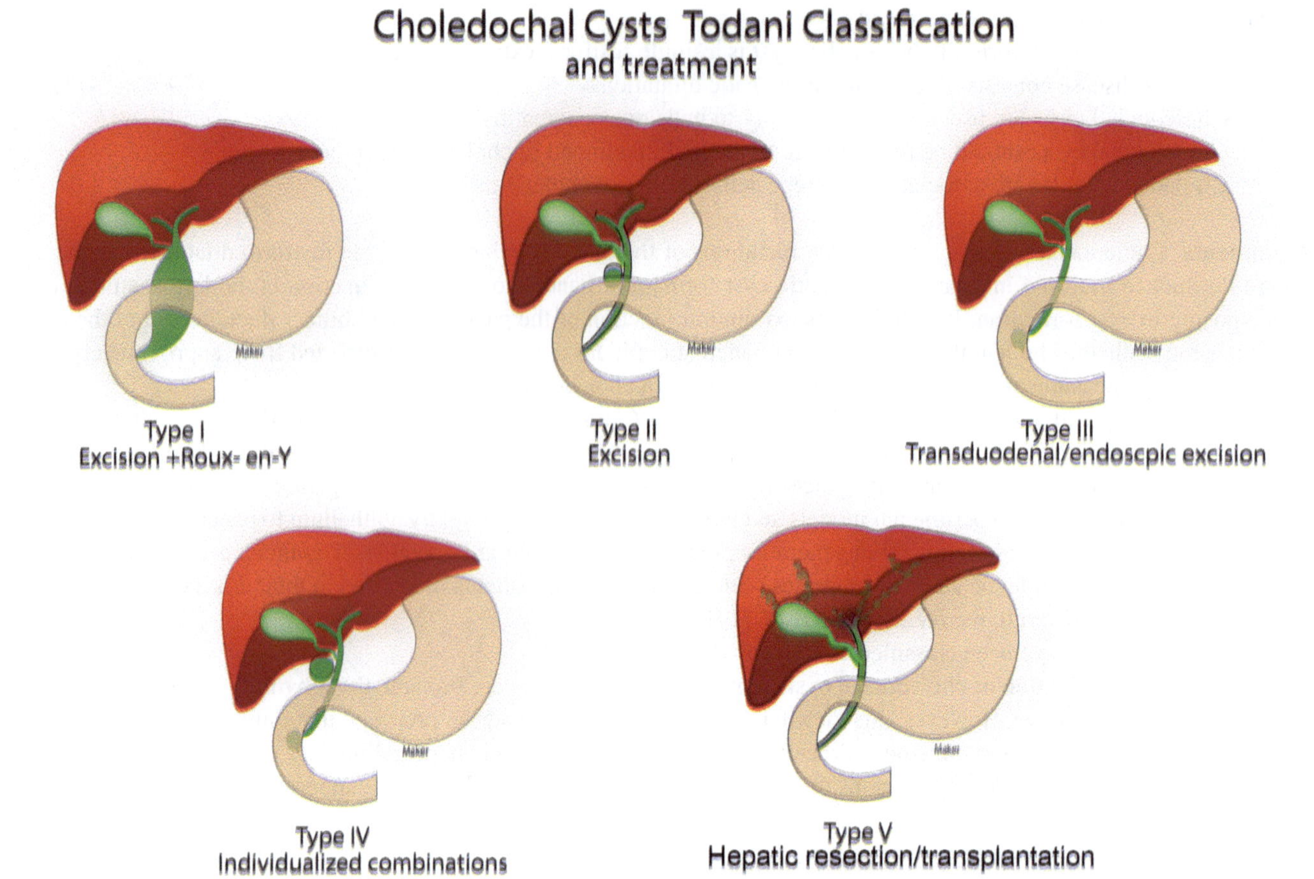

Fig. 17.4 Type 1 choledochal cysts are the most common. Risk of cancer in the cyst as well as the rest of the biliary tree is high, and hence, resection is the treatment of choice. Type 2 are basically biliary diverticula, are rare, and can be excised if symptomatic. Type 3 is choledochoceles in the wall of the duodenum and depending on size can be treated by endoscopic unroofing to operative excision. Type 4 choledochal cysts are multiple but at least one of them has to be extrahepatic. Treatment is a combination of that of type 1 and type 5. Type 5 is better known as Caroli disease. For treatment, each case needs individual consideration ranging from segmental liver excision to transplantation given the associated risk of malignancy

Answer

c

5. All of the following are correct *except*:
   (a) The average diameter of the common bile duct is 8 mm.
   (b) The supraduodenal bile duct is medial to the hepatic artery.
   (c) The portions of the common bile duct are supraduodenal, retroduodenal, pancreatic, and intramural.
   (d) There is variation in the degree of incorporation of the common bile duct to the pancreas.
   (e) The common bile duct has double arterial and venous supply.

Comments The common hepatic duct arises from the confluence of the left and right hepatic ducts, just below the liver hilum, anterior to the portal vein. It must be remembered that this classical anatomy is present only in 57–72 % of cases. The most common variation consists of the right posterior sector duct joining the left hepatic duct, with the right anterior sector duct joining them distally (16–19 % of cases). The final major variation involves a trifurcation consisting of left hepatic duct and the ducts for the right posterior and anterior sectors (11 % of cases).

The cystic duct joins the common hepatic duct to form the common bile duct (CBD). This supraduodenal CBD continues its course anterior to the vena cava along the edge of the hepaticoduodenal ligament. The hepatic artery lies medial to it. It then becomes retroduodenal, passing behind the first portion of the duodenum to reach the pancreatic groove. In its pancreatic portion, the CBD may be covered by the pancreatic parenchyma in varying degrees.

There are discrepancies in reports of the size of the common bile duct largely due to the imaging modality. The external diameter of the supraduodenal common bile duct measures 5–13 mm, with a mean of 9 mm. The internal diameter (depicted by contrast studies) varies from 4 to 12 mm, with a mean diameter of 8 mm. While the external diameter of the CBD remains fairly constant along its course, the internal diameter narrows to a mean diameter of 4 mm at the papilla.

The common bile duct may receive its blood supply from several different arteries: superior pancreaticoduodenal, gastroduodenal, hepatic artery, and cystic artery. Notwithstanding the variations in origin, fairly constant arteries arise from these tributaries and run along the common bile duct at 3 and 9 o'clock positions with stepladder collaterals that are a source of bleeding during choledochotomy. In similar fashion, multiple small venous tributaries come together to form 3 and 9 o'clock veins. Preservation of biliary blood vessels is critical, as failure to do so leads to strictures [20, 21].

Answer
b

6. All of the following are correct *except*:
   (a) Intrahepatic and proximal biliary atresia is not amenable to reconstruction and requires liver transplantation.
   (b) Distal biliary atresia may be surgically corrected.
   (c) Biliary atresia may represent an immune-mediated process.
   (d) Infants with biliary atresia present indirect hyperbilirubinemia.
   (e) The Kasai procedure (hepatoportoenterostomy) is used in the treatment of biliary atresia.

Comments Biliary atresia is a rare and deadly entity affecting the intrahepatic and extrahepatic bile ducts. It has an estimated incidence of 1 in 10,000 live births, and it is the most common indication for pediatric liver transplantation (50 % of procedures). Untreated, it reaches a near 100 % mortality by 2 years of age, with a median survival of 8 months. Death occurs due to liver failure secondary to biliary cirrhosis.

The etiology of biliary atresia remains unclear. Pathologic analysis of the affected ducts reveals inflammation and fibrosis, as well as lymphocytic infiltration, suggesting an important role of the immune system in the development of this disease. It has been postulated that a viral insult may trigger the inflammatory process and rotavirus has been implicated. Experiments in several animal models have shown that rotavirus infection in newborn specimens leads to biliary atresia. However, there is no conclusive proof in humans. Some genetic influences such as HLA type or anomalies in α-1-antitrypsin have also been found to be associated with biliary atresia. It is most likely that etiology is multifactorial [22].

Newborns with biliary atresia often appear normal at birth. They go on to develop direct jaundice, choluria, and acholic stool. The presence of direct hyperbilirubinemia beyond 2 weeks of age should raise the suspicion of biliary atresia. As the disease progresses and cirrhosis develops, patients may present hepatomegaly and stigmata of portal hypertension.

Due to the rapidly progressive nature of this disease, it is imperative that treatment be instituted promptly. Ideally, surgical correction should be performed by 60 days of age, thus preserving viable liver parenchyma.

The surgical procedure of choice is hepatoportoenterostomy also known as the Kasai procedure. This operation consists of the mobilization of the extrahepatic biliary tree as high as possible. The ducts are then sectioned, leaving open ends to which a Roux limb is approximated and sutured to the liver. This procedure is most appropriate for patients with predominantly extrahepatic disease.

The short-term success of the Kasai procedure approaches 80 %. Ten-year survival is 30 % and 20-year survival is approximately 20 %. These low numbers reflect the ongoing course of the inflammatory process affecting the biliary tree as a whole. It is expected that 70–80 % of patients undergoing a Kasai procedure will require liver transplantation. Fortunately, the long-term success of this intervention is far superior, with an 85 % 10-year survival [23, 24].

Answer
d

7. All of the following are correct *except*:
   (a) The vagus nerve initiates gallbladder emptying.
   (b) The gallbladder has peristaltic activity.
   (c) The gallbladder has a capacity of approximately 30 ml.
   (d) The gallbladder lowers the pH of the bile preventing the precipitation of calcium salts.
   (e) The gallbladder concentrates bile up to ten times in iso-osmotic fashion.

Comments The adult gallbladder commonly measures 4 cm in diameter and 7–10 cm in length. It is divided into fundus, body, and neck. The region in which the body of the gallbladder tapers into the neck is named "infundibulum." The right aspect of the neck of the gallbladder may present a recess projecting towards the duodenum. This structure is termed Hartmann's pouch and is a useful point of retraction during cholecystectomy. The capacity of the gallbladder fluctuates around 30 ml. This volume increases slightly with male sex, age, and obesity [25].

Under physiologic conditions, eating is the main stimulus for gallbladder contraction. Among the nutrients, polyunsaturated fats are the most potent in this regard, with carbohydrates and proteins playing a minor role. Peak contraction is reached 30–45 min after fat ingestion, time at which the gallbladder reaches a minimal volume of 5–10 ml. However, maximal contraction may be delayed as much as 4 h after ingestion of a mixed meal, which explains the late timing of symptoms observed in clinical practice.

Gallbladder contraction is mediated by the vagus nerve and gut-derived cholecystokinin (CCK). The right vagus nerve is responsible for maintaining muscular tone. Surgical and pharmacologic vagal blockade leads to an increase in resting volume and a decrease in the response to CCK (atonic gallbladder). CCK is the main mediator of gallbladder contraction after fat ingestion.

The gallbladder is different from the remainder of the GI tract in that it totally lacks the usual organization of its muscle layers. This explains the lack of peristalsis, which is substituted by en masse contraction. The gallbladder does exhibit a discreet bellow-like motion approximately every 2 min, both at rest and during contraction. These small fluctuations explain the nature of biliary pain, described as sustained with exacerbations [26].

The gallbladder plays an important role in modifying the composition of the bile by selective absorption and excretion. In this regard, the chief function of the gallbladder is to concentrate the bile in iso-osmotic fashion. To achieve this, sodium and water are removed from the bile proportionately, leading to a five- to tenfold concentration of bile acids. In addition, the gallbladder secretes mucus, which protects its epithelium from the detergent effects of bile. Finally, the gallbladder acidifies the bile, which prevents calcium precipitation [27].

Answer
b

8. All of the following are correct *except*:
   (a) The ducts of Luschka are communications between the gallbladder and the liver parenchyma.
   (b) The Rokitansky–Aschoff sinuses are invaginations of the gallbladder mucosa that may extend to the serosa or liver bed.
   (c) Hartmann's pouch is a dilatation of the gallbladder infundibulum.
   (d) The spiral valves of Heister may contribute to maintaining the patency of the cystic duct.
   (e) The cystic duct has sphincteric function, regulating gallbladder emptying.

Comments The ducts of Luschka, also known as subvesical ducts, were first described in 1863, as 1–2 mm ducts stemming from the wall of the gallbladder, crossing through the liver parenchyma to reach the right hepatic or common hepatic duct. Their prevalence is estimated to approximate 5 %. Their chief clinical importance is that their transection during cholecystectomy is the second most common cause of biliary leakage [28, 29].

Rokitansky–Aschoff sinuses are invaginations of the gallbladder epithelium, which may extend through the fibromuscular layer of the gallbladder into the serosa or liver bed. These sinuses become inflamed in a manner analogous to that of colonic diverticula. However, each attack of cholecystitis causes these sinuses to become deeper as they re-epithelialize from the previous attack. Some of the sinuses may reach the serosa, explaining easy leaking of bile upon grasping chronically inflamed gallbladders. Gallbladder perforations, even though rare, commonly happen at the site of the deepened Rokitansky–Aschoff sinuses from previous attacks.

Rokitansky–Aschoff may give rise to focal cholecystitis. This entity is characterized by intense gallbladder inflammation with a patent cystic duct and often times in the absence of stones [30, 31].

Adenomyosis of the gallbladder is caused by multiple submucosal sinuses, which fill with bile after the ingestion of a fatty meal. Some authors believe that these sinuses are abnormal Rokitansky–Aschoff sinuses.

As described previously, Hartmann's pouch is a dilatation of the gallbladder as it joins the cystic duct. It has been postulated that it is a zone of biliary stasis and has been positively correlated with the presence of gallstones. It exists in approximately half of gallbladders. At times, Hartmann's pouch becomes the site for a large impacted stone holding all the small stones behind, describe in the literature as a schoolmaster stone [32].

The gallbladder is unique in that it is the only hollow organ that has a common duct for filling and emptying. Serving this dual role, the cystic duct has been implicated in the genesis of multiple biliary pathologies, most importantly, cholelithiasis and biliary dyskinesia. The valves of Heister are mucosal leaflets within the cystic duct. Their function is unclear. It has been proposed that they may act as internal stents to maintain patency of the common bile duct. Detailed analyses of bile flow have concluded that they increase the resistance offered by the cystic duct to bile flow. With this in mind, it has been postulated that they may act to prevent undue increases in biliary and pancreatic pressure during gallbladder contraction. This effect, however, is most likely passive, as the cystic duct lacks intrinsic contractility or sphincter function [33, 34].

Answer
e

9. All of the following are correct *except*:
   (a) Dark green or black stones in the gallbladder are often associated with hemolytic diseases.
   (b) Shiny white or light brown stones are often mixed stones.
   (c) Stones forming in the gallbladder are smooth and rounded.
   (d) Drugs with biliary excretion may induce the formation of gallstones.
   (e) Primary choledochal stones are often light brown and crumble easily.

Comments The physical characteristic of biliary stones may provide insight into the pathophysiologic processes leading to their formation. The solubility of bile depends on the balance of cholesterol, lecithin, and bile salts. Disruption of this equilibrium leads to stone formation.

Eighty percent of gallstones are mixed stones, in which cholesterol precipitates around a calcium salt nucleus. These stones are multiple, multifaceted, and shiny white and found in three to five generations in a gallbladder packed with stones. It is believed that their shape and color are products of friction between the stones. Rarely, the nucleus of these stones can be a parasitic or bacterial. The second most common type of gallstones is dark green or black and is associated with hemolytic disease, most commonly sickle cell disease and spherocytosis.

The least common type of gallstone is the single, large, pure cholesterol stone. Interestingly enough this very often is asymptomatic, as its large size does not occlude the cystic duct [35].

The vast majority of common bile duct stones come from the gallbladder and hence are classified as secondary choledocholithiasis. Only 5 % of common duct stones are formed primarily in the duct and tend to be ovoid, light brown, solitary, and easily crushable, similar to wet sand. Like gallstones, primary common bile duct stones are thought to be a product of lithogenic bile and stasis.

Nonetheless, it is sometimes difficult to determine the origin on a common bile duct stone in the presence of a gallbladder or after the removal of said organ. For practical purposes, common bile duct stones diagnosed 2 years after cholecystectomy are considered primary. The differentiation is crucial, as treatment for primary and secondary gallstones is different. For most primary choledocholithiasis, internal drainage is preferred [36, 37].

Ceftriaxone has been implicated in the formation of biliary sludge in as many as 46 % of treated patients, with biliary symptoms arising in up to 16 % of patients receiving this drug, especially during prolonged treatments such as those for Lyme disease. Interestingly, these stones may disappear with discontinuation of this antibiotic.

Octreotide has also been implicated in the formation of gallstones, as it impedes gallbladder emptying and promotes bile concentration. Not surprisingly, gallstones are also seen in the presence of somatostatinomas, in conjunction with diabetes mellitus, steatorrhea, and gastric hypochlorhydria.

Answer

c

10. All of the following are correct *except*:
    (a) Pneumobilia is typically diagnostic of a cholecystoenteric fistula.
    (b) Air in the periphery of the liver is diagnostic of portal pylephlebitis.
    (c) The cholecystoduodenal fistula is the most common fistula caused by gallstones.
    (d) Impacted gallstones should be removed through a proximal enterotomy.
    (e) Bouveret's syndrome is the obstruction of the distal ileum.

Comments Gallstone ileus accounts for 1–4 % of all small bowel obstructions, predominantly affecting elderly females. This entity is associated with a mortality approaching 20 % due to the associated comorbidities that are often present.

Cholecystoenteric fistulas arise when bouts of gallbladder inflammation lead to adhesions between the gallbladder and the bowel, with subsequent decubitus ulceration between both organs. The first portion of the duodenum is the site most often affected, although fistulas to the colon, stomach, and other segments of the small bowel have been described. In all cases, pneumobilia is a key radiologic sign that may suggest the diagnosis. Pneumobilia is characterized by air in the central portion of the liver. In contrast, air in the periphery of the liver is formed in situ by septic emboli from portal pylephlebitis.

It is thought that most gallstones that pass through cholecystoenteric fistulas are expelled uneventfully; however, large enough stones may cause obstruction. Solitary, large gallstones are typically seen in diabetics where they may sit for years in an asymptomatic fashion leading to decubitus ulceration. These large stones lodge in the terminal ileum, which is the narrowest part of the enteric tract.

Very rarely, a gallstone may reach the intestinal tract at the level of the stomach or duodenum producing gastric outlet obstruction. This entity is termed Bouveret's syndrome [38, 39].

Principles of treatment include stone removal via enterotomy through a site proximal to that of obstruction to avoid enterotomy in compromised bowel and take advantage of the proximal dilated bowel to easily extract the stone. Another very important surgical principle is to carefully evaluate the bowel for other stones in transit. Cholecystectomy and repair of the fistula are not mandatory. Their execution is based on the stability of the patient at the time of surgery [40].

Answer

e

11. All of the following are correct *except*:
    (a) Maximal cephalad retraction of the gallbladder fundus separates the cystic duct from the hepatic duct.
    (b) Lateral retraction of the gallbladder fundus separates the cystic duct from the common bile duct.
    (c) A short cystic duct predisposes to injury of the common bile duct.
    (d) Aberrant right hepatic ducts can be mistaken for the cystic duct.
    (e) Spilled stones during cholecystectomy should be removed.

Comments Despite the all the advances in laparoscopic surgery and even with adequate experience, the incidence of laparoscopic bile duct injury continues to be higher than the rate for open laparoscopic surgery (1–2 % vs. 0.5–1 %). The etiology at present is not completely clear.

The anatomical basis for biliary injuries during laparoscopic cholecystectomy is the close approximation of the cystic duct and common bile duct, a misalignment brought about by excessive cephalad traction of the fundus of the gallbladder or insufficient lateral traction of the gallbladder infundibulum. Other aggravating factors are the multitude of anatomical variations of the biliary tract combined with the distortion caused by the inflammatory pathology. Furthermore, the limitations of laparoscopic visualization and lack of tactile dissection compound the problem.

The "infundibular technique" of cystic duct identification recommends dissecting the lateral aspect of the gallbladder until the junction to the cystic duct is reached. This junction can be identified by a flaring appearance of the duct into the gallbladder. However, in the presence of inflammation or a short cystic duct, this relation may be altered leading to common bile duct injury. To avoid this pitfall, the critical view of safety technique is recommended. This technique consists of fully dissecting the triangle of Calot, completely exposing the cystic duct and hepatic artery anterior to a clearly visualized liver in the background prior to any ligation or division [41] (Fig. 17.5).

Bismuth developed a classification of biliary strictures based on the lowest level at which healthy duct was present to perform an anastomosis. Since his original publication, his classification has been applied to the description of biliary injuries. However, caution must be taken in that subsequent strictures may extend up to one level higher than the injury at the original operation. Strasberg adapted this classification system to the injuries created during laparoscopic cholecystectomy [42, 43]. The Strasberg classification is also useful in deciding treatment (see Table 17.1).

It is extremely common (up to 50 %) to have an associated vascular injury, which at times leads to the ductal ligation during the control of bleeding. Therefore, it is imperative that any workup of biliary tract injuries include a study of the hepatic vasculature at the porta hepatis. High common duct injuries often result in three and four duct anastomoses. At this level, it is frequent to find the conventional right and left hepatic ducts, separate ducts from the caudate lobe, and ducts from the posterior sector of the right lobe [44].

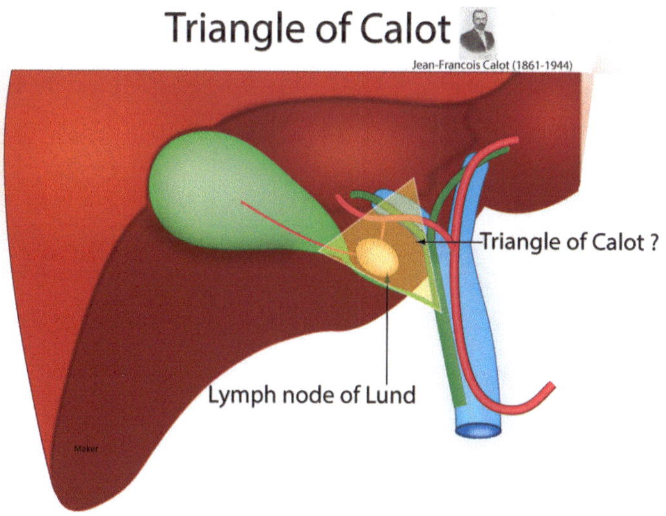

Fig. 17.5 Jean-Francois Calot described his triangle in 1890 with boundaries of the cystic duct, common hepatic duct, and cystic artery. Today, Calot's triangle is often described as the cystohepatic triangle bounded by the cystic duct, common hepatic duct, and inferior surface of the liver superiorly. It contains the lymph node of Lund often enlarged in gallbladder disease and making the dissection difficult in the area. Ligation of structures in this triangle without obtaining the critical view of safety is often the cause of common duct injury

Table 17.1 The Strasberg classification

Type of injury	Description	Treatment
A	Cystic duct or duct of Luschka leak	Intraoperative ligation or postoperative endoscopic decompression of the biliary tract
B	Occlusion of an aberrant right hepatic duct	No further treatment
C	Transection without ligation of an aberrant right hepatic duct	Drainage of the biloma with possible endoscopic decompression
D	Lateral injury to a major bile duct	Primary repair and T tube drainage or hepaticojejunostomy
E1	CBD transection >2 cm from the hilum	Hepaticojejunostomy
E2	CBD transection <2 cm from the hilum	Hepaticojejunostomy extending into the left hepatic duct
E3	Transection at the hilum preserving the superior wall	Hepaticojejunostomy extending into the left hepatic duct with lowering of the hilar plate
E4	Separation of major bile ducts	Lowering of the hilar plate, reconstruction of the hepatic confluence, or separate anastomosis
E5	Type C + E1–E4	Anastomosis or ligation of the right hepatic duct in addition to repairs described for E1–E4

Answer

a

12. All of the following are correct *except*:
    (a) Primary sclerosing cholangitis may affect bile ducts of any caliber.
    (b) Intrahepatic strictures are amenable to surgical management.
    (c) Liver transplantation is the most definitive treatment for primary sclerosing cholangitis.
    (d) Ascending cholangitis is caused by biliary obstruction.
    (e) Cholangiohepatitis is often caused by parasitic disease.

Comments Primary sclerosing cholangitis (PSC) presents as recurrent fever, pain, and jaundice from progressive immune-mediated fibrosis of the biliary system. The natural history of this disease is to progress to biliary cirrhosis, portal hypertension, liver failure, and death. The incidence of this condition is estimated to be 1.3 cases per 100,000. It predominantly affects males in the fifth decade of life. There is a clear association with inflammatory bowel disease (IBD): 70–80 % of patients with PSC have IBD, and 2–4 % of patients with IBD will develop PSC. PSC is also considered a precancerous lesion leading to cholangiocarcinoma. Autopsy studies have established a 20–40 % prevalence of cholangiocarcinoma in patients with PSC. Surgical treatment is twofold. In early stages, attempts are made at correcting extrahepatic strictures. As the disease progresses and liver failure ensues, liver transplantation becomes necessary [45].

Acute ascending cholangitis is the most common cause of infection of the biliary tree in the United States. It results from biliary obstruction, most often due to stones. Presentation can vary from mild to fulminant (i.e., acute suppurative cholangitis, which is a surgical emergency). A key pathophysiologic factor is increases in biliary pressure leading to disruption of hepatocellular junctions and reflux of bacteria and toxins into the systemic circulation. Charcot recognized the triad of fever, right upper quadrant pain, and jaundice that occurs in 60–70 % of patients with cholangitis. Reynolds' pentad, which adds hypotension and mental status changes, is present in 5–7 % of cases. While the original treatment of ascending cholangitis involved surgical drainage via choledochotomy and T tube placement, this approach has been largely replaced by ERCP or percutaneous biliary drainage. Surgical intervention is reserved for patients in whom less invasive techniques are not feasible or have failed. Of note, due to the instability of the patients, cholecystectomy is usually deferred for a second operation [46].

Cholangiohepatitis is the inflammation of both the liver parenchyma and the ductal system. It is endemic in Southeast Asia, where it is a major cause of abdominal pain, fever, and jaundice. Intra- and extrahepatic biliary dilatation and soft pigment stones with pus in the biliary system are characteristic. The cause is not fully understood, but it is thought to depend on bacterial superinfection in association with clonorchiasis and ascariasis. Bacteria deconjugate bile salts, which explain the formation of stones by precipitation around a parasitic nucleus. The main diagnostic modalities are percutaneous transhepatic cholangiography and magnetic resonance cholangiography. Treatment involves treatment of the parasitic infestation, together with cleansing of the biliary system and hepaticojejunostomy [47, 48].

Answer

e

13. All of the following are correct *except*:
    (a) Radical cholecystectomy involves the resection of liver segments IVb and V.
    (b) Intrahepatic cholangiocarcinomas are managed with liver resection.
    (c) Right or left hepatic duct occlusion produces jaundice.
    (d) The best survival in gallbladder carcinoma is observed in cases of incidentally found malignancy on pathology.
    (e) Pruritus is a salient finding in obstructive jaundice.

Comments Gallbladder cancer is a relatively rare malignancy with poor prognosis. Approximately 5,000 new cases are diagnosed each year in the United States. It is seen with more frequency in China, India, and Chile. Most curable gallbladder cancers are asymptomatic, and the diagnosis is made at the time of laparoscopic cholecystectomy or upon pathologic review of the specimen. This malignancy is most frequent in elderly females. It is associated with a history of gallstones in up to 80 % of the cases. Gallbladder polyps are also a risk factor, especially those that are large (>1 cm) and sessile. There is no specific presentation of gallbladder cancer. Manifestations of the disease may include biliary symptoms, weakness, fatigue, weight loss, and occasionally hemobilia. While ultrasound is very sensitive for the detection of gallstones (>95 %), it only recognizes 50–85 % of gallbladder cancers. Upon radiologic diagnosis, CT scanning is useful in determining the local extent of disease. Alternatively, endoscopic ultrasound can be used.

Surgical treatment aims at the complete removal of the gallbladder with clear bile duct margins and en bloc resection of any affected liver parenchyma and lymph nodes. For incidentally found tumors that do not invade past the lamina propria (T1a), laparoscopic cholecystectomy is sufficient, provided no biliary spillage has occurred. Deeper tumors require open radical cholecystectomy, in which segments IVb and V are excised. Cases in which the gallbladder was extracted laparoscopically and later found to have a tumor greater than T1a should have a secondary liver resection. Excision of port sites has been recommended due to the high incidence of seeding and local recurrence, especially if there has been spillage during laparoscopic surgery, but is not required (Fig. 17.6) [49].

While patients with smaller T1a tumors are considered cured after cholecystectomy, the prognosis for more advanced lesions is dismal. Overall 5-year survival ranges from 25 to 45 %. This rate decreases to 16 % in those with nodal metastasis. Unresectable disease carries a life expectancy of 6–8 months [38, 50–52].

Cholangiocarcinoma has a similar incidence to that of gallbladder cancer. While it remains a disease of the elderly population, it is slightly more frequent in males. Histologically, these tumors are adenocarcinomas, showing moderate to good differentiation in 90 % of cases. From an anatomical standpoint, they are divided into intrahepatic and extrahepatic. Risk factors include sclerosing cholangitis, liver fluke infestation, hepatolithiasis, choledochal cysts, and liver cirrhosis. Exposure to the radiologic contrast thorotrast was associated with a 300-fold risk increase. Cholangiocarcinomas have local spread along the mucosa and submucosa and radially into adjacent structures such as the liver parenchyma.

While most tumors are asymptomatic or present with nonspecific symptoms, persistent, progressive painless jaundice suggests the diagnosis. Pruritus due to skin deposition of bile salts is also a salient finding. Cholestyramine is used for the treatment of this symptom, as it impedes enterohepatic recycling of bile acids [53].

In cases in which one of the main bile ducts remains patent, an elevation in alkaline phosphatase without an elevation in bilirubin may suggest the diagnosis; in this setting, pruritus may also be present. Unilateral main bile duct involvement leads to atrophy of the affected site and contralateral compensatory hypertrophy. Ultrasound, CT scanning, and MRI are all useful noninvasive imaging modalities. ERCP is limited in its assessment of the proximal biliary tree. Bile duct margins of 2 cm or greater are recommended for tumors with mucosal spread, while 1 cm margins are adequate for submucosal spread.

Surgical therapy is an option for medically fit patients with no extrahepatic disease or lymphadenopathy beyond the porta hepatis. Intrahepatic cholangiocarcinoma is treated with anatomical liver resection. Extrahepatic infraduodenal cholangiocarcinomas are treated with a Whipple procedure. In other words, intrahepatic cholangiocarcinomas are managed as hepatocellular carcinomas; extrahepatic infraduodenal cholangiocarcinomas are managed like pancreatic adenocarcinomas. Tumors involving the extrahepatic common bile duct (Klatskin) and supraduodenal common bile duct are typically treated with distal resection and hepaticojejunostomy [50, 54]. Extensive lymphadenectomy for biliary tumors has not been shown to increase survival. However, lymphadenectomy may help achieve local control and has prognostic implications, given the effect of lymph node status and survival (Fig. 17.7).

Klatskin tumors are cholangiocarcinomas located at the level of the biliary bifurcation (Bismuth class IV). Their natural history is to cause progressive biliary obstruction, leading to liver failure and death. Surgical management of these tumors is very challenging, requiring excision of the extrahepatic bile duct, cholecystectomy, and usually partial hepatectomy as directed by the areas of tumor invasion. Biliary drainage is restored through Roux-en-Y hepaticojejunostomy. On occasion, vascular resection and subsequent reconstruction is also necessary [55].

Liver transplantation is emerging as an option for patients that would require a total hepatectomy for clear margins or for those whose liver function does not allow a more limited resection. Palliative treatments are aimed at diverting bile flow through internal and external drainage procedures, as well as at reducing tumor burden with chemotherapy, radiotherapy, radiofrequency ablation, and embolization.

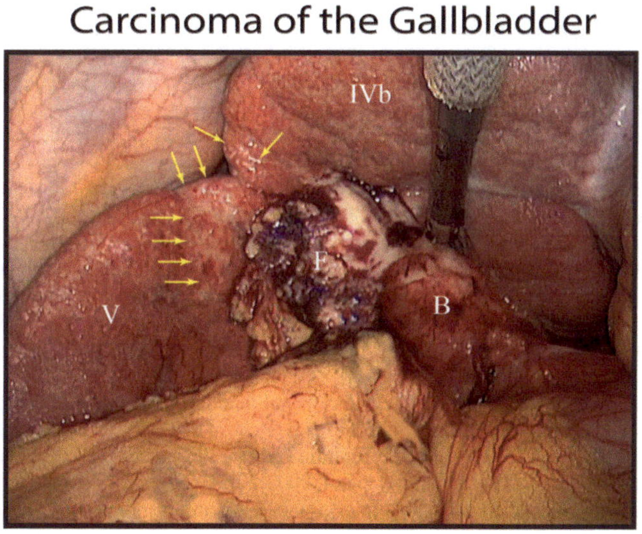

Fig. 17.6 Carcinoma is visible in the fundus of the gallbladder and invading segments 5 and 4b as marked by the *yellow arrows*. With adequate liver function and without evidence of metastatic disase or medical contraindications, this patient will qualify for en bloc segment 5 and 4b resection with portal lymph node dissection. *F* fundus of the gallbladder, *B* body of the gallbladder; *yellow arrows* mark the direct carcinoma infiltration in the cirrhotic liver

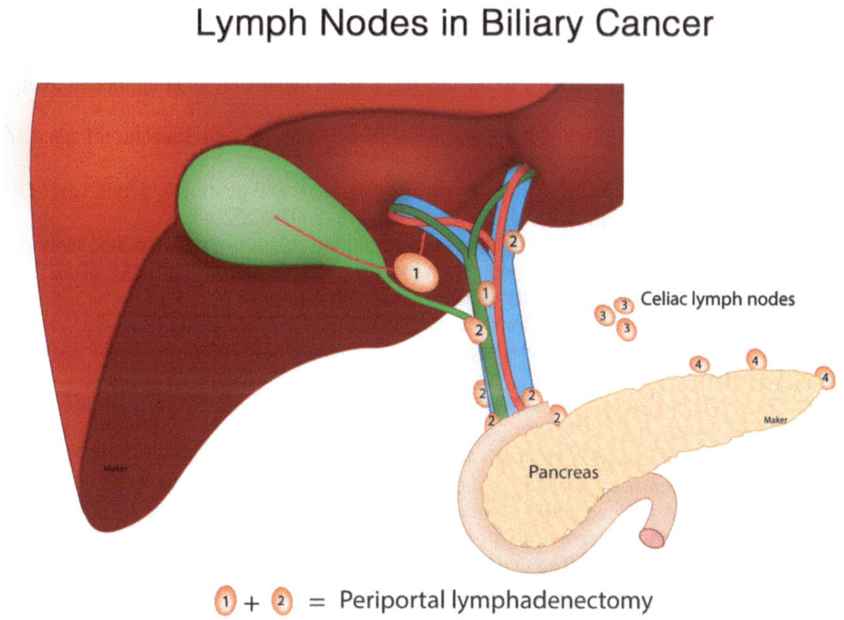

Fig. 17.7 Periportal lymphadenectomy consists of 360° removal of the lymph node basin around the portal system in the hepatoduodenal ligament starting superiorly at the porta hepatis and continuing inferiorly to the superior and posterior aspect of the pancreas (stations 1 and 2 in this figure). This is recommended in selected resectable gallbladder and biliary duct cancers to achieve an R0 resection and for appropriate staging

Answer

c

References

1. Noto M, Miwa K, Kitagawa H, et al. Pancreas head carcinoma: frequency of invasion to soft tissue adherent to the superior mesenteric artery. Am J Surg Pathol. 2005;29:1056–61.
2. Bergamaschi R, Ignjatovic D. More than two structures in Calot's triangle. A postmortem study. Surg Endosc. 2000;14:354–7.
3. Hiatt JR, Gabbay J, Busuttil RW. Surgical anatomy of the hepatic arteries in 1000 cases. Ann Surg. 1994;220:50–2.
4. Neilan RE, Groce JR, Jalil S, Raju GS. White bile (with video). Gastrointest Endosc. 2007;66:180–1; discussion 181.
5. Hashmonai M, Kam I, Schramek A. The etiology of "white bile" in the biliary tree. J Surg Res. 1984;37:479–86.
6. Munoz C, Fernandez M, Brahm J. Traumatic hemobilia: a case report and literature review. Gastroenterol Hepatol. 2008;31:79–81.
7. Massoumi H, Kiyici N, Hertan H. Bile leak after laparoscopic cholecystectomy. J Clin Gastroenterol. 2007;41:301–5.
8. Singh B, Ramsaroop L, Allopi L, Moodley J, Satyapal KS. Duplicate gallbladder: an unusual case report. Surg Radiol Anat. 2006;28:654–7.
9. Dhulkotia A, Kumar S, Kabra V, Shukla H. Aberrant gallbladder situated beneath the left lobe of liver. HPB (Oxford). 2002;4:39–42.
10. Blanton DE, Bream CA, Mandel SR. Gallbladder ectopia. A review of anomalies of position. Am J Roentgenol Radium Ther Nucl Med. 1974;121:396–400.
11. de Csepel J, Carroccio A, Pomp A. Soft-tissue images. "Phrygian cap" gallbladder. Can J Surg. 2003;46:50–1.
12. Freeman ME, Rose JL, Forsmark CE, Vauthey J. Mirizzi syndrome: a rare cause of obstructive jaundice. Dig Dis. 1999;17:44–8.
13. Kochar K, Vallance K, Mathew G, Jadhav V. Intrahepatic perforation of the gall bladder presenting as liver abscess: case report, review of literature and Niemeier's classification. Eur J Gastroenterol Hepatol. 2008;20:240–4.
14. Franko J, Nussbaum ML, Morris JB. Choledochal cyst cholangiocarcinoma arising from adenoma: case report and a review of the literature. Curr Surg. 2006;63:281–4.
15. Okada A, Hasegawa T, Oguchi Y, Nakamura T. Recent advances in pathophysiology and surgical treatment of congenital dilatation of the bile duct. J Hepatobiliary Pancreat Surg. 2002;9:342–51.
16. Edil BH, Cameron JL, Reddy S, et al. Choledochal cyst disease in children and adults: a 30-year single-institution experience. J Am Coll Surg. 2008;206:1000–5; discussion 1005–8.
17. Iwai N, Yanagihara J, Tokiwa K, Shimotake T, Nakamura K. Congenital choledochal dilatation with emphasis on pathophysiology of the biliary tract. Ann Surg. 1992;215:27–30.
18. Lipsett PA, Pitt HA, Colombani PM, Boitnott JK, Cameron JL. Choledochal cyst disease. A changing pattern of presentation. Ann Surg. 1994;220:644–52.
19. Visser BC, Suh I, Way LW, Kang SM. Congenital choledochal cysts in adults. Arch Surg. 2004;139:855–60; discussion 860–2.
20. Vakili K, Pomfret EA. Biliary anatomy and embryology. Surg Clin North Am. 2008;88:1159–74.
21. Ohkubo M, Nagino M, Kamiya J, et al. Surgical anatomy of the bile ducts at the hepatic hilum as applied to living donor liver transplantation. Ann Surg. 2004;239:82–6.
22. Zheng S, Luo Y, Wang W, Xiao X. Analysis of the pathomorphology of the intra- and extrahepatic biliary system in biliary atresia. Eur J Pediatr Surg. 2008;18:98–102.
23. Bates MD, Bucuvalas JC, Alonso MH, Ryckman FC. Biliary atresia: pathogenesis and treatment. Semin Liver Dis. 1998;18:281–93.
24. Bassett MD, Murray KF. Biliary atresia: recent progress. J Clin Gastroenterol. 2008;42:720–9.
25. Caroli-Bosc FX, Pugliese P, Peten EP, et al. Gallbladder volume in adults and its relationship to age, sex, body mass index, body surface area and gallstones. An epidemiologic study in a nonselected population in France. Digestion. 1999;60:344–8.
26. O'Donnell LJ, Fairclough PD. Gall stones and gall bladder motility. Gut. 1993;34:440–3.
27. Wood JR, Svanvik J. Gall-bladder water and electrolyte transport and its regulation. Gut. 1983;24:579–93.
28. Jahan M, Xiao P, Go A, Cheema M, Hameed A. Intraductal and invasive adenocarcinoma of duct of Luschka, mimicking chronic cholecystitis and cholelithiasis. World J Surg Oncol. 2009;7:4.
29. Ko K, Kamiya J, Nagino M, et al. A study of the subvesical bile duct (duct of Luschka) in resected liver specimens. World J Surg. 2006;30:1316–20.
30. Terada T. Gallbladder adenocarcinoma arising in Rokitansky-Aschoff sinus. Pathol Int. 2008;58:806–9.
31. Warshauer D, Scott G, Gottschalk A. Focal acute acalculous cholecystitis. AJR Am J Roentgenol. 1987;149:505–6.
32. van Eijck FC, van Veen RN, Kleinrensink GJ, Lange JF. Hartmann's gallbladder pouch revisited 60 years later. Surg Endosc. 2007;21:1122–5.
33. Dasgupta D, Stringer MD. Cystic duct and Heister's "valves". Clin Anat. 2005;18:81–7.
34. Ooi RC, Luo XY, Chin SB, Johnson AG, Bird NC. The flow of bile in the human cystic duct. J Biomech. 2004;37:1913–22.
35. Ko CW, Lee SP. Gallstone formation. Local factors. Gastroenterol Clin North Am. 1999;28:99–115.
36. Madden JL. Primary common bile duct stones. World J Surg. 1978;2:465–71.
37. Saharia PC, Zuidema GD, Cameron JL. Primary common duct stones. Ann Surg. 1977;185:598–604.
38. Ariche A, Czeiger D, Gortzak Y, Shaked G, Shelef I, Levy I. Gastric outlet obstruction by gallstone: Bouveret syndrome. Scand J Gastroenterol. 2000;35:781–3.
39. O'Neill C, Colquhoun P, Schlachta CM, Etemad-Rezai R, Jayaraman S. Gastric outlet obstruction secondary to biliary calculi: 2 cases of Bouveret syndrome. Can J Surg. 2009;52:E16–8.
40. Zaliekas J, Munson JL. Complications of gallstones: the Mirizzi syndrome, gallstone ileus, gallstone pancreatitis, complications of "lost" gallstones. Surg Clin North Am. 2008;88:1345–68.
41. Strasberg SM. Avoidance of biliary injury during laparoscopic cholecystectomy. J Hepatobiliary Pancreat Surg. 2002;9:543–7.
42. McPartland KJ, Pomposelli JJ. Iatrogenic biliary injuries: classification, identification, and management. Surg Clin North Am. 2008;88:1329–43.
43. Bismuth H, Majno PE. Biliary strictures: classification based on the principles of surgical treatment. World J Surg. 2001;25:1241–4.
44. Tsalis K, Zacharakis E, Vasiliadis K, et al. Bile duct injuries during laparoscopic cholecystectomy: management and outcome. Am Surg. 2005;71:1060–5.
45. Gordon FD. Primary sclerosing cholangitis. Surg Clin North Am. 2008;88:1385–407.

46. Attasaranya S, Fogel EL, Lehman GA. Choledocholithiasis, ascending cholangitis, and gallstone pancreatitis. Med Clin North Am. 2008;92:925–60.
47. Lim JH. Oriental cholangiohepatitis: pathologic, clinical, and radiologic features. AJR Am J Roentgenol. 1991;157:1–8.
48. Thinh NC, Breda Y, Faucompret S, Farthouat P. Louis C [Oriental biliary lithiasis. Retrospective study of 690 patients treated surgically over 8 years at Hospital 108 in Hanoi (Vietnam)]. Med Trop (Mars). 2001;61:509–11.
49. Maker AV, Butte JM, Oxenberg J, et al. Is port site resection necessary in the surgical management of gallbladder cancer? Ann Surg Oncol. 2012;19:409–17.
50. Brown KM. Multidisciplinary approach to tumors of the pancreas and biliary tree. Surg Clin North Am. 2009;89:115–31.
51. Lai CH, Lau WY. Gallbladder cancer–a comprehensive review. Surgeon. 2008;6:101–10.
52. Misra S, Chaturvedi A, Misra NC, Sharma ID. Carcinoma of the gallbladder. Lancet Oncol. 2003;4:167–76.
53. Mashima H. Studies on pruritus in obstructive jaundice cases with special references to serum bile acid fractions. Fukuoka Igaku Zasshi. 1991;82:445–57.
54. Ustundag Y, Bayraktar Y. Cholangiocarcinoma: a compact review of the literature. World J Gastroenterol. 2008;14:6458–66.
55. Akoad M, Jenkins R. Proximal biliary malignancy. Surg Clin North Am. 2008;88:1409–28.

18 Pancreas

1. All of the following are correct *except*:
   (a) The islets of Langerhans are found throughout the pancreas.
   (b) The minor papilla, when present, is proximal to the major papilla.
   (c) The ventral anlage forms the uncinate process and part of the head of the pancreas.
   (d) The dorsal anlage forms the neck, body, tail, and part of the head of pancreas.
   (e) The ventral and dorsal pancreatic buds preserve their independent duct systems.

Comments Please see the discussion for question 4

Answer
e

V.K. Maker, E.D. Guzman-Arrieta, *Cognitive Pearls in General Surgery*,
DOI 10.1007/978-1-4939-1850-8_18, © Springer Science+Business Media New York 2015

2. The following are normally found in the islets of Langerhans *except*:
   (a) α cells – Glucagon
   (b) β cells – Insulin
   (c) δ cells – Somatostatin
   (d) PP cells – Pancreatic polypeptide
   (e) G cells – Gastrin

Comments Please see the discussion for question 4

Answer
e

3. All of the following are correct *except*:
   (a) Pancreas divisum represents the failure of the ventral and dorsal anlagen to fuse.
   (b) Pancreas divisum increases the risk of acute pancreatitis.
   (c) The minor papilla is unable to accommodate pancreatic flow in pancreas divisum.
   (d) Pancreas divisum is treated with stenting or sphincteroplasty of both ducts.
   (e) The ventral anlage may atrophy in pancreas divisum.

Comments Please see the discussion for question 4

Answer
e

4. All of the following are correct *except*:
   (a) Annular pancreas compresses the second portion of the duodenum.
   (b) Annular pancreas may be treated with duodenoduodenostomy.
   (c) Annular pancreas may be treated with division of the annulus.
   (d) The tissue found in annular pancreas is identical to normal pancreatic tissue.
   (e) Annular pancreas may present with the double bubble sign.

Comments Pancreatic development is a complex process in which primitive endodermal cells give rise to highly differentiated ductal, endocrine, and exocrine tissues.

Human pancreatic development starts on the 26th day of gestation, with the formation of the dorsal pancreatic bud, arising from the dorsal foregut. Six days after, the ventral pancreatic bud develops from a more caudal position in the foregut. Once formed, the ventral bud rotates approximately 180° in clockwise direction to fuse with the dorsal bud. Remnants of this migration give rise to annular pancreas. In the fully developed pancreas, the dorsal bud contribution consists of the superior and anterior portion of the pancreatic head, the neck, body, and tail of the pancreas. The ventral bud contributes to the inferior and posterior part of the pancreatic head as well as the uncinate process. As noted above, it is interesting that the dorsal anlage gives rise to anterior elements, while the opposite holds true for [1] the ventral anlage (Fig. 18.1).

Annular pancreas is often associated with other congenital malformations such as Down's syndrome, intestinal malrotation, duodenal and esophageal atresia, and tracheoesophageal fistulas. This condition becomes symptomatic by causing duodenal obstruction. While presentation is most common in early life, there have been cases reported in adults. Treatment involves surgical bypass of the obstruction. Division of the constricting annulus is not advised due to the frequent presence of pancreatic ductal structures [2] (Fig. 18.2).

Originally, the dorsal bud is drained by its own duct (Santorini) which opens into the more cephalad minor pancreatic papilla in the duodenum. In similar fashion, the ventral bud is drained by the duct of Wirsung into the ampulla of Vater. However, as both pancreatic buds fuse, their ductal systems are rearranged. The distal part of the duct of Santorini (draining the body and tail) fuses with the duct of Wirsung, giving rise to a main pancreatic duct that runs along the entire length of the gland. Meanwhile, the proximal part of the duct of Santorini may regress completely or drain the upper portion of the pancreatic head independently.

Failure of this ductal fusion results in pancreas divisum, an entity in which the original ductal systems for the ventral and dorsal buds are maintained. This anomaly is found in up to 10 % of the population. It is thought that the minor pancreatic papilla is too small to accommodate the exocrine output of the upper head, body, and tail of the pancreas, giving rise to increased ductal pressure and recurrent pancreatitis. Over time, the elements derived from the dorsal bud atrophy, giving a typical non-enhancing appearance on CT scanning and ultrasound, in contrast with the normal texture of the ventral anlage. ERCP and MRCP are the main diagnostic modalities. Treatment involves enlarging the minor papilla to facilitate flow. While surgical sphincterotomy and sphincteroplasty were performed in the past, endoscopic sphincterotomy and stenting are currently more widely practiced [3, 4].

It has been well established that the endocrine pancreas is also derived from the foregut endoderm. The first pancreatic endocrine cells to appear are glucagon positive. These cells are integrated among the exocrine pancreas and in contact with the ductal lumen. There is a period of "secondary transition" in which the endocrine cells of the pancreas undergo exponential expansion and the β cells become the dominant type. Around this period, the endocrine cells of the pancreas detach themselves from the ductal margins and group in cords along the blood vessels to form the islets of Langerhans. Differentiation yields specialized glucagon-producing α-cells, insulin-producing β-cells, somatostatin-producing δ-cells, ghrelin-producing ε-cells, and pancreatic polypeptide-producing PP cells. While the islets of Langerhans are distributed throughout the pancreas, there are regional variations within the predominant cell type within the islets [5–9].

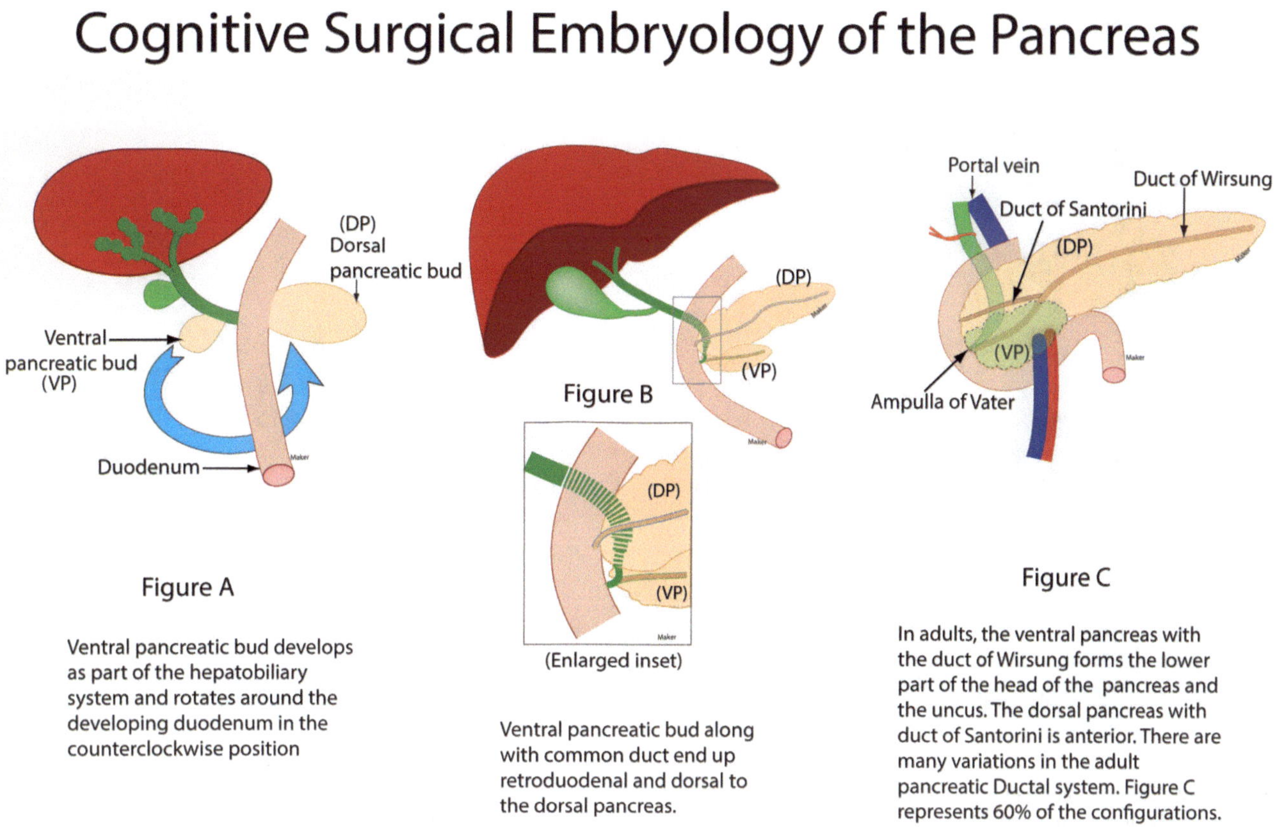

Fig. 18.1 Apart from obvious embryology-based diseases like annular pancreas and pancreas divisum, thorough knowledge of the fundamental developmental anatomy shown above forms the backbone of understanding for the pancreatic surgeon, e.g., why a penetrating peptic ulcer affects the duct of Santorini, the various diagnostic challenges of pancreatic cancer, and the complex critical steps of a pancreaticoduodenectomy

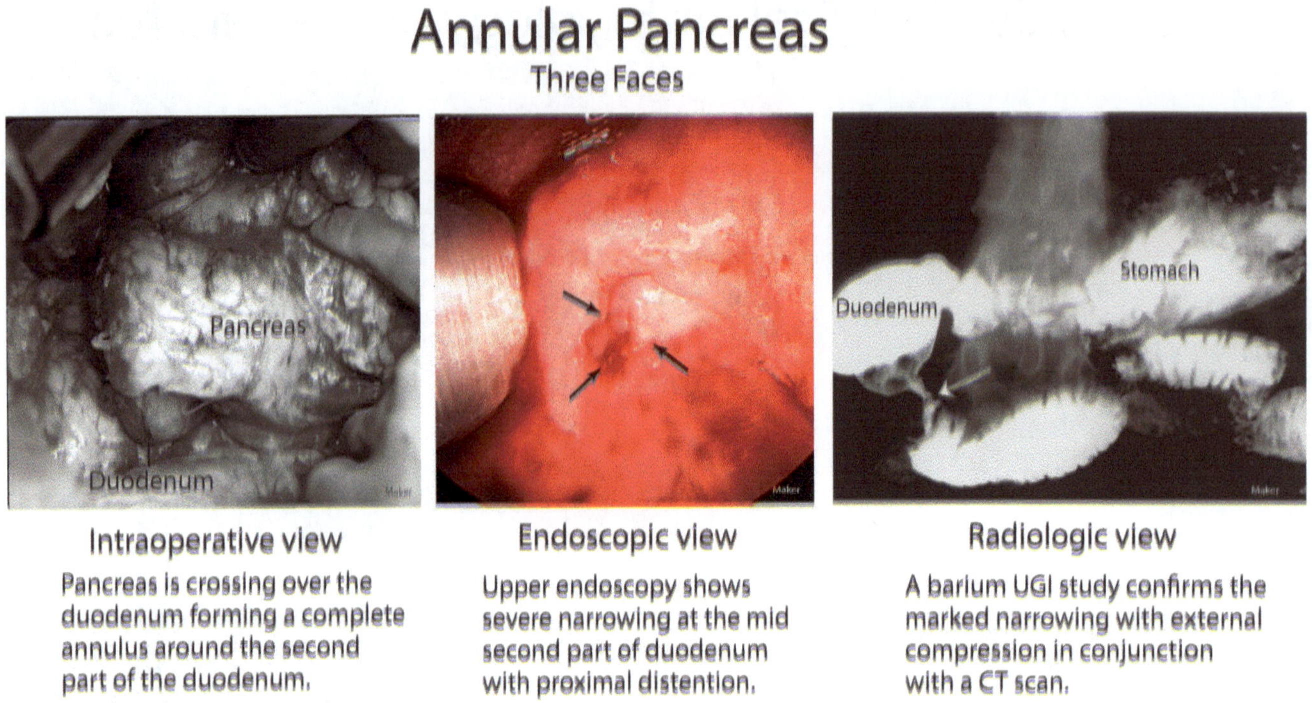

Fig. 18.2 The pancreas had a complicated embryological upbringing starting with the fusion of two buds, two separate ducts, and responsibility for a variety of exocrine and endocrine functions. Annular pancreas is the direct result of persistent fusion of the two buds forming a choking annulus around the second part of the duodenum. Arrows in the endoscopic and the radiologic view show the very narrow lumen at the site of the annulus

Answer

c

5. All of the following are correct *except*:
   (a) Gastrinomas are most frequent to the right of the superior mesenteric vein.
   (b) Insulinomas are the most common endocrine tumors of the pancreas.
   (c) Insulinomas are the most common pancreatic tumor in MEN I.
   (d) Insulinomas are most often solitary and benign.
   (e) Gastrinomas are most often multiple and malignant.

Comments Please see the discussion for question 6

Answer
c

6. All of the following are correct *except*:
   (a) Glucagonomas produce watery diarrhea, hypokalemia, and metabolic alkalosis.
   (b) Secretin blocks normal gastrin secretion but exerts a paradoxical effect upon gastrinomas.
   (c) Somatostatinomas produce diabetes, diarrhea, cholelithiasis, and achlorhydria.
   (d) Zollinger–Ellison syndrome causes peptic ulcers in atypical locations.
   (e) Intraoperative ultrasonography is the most sensitive method for localizing functional pancreatic tumors.

Comments Islet cell tumors, also known as neuroendocrine tumors, are rare malignancies that arise from the endodermal cells that give rise to the islets of Langerhans. They were previously classified as APUD tumors, based on their ability to uptake and decarboxylate amine precursors. Their incidence is 1–1.5 cases per 100,000. They account for 1–2 % of all pancreatic malignancies.

As a group, they are recognizable by the presence of neurosecretory granules as well as markers such as chromogranin, synaptophysin, and neuron-specific enolase. Clinically, they can be divided into functioning and nonfunctioning, based on hormone production and associated endocrine derangements. Nonfunctioning tumors are the most frequent type. Due to their uncommon presentations, these tumors are often diagnosed in late stages. Even though gastrinomas are relatively more malignant than other pancreatic endocrine tumors, their prognosis is far more benign than that of pancreatic adenocarcinoma. Approximately half of pancreatic neuroendocrine tumors have endocrine activity and are classified by the hormone they produce, although it must be kept in mind that many produce more than one hormone.

Neuroendocrine tumors express a high concentration of somatostatin receptors. This allows diagnosis via scintigraphy with indium-labeled octreotide (a somatostatin analogue). This trait may also allow palliative treatment with somatostatin analogues, which may reduce hormone production and the clinical manifestations thereof.

Intraoperative ultrasound is the most sensitive diagnostic modality for localization as well as for the diagnosis of lesions that might have escaped noninvasive imaging modalities. Endoscopic ultrasound has also proven to be an excellent modality especially in the tumors of the head and body of the pancreas. The tail of the pancreas is out of the range of this technique [10, 11].

Among the functional tumors, insulinomas are the most common type. They present in older females. The main manifestations are associated with hypoglycemia, made worse with fasting. Common symptoms include fatigue, weakness, tremors, and hunger. Whipple described the triad of symptoms of hypoglycemia, measured low blood glucose levels (less than 50 mg/dl), and relief of symptoms with administration of glucose. Most insulinomas are benign, 1–2 cm in size, solitary, and equally distributed through the pancreas. Specific diagnostic tests include measurements of serum insulin, proinsulin, and C-peptide levels. Enucleation is the preferred form of surgical treatment for lesions that do not involve major ductal structures (i.e., small tumors or those close to the edge of the pancreas). Pancreatic resection is reserved for cases in which enucleation is not possible.

Insulinomas may be associated with MEN-1 syndrome, in which case they tend to be multiple, and appear during the third decade of life. Of note, the most common type of neuroendocrine pancreatic tumor in MEN-1 is nonfunctional tumor, followed by gastrinomas and insulinomas [12].

Gastrinomas are the second most common type of neuroendocrine tumor of the pancreas. They are different from the others in that G cells are not normally present in the islets of Langerhans. Ectopic G cells can be found outside their normal location in the antrum and duodenum, in an area that has been termed gastrinoma triangle. This is defined as the space between the junction of the neck and body of the pancreas, the cystic to common bile duct junction and the duodenum. Gastrinomas are present in 0.1 % of patients with peptic ulcer disease and in 2 % of those with recurrent ulcer disease. Gastrinomas exhibit a paradoxical response to secretin administration. While this hormone normally abolishes gastrin production, gastrinomas respond to it by an increase in production. This trait is useful in establishing the diagnosis [13].

Gastrinomas are the cause of Zollinger–Ellison syndrome, characterized by hypergastrinemia and multiple peptic ulcers in classic and atypical locations (e.g., postbulbar duodenum, esophagogastric junction, and proximal small bowel). Surgical exploration for gastrinoma should always include duodenotomy, as the duodenum is the most common site for this tumor. In 5 % of cases, it is not possible to locate the tumor. Under this circumstance, antrectomy with vagotomy is advised. Finally, when gastrinomas are associated with primary hyperparathyroidism as part of MEN-1 syndrome, it is advisable to perform a parathyroidectomy before resection of the gastrinoma. This recommendation is based on the fact that calcium is a potent gastric secretagogue by itself [14].

VIPomas are the cause of Verner–Morrison syndrome also known as pancreatic cholera. Hypersecretion of vasoactive intestinal peptide induces secretory diarrhea (rich in bicarbonate), hypokalemia, and achlorhydria. Stool output is as high as

5–10 l per day. Most VIPomas are located in the tail of the pancreas. VIP-induced diarrhea responds dramatically to octreotide administration. This drug is very useful as an adjunct during preoperative fluid resuscitation [15].

Glucagonomas are very rare tumors that cause the four "Ds" of diabetes mellitus type 2, DVT, depression, and dermatitis (necrolytic migratory erythema). Due to their nonspecific presentation, diagnosis is usually delayed, and tumors are large (>5 cm) at the time of presentation. Like with VIPomas, these tumors are more commonly found in the tail of the pancreas.

Somatostatinomas produce steatorrhea, cholelithiasis, diabetes mellitus type 2, and hypochlorhydria. Most tumors are malignant and located within the head of the pancreas, making pancreaticoduodenectomy necessary. Fortunately, these tumors follow a rather indolent course, with 100 % 5-year survival after R0 resection and 60 % survival in the presence of metastatic disease.

Ghrelin is a relatively newly discovered hormone whose main role appears to be the induction of hunger. However, multiple functions of this hormone have been identified. It induces gastric secretion and contractility. Interestingly, it also seems to play a role in neurological development, learning, memory, and depression. While its main site of production is the stomach, it is also produced in the pancreas. A case of pancreatic ghrelinoma and another of gastric ghrelinoma are reported in the literature. In both cases, no particular clinical syndrome was identified [16].

As would be expected from the portal drainage of pancreatic venous blood, the liver is the primary site of metastasis for neuroendocrine tumors of the pancreas. When feasible, anatomic liver resection with curative intent should be attempted. More limited resections or angiographic hepatic embolization are useful palliative techniques.

Carcinoid tumors, while not particular to the pancreas, are presumed neuroendocrine tumors, being diagnosed with increasing frequency in the wall of the duodenum as well as pancreas.

Answer

a

7. All of the following are correct *except*:
   (a) The dorsal aspect of the pancreatic head together with the ventral aspect of the uncinate process cradle the superior mesenteric vessels.
   (b) The posterior superior pancreaticoduodenal artery may be injured during papillotomy.
   (c) The neck of the pancreas is defined by the location of the superior mesenteric vessels.
   (d) The splenic artery may be sacrificed without consequence to the pancreas.
   (e) Ligation of the splenic artery requires splenectomy.

Comments Please see the discussion for question 8

Answer
d

8. All of the following are correct *except*:
   (a) The head of the pancreas is supplied both by the celiac and superior mesenteric arteries.
   (b) The splenic artery supplies the body and tail of the pancreas.
   (c) The pancreatica magna artery should be preserved when ligating the splenic artery.
   (d) The portal vein forms behind the superior aspect of the pancreatic neck.
   (e) It is *not* possible to separate the vascular supplies of the duodenum and pancreatic head.

Comments The vascular anatomy of the head of the pancreas is classically based on four vessels: the celiac trunk derived anterior superior pancreaticoduodenal artery (ASPDA) and posterior superior pancreaticoduodenal artery (PSPDA) and the superior mesenteric artery derived anterior inferior pancreaticoduodenal artery (AIPDA) and posterior inferior pancreaticoduodenal artery (PIPDA). Anteriorly and posteriorly the superior and inferior PDA's anastomose forming two vascular arcades (anterior and posterior), which supply the head of the pancreas and C-loop of the duodenum. These four arteries are described as having matching veins [17, 18].

However, the abovementioned pattern is subject to multiple variations, the more frequent being absence of an arcade, presence of vessels communicating and interrupting the anterior and posterior arcades, and missing veins [19].

While it was originally thought that due to their common blood supply the duodenum and pancreatic head were indivisible, it has been shown that it is possible to separate both structures through careful dissection and ligation of the branches supplying the pancreas while preserving the vascular arcades and branches to the duodenum. In this process, the area of greatest difficulty is in the vicinity of the papillae [20]. It must be noted that this procedure is indicated only for benign pathology [21–23].

Branches of the splenic artery supply the body and tail of the pancreas. The splenic artery gives rise to the pancreatica magna artery near the junction of the body and tail. The importance of recognizing this artery lies in that ligation of the splenic artery proximal to its emergence may lead to pancreatitis and necrosis of the pancreatic tail. This concept must also be applied when performing angiographic splenic embolization.

The superior mesenteric vein courses to the right of the superior mesenteric artery. Both structures are cradled between the uncinate process of the pancreas posteriorly and the neck of the pancreas anteriorly. In normal conditions, the space between these structures is filled by loose areolar tissue, which may become replaced in the presence of pancreatic cancer rendering the tumor unresectable. Interestingly, most often there are no tributaries draining to the SMV as it courses through the pancreatic tunnel.

The portal vein is formed by the confluence of the splenic and superior mesenteric veins, which occurs behind the superior aspect of the pancreatic neck. As is the case with the superior mesenteric vessels, a thin plane of loose areolar tissues exists between the pancreas and the porta, allowing surgical separation of both structures [24].

Answer
e

9. The following are procedures for the treatment of pancreatic pseudocyst *except*:
   (a) Cystoduodenostomy
   (b) Cystogastrostomy
   (c) Cystojejunostomy
   (d) Cystocolostomy
   (e) Biliary stenting

Comments By definition, a pseudocyst is a fluid collection surrounded by fibrous and granulation tissue rather than epithelium, with walls being formed by adjacent organs. In the case of the pancreas, these walls are the boundaries of the lesser peritoneal sac. In the case of true cysts, the walls make the content; while in a pseudocyst, the contents make the walls (Fig. 18.3).

Pancreatic pseudocysts contain pancreatic fluid and result from pancreatic duct disruptions due to increase in intraductal pressure coupled with tissue necrosis as seen in acute pancreatitis (most often alcoholic). Pseudocysts classically occupy the lesser peritoneal sac but may extend beyond its boundaries as illustrated (Fig. 18.4).

As discussed previously, the lesser sac is the adult remnant of the left celomic cavity in the embryo and can be conceptualized as a balloon inside a balloon, communicating via the foramen of Winslow (Fig. 18.5).

The lesser sac is largely a potential space, bound by the elements illustrated in Figs. 18.6 and 18.7. As such, lacking a defined wall, its limits may vary. Particularly, the lesser sac may extend into the mesocolon (Figs. 18.6 and 18.7).

Small pseudocysts are often asymptomatic, while larger ones cause early satiety as well as biliary or enteric obstruction through a mass effect. Pseudocysts may also undergo bleeding, infection, and rupture.

Fortunately, most pancreatic pseudocysts resolve with nonoperative management, consisting of pain control and nutritional support. In general, the larger and older a pseudocyst is, the less likely it is to spontaneously resolve. However, size or age alone is not mandatory indication for drainage. Rather, drainage should be performed in patients with symptoms or complications.

There are three surgical modalities for mature pseudocyst drainage: laparoscopic, endoscopic, and open surgical. There are no trials comparing these modalities; hence, the choice of one over another is largely based on technical feasibility and local expertise. In cases in which the pseudocyst communicates with the pancreatic duct, it may be possible to facilitate resolution of the collection with endoscopic transpapillary drainage (ERCP).

Open surgical drainage is currently reserved for patients in whom laparoscopic and endoscopic drainage are not possible or have failed. Other indications include infection, necrosis, suspicion of neoplasia, or stricture of the pancreatic duct. The key principle is to create a stoma between the pseudocyst and the enteric tract over the most dependent part of the pseudocysts in order to facilitate drainage. Depending on the anatomy of the collection, cystogastrostomy, cystoduodenostomy, or cystojejunostomy (often with a Roux-en-Y loop) are viable options. The laparoscopic approach has been successfully used for these operations. Endoscopic drainage is becoming increasingly popular in patients where the cyst wall is attached to the posterior gastric wall and an endoscopic transgastric cystogastrostomy is feasible. Distal pancreatectomies are performed for small pseudocysts or when a question of neoplasia is entertained [25, 26].

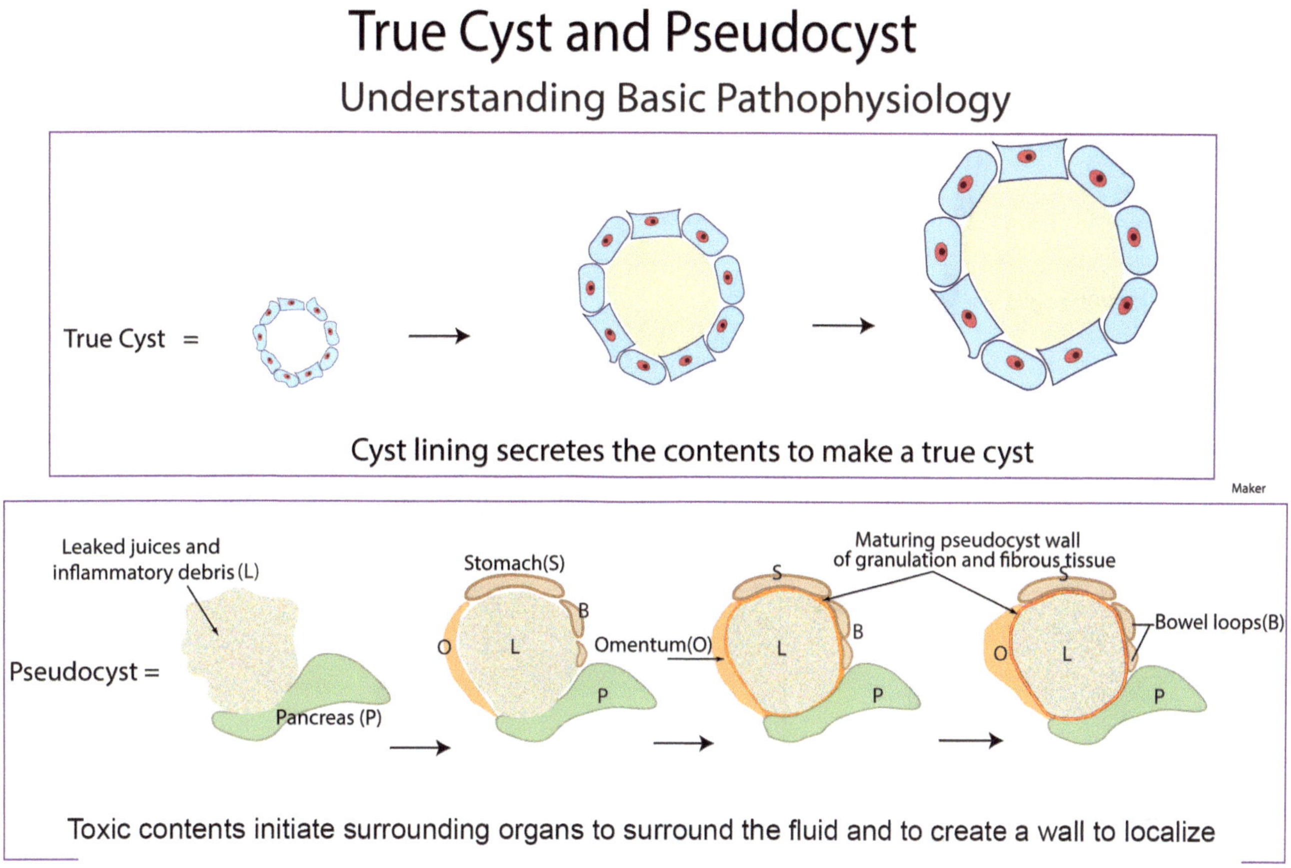

Fig. 18.3 True cyst and pseudocyst. Understanding basic pathophysiology

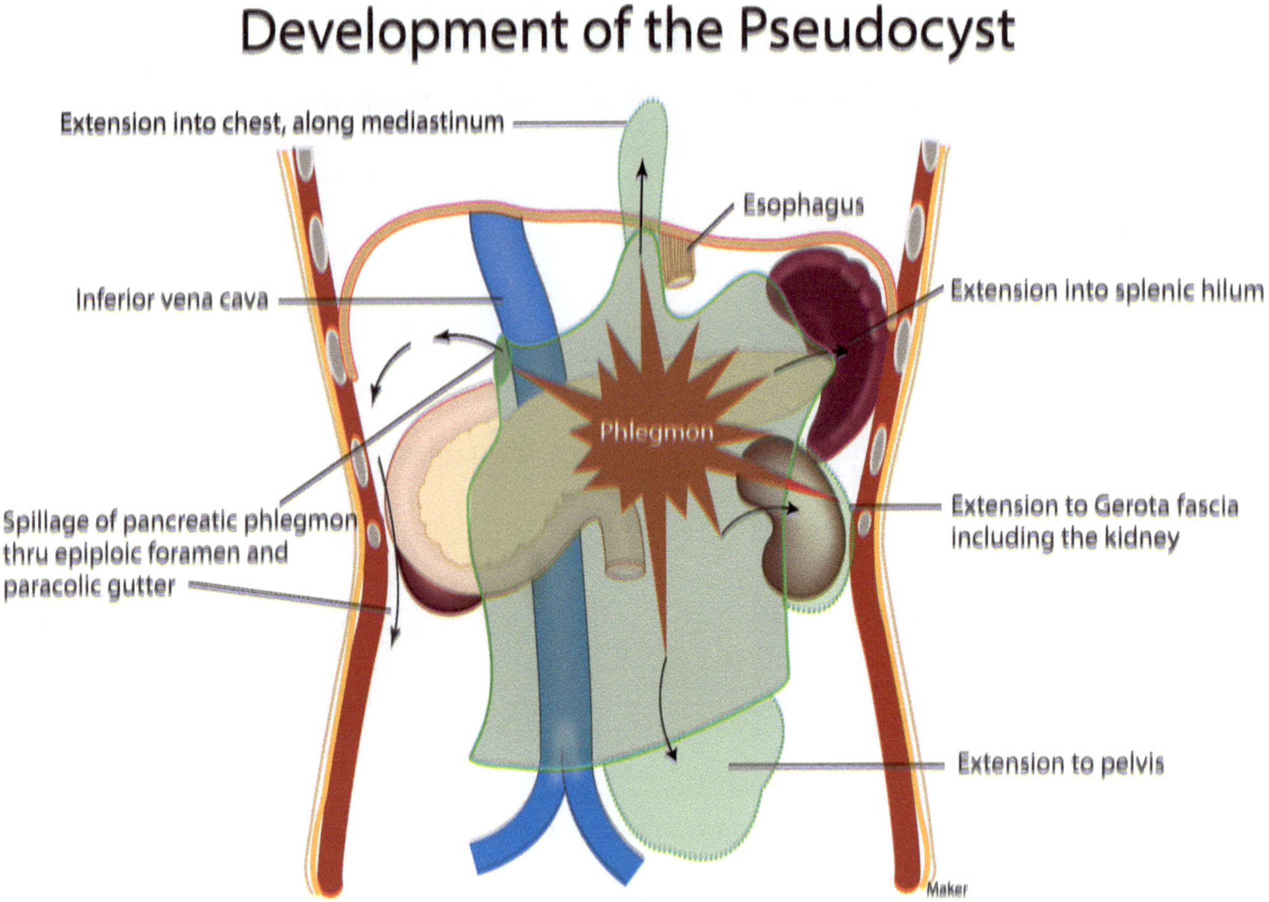

Fig. 18.4 In pancreatitis, caustic pancreatic juice and the resulting phlegmon become the contents of the lesser sac. These contents may then extend in any direction inside the anatomical lesser sac or can dissect outside the lesser sac. Uncommon but classically described extensions are superior in the mediastinum, lateral to the splenic hilum, and around Gerota's fascia engulfing the left kidney. Inferiorly, it may extend into the lower abdomen and pelvis. On the right side, the pancreatic phlegmon can spill out of the epiploic foramen and gain access to the right paracolic gutter. Each location described presents with distinct symptoms and clinical implications, and if not resolved, determines the future development and the locations of the developing pseudocyst

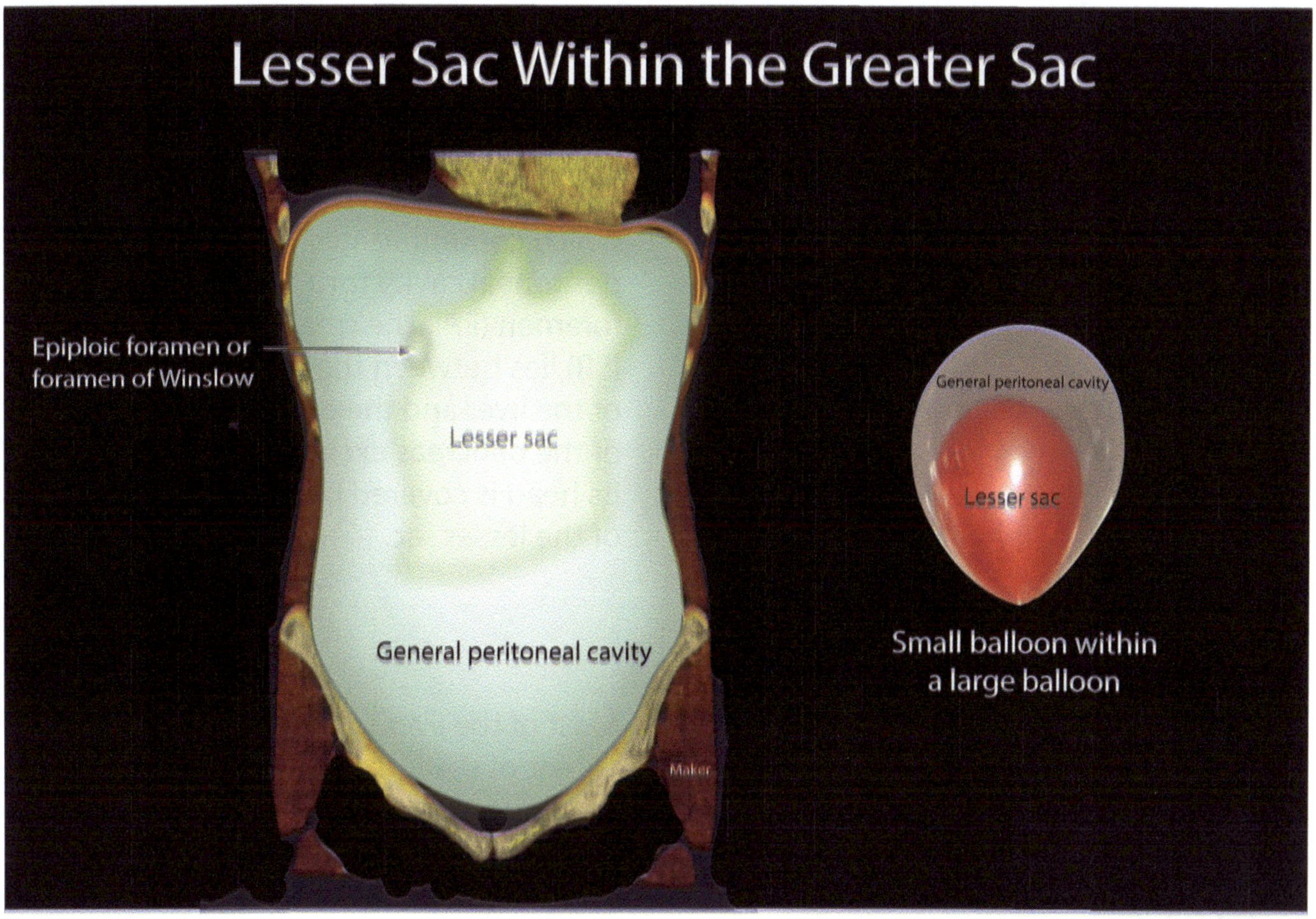

Fig. 18.5 The general peritoneal cavity, or the greater sac, is a potential space between the parietal peritoneum, which lines the entire abdominal wall including the back, and the visceral peritoneum, which lines all of the intra-abdominal organs, mesenteries, and the ligaments. Embyologically, the abdominal contents are herniated and then return intraabdominally and rotate. In this process, a part of the greater sac gets pinched posterior to the stomach and transverse colon. This pinched off peritoneal lined space is the lesser sac. The greater and lesser sac communicate thru the epiploic foramen

Sequential Applied Anatomy of the Lesser Sac

(From Posterior to Anterior)

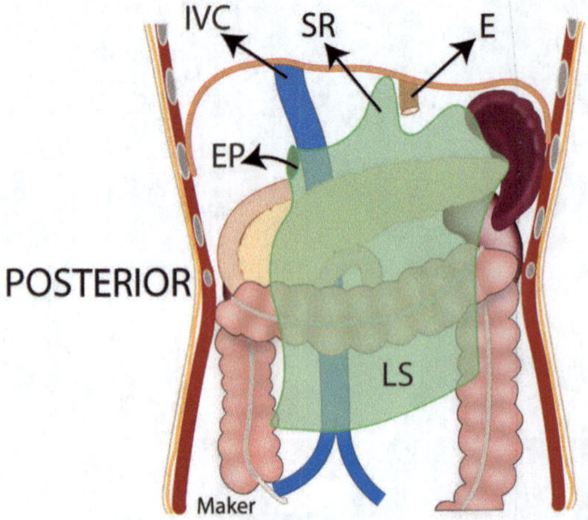

Lesser sac (LS) is a potential space which communicates with the general peritoneal cavity thru the epiploic foramen (EP). The small superior recess (SR) lies between the umbilical fissure of the liver and the esophagus (E). Most of the pancreas except a small part of its head is covered by the post. layer of the lesser sac.

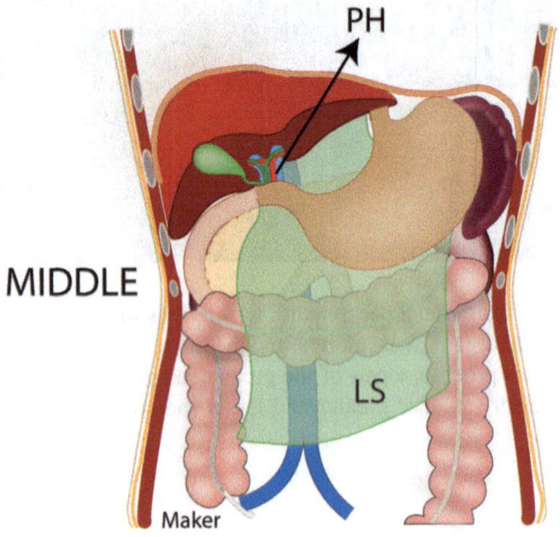

Most of the liver forms the superior extent of the lesser sac except the small sup. recess which is posterior to the caudate lobe. Stomach is the most consistent anterior boundary of the lesser sac. Structures of the Porta Hepatis (PH) form the anterior boundry of the epiploic foramen and the Inferior Vena Cava (IVC) forms the posterior boundary.

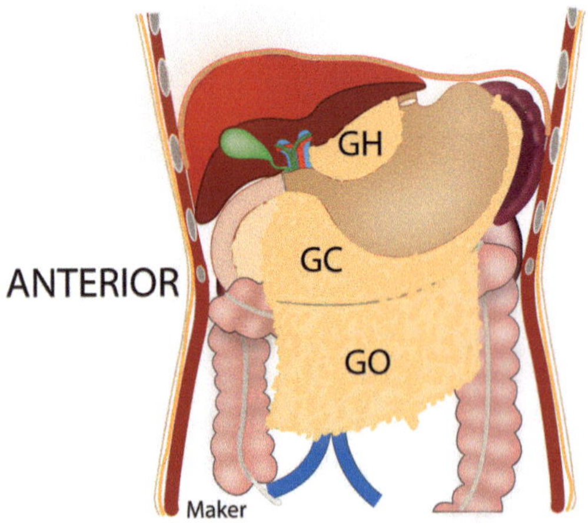

The anterior borders of the lesser sac are the posterior aspect of the caudate lobe, the gastrohepatic ligament (GH), stomach, gastrocolic ligament (GC), and its continuation under the anterior layer of the greater omentum (GO) (see Fig 18.7).

Fig. 18.6 Sequential applied anatomy of the lesser sac (from posterior to anterior)

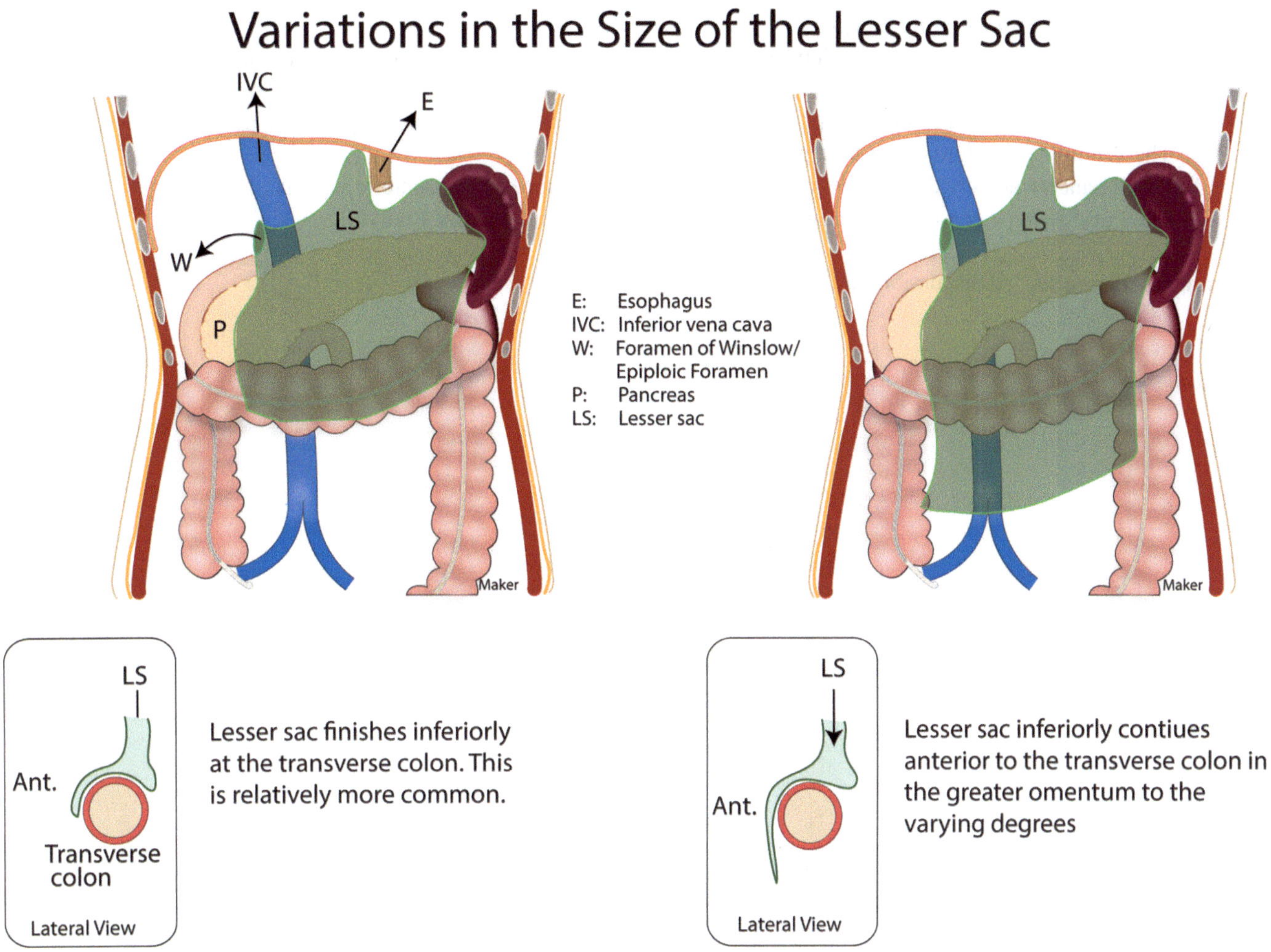

Fig. 18.7 Lesser sac is a potential, pinched off space from the greater sac. While its extent behind the gastrohepatic ligament, stomach, and gastrocolic ligament is fairly constant, its inferior extent is variable. The lesser sac may continue inside the greater omentum for varying lengths explaining the common sites for the extention and location of pseudocysts. *E* esophagus, *IVC* inferior vena cava, *W* foramen of Winslow/epiploic foramen, *P* pancreas, *LS* lesser sac

Answer
d

10. All of the following are correct *except*:
    (a) 95 % pancreatectomies spare the duodenum along with the pancreaticoduodenal arteries and a rim of attached pancreatic tissue.
    (b) Enucleation of well-differentiated pancreatic adenocarcinomas is an acceptable palliative procedure.
    (c) The Whipple procedure divides the pancreas at the neck.
    (d) Distal pancreatectomy divides the pancreas to the left of the superior mesenteric vessels.
    (e) The Puestow-type procedure consists of a longitudinal pancreaticojejunostomy.

Comments Please see the discussion for question 11

Answer
b

11. The following criteria must be met to perform a Whipple procedure *except*:
    (a) Pathologic confirmation of the pancreatic head tumor.
    (b) Absence of celiac and superior mesenteric lymph nodes.
    (c) Absence of liver metastasis.
    (d) Absence of gross invasion of the superior mesenteric vessels and porta.
    (e) Absence of malignant ascites.

Comments The Whipple procedure, also known as pancreaticoduodenectomy, is most often carried out to treat adenocarcinomas of the head of the pancreas, ampullary carcinoma, cystic neoplasms, and neuroendocrine tumors. Rarely it is also performed in the setting of chronic pancreatitis involving the head [27]. It consists of excision of the pancreatic head (the pancreas is transected at the level of the SMV) en bloc with the duodenum and pylorus. This is classically followed by reconstruction via pancreaticojejunostomy, hepaticojejunostomy, and gastrojejunostomy. Modifications to this procedure include preservation of the pylorus, creation of a pancreaticogastrostomy, and stapled transection rather than anastomosis of the pancreatic duct [28–30].

Perhaps the most important intraoperative step in a Whipple procedure for adenocarcinoma of the pancreas is determining the respectability of the tumor. This is accomplished by methodical evaluation of abdominal contents, often with the aid of intraoperative ultrasound. In order for the procedure to be undertaken, there must not be evidence of peritoneal invasion, liver metastasis, involvement of celiac and SMA nodes, or invasion of the SMV, portal vein, SMA, and vena cava. Contrary to other tumors, tissue diagnosis is not necessary to proceed with a radical resection of the pancreas. This is due to the high rate of false-negative biopsies coupled with the high sensitivity and specificity of imaging findings. Figure 18.8a–g highlights key steps in the execution of a pancreaticoduodenectomy.

Periampullary carcinoma of the pancreas deserves special mention. In contrast with carcinomas of the pancreas proper, these lesions tend to carry better prognosis due to their tendency to become symptomatic by causing jaundice early in the disease process, thus allowing early diagnosis and treatment (Fig. 18.9).

Enucleation of a lesion suspicious for adenocarcinoma is never to be performed. It offers no oncologic yield and predisposes to surgical complications. Palliative surgical treatment for adenocarcinoma of the pancreas attempts to achieve biliary and enteric diversion and provide pain control. Diversion may be achieved endoscopically through biliary and duodenal stenting or surgically by hepaticojejunostomy and gastroenterostomy. Whipple procedures with the intent to control pain are highly controversial [31].

Ninety-five percent pancreatectomy was developed as a treatment of chronic calcific pancreatitis with a small pancreatic duct to minimize the complications of total pancreatectomy. This operation preserves a rim of pancreatic tissue together with the duodenum and the four pancreaticoduodenal vessels. It is currently seldom performed in the treatment of congenital hyperinsulinism [32].

Distal pancreatectomy consists of the excision of the pancreas to the left of the superior mesenteric artery. The most common indications for this procedure are chronic pancreatitis, pancreatic cystoadenoma, neuroendocrine tumors, pancreatic pseudocysts, and cystadenocarcinomas. Whenever possible, the spleen and its blood supply should be preserved, especially in the setting of benign disease. Closure of the pancreatic duct and avoidance of subsequent leaks is the main challenge. Usually, a combination of staples and biologic sealants are used [30, 33, 34].

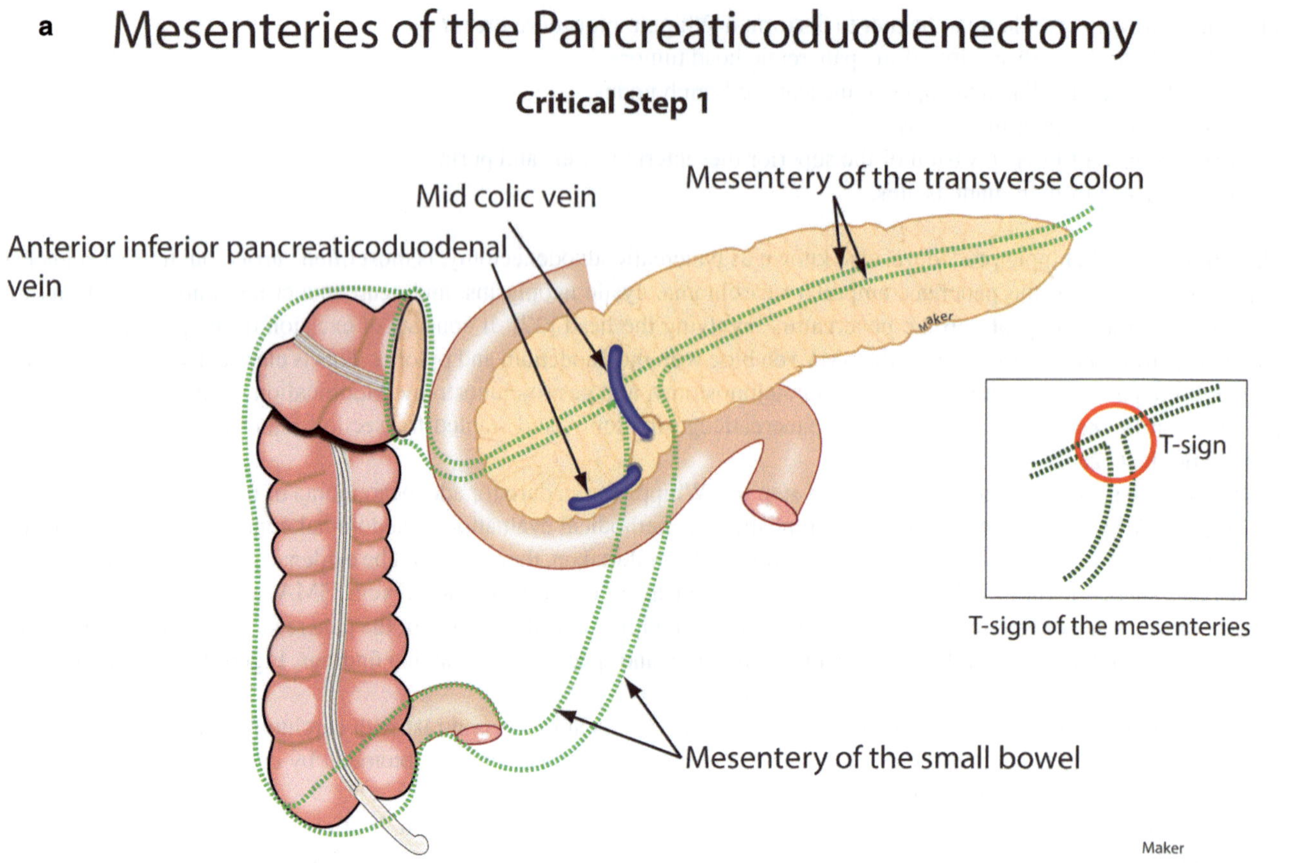

Fig. 18.8 (**a**) Critical Step 1: the transverse mesocolon and small bowel mesenteries meet, forming a "T" where multiple veins drain the pancreas, transverse colon, and small bowel into the superior mesenteric vein (SMV). As one mobilizes the hepatic flexure early on in the surgery and the SMV is not yet fully exposed, these veins can get inadvertently avulsed

b

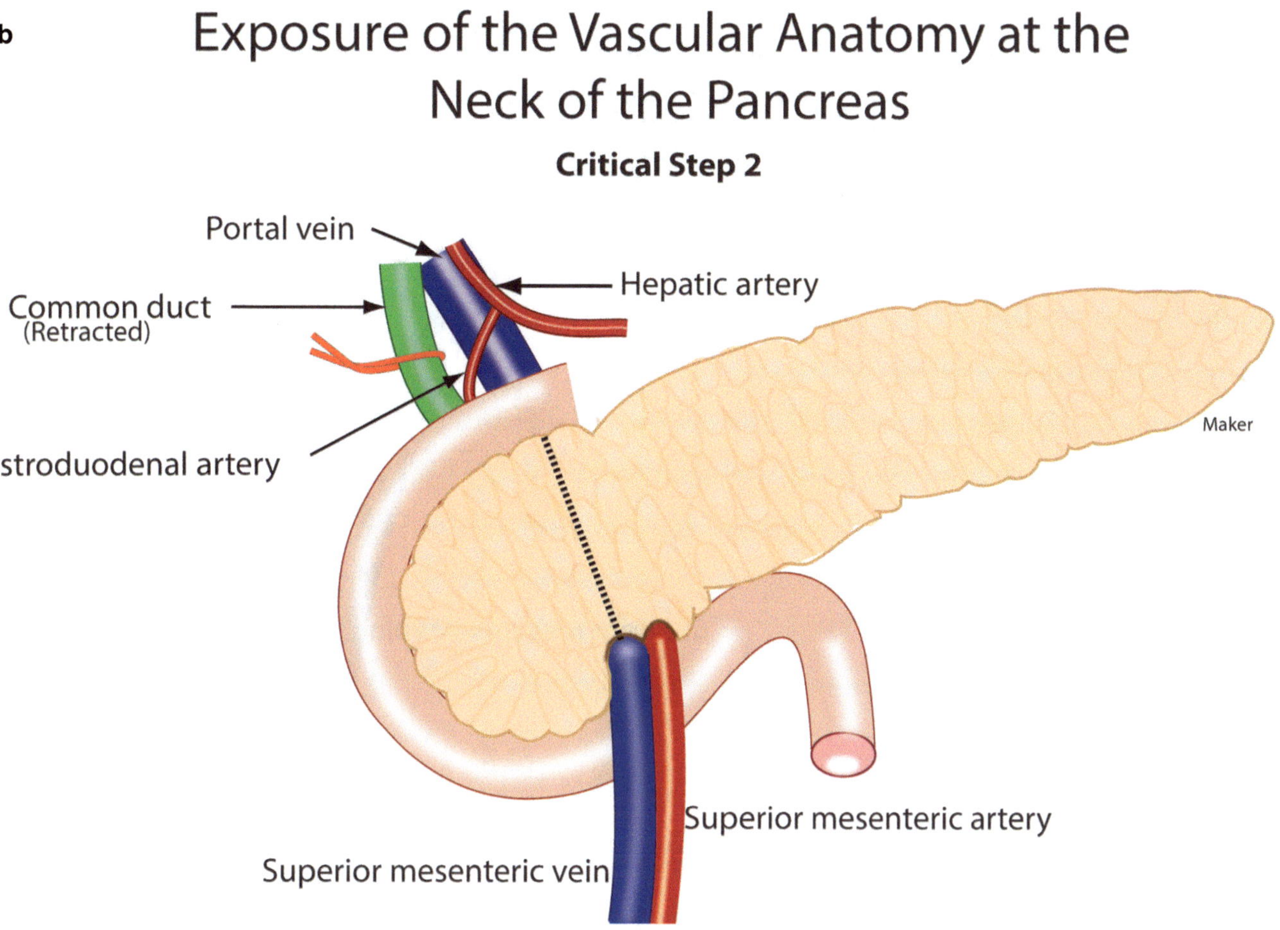

Fig. 18.8 (continued) (**b**) Critical Step 2: the vascular anatomy of the porta hepatis is defined and any anomalies identified and dissected. As the Kocherization is completed, the first structures to cross anterior to the duodenum are the superior mesenteric vessels. The *Dotted line* represents the neck of the pancreas anterior to the superior mesenteric/portal venous axis

c

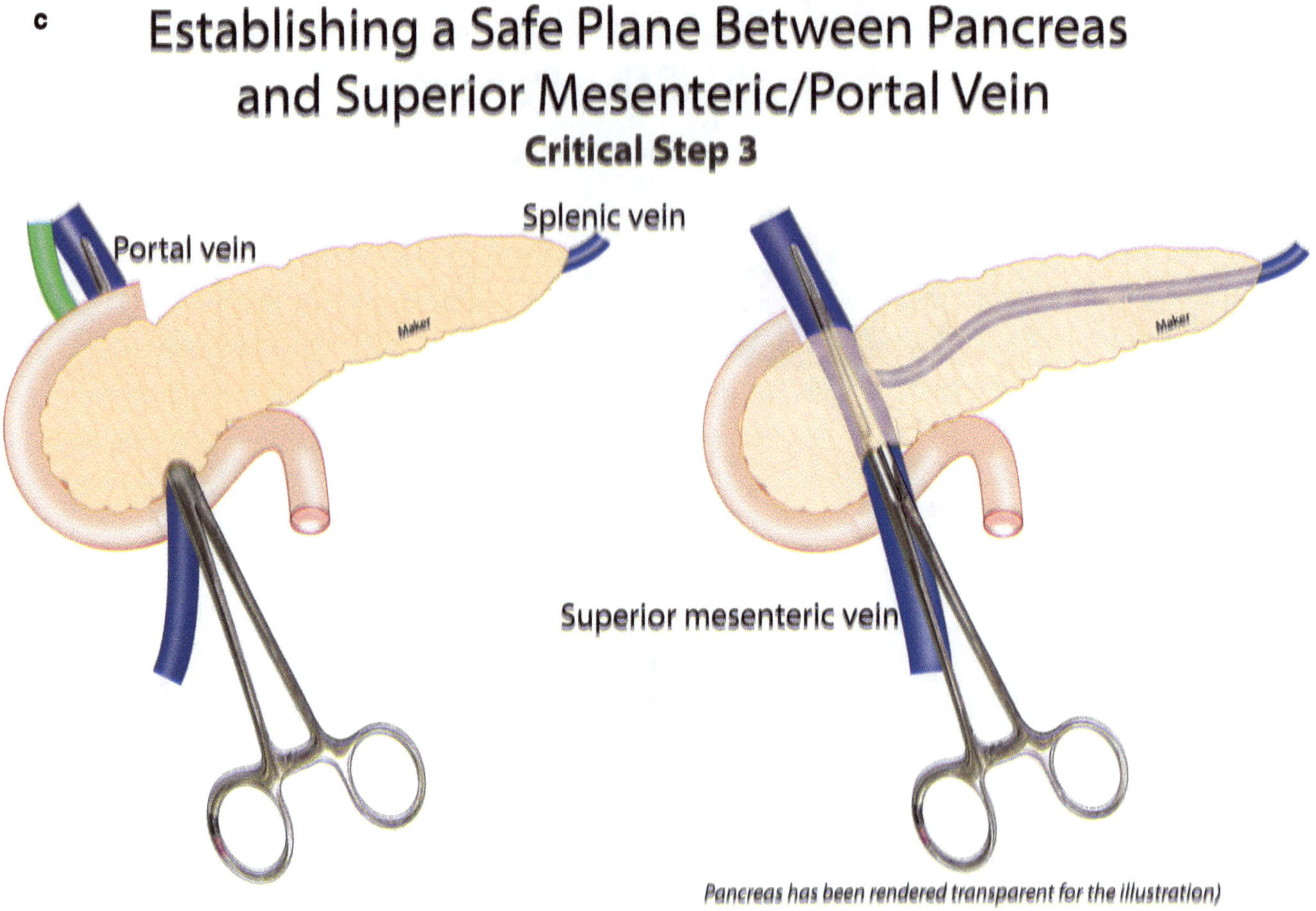

Fig. 18.8 (continued) (**c**) Critical Step 3: the superior mesenteric vein and the portal vein confluence must be fully exposed at the neck of the pancreas. Normally, no venous tributaries enter the pancreas from the anterior aspect of these veins in this area. Using a blunt-tipped instrument or fingertips, a safe plane/tunnel is developed at the neck of the pancreas. Absence of a clear plane may in some cases be regarded as invasion by the tumor

d Ligation of Multiple Pancreatic Veins Draining into the Superior Mesenteric Vein, at Site of Pancreatic Transaction

Critical Step 4

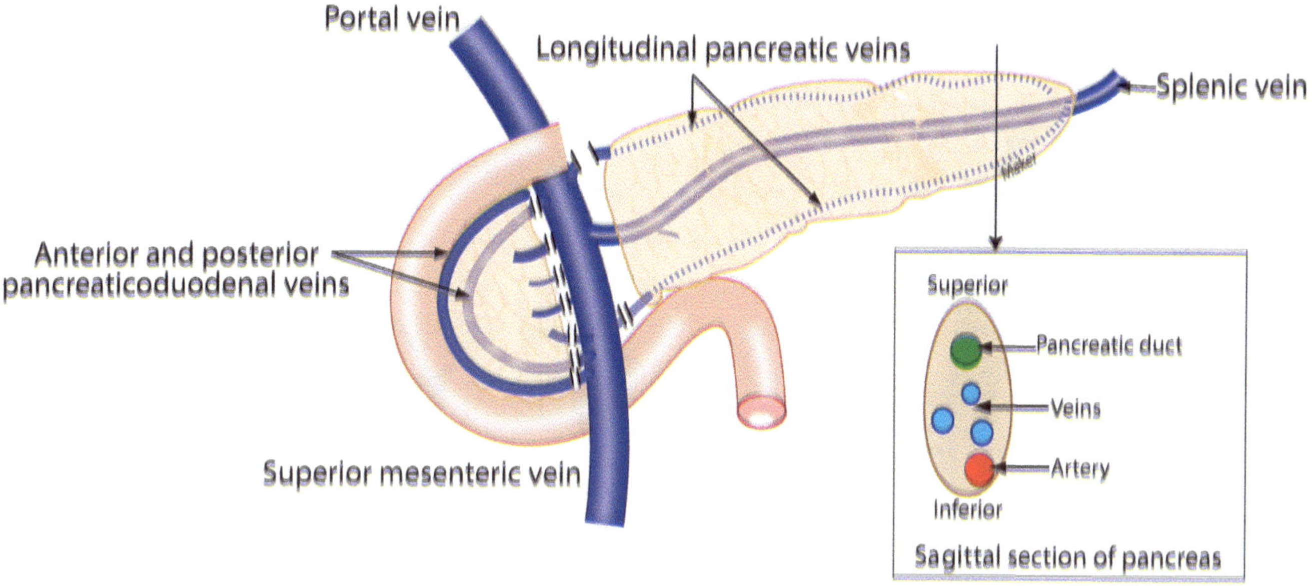

Fig. 18.8 (continued) (**d**) Critical Step 4: multiple veins drain the head of the pancreas into the right lateral aspect of the superior mesenteric vein (*SMV*). These veins are typically 1–4 mm in size and very fragile. Few veins drain into the left side of the SMV and are often from the uncus and proximal jejunum. Multiple small arteries are also encountered, but these are fewer in number and easier to identify and control

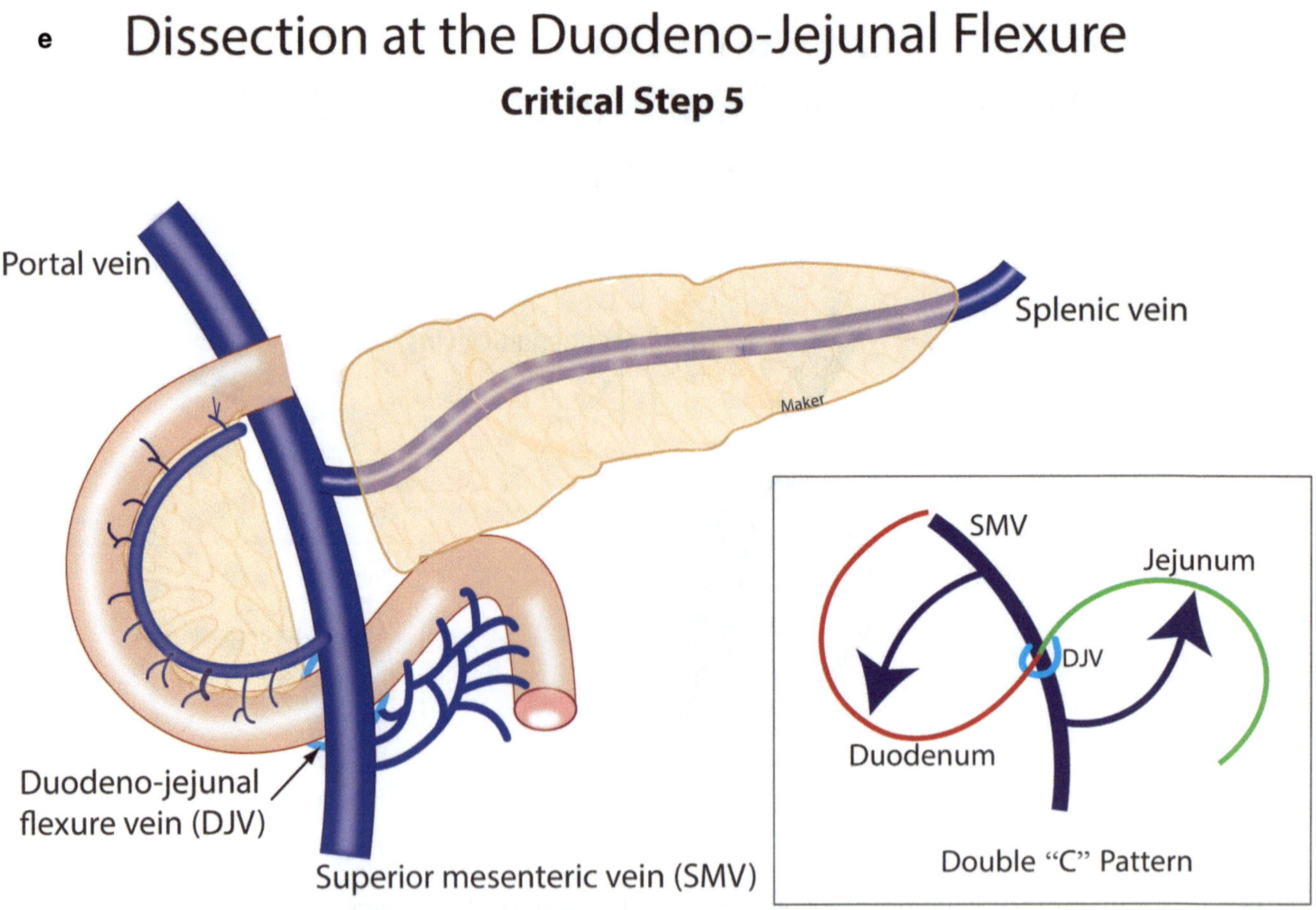

Fig. 18.8 (continued) (**e**) Critical Step 5: the duodenojejunal junction at the ligament of Treitz represents a double C pattern. The blood supply to both "C" curves comes from their concave sides. The junctional area of the duodenum and jejunum represent a challenging vascular dissection. One or two jejunal vessels (*DJV*) may actually come from the right, or duodenal, side of the superior mesenteric vessels and cross back underneath to enter the jejunum. These jejunal vessels are very short and prone to avulsion. Bothersome and brisk bleeding can occur from injury to these small vessels and care must be taken not to cause narrowing of the parent vessel during repair

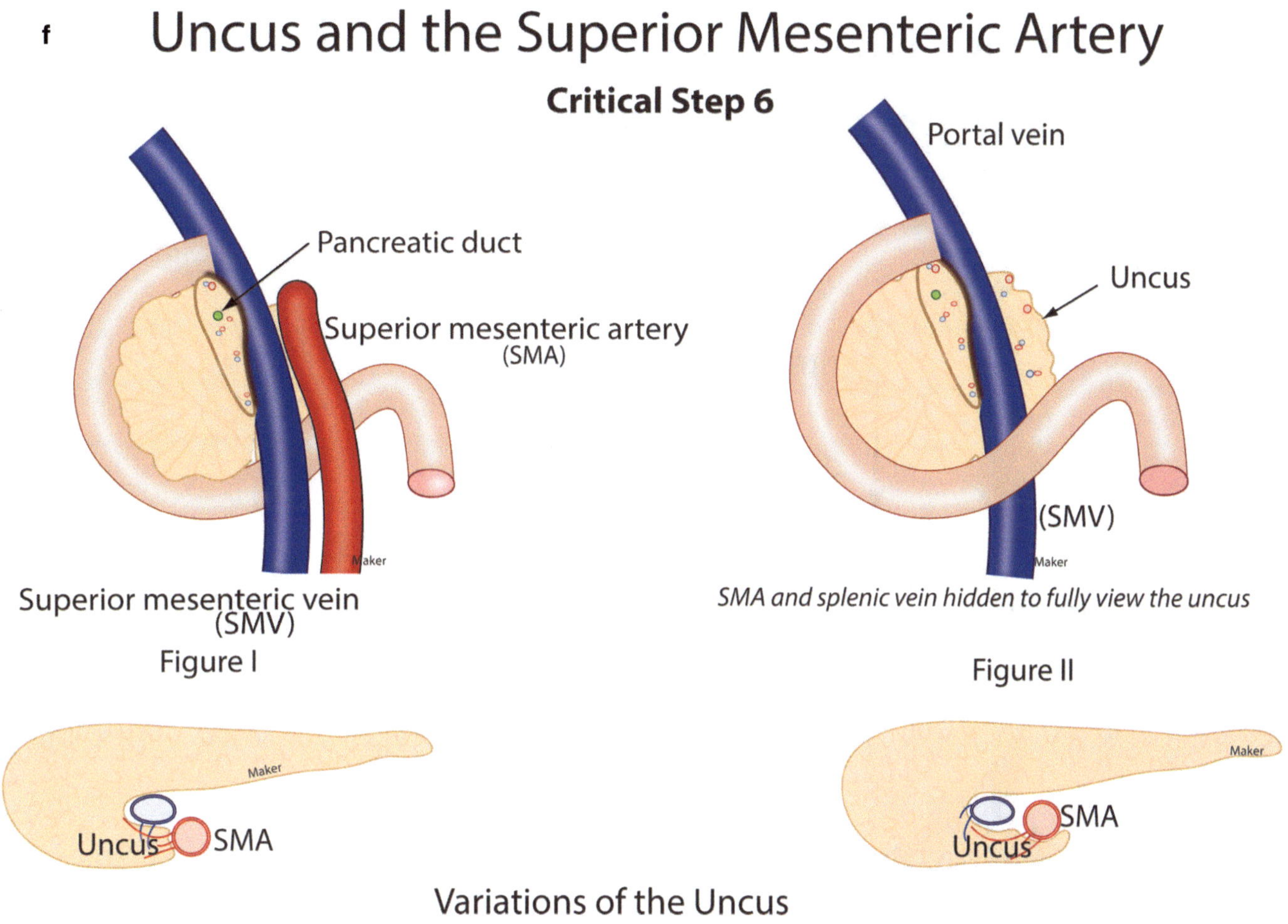

Fig. 18.8 (continued) (**f**) Critical Step 6: the uncus is the dorsal part of the pancreas, a paradoxical remnant of the ventral pancreatic bud, which lies behind the SMV and extends to varying distances laterally up to SMA and at times beyond it as shown above. The uncus also receives its vascular supply from the SMA and SMV, branches of which must be carefully ligated

g

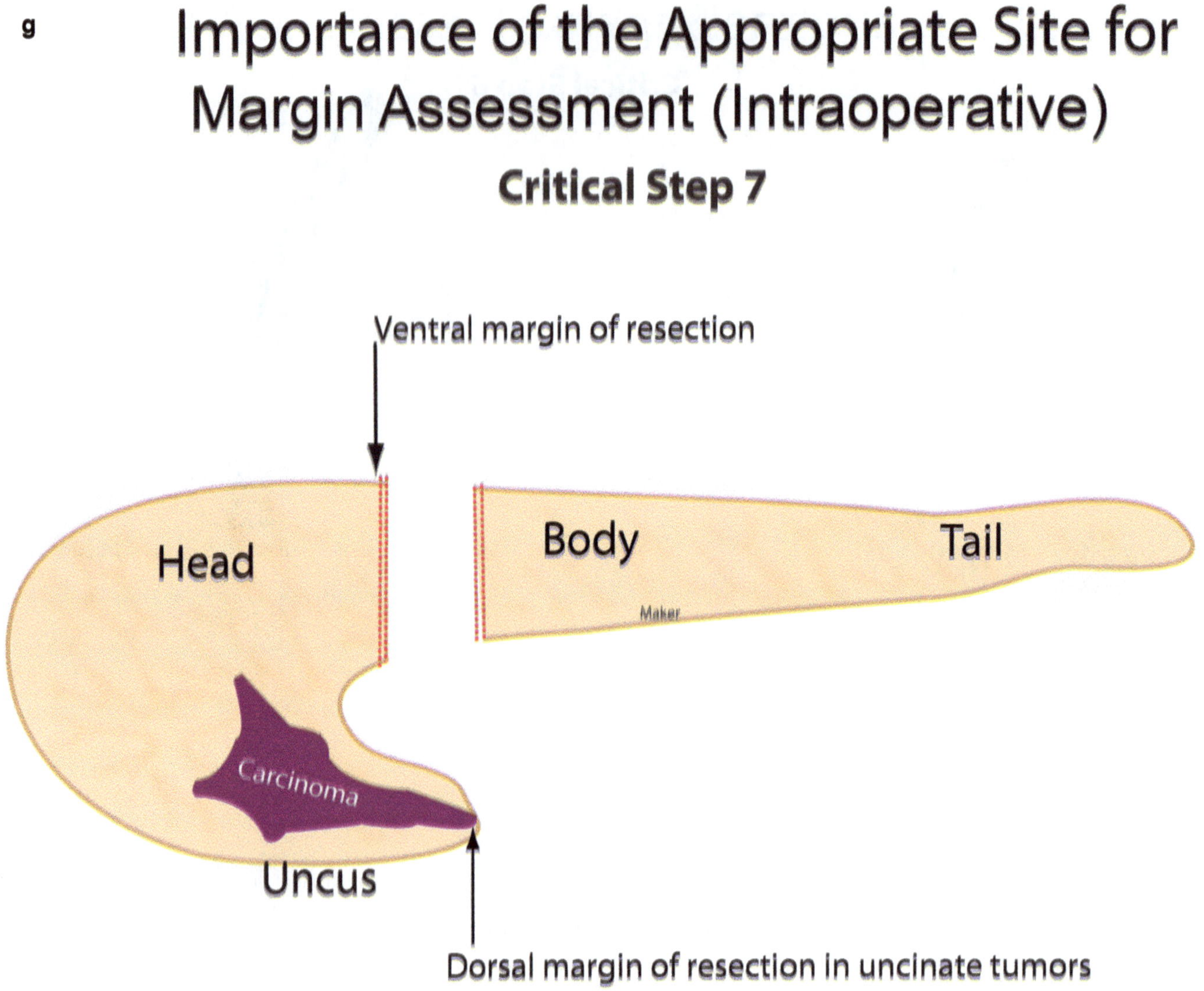

Fig. 18.8 (continued) (**g**) Critical Step 7: for most resectable cases of pancreatic cancer, if necessary, frozen section is sent from the transection margin at the neck of the pancreas. However, in cases of tumors involving uncus, the critical margin is rather the dorsal margin of the resection of uncus as illustrated. This margin on the SMA is the true margin of resection for these tumors

Periampullary Carcinoma of the Pancreas

Better Prognosis

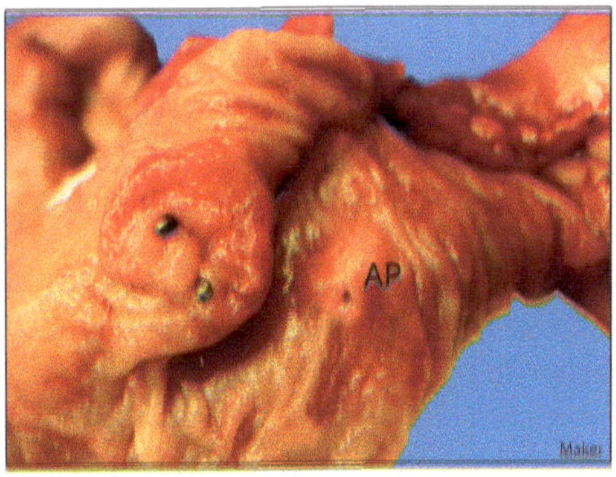

View of the open duodenum with ampullary carcinoma. Pancreatic duct as well as common duct are obstructed, each with a probe in it for illustration. This produces classic dilated double duct sign on imaging. Accessory pancreatic duct (AP) is visualized as well.

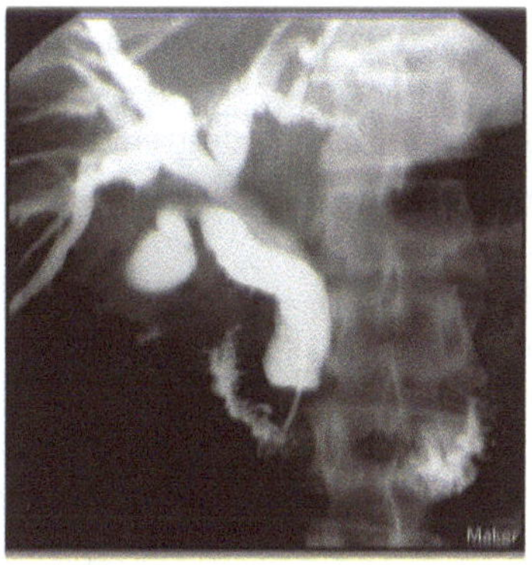

Transhepatic cholangiogram revealing a filling defect with abrupt cut off consistent with distal common duct carcinoma. Dilated proximal ducts are seen.

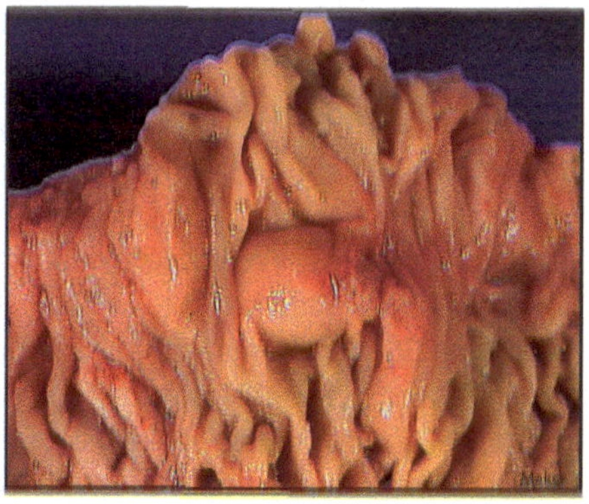

Very early invasive ampullary carcinoma discovered on upper endoscopy for vague right upper quadrant pain. Patient had minimal increase in bilirubin and alkaline phosphatase. Above is the view of the duodenum from a pancreaticoduodenectomy specimen

Fig. 18.9 Periampullary cancers generally have higher rate of resectability and survival because of the early diagnosis as these tumors develop symptoms and signs of the obstructive jaundice much earlier than cancers in the head of pancreas. Also rates of superior mesenteric vein involvement are much lower

Answer

a

12. All of the following are correct *except*:
    (a) Longitudinal pancreaticojejunostomy should be performed along the entire length of the diseased duct.
    (b) The Frey procedure involves partial excision of the pancreatic head.
    (c) The Puestow-type procedures are ideal for small duct pancreatitis.
    (d) Chronic pancreatitis is often associated with splenic vein thrombosis.
    (e) The objective of pancreatic resections is effective pain control.

Comments Chronic pancreatitis represents the progressive destruction of pancreatic acinar cells as well as the islets of Langerhans, leading to exocrine failure and delayed endocrine dysfunction. Clinical manifestations include chronic intractable abdominal pain, nutrient malabsorption, and diabetes. While there is a strong association with alcohol consumption, this disease process is most likely multifactorial.

Alcohol has been shown to induce an inflammatory response mediated by the macrophage-derived pancreatic stellate cells. In addition, it stimulates the secretion of a pancreatic juice, which is rich in protein but low in volume and bicarbonate concentration, making it prone to stone formation. Repeated bouts of inflammation lead to gland calcification and ductal strictures. In turn, strictures lead to ductal hypertension transmitted to the gland as a whole. It is thought that increased ductal pressure generates conditions of ischemia within the gland, furthering pain and injury [35, 36].

For unknown reasons, some patients with chronic pancreatitis develop dilated ducts, while others present normal or strictured ducts. There are also patients who develop a combination of dilated and strictured segments, in what is called a "chain of lakes" or "string of pearls" pattern [37]. Often, these ductal dilatations are filled with pancreatic duct stones (Fig. 18.10).

Surgery for chronic pancreatitis is performed with the intent to control intractable pain and also when there is suspicion of malignancy, given that pancreatic cancer and chronic pancreatitis are associated. It is estimated that 1.8 % of patients with chronic pancreatitis will develop pancreatic adenocarcinoma within 10 years of diagnosis [38–40].

Surgical ductal decompression may not only alleviate pain but also preserve glandular function. The main factor influencing the choice of surgical procedure is duct size. Patients with larger ducts are best served by direct decompression into the bowel via longitudinal pancreaticojejunostomy, while patients with chronic calcific pancreatitis and small ducts are candidates for pancreatic resections of varying degrees [41].

In the late 1980s, Frey proposed a combination of longitudinal pancreaticojejunostomy and duodenum preserving coring of the diseased pancreatic head. In the operation that bears his name, the pancreatic duct is opened in all its length and the pancreatic parenchyma of the head is cored out, leaving only the posterior capsule of the pancreatic head. This procedure not only achieves complete ductal decompression but also eliminates the chronic inflammatory tissue in the head of the pancreas, which is thought to be an important source of pain for these patients [42]. Another surgical option popularized by Hans Beger in Ulm, Germany, is the duodenum-preserving pancreatic head resection, also known as Beger procedure. In this operation, the pancreatic head is resected together with the diseased duct, while the stomach, duodenum, and bile duct are preserved. Reconstruction is via a Roux-en-Y loop [43].

Chronic Pancreatitis
Chain o' Lakes

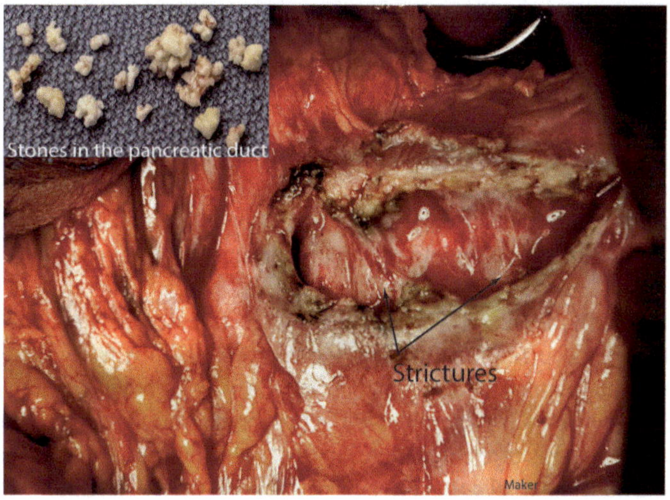

Fig. 18.10 Chain of lakes pattern of chronic pancreatitis reveals multiple strictures in the pancreatic duct with dilated areas, "lakes," in between. Often the ducts are full of inspissated calcium stones

Answer
c

13. All of the following are correct *except*:
    (a) Pancreatic necrosis may extend into adjacent retroperitoneal structures.
    (b) Viable pancreatic tissue should be preserved during pancreatic necrosectomy.
    (c) Pancreatic necrosectomy should be followed by wide drainage.
    (d) Endoscopic pancreatic necrosectomy is an emerging treatment modality for infected pancreatic necrosis.
    (e) Infected pancreatic necrosis is primarily approached by percutaneous drainage.

Comments Surgical therapy for acute pancreatitis is currently limited to the treatment of infected necrosis and the control of hemorrhage. Due to the thick and tenacious consistency of pancreatic abscesses, percutaneous drainage is often ineffective. There are two main approaches to surgical drainage: necrosectomy and closed drainage vs. necrosectomy followed with serial abdominal packing. The former is more widely practiced currently, while the latter has been associated with higher morbidity and mortality.

Necrosectomy is usually performed though the lesser sac, which is accessed between the stomach and colon. Due to the delayed nature of the procedure in the course of the disease, the necrotic tissue is fairly well demarcated and is amenable to blunt finger dissection. Necrosis may extend into the retroperitoneal tissues beyond the pancreas and into the mesentery. Gentle debridement of all devitalized tissue is recommended. After the necrotic tissue has been removed, several large-bore sump drains are placed and the abdomen is often closed. A laparoscopic version of this procedure has been developed [44].

Endoscopic necrosectomy is a novel approach that has been successfully used in patients with infected pancreatic necrosis who were not candidates for surgical drainage. This procedure consists of transgastric drainage of the pancreatic cell under ultrasound guidance. Initial access is obtained by needle puncture, followed by balloon dilatation. A guidewire is introduced and allows guidance of an upper GI endoscope into the abscess cavity. There, debridement is performed with a combination of irrigation, suction, and endoscopic snares [45].

Answer
b

References

1. Gittes GK. Developmental biology of the pancreas: a comprehensive review. Dev Biol. 2009;326:4–35.
2. Maker V, Gerzenshtein J, Lerner T. Annular pancreas in the adult: two case reports and review of more than a century of literature. Am Surg. 2003;69:404–10.
3. Klein SD, Affronti JP. Pancreas divisum, an evidence-based review: part I, pathophysiology. Gastrointest Endosc. 2004;60:419–25.
4. Klein SD, Affronti JP. Pancreas divisum, an evidence-based review: part II, patient selection and treatment. Gastrointest Endosc. 2004;60:585–9.
5. Baetens D, Malaisse-Lagae F, Perrelet A, Orci L. Endocrine pancreas: three-dimensional reconstruction shows two types of islets of langerhans. Science. 1979;206:1323–5.
6. Bocian-Sobkowska J, Zabel M, Wozniak W, Surdyk-Zasada J. Polyhormonal aspect of the endocrine cells of the human fetal pancreas. Histochem Cell Biol. 1999;112:147–53.
7. Oliver-Krasinski JM, Stoffers DA. On the origin of the beta cell. Genes Dev. 2008;22:1998–2021.
8. Baetge EE. Production of beta-cells from human embryonic stem cells. Diabetes Obes Metab. 2008;10 Suppl 4:186–94.
9. Wolfe-Coote SA, Du Toit DF. Distribution of cell types of the islets of Langerhans throughout the pancreas of the Chacma baboon. Anat Rec. 1987;217:172–7.
10. Abood GJ, Go A, Malhotra D, Shoup M. The surgical and systemic management of neuroendocrine tumors of the pancreas. Surg Clin N Am. 2009;89:249–66, x.
11. Alexakis N, Neoptolemos JP. Pancreatic neuroendocrine tumours. Best Pract Res Clin Gastroenterol. 2008;22:183–205.
12. Abboud B, Boujaoude J. Occult sporadic insulinoma: localization and surgical strategy. World J Gastroenterol. 2008;14:657–65.
13. Stabile BE, Morrow DJ, Passaro Jr E. The gastrinoma triangle: operative implications. Am J Surg. 1984;147:25–31.
14. Ellison EC, Johnson JA. The Zollinger-Ellison syndrome: a comprehensive review of historical, scientific, and clinical considerations. Curr Probl Surg. 2009;46:13–106.
15. Ghaferi AA, Chojnacki KA, Long WD, Cameron JL, Yeo CJ. Pancreatic VIPomas: subject review and one institutional experience. J Gastrointest Surg. 2008;12:382–93.
16. Corbetta S, Peracchi M, Cappiello V, et al. Circulating ghrelin levels in patients with pancreatic and gastrointestinal neuroendocrine tumors: identification of one pancreatic ghrelinoma. J Clin Endocrinol Metab. 2003;88:3117–20.
17. Skandalakis LJ, Rowe Jr JS, Gray SW, Skandalakis JE. Surgical embryology and anatomy of the pancreas. Surg Clin N Am. 1993;73:661–97.
18. Reichardt W, Cameron R. Anatomy of the pancreatic veins. A post mortem and clinical phlebographic investigation. Acta Radiol Diagn (Stockh). 1980;21:33–41.
19. Chong M, Freeny PC, Schmiedl UP. Pancreatic arterial anatomy: depiction with dual-phase helical CT. Radiology. 1998;208:537–42.
20. Nimura Y. Pancreatic surgery: cutting-edge developments and technology. Pancreas. 1998;16:227–32.
21. McClusky 3rd DA, Skandalakis LJ, Colborn GL, Skandalakis JE. Harbinger or hermit? Pancreatic anatomy and surgery through the ages–part 3. World J Surg. 2002;26:1512–24.
22. McClusky 3rd DA, Skandalakis LJ, Colborn GL, Skandalakis JE. Harbinger or hermit? Pancreatic anatomy and surgery through the ages–part 2. World J Surg. 2002;26:1370–81.
23. McClusky 3rd DA, Skandalakis LJ, Colborn GL, Skandalakis JE. Harbinger or hermit? Pancreatic anatomy and surgery through the ages–part 1. World J Surg. 2002;26:1175–85.
24. Murakami G, Hirata K, Takamuro T, Mukaiya M, Hata F, Kitagawa S. Vascular anatomy of the pancreaticoduodenal region: a review. J Hepatobiliary Pancreat Surg. 1999;6:55–68.
25. Aghdassi A, Mayerle J, Kraft M, Sielenkamper AW, Heidecke CD, Lerch MM. Diagnosis and treatment of pancreatic pseudocysts in chronic pancreatitis. Pancreas. 2008;36:105–12.
26. Habashi S, Draganov PV. Pancreatic pseudocyst. World J Gastroenterol. 2009;15:38–47.
27. Rios G, Conrad A, Cole D, et al. Trends in indications and outcomes in the Whipple procedure over a 40-year period. Am Surg. 1999;65:889–93.
28. Wente MN, Shrikhande SV, Muller MW, et al. Pancreaticojejunostomy versus pancreaticogastrostomy: systematic review and meta-analysis. Am J Surg. 2007;193:171–83.
29. Diener MK, Heukaufer C, Schwarzer G, et al. Pancreaticoduodenectomy (classic Whipple) versus pylorus-preserving pancreaticoduodenectomy (pp Whipple) for surgical treatment of periampullary and pancreatic carcinoma. Cochrane Database Syst Rev. 2008;(2):CD006053.
30. Marczell AP, Stierer M. Partial pancreaticoduodenectomy (Whipple procedure) for pancreatic malignancy: occlusion of a non-anastomosed pancreatic stump with fibrin sealant. HPB Surg. 1992;5:251–9; discussion 259–60.
31. Mann O, Strate T, Schneider C, Yekebas EF, Izbicki JR. Surgery for advanced and metastatic pancreatic cancer–current state and perspectives. Anticancer Res. 2006;26:681–6.
32. Mazor-Aronovitch K, Landau H, Gillis D. Surgical versus non-surgical treatment of congenital hyperinsulinism. Pediatr Endocrinol Rev. 2009;6:424–30.
33. Lillemoe KD, Kaushal S, Cameron JL, Sohn TA, Pitt HA, Yeo CJ. Distal pancreatectomy: indications and outcomes in 235 patients. Ann Surg. 1999;229:693–8; discussion 698–700.
34. Kimura W, Moriya T, Ma J, et al. Spleen-preserving distal pancreatectomy with conservation of the splenic artery and vein. World J Gastroenterol. 2007;13:1493–9.
35. Behrman SW, Fowler ES. Pathophysiology of chronic pancreatitis. Surg Clin N Am. 2007;87:1309–24, vii.
36. Conwell DL, Banks PA. Chronic pancreatitis. Curr Opin Gastroenterol. 2008;24:586–90.
37. Kim DH, Pickhardt PJ. Radiologic assessment of acute and chronic pancreatitis. Surg Clin N Am. 2007;87:1341–58, viii.
38. Mihaljevic AL, Kleeff J, Friess H, Buchler MW, Beger HG. Surgical approaches to chronic pancreatitis. Best Pract Res Clin Gastroenterol. 2008;22:167–81.

39. Lowenfels AB, Maisonneuve P, Cavallini G, et al. Pancreatitis and the risk of pancreatic cancer. International Pancreatitis Study Group. N Engl J Med. 1993;328:1433–7.
40. O'Neil SJ, Aranha GV. Lateral pancreaticojejunostomy for chronic pancreatitis. World J Surg. 2003;27:1196–202.
41. Han SL, Chen J, Zhou HZ, Lan SH, Zhang PC, Zhu GB. Indications and surgical treatment of chronic pancreatitis. Hepatobiliary Pancreat Dis Int. 2008;7:638–42.
42. Frey CF, Reber HA. Local resection of the head of the pancreas with pancreaticojejunostomy. J Gastrointest Surg. 2005;9:863–8.
43. Beger HG, Kunz R, Poch B. The Beger procedure–duodenum-preserving pancreatic head resection. J Gastrointest Surg. 2004;8:1090–7.
44. Haney JC, Pappas TN. Necrotizing pancreatitis: diagnosis and management. Surg Clin N Am. 2007;87:1431–46.
45. Mathew A, Biswas A, Meitz KP. Endoscopic necrosectomy as primary treatment for infected peripancreatic fluid collections (with video). Gastrointest Endosc. 2008;68:776–82.

19 Spleen

1. All of the following are correct *except*:
   (a) The spleen is a site of prenatal erythropoiesis.
   (b) The spleen is the largest secondary lymphatic organ.
   (c) The spleen arises between the two leaves of the dorsal mesogastrium.
   (d) The spleen is derived from the endoderm.
   (e) The spleen is formed by the fusion of several splenicules represented by the notches on the spleen.

Comments In common with lymphoid tissue, the spleen is derived from the mesodermal cells found between the two layers of the dorsal mesogastrium. These cells proliferate in clusters known as splenicules, that later fuse to form the adult spleen. This developmental pattern explains the frequency of accessory spleens (splenicules that failed to fuse) as well as the segmental nature of splenic blood supply, which allows partial resections [1, 2].

While it does not share the architecture of a lymph node, it is the largest secondary lymphoid organ and hosts lymphocyte maturation and antibody production. In addition to its role in the immune system, the spleen is also the chief site of hemocatheresis and serves as a reservoir of neutrophils and platelets. In some species, the spleen possesses a contractile capsule that allows it to release a hemodynamically significant volume of blood, resulting in an autotransfusion. While the spleen serves an important role on in prenatal erythropoiesis, this function is absent in the adult, returning only in pathologic circumstances [3, 4].

Answer
d

V.K. Maker, E.D. Guzman-Arrieta, *Cognitive Pearls in General Surgery*,
DOI 10.1007/978-1-4939-1850-8_19, © Springer Science+Business Media New York 2015

2. All of the following are correct *except*:
   (a) Wandering and accessory spleens are susceptible to infarction and torsion.
   (b) The most common site for an accessory spleen is the splenic hilum.
   (c) The prevalence of accessory spleens is approximately 25 %.
   (d) Congenital asplenia carries no immunologic consequences.
   (e) Splenosis (ectopic implantation of splenic tissue) is usually secondary to splenic rupture.

Comments The spleen is normally fixed in the left upper quadrant by at least five major ligamentous structures: splenophrenic, gastrosplenic, pancreaticosplenic, splenocolic, and splenorenal ligaments. Wandering spleens are characterized by their lack of peritoneal attachments. They are also termed displaced or ectopic, with the term dislocated reserved for instances in which the spleen is attached in an abnormal location. While commonly asymptomatic, this condition predisposes to splenic torsion. Said torsion may be intermittent, causing pain, but it may also be sustained, leading to infarction. In addition, wandering spleens have been associated with hypersplenism and gastric varices (when the splenic vein is thrombosed). While the traditional approach to the management of wandering spleens was splenectomy, currently splenopexy is preferred. This operation consists of raising peritoneal flaps in the splenic fossa and suturing the splenic capsule to these flaps. Alternatively, synthetic materials have been used to the same end [5–7] (Fig. 19.1).

Accessory spleens are fully vascularized and functional collections of splenic tissue. As mentioned earlier, they represent a failure of fusion of the splenicules. They are the most common splenic anomaly, present in 10–30 % of autopsy cases and 10 % in CT imaging series. Accessory spleens are most often solitary and located in the splenic hilum. Other sites include the omentum, mesentery, lesser sac, and also within the pancreatic tissue. Their importance lies in that they may be mistaken for lymphoid tumors, but more importantly, when unrecognized they may lead to the failure of splenectomy as therapy for hematologic conditions [8].

Congenital asplenia is a rare condition associated with cardiac and pulmonary malformations. It is present in up to 3 % of neonates with cardiac malformations. Cases of isolated asplenia have also been reported. Highlighting the immune function of the spleen, congenitally asplenic patients are vulnerable to overwhelming sepsis by encapsulated bacteria. The diagnosis of asplenia can be suspected by the presence of Howell–Jolly bodies and can be easily confirmed by imaging. These patients should be treated as their surgical asplenic counterparts [9–11].

Splenosis is the result of autotransplantation of viable splenic tissue after trauma to the spleen. In contrast with accessory spleen, splenosis is often multiple. The ectopic tissue lacks independent blood supply and is devoid of its normal immunological function and may be located in remote locations from the spleen. Splenosis has been reported in as many as 65 % of gross splenic rupture. While most commonly asymptomatic, splenosis may also present as a mass or as a source of pain from recurrent hemorrhage and adhesions. The diagnosis can be established with technetium 99 sulfur colloid scan, which is also the test of choice to locate accessory spleens [12].

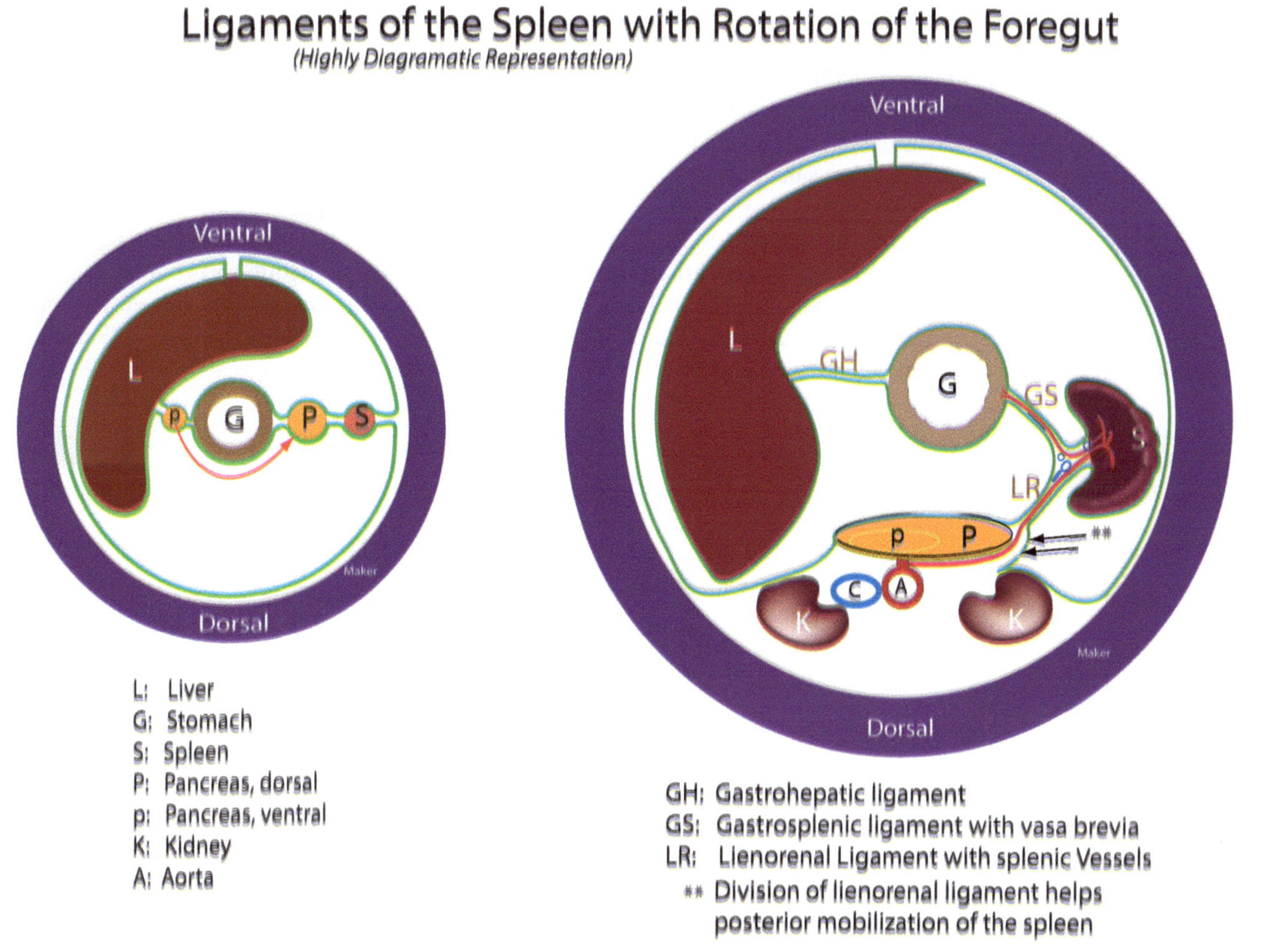

Fig. 19.1 As the embryonic foregut mesentery rotates from a vertical midline to the horizontal position (see Fig. 9.1), the ventral pancreas moves to its new position in the dorsal area, and the spleen is left attached to the parietal peritoneum by lienorenal and lienophrenic ligaments. These are clinically the same ligament with two names depending on reflection from the spleen to the kidney or to the diaphragm. The splenic artery and vein course thru the lienorenal ligament while the vasa brevia (short gastric vessels) travel through gastrosplenic ligament. The splenocolic ligament is generally avascular. *L* liver, *G* stomach, *S* spleen, *P* pancreas, dorsal, *p* pancreas, ventral, *K* kidney, *A* aorta, *C* cava, inferior vena, *GH* gastrohepatic ligament, *GS* gastrosplenic ligament with vasa brevia, *LR* lienorenal ligament with splenic vessels; **division of lienorenal ligament helps posterior mobilization of the spleen

Answer

d

3. All of the following are correct *except*:
   (a) The pediatric spleen is more resistant to trauma than the adult spleen.
   (b) The adult spleen holds sutures better than the pediatric spleen.
   (c) The success rate of conservative management of traumatic splenic injuries is higher in children than in adults.
   (d) Splenic embolization is a feasible option for pediatric trauma.
   (e) Children have relatively larger spleens than adults.

Comments When compared to the adult, the pediatric spleen presents a thicker capsule and a higher proportion of myoepithelial cells. In addition the arterioles found in the pediatric spleen exhibit more efficient retraction and contraction. These factors determine that the pediatric spleen is more likely to achieve hemostasis after trauma than the adult spleen. The failure rate of nonoperative management for splenic injuries in children is 5 %, compared to 15 % in adults. Due to its thicker capsule, splenorrhaphy is more easily accomplished in children [13, 14].

Answer
b

4. All of the following are correct *except*:
   (a) The most frequent causative organisms of overwhelming postsplenectomy infection (OPSI) are S. *pneumoniae*, *H. influenzae*, *N. meningitides*, and group A *Streptococcus*.
   (b) The fraction of spleen required to prevent OPSI is 30–50 %.
   (c) Immunizations against encapsulated bacteria should be administered 2 weeks prior to elective splenectomy.
   (d) Immunizations after splenectomy for trauma are best administered immediately after surgery.
   (e) Booster pneumococcal vaccine should be administered every 5 years.

Comments Please see the discussion for question 5.

Answer
d

5. All of the following are correct except:
   (a) Splenectomized patients have increased vulnerability to *Babesia microti* and *Plasmodium* infections.
   (b) The lifetime incidence of OPSI is greater in children than in adults.
   (c) OPSI most often occurs during the first 2 years postsplenectomy.
   (d) The risk of OPSI is highest if the indication for splenectomy is trauma.
   (e) 50 % of patients with OPSI die within 48 h of admission to the hospital.

Comments Overwhelming postsplenectomy infection is perhaps the most devastating complication of splenectomy. While its lifetime incidence is relatively low (3 %), it carries a morality of 50–70 %. It has been established that its incidence is higher after splenectomy for hematologic or malignant disease as opposed to trauma and in children when compared to adults. Moreover, the majority of cases occur in the first two years following surgery.

The bacteria causing OPSI have a polysaccharide capsule, which helps them evade phagocytosis outside the spleen. The presence of antibodies against the capsule allows bacterial clearance by the Kupffer cells of the liver. Antibodies are not necessary for phagocytosis within the spleen due to its unique sinusoidal vascular pattern that acts as a filter to blood-borne pathogens. This pattern of circulation also makes the spleen vulnerable to septic and metastatic emboli. The bacteria most often involved in OPSI are *Streptococcus pneumoniae*, *Neisseria meningitides*, and *Haemophilus influenzae*.

Clinical features include the presence of a short prodromal phase with fevers, chills, malaise, and GI complaints often without an obvious source of infection. This is followed by a rapid deterioration with hypotension, disseminated intravascular coagulation, respiratory distress, coma, and death within hours of presentation. Survivors often have sequelae from multiple organ failure, as well as peripheral gangrene, bacterial endocarditis, and cardiac valve injuries.

The main line of therapy against OPSI is prevention. Attempts to salvage the spleen should always be made. Additionally, it must be remembered that intact vascular supply. At least 20–30 % of normally vascularized splenic tissue is required to serve the immunological function of this organ. As such, splenic embolization, while physically preserving the spleen, may impair splenic function.

Vaccination against encapsulated pathogens is mandatory. It should be performed 2 weeks before elective splenectomy. In trauma cases, immunization is best given 2 weeks postsplenectomy. In practice immunization is given upon discharge as this allows time for some recovery of the immune system after injury and guarantees 100 % compliance. Boosters must be given every 5 years. In addition, patients should be educated regarding this syndrome. Continuous prophylaxis with penicillin has not proven to be effective. The preferred strategy involves providing patients with antibiotics such as amoxicillin to be taken upon the onset of fevers and rigors, with clear instructions to seek urgent medical care where these symptoms to appear [15, 16].

Due to its role in the destruction of red blood cells, splenectomized patients are at a disadvantage when infected with erythrocyte pathogens such as *Plasmodium* and *Babesia* species. The encapsulated bacteria *Capnocytophaga canimorsus* has been linked to OPSI after dog bites [17, 18].

Answer

d

6. Splenectomy is indicated in the treatment of:
   (a) Cold antibody hemolytic anemia
   (b) Disseminated intravascular coagulation
   (c) Sickle cell anemia
   (d) Thalassemia major
   (e) Acute lymphocytic leukemia

Comments Excluding trauma, splenectomies are carried out with the goal of reducing the splenic elimination of corpuscular elements of the blood, treating symptoms derived from splenomegaly, and for staging purposes. While splenectomy has traditionally been carried out through a laparotomy; currently, laparoscopy is feasible in most cases in which the spleen does not exceed 20 cm in length [19].

The most prominent indication for splenectomy is idiopathic thrombocytopenic purpura, when treatment with corticosteroids has failed or is not possible due to unacceptable side effects. In this setting, splenectomy is 80 % successful in alleviating the disease process. With much less frequency, splenectomy is indicated in thrombotic thrombocytopenic purpura, in instances in which plasma exchange is unsuccessful or not tolerated.

Splenectomy is indicated in red blood cell disorders such as spherocytosis, thalassemia with high transfusion requirements (>200 ml/kg/year), and warm antibody hemolytic anemia refractory to steroids. Splenectomy may also be helpful in reducing transfusion requirements in patients with glucose-6-phosphate dehydrogenase deficiency as well as those with pyruvate kinase deficiency.

While sickle cell anemia results in splenic infarction and functional splenectomy, it is not an indication for splenectomy. However, splenectomy may be indicated for hypersplenism as well as for sickle cell sequestration crisis.

Splenectomy is indicated in the setting of multiple hematologic disorders causing splenomegaly and hypersplenism. It is of benefit in acute and chronic myelocytic leukemia as well as in chronic lymphocytic leukemia. However, it is not indicated in acute lymphocytic leukemia.

In the past, splenectomy was indicated for staging of Hodgkin and non-Hodgkin lymphoma, but this is no longer the case. The only current indication in these setting is to treat the symptomatic splenomegaly that is often present [20].

Answer
d

7. All of the following are correct *except*:
   (a) Primary hypersplenism is more common than secondary hypersplenism.
   (b) Hypersplenism is accompanied by increased bone marrow activity.
   (c) Hypersplenism may be treated with splenectomy.
   (d) Less than 10 % of patients with splenomegaly have hypersplenism.
   (e) Hypersplenism causes anemia, leucopenia, and/or thrombocytopenia.

Comments Hypersplenism is defined as splenomegaly, any combination of anemia, leucopenia, and thrombocytopenia, compensatory bone marrow hyperplasia, and improvement after splenectomy. Portal hypertension secondary to cirrhosis is the most common cause of hypersplenism in the United States. With less frequency, sinistral (left-sided) portal hypertension due to splenic vein thrombosis is seen. Other causes include neoplastic disorders, myeloid metaplasia, metabolic storage disorders, and infectious conditions such as tuberculosis. Rarely, hypersplenism may occur primarily. While this diagnosis was more common in the past, diagnostic advances have led to identify lymphoma or leukemia as the underlying cause. Splenectomy is indicated in order to relieve the mass and hematologic effects when treatment of the primary cause is ineffective or not possible [20, 21].

Answer

a

8. All of the following are correct *except*:
   (a) The splenic artery follows two patterns: distributed (70 %) and bundled or magistral (30 %).
   (b) Ligation of the splenic artery should precede ligation of the splenic vein when possible.
   (c) En bloc ligation of the splenic artery and veins predisposes to the formation of AV fistulas.
   (d) Partial splenectomy is possible because of the segmental distribution of the splenic vasculature.
   (e) Drainage of the splenic bed is mandatory.

Comments The performance of a successful open splenectomy begins with an adequate mobilization. The initial maneuver is to divide the splenorenal and splenophrenic ligaments while exerting dorsal and medial traction. Attempts to traction the spleen ventrally prior to lateral mobilization often result in capsular tears. Once the spleen has been free from its lateral attachments, it may be elevated and tractioned laterally in order to divide the splenocolic and splenogastric ligaments, together with the associated short gastric vessels (Fig. 19.2).

This last maneuver exposes the splenic vessels. The splenic artery may follow one of two main patterns: distributed splenic arteries branch away from the splenic parenchyma, while bundled or magistral arteries do so very close to the spleen or within its parenchyma. This anatomical distinction becomes important to avoid injury to the pancreatic tail, more so during laparoscopic splenectomy (Fig. 19.3).

Laparoscopic splenectomy relies on gravity for traction and exposure. The spleen is left attached to the body wall via intact splenophrenic and splenorenal ligaments. The patient is placed in right lateral decubitus position, and the splenocolic ligament and the medial attachments of the spleen are divided first.

It is recommended to divide the splenic artery first, to avoid engorgement of the organ. En bloc ligation of the artery and vein may lead to the formation of AV fistulas and is not recommended.

While it is true that the splenic bed is the most frequent site of abscess formation after splenectomy, routine drainage of this area is not recommended, as it increases rather than decreases the incidence of this complication.

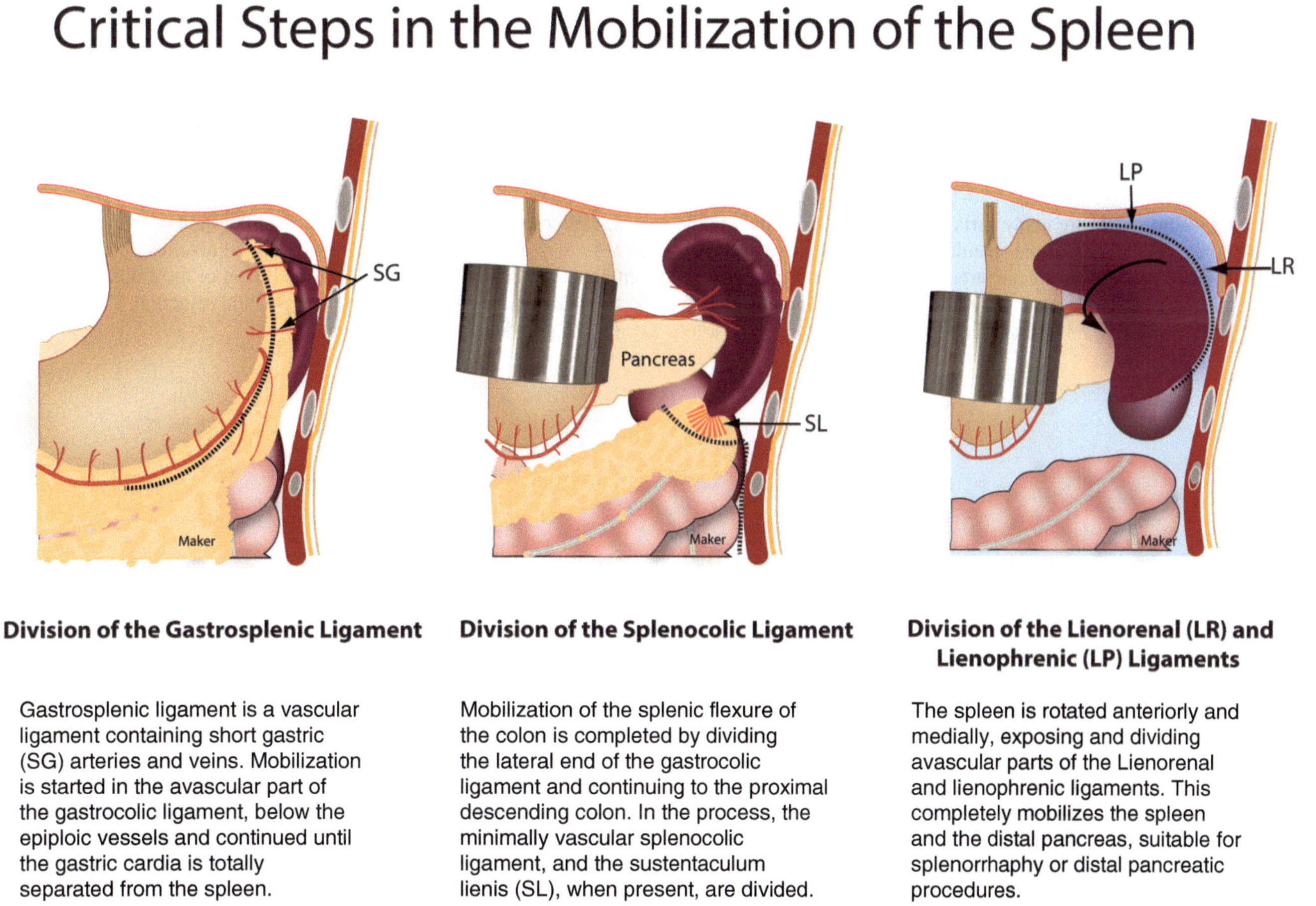

Fig. 19.2 Technique described is for open procedures and the order can be modified for a laparoscopic approach. For removing massive spleens, it is appropriate to ligate the splenic artery in the lesser sac, mobilize the spleen, and ligate splenic vein at the end. This sequence causes the spleen to shrink during mobilization with autotransfusion of blood from the spleen

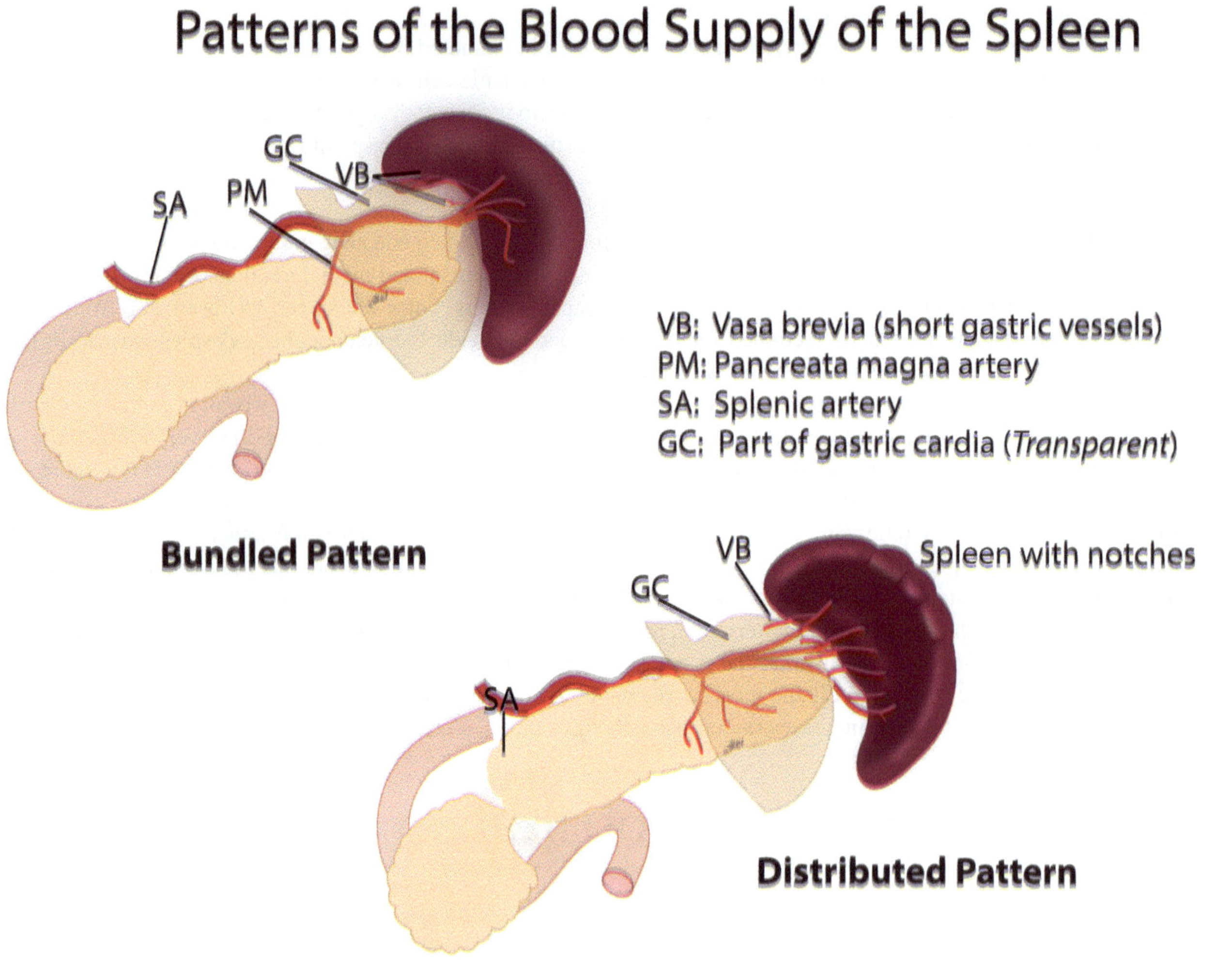

Fig. 19.3 While there are many variations in the blood supply to the spleen, two common patterns are seen at the hilar area of the spleen. In the bundled pattern, division of the splenic artery into hilar branches is within 2–4 cm, and often there are not well-defined notches on the spleen. In the distributed pattern, the splenic artery divides more proximally and prominent splenic notches likely mark the fusion of the embryonic splenic segments. Surgical applications are endless, including and not limited to the surgical approach to the hilum and segmental resection. *VB* vasa brevia (short gastric vessels), *PM* pancreatica magna artery, *SA* splenic artery, *GC* part of gastric cardia (transparent)

Answer

e

9 All of the following are correct *except:*
(a) Splenic artery aneurysms have an overall rupture rate of 2 %.
(b) Splenic artery aneurysms are more common in men.
(c) Splenic artery aneurysms are usually asymptomatic.
(d) Splenic artery pseudoaneurysms are most often secondary to pancreatitis and trauma.
(e) Women with known splenic artery aneurysm should be treated electively if pregnancy is planned.

Comments Please see the discussion for question 10.

Answer
b

10. All of the following are correct *except*:
    (a) The splenic artery is the most common site for visceral aneurysm.
    (b) Bleeding splenic artery aneurysms exhibit a double rupture phenomenon.
    (c) Splenic artery aneurysms are most frequent in multiparous women.
    (d) Splenectomy is always part of the surgical management of splenic artery aneurysms.
    (e) An asymptomatic splenic artery aneurysm should be removed if it is larger than 2 cm.

Comments Visceral artery aneurysms are infrequent but potentially lethal. Approximately 60 % are found in the splenic artery and 20 % in the hepatic artery, and the remainder is divided between the SMA, IMA, and other visceral arteries [22].

Diagnosis is made through imaging studies, in which a classic eggshell calcification is seen. Splenic artery aneurysms are four times more frequent in women and are particularly prone to rupture during pregnancy. Multiparity is an important risk factor. Splenic artery aneurysms have also been associated with liver transplantation [23].

Aneurysm rupture usually occurs in two stages, the first of which involves bleeding into the lesser sac with some degree of hemodynamic compensation. Following this, free rupture into the peritoneal cavity and shock ensue.

Indications for repair of splenic artery aneurysms include rupture, the presence of symptoms (abdominal pain), size over 2 cm, and the intention to become pregnant. Treatment of proximal aneurysms involves proximal and distal ligation, relying on collateral circulation for spleen preservation. Distal aneurysms may be treated by ligation and splenectomy or bypass with spleen preservation. Endovascular interventions have also been proposed as a form of treatment. However, infarction, coil migration, and delayed ruptured are valid concerns [24]. In contrast splenic artery pseudoaneurysms are seen in pancreatitis and are amenable to observation [25].

Answer

d

11. All of the following are correct *except*:
    (a) The heart is the most common source of splenic abscesses.
    (b) Splenic abscesses are amenable to percutaneous drainage.
    (c) Splenitis most often affects immunocompromised hosts.
    (d) Splenectomy in contraindicated in splenitis.
    (e) Crohn's disease is associated with aseptic splenic abscesses.

Comments Due to its relatively high blood flow, the spleen may be affected by septic emboli that may develop into splenic abscesses. The most common cause of splenic abscesses is infectious endocarditis; however, any source of bacteremia may be the culprit. Cases associated with colon perforations and extremity wounds have been reported. Manifestations include fever, leukocytosis, left upper quadrant pain, and left-sided pleural effusion. Splenic abscesses do not respond to antibiotic therapy. Percutaneous drainage has emerged as a viable treatment modality. Splenectomy may be necessary in select cases [26–28].

Splenitis, also known as acute splenic tumor or septic spleen, is pathologically defined as vascular congestion and neutrophilic infiltration of the red pulp of the spleen. This condition was seen in association with severe sepsis in the pre-antibiotic era. It is currently seen with less frequency, and the pathogens associated with this condition have changed to agents not commonly covered with standard antibiotics. Examples in the United States include *Bartonella henselae*, *Trypanosoma cruzi*, *Treponema pallidum*, *Borrelia burgdorferi*, and *Plasmodium* sp. Patients who develop splenitis tend to be affected by immunosuppressive pathologies such as HIV/AIDS, end-stage renal disease, and terminal malignancies such as lymphoma. Splenectomy may be indicated to control the source of sepsis or also in cases of massive splenomegaly with impending rupture. Splenectomy after resolution of splenitis is challenging due to obliteration of the avascular ligamentous planes. In this setting, the spleen is removed with portions of the parietal peritoneum to which it is attached [29–31].

Splenic abscesses may be associated Crohn's disease and much more rarely with ulcerative colitis. In this setting, the abscesses are most commonly sterile and are thought to be a systemic manifestation of the disease rather than the consequence of an infectious process [32, 33].

Answer
d

References

1. McClusky 3rd DA, Skandalakis LJ, Colborn GL, Skandalakis JE. Tribute to a triad: history of splenic anatomy, physiology, and surgery-part 2. World J Surg. 1999;23:514–26.
2. McClusky 3rd DA, Skandalakis LJ, Colborn GL, Skandalakis JE. Tribute to a triad: history of splenic anatomy, physiology, and surgery–part 1. World J Surg. 1999;23:311–25.
3. Poulin EC, Thibault C. The anatomical basis for laparoscopic splenectomy. Can J Surg. 1993;36:484–8.
4. Skandalakis PN, Colborn GL, Skandalakis LJ, Richardson DD, Mitchell Jr WE, Skandalakis JE. The surgical anatomy of the spleen. Surg Clin N Am. 1993;73:747–68.
5. Misawa T, Yoshida K, Shiba H, Kobayashi S, Yanaga K. Wandering spleen with chronic torsion. Am J Surg. 2008;195:504–5.
6. Soleimani M, Mehrabi A, Kashfi A, Fonouni H, Buchler MW, Kraus TW. Surgical treatment of patients with wandering spleen: report of six cases with a review of the literature. Surg Today. 2007;37:261–9.
7. Wani S, Abdulkarim AB, Buckles D. Gastric variceal hemorrhage secondary to torsion of wandering spleen. Clin Gastroenterol Hepatol. 2008;6:A24.
8. Gayer G, Hertz M, Strauss S, Zissin R. Congenital anomalies of the spleen. Semin Ultrasound CT MR. 2006;27:358–69.
9. Gilbert B, Menetrey C, Belin V, Brosset P, de Lumley L, Fisher A. Familial isolated congenital asplenia: a rare, frequently hereditary dominant condition, often detected too late as a cause of overwhelming pneumococcal sepsis. Report of a new case and review of 31 others. Eur J Pediatr. 2002;161:368–72.
10. Phoon CK, Neill CA. Asplenia syndrome: insight into embryology through an analysis of cardiac and extracardiac anomalies. Am J Cardiol. 1994;73:581–7.
11. Thiruppathy K, Privitera A, Jain K, Gupta S. Congenital asplenia and group B streptococcus sepsis in the adult: case report and review of the literature. FEMS Immunol Med Microbiol. 2008;53:437–9.
12. Fremont RD, Rice TW. Splenosis: a review. South Med J. 2007;100:589–93.
13. Cloutier DR, Baird TB, Gormley P, McCarten KM, Bussey JG, Luks FI. Pediatric splenic injuries with a contrast blush: successful nonoperative management without angiography and embolization. J Pediatr Surg. 2004;39:969–71.
14. Hilmes MA, Strouse PJ. The pediatric spleen. Semin Ultrasound CT MR. 2007;28:3–11.
15. Okabayashi T, Hanazaki K. Overwhelming postsplenectomy infection syndrome in adults - a clinically preventable disease. World J Gastroenterol. 2008;14:176–9.
16. Brigden ML, Pattullo AL. Prevention and management of overwhelming postsplenectomy infection–an update. Crit Care Med. 1999; 27:836–42.
17. Demar M, Legrand E, Hommel D, Esterre P, Carme B. Plasmodium falciparum malaria in splenectomized patients: two case reports in French Guiana and a literature review. Am J Trop Med Hyg. 2004;71:290–3.
18. Rosner F, Zarrabi MH, Benach JL, Habicht GS. Babesiosis in splenectomized adults. Review of 22 reported cases. Am J Med. 1984; 76:696–701.
19. Uranues S, Alimoglu O. Laparoscopic surgery of the spleen. Surg Clin N Am. 2005;85:75–90. ix.
20. Katz SC, Pachter HL. Indications for splenectomy. Am Surg. 2006;72:565–80.
21. Eichner ER. Splenic function: normal, too much and too little. Am J Med. 1979;66:311–20.
22. Stanley JC, Wakefield TW, Graham LM, Whitehouse Jr WM, Zelenock GB, Lindenauer SM. Clinical importance and management of splanchnic artery aneurysms. J Vasc Surg. 1986;3:836–40.
23. Annicchiarico BE, Avolio AW, Caracciolo G, et al. Late development of splenic artery aneurysm after orthotopic liver transplantation: a case report. Transplant Proc. 2009;41:1383–5.
24. Kim MK, Kwak BK, Shim HJ, Park SJ. Endovascular treatment of a distal splenic artery aneurysm with use of a stent-graft. J Vasc Interv Radiol. 2009;20:687–9.
25. Berceli SA. Hepatic and splenic artery aneurysms. Semin Vasc Surg. 2005;18:196–201.
26. Delis SG, Maniatis PN, Triantopoulou C, Papailiou J, Dervenis C. Splenic abscess in a patient with fecal peritonitis. World J Gastroenterol. 2007;13:1626–7.
27. Escamilla-Lopez M, de la O-cavazos ME, Hinojosa-Lezama M, Gonzalez-Velazco RN, Abrego-Moya V. Splenic abscesses. A case report and review of the literature. Bol Med Hosp Infant Mex. 1992;49:502–5.
28. Thanos L, Dailiana T, Papaioannou G, Nikita A, Koutrouvelis H, Kelekis DA. Percutaneous CT-guided drainage of splenic abscess. AJR Am J Roentgenol. 2002;179:629–32.
29. Bynum B. Splenitis. Lancet. 2002;359:1953.
30. El Tayar AR, Labruzzo C, Haritopoulos K, Papalois V, Hakim NS. Perisplenitis as a cause of acute abdomen: a case report. Int Surg. 2002;87:205–7.
31. Feig JA, Cina SJ. Evaluation of characteristics associated with acute splenitis (septic spleen) as markers of systemic infection. Arch Pathol Lab Med. 2001;125:888–91.
32. Coyne JD. Crohn's disease with inflammatory splenic granuloma. J Clin Pathol. 2006;59:889.
33. Coat N, Le Berre-Heresbach N, Poinsignon Y, et al. Crohn's disease complicated by multiple and recurrent aseptic splenic abscesses. Gastroenterol Clin Biol. 2001;25:425–8.

20 Urinary System

1. All of the following are correct *except*:
   (a) The kidneys are derived from the mesoderm.
   (b) The pronephros gives rise to the collecting system.
   (c) The metanephros gives rise to the nephrons.
   (d) The kidneys develop in the pelvis and later ascend to the lumbar region.
   (e) Ectopic kidneys may be found anywhere along the normal path of kidney ascent.

Comments The kidney arises from the mesoderm. The mesonephros will give rise to the mesonephric ducts, also known as Wolffian ducts. By week 5 of development, the metanephros forms caudal to the mesonephros, in close vicinity to the bladder, in the pelvis. The key step in renal organogenesis is the invasion of the metanephros by the ureteric bud, a derivative of the Wolffian duct. This interaction induces the formation of glomeruli within the metanephros as well as the differentiation of the ureteric bud into the renal collecting system, starting with the collecting ducts and ending with the ureters and trigone of the bladder. Failure in this relationship is responsible for multiple congenital anomalies.

Renal development occurs as the embryo elongates, making the kidneys ascend from the pelvis (S1–S2) into their adult location in the lumbar region. As they ascend, they rotate medially, with the renal pelvis passing from an anterior to a posterior location. Finally, there is a change in blood supply to the kidney. Vessels arising from the abdominal aorta and inferior vena cava substitute the original supply arising from the distal aorta and iliac vessels (Fig. 20.1).

The process of relocation of the kidneys may be arrested at any stage. As the name implies "pelvic" kidneys fail to ascend and rotate medially (the renal pelvis remains in an anterior position). These kidneys also preserve their original blood supply. Due to their flattened shape, they are also called pancake kidneys. As the kidney ascends along the vascular ladder from the pelvis to the perilumbar position, the gonads descend along the same ladder in the vascular axis taking blood vessels from the high lumbar area into the pelvis [1–3].

V.K. Maker, E.D. Guzman-Arrieta, *Cognitive Pearls in General Surgery*,
DOI 10.1007/978-1-4939-1850-8_20,

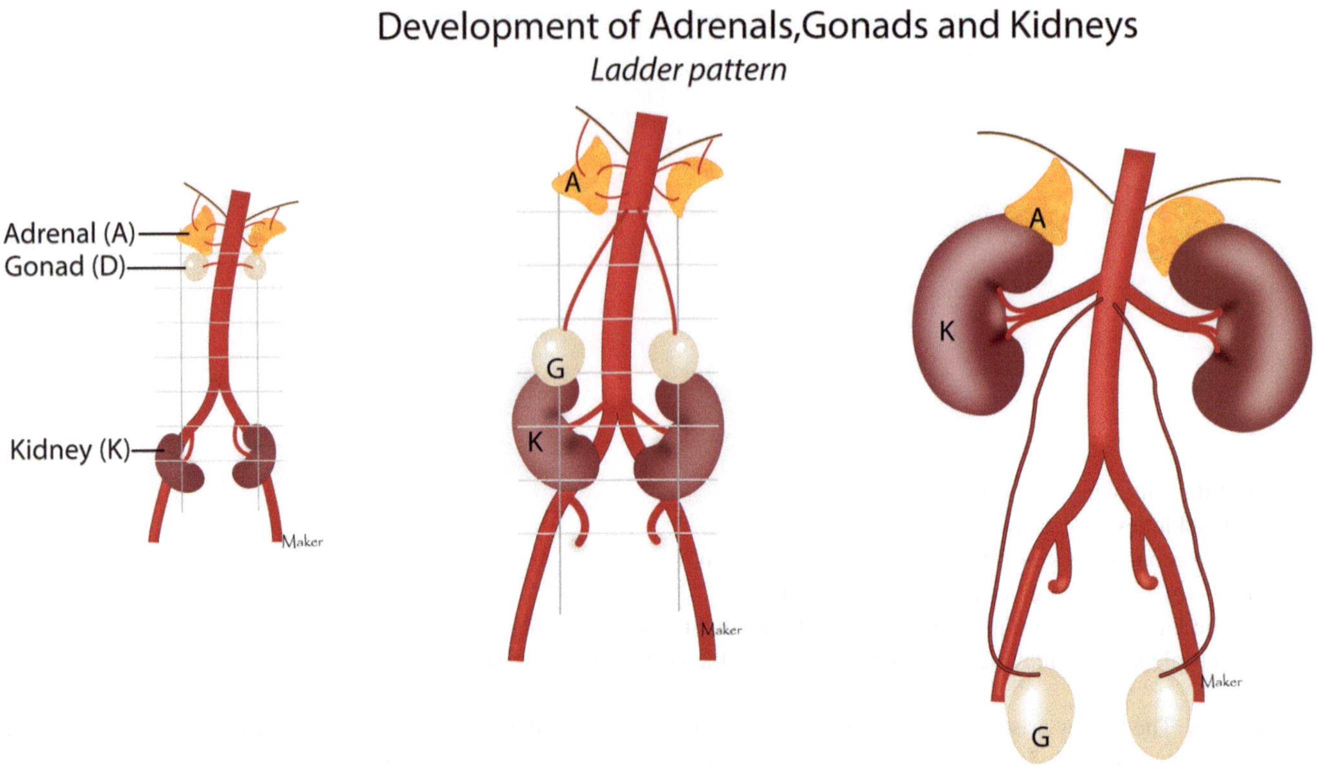

Fig. 20.1 The adrenals, gonads, and kidneys develop in the retroperitoneal paravertebral area. The kidneys ascend up the ladder and keep on getting a new blood supply until their final destination below the adrenal at lumbar 1 to 4th (L1–L4) vertebra. The gonads, on the other hand, start at L1 and descend down the ladder keeping their blood supply from L1. Adrenals stay on the ladder and maintain their blood supply. This explains the multiple anomalies dealing with these organs

Answer
b

2. All of the following are correct *except*:
   (a) Horseshoe kidneys are fused by their caudal poles.
   (b) Horseshoe kidneys get "hung up" on the inferior mesenteric artery.
   (c) Horseshoe kidneys require division and replacement in an anatomically correct position.
   (d) The ureters cross anterior to the fused portion of a horseshoe kidney.
   (e) Aberrant branches arising directly from the aorta may supply the isthmus of a horseshoe kidney.

Comments Horseshoe kidneys are the most common fusion abnormality of the kidneys. They arise from the fusion of the inferior renal poles while they still reside in the pelvis. This union impedes subsequent medial rotation and ascent of the kidneys, as the area of fusion cannot progress cephalad to the inferior mesenteric artery. The lack of medial rotation determines that the ureters remain in an anterior location. Vascular development is also hindered, and horseshoe kidneys often preserve their primitive blood supply arising from the distal aorta and iliac vessels [4].

While up to one third of horseshoe kidneys remain asymptomatic and are discovered incidentally, the abnormal blood supply and ureteral implantation predispose to urinary stasis and reflux, leading to nephrolithiasis and urinary tract infections.

Horseshoe kidneys are more vulnerable to trauma due to their lack of protection by the ribs. In addition, the isthmus may be compressed against the spinal column. There have been reports of tumors arising from horseshoe kidneys, and it is unclear whether horseshoe kidney is a predisposing factor for renal cell carcinoma. Finally, horseshoe kidneys represent an obstacle in the repair of abdominal aortic aneurysms. This obstacle can be circumvented by the use of endovascular or retroperitoneal approaches.

Horseshoe kidneys do not require any specific treatment. Division of the isthmus and attempts at relocation are contraindicated. However, surgery may be undertaken to address urinary reflux and stones [5].

Answer

c

3. All of the following are correct *except*:
   (a) Simple renal cysts are more common with increasing age.
   (b) Infantile polycystic disease is associated with biliary ectasia and hepatic fibrosis.
   (c) Infantile polycystic disease follows a more benign course than the adult type.
   (d) Adult polycystic disease is autosomal dominant.
   (e) Adult polycystic disease is associated with cysts in the liver, pancreas, and spleen.

Comments Simple renal cysts are commonly seen as acquired lesions. They are epithelium-lined, urine-containing cavities thought to constitute the diverticula of the distal convoluted or collecting tubules due to an age-related weakening of the basement membrane. They are typical of the elderly population and tend to increase in number and size with time. They are not considered a premalignant lesion and require no specific therapy [6–8].

Adult (autosomal dominant) polycystic kidney disease (PKD) is the most common genetically transmitted renal cystic disease, occurring in 2 per 1,000 live births. It is caused by mutations in the PDK1, PDK2, and PDK3 genes. Although it may become manifest at any age, it is most often detected between the fourth and fifth decades of life, when a multitude of cysts of varying size throughout the renal parenchyma have developed [9].

Patients with adult PKD are at increased risk for developing renal carcinoma. They may also develop hepatic, pancreatic, and splenic cysts. Another noteworthy association is that with cerebral aneurysms, which occur with an 8 % incidence. Hypertension, hematuria, and recurrent urinary tract infections are often present. This disease causes progressive loss of renal mass leading to end-stage renal disease.

Infantile (autosomal recessive) PKD is 40 times less common than the adult variety (1 per 20,000 live births). It is caused by a mutation in the PKDH1 gene. The infantile variety of PDK is consistently associated with hepatic cysts. Thirty percent of affected patients die in the perinatal period due to lung hypoplasia. Survivors develop hypertension, with up to 50 % of cases developing end-stage renal disease by age 15. Cyst morphology is distinct, with multiple, homogeneous dilatations of the collecting ducts, with radial orientation. Liver involvement consists of portal ectasia leading to cirrhosis [10].

Answer

c

4. All of the following are correct *except*:
   (a) The renal arteries arise at the L1–L2 level, caudal to the superior mesenteric artery.
   (b) Renal arteries are end arteries without any collateral circulation.
   (c) The vasa recta supplying the renal tubules are branches of the efferent arteriole.
   (d) The renal tubules have a blood supply independent from that of the glomerulus.
   (e) Accessory renal arteries are a normal anatomic variant.

Comments The renal arteries are typically single and arise from the abdominal aorta, between L1 and L2, inferior to the superior mesenteric artery. The right renal artery originates slightly more cephalad than the left and follows a downward course behind the inferior vena cava towards the kidney. In contrast, the left renal artery has a more caudal origin and follows a short straight course towards the kidney. Both arteries travel from anterior to posterior to reach the kidney. At the level of the renal hilum, they occupy an intermediate plane, in front of the renal pelvis and ureter, but behind the renal vein. The renal arteries are considered the sole end artery supply of the kidney, although accessory renal arteries may be present in about 2 % of the population. Ligation of the renal artery or an accessory branch will lead to an area of infarction. However, renal veins can be ligated in exceptional traumatic injuries. In this setting, venous drainage occurs through collaterals through the adrenal veins. The renal veins course parallel and slightly inferior and anterior to the renal arteries. These relationships are important as instrumentation of the inferior vena cava and aorta is usually performed below the level of the renal vessels to preserve kidney perfusion and protect the superior mesenteric artery (Fig. 20.2).

At the renal hilum, the renal artery starts branching into progressively smaller vessels becoming the afferent arterioles that supply the glomerulus. The efferent arterioles collect the blood from the glomerular tufts and channel it towards the renal tubules via the vasa recta. In low-perfusion states, renal tubules are particularly vulnerable to acute tubular necrosis because of this arrangement [11, 12] (Fig. 20.3).

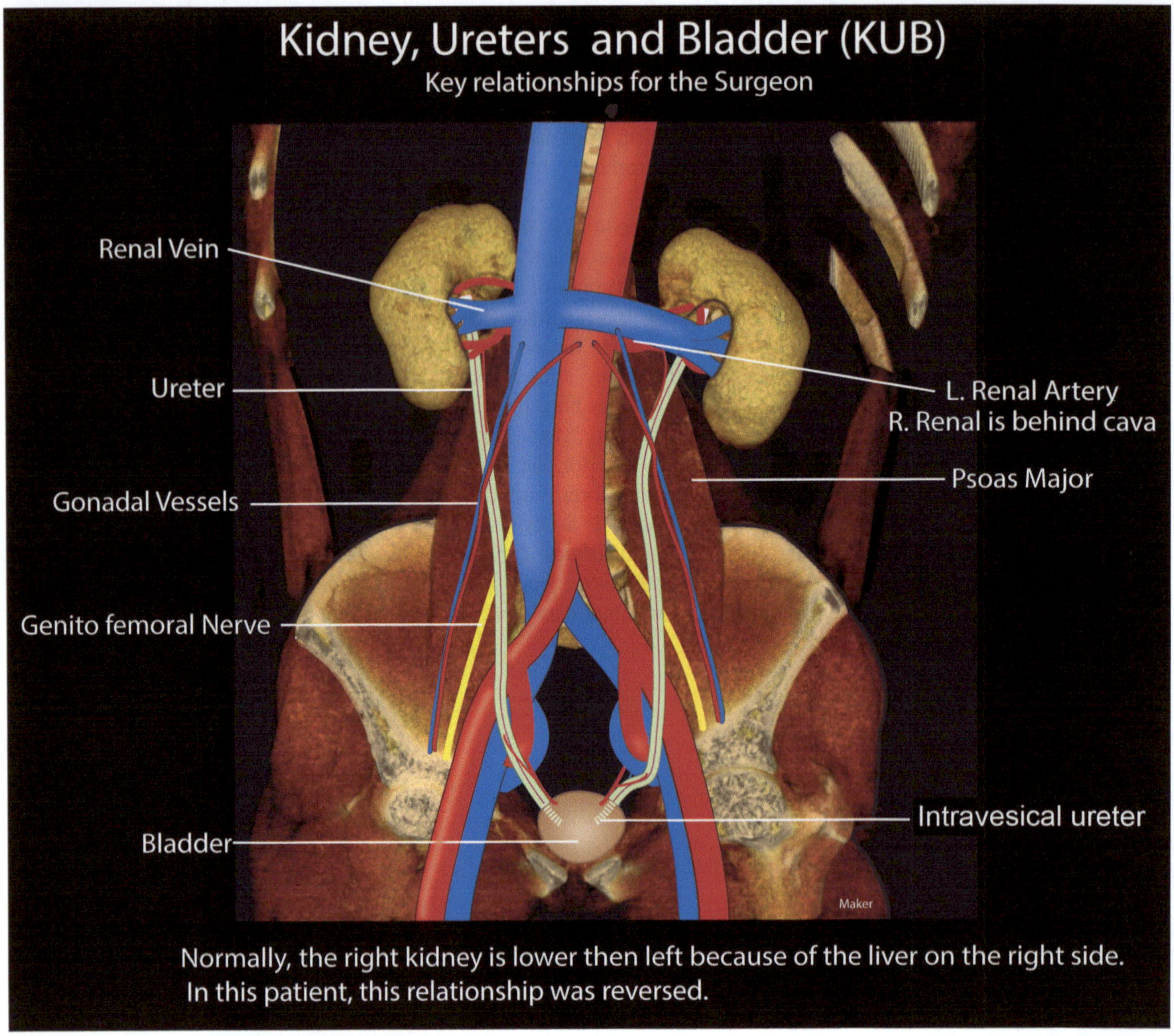

Fig. 20.2 The inferior vena cava stands with both arms (renal veins) stretched out in front of the aorta and then it gradually travels inferiorly hiding behind the aorta and iliacs in the pelvis. Ureters collecting the waste of the body are appropriately at the back of the hilum of the kidney, travel posteriorly behind the gonadal vessels, and then detour anterior to the iliac vessels to get to the anteriorly located urinary bladder. The right gonadal veins drain into the inferior vena cava already located on the right, but on the left find ease to drain into the left renal vein. Both gonadal arteries, however, originate directly from the aorta. The psoas major, the filet mignon, is the only intra-abdominal muscle and it provides a posterior cushion for vessels, ureters, and most intimately for the genitofemoral nerve. As the embryonic kindeys migrate cephalad from the pelvis to their adult position, the ureters derive their blood supply from the vesical arteries, internal iliac arteries, common iliac arteries, aorta, gonadal arteries and renal arteries.

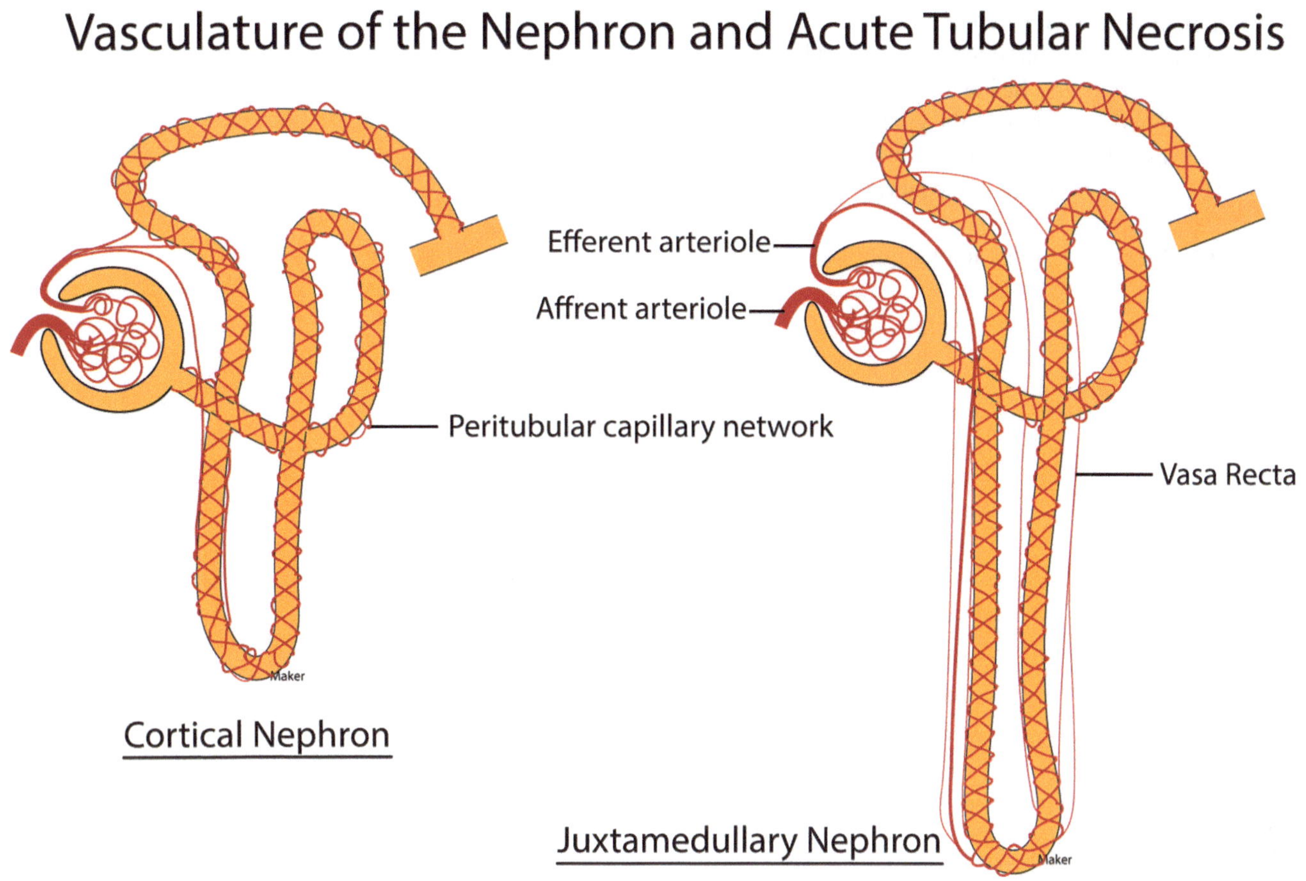

Fig. 20.3 Renal blood flow is about 1,200 ml/min representing 20 % of the cardiac output. Renal vasculature has two distinct capillary beds in series. The glomerular capillary bed finishes with the smaller efferent arteriole that feeds the entire peritubular capillary bed. The peritubular capillary bed includes the vasa recta that feeds Henle's loop in the juxtamedullary glomeruli. Because of the above arrangement, in conditions resulting in renal hypotension, the tubules are at a distinct disadvantage and may undergo acute tubular necrosis, especially if the glomeruli have also filtered in nephrotoxins like free hemoglobin or myoglobin

Answer

d

5. All of the following are correct *except*:
   (a) The ureters are ventral to the iliac vessels.
   (b) The ureters course inside the peritoneal cavity.
   (c) The ureters are dorsal to the gonadal vessels.
   (d) The vas deferens is ventral to the ureter.
   (e) The ureters are dorsal to the uterine vessels.

Comments Please see discussion for question 6.

Answer
d

6. All of the following are correct *except*:
   (a) The ureter has three points of narrowing: ureteropelvic junction, crossing of the iliac vessels, and ureterovesical junction.
   (b) The narrowest point of the ureter is the ureterovesical junction, causing most renal stones to become impacted in this location.
   (c) The ureter has a segmental blood supply from multiple vessels closely wrapped around it.
   (d) The ureters should be widely skeletonized to ensure a watertight anastomosis.
   (e) The ureter has a subadventitial anastomotic network.

Comments A clear knowledge of ureteral anatomy is essential to those operating in the abdomen, retroperitoneum, pelvis, and perineum, where the incidence of injury to these structures ranges from 0.3 to 1.5 %. This high incidence is explained by the presence of hostile surgical conditions as well as to the multiple anatomical variations.

The adult ureters are 25–30 cm in length, with a diameter of 1.5–6 mm. The ureters remain extraperitoneal throughout their course. They course lateral to the lumbar vertebrae and anterior to the psoas muscles as they descend into the pelvis. Through their course, they come in relation with multiple structures.

The ureters are crossed anteriorly by the gonadal vein and artery (bridge over water). This happens as the ureters go from lateral to medial, while the gonadal vessels go from medial to lateral en route to their target organs. Posteriorly they cross over the genitofemoral nerve. Both ureters cross anterior to the iliac vessels as they enter the pelvis to reach the bladder. On the right side, the duodenum covers the proximal aspect of the ureter. On the left, the ureter is covered by the descending and sigmoid mesocolon and is at times injured with medial mobilization of the left colon, especially in cases of diverticulitis or advanced left colon cancers. In the male, the ureters lie dorsal to the vas deferens and are vulnerable during the perineal rectal dissection. In the female, the ureters are dorsal to the round ligament, ovaries, fallopian tubes, and uterine vessels.

The blood supply of the ureters is segmental, derived from adjacent arteries, namely, renal, gonadal, distal aorta, iliac, and cystic arteries. The uterine arteries also contribute to the ureteral blood supply in the female. All these tributaries form an extensive periureteral anastomotic vascular network that must be preserved by avoiding skeletonization in order to maintain ureteral viability. Ureteral repair follows three key principles: watertight closure with interrupted reabsorbable sutures, lack of tension, and spatulation with internal stenting.

The ureter has three points of narrowing where renal stone impaction may occur. They are the ureteropelvic junction, the crossing of the iliac vessels, and the ureterovesical junction. The latter one is the smallest in diameter and the most common site of stone impaction. At this location, symptoms may be confused with those of acute appendicitis, especially in pregnancy, where a hydroureter is at times physiologically present.

The right ureter may occupy a retrocaval location, in which case it wraps around the cava. This anomaly has an incidence of 1 in 1,500, with a 3:1 male predominance. It can manifest as right ureteric obstruction. Other malformations include complete and partial duplication as well as ureteral crossing. Preoperative knowledge of ureteral anatomy is key in preventing intraoperative injuries [13].

Answer
d

7. All of the following are correct *except*:
   (a) The adrenal glands lie within Gerota's fascia.
   (b) Gerota's fascia allows the contralateral spread of perirenal collections.
   (c) Gerota's fascia is fused with the peritoneum anteriorly.
   (d) Gerota's fascia is weakest in its inferior aspect.
   (e) Gerota's fascia is excised during a radical nephrectomy.

Comments Gerota's fascia is a condensation of retroperitoneal connective tissue forming a sheath that envelops the kidney, adrenal gland, and perinephric fat on either side of the midline. Anteriorly, Gerota's fascia is loosely attached to the parietal peritoneum. Posteriorly, it is a more defined structure that can be separated from the muscular elements of the posterior body wall. Medially, it reflects along the elements of the renal hilum.

Although there is some controversy regarding the limits of Gerota's fascia, it is clear that this structure contains collections of blood, pus, and urine impeding their spread to the opposite side of the retroperitoneum. It appears that the weakest part of this fascia is the inferior pole, as this is the route through which perinephric collections erode to extend into the retroperitoneum.

Gerota's fascia also acts as an anatomical barrier relevant to the spread of renal tumors as well as urine and blood collections caused by trauma. The integrity of Gerota's fascia forms the anatomical basis for the nonoperative management of most renal injuries. For the same reason, oncologic control of renal malignancies requires the en bloc resection of the kidneys, perirenal fat, and Gerota's fascia [14, 15].

Answer
b

8. All of the following are correct *except*:
   (a) Bladder detrusor function is controlled by the parasympathetic system.
   (b) The internal sphincter of the bladder is controlled by the sympathetic system.
   (c) The external sphincter is under somatic control by the pudendal nerve.
   (d) The advantage of radiation therapy for prostate cancer is that it preserves nerve function.
   (e) Autonomic nerve preservation is achieved by dissecting close to the visceral planes.

Comments The bladder, pelvic floor, and urethra function in concert to allow the low-pressure storage of urine and its periodic expulsion. Regulation of this function is subject to the actions of the somatic and autonomic nervous system acting upon a complex anatomical substrate.

The bladder has a storage capacity of 300–500 ml, but is often emptied at smaller filling volumes (100–150 ml) between five and seven times a day. It occupies the retropubic space of Retzius to different extents depending on its degree of filling.

In line with the fight-or-flight response, activation of the sympathetic system impedes bladder emptying through contraction of the smooth muscle of the vesical neck (T11–L2). Interestingly, this sympathetic pathway is also responsible for the prevention of retrograde ejaculation. In contrast, bladder emptying is mediated by the parasympathetic system (S2–S4). The actions of the two branches of the autonomic nervous system are modulated through voluntary efferent somatic pathways acting on the external vesical sphincter (S2–S4) [16].

It is interesting to note that the autonomic nerve supply of the bladder coincides with its embryologic origin. The bladder detrusor muscle is derived from the cloaca, which is in turn derived from the endodermal hindgut. It is supplied by the parasympathetic system. In contrast, the bladder trigone is derived from the mesonephros (mesoderm) and receives sympathetic nerve supply.

The micturition reflex is triggered by bladder filling, which induces parasympathetic-mediated contraction of the detrusor muscle in concert with relaxation of the internal and external sphincters. Voluntary control of the external sphincter may override this reflex.

The mechanism that controls bladder filling and emptying is vulnerable to injury at many levels, leading to incontinence, urinary retention, and incomplete evacuation. The pelvic splanchnic nerves, also known as nervi erigentes, carry the parasympathetic fibers arising from S2 to S4 that will regulate the emptying of the urinary bladder and rectum and are also responsible for erection. These nerves travel along the pelvic sidewalls beneath the endopelvic fascia to reach their target organs. This location makes them vulnerable to injury during rectal and prostatic surgery, leading to bladder dysfunction. Nerve-sparing surgery of the rectum and prostate avoids injury to these nerves by dissecting along a plane that is adjacent to the organ. Radiation therapy does not protect the nerves and may lead to their dysfunction [17].

Spinal cord injuries lead to bladder dysfunction. In general, spinal cord lesions above S2 spare parasympathetic function while interrupting inhibitory influences from higher centers, leading to bladder spasticity. In contrast, lesions to levels S2–S4 or to the cauda equina disrupt afferent fibers from the bladder, destroying the reflex responsible for bladder contraction in response to filling. This leads to an atonic neurogenic bladder [18].

Answer
d

9. All of the following are correct *except*:
   (a) The bladder is an abdominal organ in the child.
   (b) The bladder enters the true pelvis after puberty.
   (c) In cases of severe urinary retention the dome of the bladder may ascend above the umbilicus.
   (d) A full bladder provides an excellent window for the ultrasonographic examination of the pelvis.
   (e) The bladder must be emptied before any infraumbilical midline peritoneal puncture.

Comments While the dome of the bladder is covered by peritoneum, the bladder itself is considered an extraperitoneal organ. In the adult, it resides within the true pelvis, between the pubic bones and the rectum or vagina. Laterally, it extends towards the pelvic sidewalls. Inferiorly, it rests upon the pelvic diaphragm. As the bladder fills and rises outside the true pelvis, it comes to occupy the space of Retzius. This space is continuous with the preperitoneal space of Bogros as well as with the retroperitoneal space. All of these spaces may be occupied with urine in cases of extraperitoneal bladder rupture. The bladder cannot extend above the umbilicus, even in the most severe cases of urinary retention. In effect, the umbilicus is the apex of the space of Retzius (Fig. 20.4).

The ultrasonographic examination of the pelvis is an integral part of the FAST exam (Focused Assessment with Sonography in Trauma) as well as the evaluation of pelvic organs. In this setting, the bladder is allowed to fill and exit the true pelvis, providing a window for the ultrasonic waves to reach pelvic organs. On the same note, the bladder must be emptied before any infraumbilical peritoneal punctures such as those carried out for peritoneal lavage or blind laparoscopic trocar placement.

In the infant, the bladder is an abdominal organ, occupying the preperitoneal space below the umbilicus. Towards the 5th–6th year of age, it begins its descent into the true pelvis. This determines that the pediatric bladder is susceptible to injury during blunt abdominal trauma.

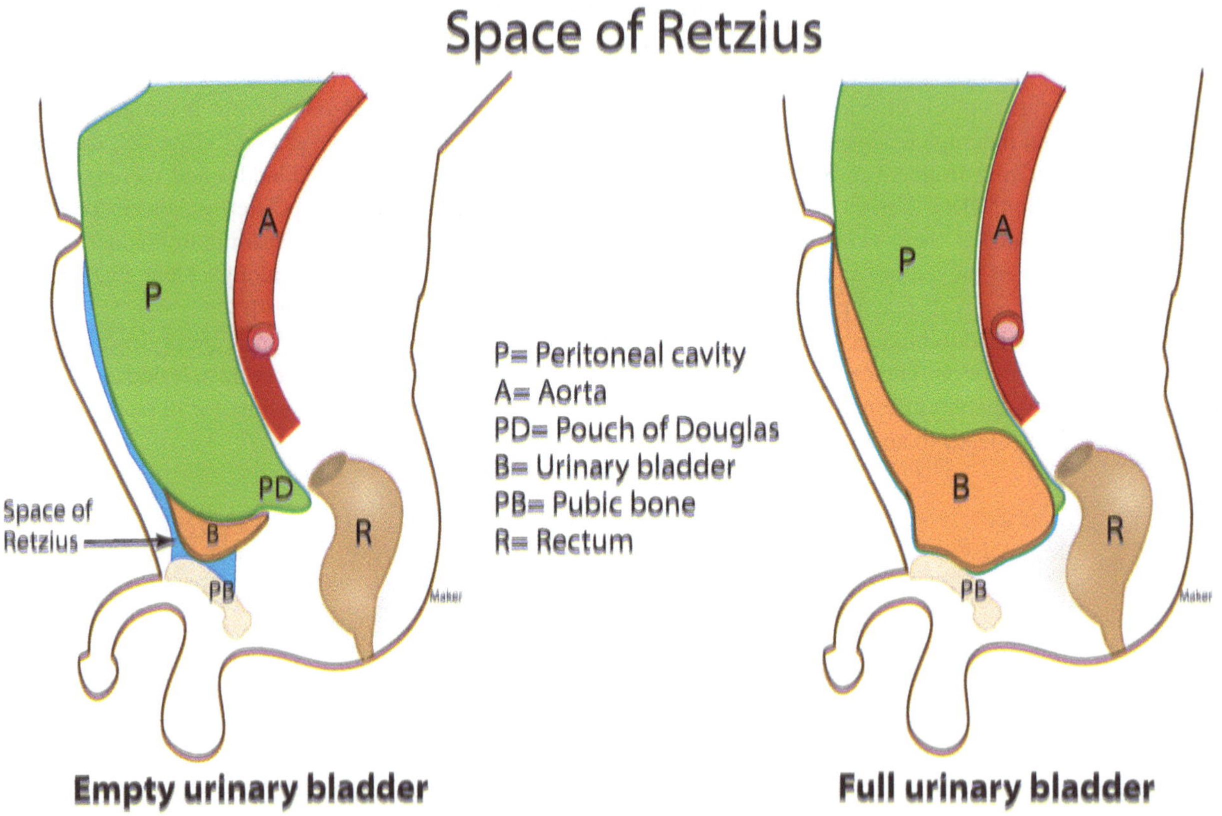

Fig. 20.4 Retropubic space is a part of the extraperitoneal or preperitoneal space which is between the pubic bone and the urinary bladder. This space can potentially extend superiorly up to the umbilicus, laterally to the medial umbilical ligaments, and inferiorly to pubovesical or puboprostatic ligaments. *P* peritoneal cavity, *A* aorta, *PD* pouch of Douglas, *B* urinary bladder, *PB* pubic bone, *R*, rectum

Answer
e

10. All of the following are correct *except*:
    (a) Exstrophy of the bladder is the pathologic opening of the bladder to the exterior through the abdominal wall.
    (b) Exstrophy of the bladder is accompanied by epispadias and failure of midline fusion.
    (c) Exstrophy of the bladder represents the nonfusion of the lateral folds forming the anterior abdominal wall.
    (d) Exstrophy of the bladder extends above the umbilicus.
    (e) After repair, patients with exstrophy of the bladder experience a high rate of vesicoureteral reflux.

Comments Bladder exstrophy is an uncommon condition, occurring in 1 of every 20,000–40,000 live births. It represents a failure in the fusion of the midline structures (lateral abdominal folds) below the umbilicus, also involving the pubic bones and genitals. In this condition, the anterior wall of the bladder is nonexistent, and the posterior bladder wall can be seen through a defect in the lower anterior abdominal wall spanning the distance from the umbilicus to the anus [19].

Even though this malformation is impressive, patients seldom have associated life-threatening conditions. Initial treatment consists of protection of the exposed urothelium. Repair of the defect involves pelvic osteotomies to correct the pubic diastasis, followed by bladder closure, repair of the anterior abdominal wall, placement of the bladder in the pelvis, and repair of the epispadias. Of note, patients with bladder exstrophy have an increased risk of developing latex allergy as do patients with myelomeningocele [20].

Answer
d

11. All of the following are correct *except*:
    (a) Extraperitoneal bladder ruptures are treated with Foley catheter drainage.
    (b) Intraperitoneal bladder ruptures require surgical repair and drainage.
    (c) Bladder injuries must be ruled out in the presence of pelvic fractures.
    (d) The diagnostic test of choice to rule out bladder injuries is cystourethrography.
    (e) Bladder injuries most commonly present in isolated fashion.

Comments The bladder is exposed to two distinct mechanisms of injury. When empty, it rests within the pelvis and may be injured by the shearing forces or bone fragments generated in pelvic fractures. As the bladder fills and becomes intra-abdominal, it becomes vulnerable to direct dome injuries. The former mechanism commonly leads to extraperitoneal bladder ruptures, while the latter gives rise to intraperitoneal ruptures. Missiles may cause both intra- and extraperitoneal bladder ruptures.

Hematuria is the main presenting sign of bladder rupture, but it may be absent. Other manifestations include pelvic pain and inability to void. The test of choice to diagnose a bladder rupture is a retrograde cystogram. For this test to be adequate, the bladder must be distended with contrast to approximately 300 ml, and later emptied to check for posterior ruptures that may have been obscured by the full bladder. In males, this test must be preceded by a retrograde urethrogram, due to the association with urethral injury.

Extraperitoneal bladder rupture is most commonly associated with pelvic injuries. Cystography may demonstrate a bladder that is displaced by a pelvic hematoma, giving it a classic pear shape. Extravasated urine may extend along the retroperitoneum and preperitoneal spaces. In addition, it may reach the scrotum through the inguinal canal or the thigh through the obturator foramen. Primary treatment consists of drainage with a large-bore urinary catheter. Surgical repair should be undertaken if drainage is not possible, if there is injury to other organs or injury to the bladder neck. In these instances, the bladder is entered through the dome, and the repair is performed from within the bladder.

Intraperitoneal bladder injuries often result from bursting of the bladder due to sudden increases in pressure. A common mechanism is through pressure exerted on a full bladder by seat belts in motor vehicle collisions. The area of injury is the dome because this is the thinnest and most mobile part of the bladder. Immediate watertight layered bladder repair is indicated. Reabsorbable sutures are employed to avoid later urinary stone formation. The bladder must then be drained with a large-bore Foley catheter. When undertaking surgical repair, it is imperative to fully inspect the inside of the bladder for other injuries that may not be initially apparent. This is usually accomplished through the injury itself, which may be enlarged to allow better visualization [21] (Fig. 20.5).

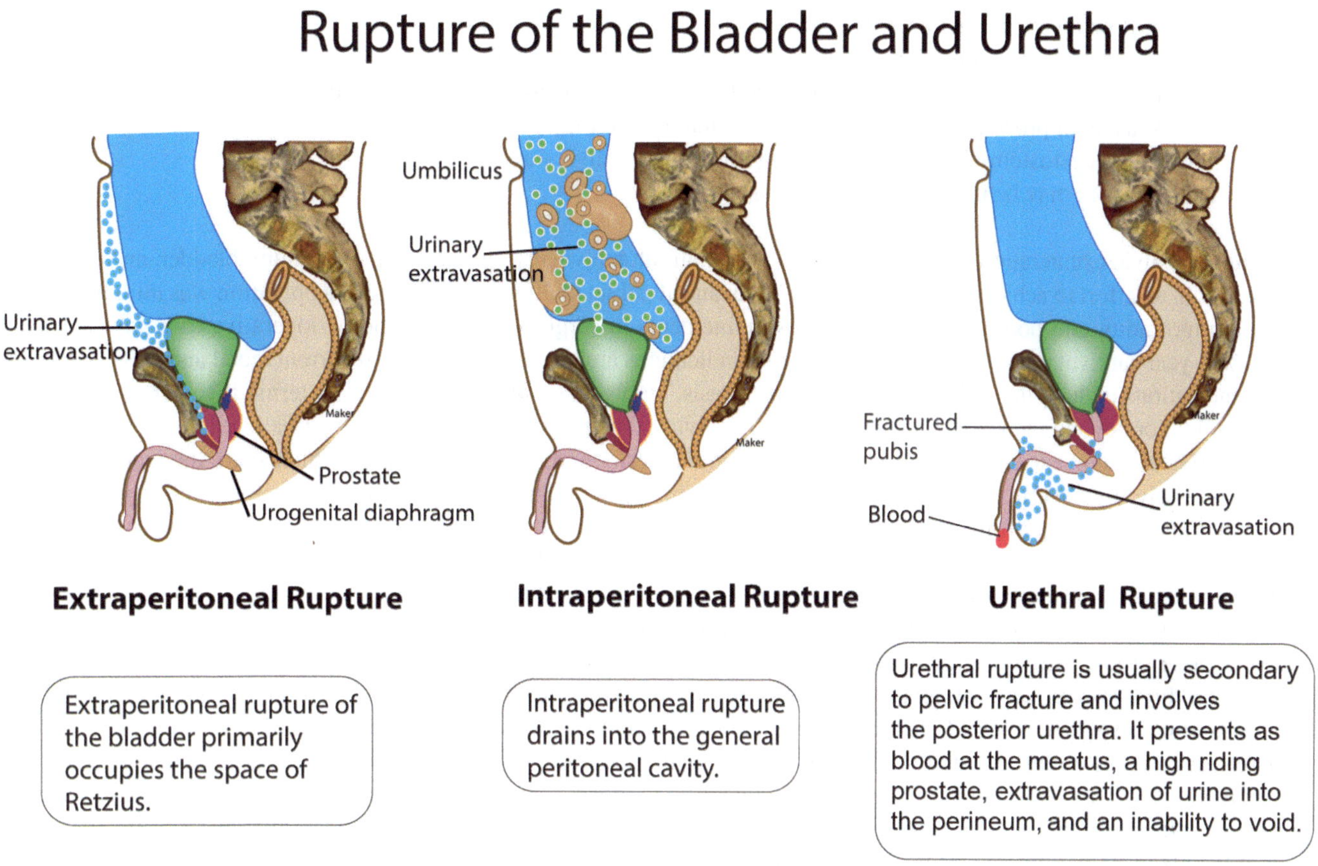

Fig. 20.5 Rupture of the bladder and urethra is a common scenario in multiorgan blunt trauma, specifically when associated with pelvic fractures. Diagnosis of each of the three types is important as the treatment strategies and the urgency changes

Answer

e

12. All of the following are correct *except*:
    (a) Pelvic exenteration is contraindicated in the presence of metastatic disease.
    (b) Urinary diversion after cystectomy is preferably achieved through a segment of defunctionalized small intestine.
    (c) The psoas hitch procedure is indicated for proximal ureteral injury.
    (d) Suprapubic cystostomy is indicated for long-term urinary diversion.
    (e) The appendix may be used for urinary diversion.

Comments Pelvic exenteration consists of the removal of all intrapelvic organs including the rectum, bladder, and reproductive organs in an effort to achieve en bloc resection of advanced pelvic malignancies. While this operation was initially fraught with high morbidity and poor oncologic outcomes, refinements in surgical technique and perioperative care have achieved 20–60 % 5-year survival rates. The main contemporary indications are locally advanced or recurrent rectal and cervical cancer. Contraindications include the presence of distant metastasis, involvement of the common or external iliac vessels, and local extension into or beyond the walls of the pelvis. Rarely pelvic exenteration is performed with palliative intent.

The classical pelvic exenteration has been modified into anterior and posterior varieties, which spare the rectum or bladder, respectively. Reconstruction after pelvic exenteration includes creation of a permanent colostomy, urostomy, vaginal reconstruction, and filling of the pelvic dead space. This last step is particularly important as it impedes the descent of the bowel into the pelvis, which may result in delayed bowel obstruction and may limit postoperative radiation therapy [22].

Initial attempts at urinary diversion after cystectomy consisted of ureteroileostomies and ureterocolostomies. However, these operations lead to a high rate of urinary tract infection, renal impairment, and fluid and electrolyte imbalances. In order to avoid these problems, reconstruction shifted into diversions into defunctionalized segments of the bowel (ileum or sigmoid colon) brought out as incontinent stomas. Since the 1980s, several techniques for the creation of continent, non-refluxing urostomies have been reported, including creation of neo-bladders and artificial sphincters [23] (Fig. 20.6).

Ureteral continuity may be compromised as a result of trauma and planned or unplanned surgical division. When the injury is limited to the lower ureter and yet is severe enough to make a primary repair unfeasible, the bladder may be used for reconstruction. In this setting, a psoas hitch ureteral implantation is performed. This operation consists of the mobilization of the bladder (by division of the obliterated umbilical arteries), elevation and lateral traction of the bladder by fixation to the psoas tendon, and creation of a tension-free non-refluxing ureterocystostomy over a stent [24] (Fig. 20.7).

Bladder drainage is most commonly achieved through the urethra with the use of a Foley catheter. However, in instances where this is not possible, or when long-term drainage is desired, a suprapubic cystostomy may be performed. Common indications for this procedure include urethral injury, severe neurologic impairment, neurogenic bladder in patients unable to self-catheterize, and Fournier's gangrene. Suprapubic cystostomy is performed through a suprapubic incision. The bladder wall is opened to allow passage of a catheter and then closed over it in watertight fashion [25].

The Mitrofanoff procedure is an alternative to suprapubic cystostomy. It may be used in the setting of neuropathic bladder, advanced malignancies, and congenital malformations of the genitourinary tract. This operation consists of isolating the appendix with its intact blood supply, and using it as a continent conduit between the bladder and the skin. The umbilicus is often chosen as the site of implantation, as it allows the shortest distance to the bladder. The bladder can then be accessed through intermittent catheterization [26].

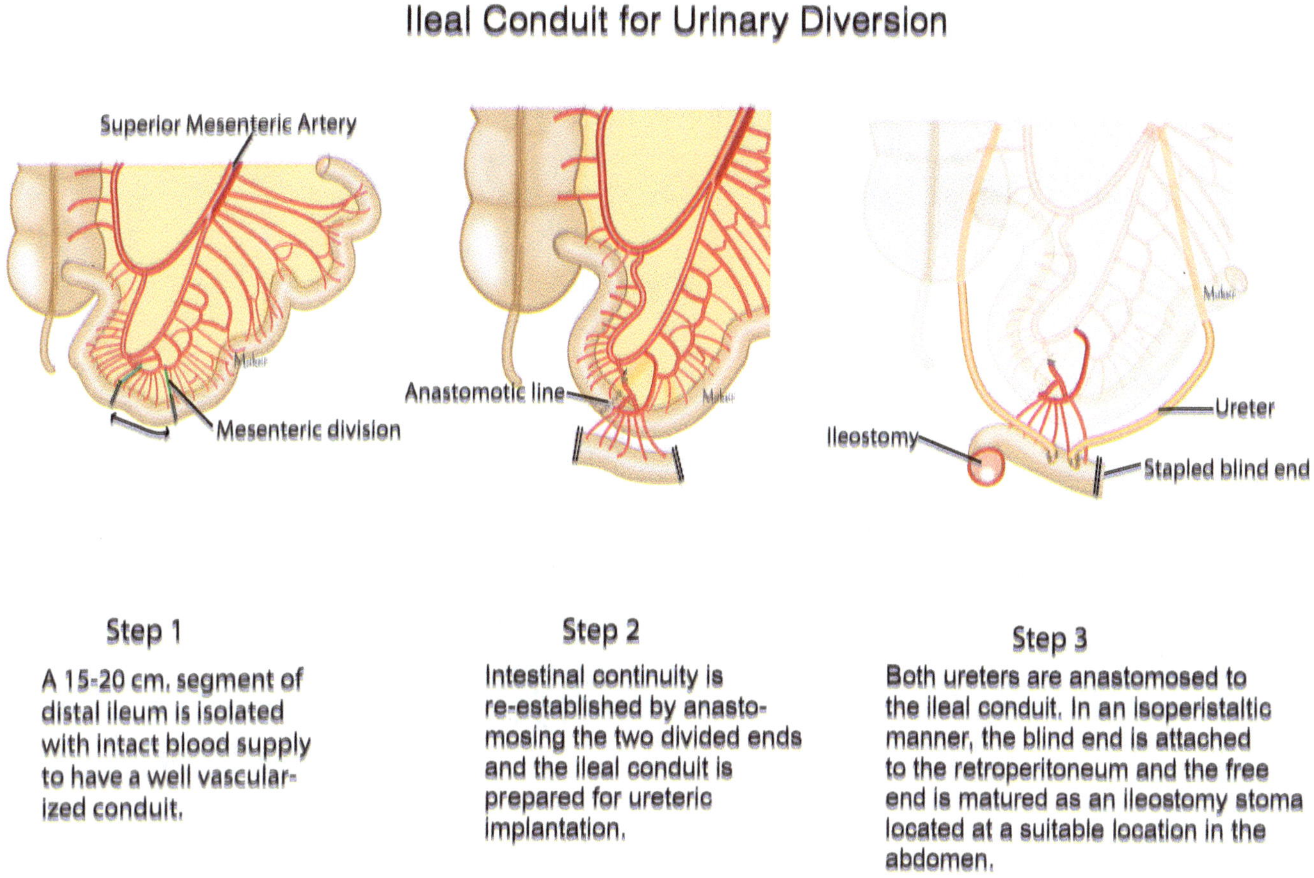

Fig. 20.6 An ileal conduit is an old, time-proven option for providing an external stoma for the ureters when other options are not available or contraindicated

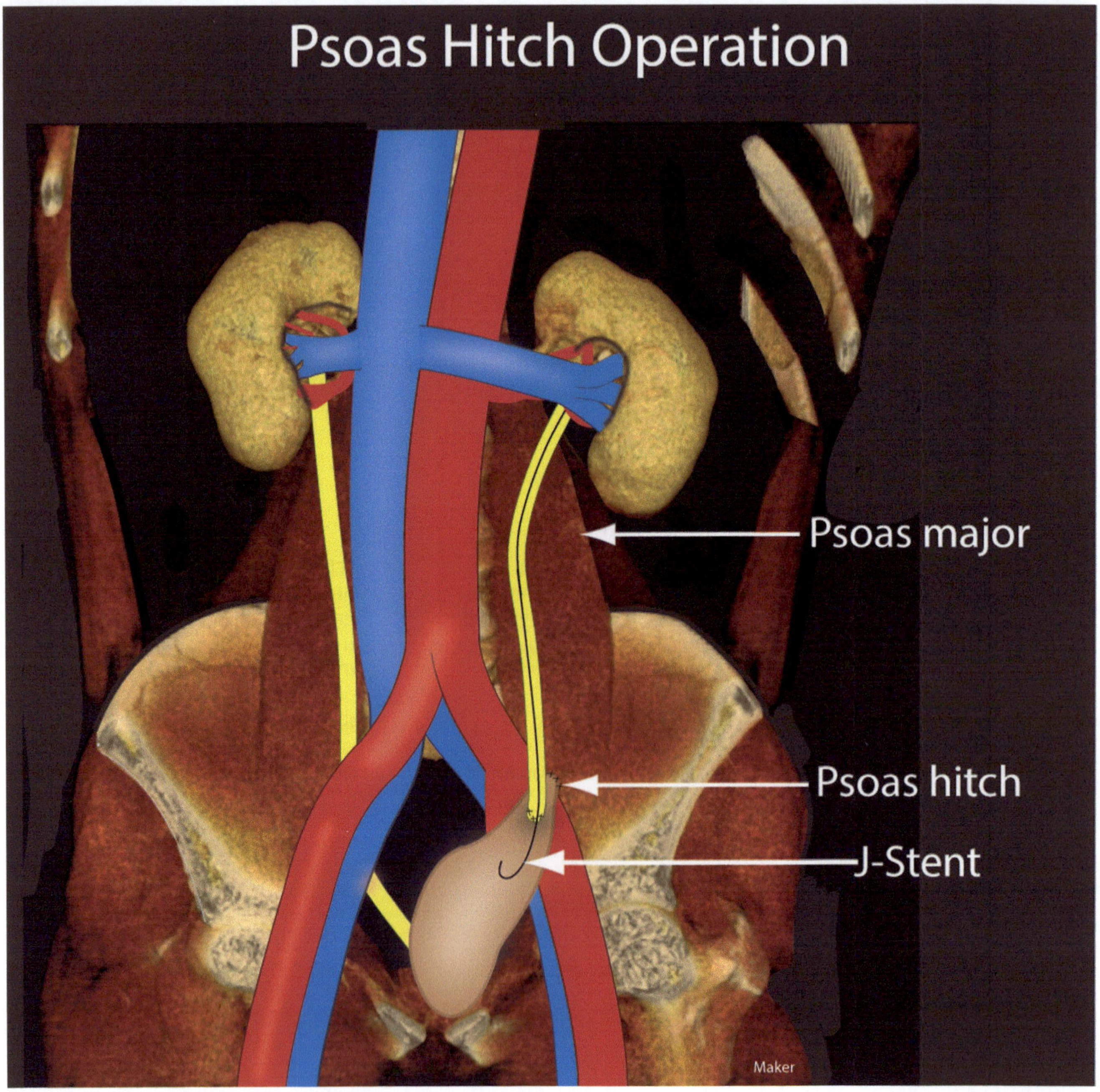

Fig. 20.7 In a lower ureteral injury, the bladder is mobilized and attached to the psoas muscle so that a shortened injured ureter can be reimplanted over a double J stent without tension

Answer

c

References

1. Baker LA, Gomez RA. Embryonic development of the ureter. Semin Nephrol. 1998;18:569–84.
2. Lechner MS, Dressler GR. The molecular basis of embryonic kidney development. Mech Dev. 1997;62:105–20.
3. Marshall FF. Embryology of the lower genitourinary tract. Urol Clin N Am. 1978;5:3–15.
4. O'Brien J, Buckley O, Doody O, Ward E, Persaud T, Torreggiani W. Imaging of horseshoe kidneys and their complications. J Med Imaging Radiat Oncol. 2008;52:216–26.
5. Stein RJ, Desai MM. Management of urolithiasis in the congenitally abnormal kidney (horseshoe and ectopic). Curr Opin Urol. 2007;17:125–31.
6. Terada N, Arai Y, Kinukawa N, Terai A. The 10-year natural history of simple renal cysts. Urology. 2008;71:7–11; discussion 11–2.
7. Terada N, Ichioka K, Matsuta Y, Okubo K, Yoshimura K, Arai Y. The natural history of simple renal cysts. J Urol. 2002;167:21–3.
8. Bisceglia M, Galliani CA, Senger C, Stallone C, Sessa A. Renal cystic diseases: a review. Adv Anat Pathol. 2006;13:26–56.
9. Grantham JJ. Clinical practice. Autosomal dominant polycystic kidney disease. N Engl J Med. 2008;359:1477–85.
10. Turkbey B, Ocak I, Daryanani K, et al. Autosomal recessive polycystic kidney disease and congenital hepatic fibrosis (ARPKD/CHF). Pediatr Radiol. 2009;39:100–11.
11. Gupta A, Tello R. Accessory renal arteries are not related to hypertension risk: a review of MR angiography data. AJR Am J Roentgenol. 2004;182:1521–4.
12. Urban BA, Ratner LE, Fishman EK. Three-dimensional volume-rendered CT angiography of the renal arteries and veins: normal anatomy, variants, and clinical applications. Radiographics. 2001;21:373–86; questionnaire 549–55.
13. Frober R. Surgical anatomy of the ureter. BJU Int. 2007;100:949–65.
14. Amin M, Blandford AT, Polk Jr HC. Renal fascia of Gerota. Urology. 1976;7:1–3.
15. Chesbrough RM, Burkhard TK, Martinez AJ, Burks DD. Gerota versus Zuckerkandl: the renal fascia revisited. Radiology. 1989; 173:845–6.
16. Roberts MM. Neurophysiology in neurourology. Muscle Nerve. 2008;38:815–36.
17. Chai TC, Steers WD. Neurophysiology of micturition and continence. Urol Clin N Am. 1996;23:221–36.
18. Samson G, Cardenas DD. Neurogenic bladder in spinal cord injury. Phys Med Rehabil Clin N Am. 2007;18:255–74, vi.
19. Eeg KR, Khoury AE. The exstrophy-epispadias complex. Curr Urol Rep. 2008;9:158–64.
20. Kiddoo DA, Carr MC, Dulczak S, Canning DA. Initial management of complex urological disorders: bladder exstrophy. Urol Clin N Am. 2004;31:417–26, vii–viii.
21. Corriere Jr JN, Sandler CM. Diagnosis and management of bladder injuries. Urol Clin N Am. 2006;33:67–71, vi.
22. Pawlik TM, Skibber JM, Rodriguez-Bigas MA. Pelvic exenteration for advanced pelvic malignancies. Ann Surg Oncol. 2006;13:612–23.
23. Mirhashemi R, Im S, Yazdani T. Urinary diversion following radical pelvic surgery. Curr Opin Obstet Gynecol. 2004;16:419–22.
24. Ahn M, Loughlin KR. Psoas hitch ureteral reimplantation in adults–analysis of a modified technique and timing of repair. Urology. 2001;58:184–7.
25. Feifer A, Corcos J. Contemporary role of suprapubic cystostomy in treatment of neuropathic bladder dysfunction in spinal cord injured patients. Neurourol Urodyn. 2008;27:475–9.
26. Mhiri MN, Bahloul A, Chabchoub K. Mitrofanoff appendicovesicostomy in children: indication and results. Prog Urol. 2007;17: 245–9.

21 Genital System

1. All of the following are correct *except*:
   (a) Cryptorchidism results from an arrest in testicular descent.
   (b) The gubernaculum testis pulls the testicle into the scrotum.
   (c) The round ligament is the female equivalent of the gubernaculum testis.
   (d) The incidence of undescended testicles is higher in premature neonates.
   (e) Surgical correction of an undescended testicle always involves repair of an indirect inguinal hernia.

Comments Incomplete testicular descent affects 2–8 % of male newborns. Testicles located in the abdomen and inguinal canal are subject to a 2–3 °C temperature increase, which inhibits spermatogenesis and increases the risk of malignant transformation. Endocrine function, including testosterone production, is normal in undescended testicles. In cases of unilateral cryptorchidism, the contralateral testis has normal function and no increased risk of developing cancer. Approximately 20 % of undescended testicles are non-palpable. While ultrasound may be useful in identifying testicles in the inguinal canal, the gold standard for the diagnosis of intra-abdominal testicles is laparoscopy. In the past, it had been thought that intra-abdominal testicles carried a particularly elevated risk of malignant transformation when compared to more caudal locations; however, this has not been proven to be the case.

The testicles originate from the urogenital ridge. Initially, they are attached to the abdominal surface of the diaphragm by the cranio-suspensory ligament, which degenerates to allow testicular descent. Caudally, the testicles are attached to the gubernaculum testis, which guides the testicles into the scrotum. In the female, the cranio-suspensory ligament persists, forming the ovarian ligament, while the gubernaculum becomes the round ligament.

During testicular migration, the gubernaculum thickens considerably and widens the inguinal canal to allow testicular passage. The forces driving testicular descent appear to be an increase in intra-abdominal pressure as well as lengthening of the embryo while the gubernaculum remains with a fixed length. The idea that the gubernaculum "pulls" the testicle into the scrotum is no longer considered accurate. Testicular descent is an androgen-mediated process [1, 2].

Undescended testicles are at risk of malignant transformation, with a relative risk of 2.75–8 in relation to the normal population. Orchiopexy after puberty carries a two to sixfold risk of malignancy in comparison to prepubertal orchiopexy [3]. Surgically descended testicles have an increased risk of developing non-seminomatous tumors, while undescended testicles tend to develop seminomas [4]. Optimal treatment of cryptorchidism consists of orchiopexy, ideally between 6 and 12 months of age, and at worse before puberty in cases of delayed diagnosis. Cryptorchidism is always associated with a patent processus vaginalis that must be ligated at the time or orchiopexy. Undescended testicles diagnosed later in life should be removed. Occasionally observation may be acceptable in patients with high anesthesia risk or those older than 50 years [5, 6].

V.K. Maker, E.D. Guzman-Arrieta, *Cognitive Pearls in General Surgery*,
DOI 10.1007/978-1-4939-1850-8_21, © Springer Science+Business Media New York 2015

Treatment with human chorionic gonadotropin (hCG) has an efficacy of approximately 20 %, as compared to a 95 % success rate of surgery. In addition, there is evidence to suggest that hCG treatment may induce germinal cell apoptosis, leading to testicular atrophy and dysfunction later in life.

Another entity of interest is retractile testicle. They are defined as suprascrotal testis that can be easily manipulated into the scrotum and remain there without tension, until they ascend due to the cremasteric reflex. They carry no risk of infertility or malignancy. However, follow-up is recommended because up to one third of cases may become fixed in a suprascrotal position (acquired undescended testicles) [7].

Answer

b

2. All of the following are correct *except*:
   (a) The processus vaginalis is an extension of the peritoneum into the scrotum in the fetus.
   (b) The tunica vaginalis envelops the whole testis except at its posterior border and superior pole.
   (c) The testicle is intraperitoneal.
   (d) The canal of Nuck is the female equivalent of the processus vaginalis and may develop a hydrocele.
   (e) Congenital indirect hernias are a consequence of a patent processus vaginalis.

Comments As the testicles descend into the scrotum, they are preceded by the gubernaculums as well as by a fingerlike projection of peritoneum, which forms the processus vaginalis. The processus vaginalis normally becomes obliterated by the 36th–40th week of gestation (except for the portion that becomes the tunica vaginalis), thereby closing the internal inguinal ring. Frequently, the processus vaginalis is patent at birth and closes in early life. The left processus vaginalis becomes obliterated before the right, owing to the earlier descent of the left testicle [1].

Patency of the processus vaginalis is necessary for, but not synonymous with, the occurrence of indirect inguinal hernias and communicating hydroceles. It has been shown that inguinal hernias occur in only 8–12 % of patients with a patent processus vaginalis. Given the central role of patency of the processus vaginalis in pediatric inguinal hernias, treatment consists of high ligation of the hernial sac. In females, the processus vaginalis becomes the canal of Nuck, which normally becomes obliterated. However, the canal of Nuck may give rise to hydroceles, which manifest as inguinolabial masses [8–10].

In the adult, the tunica vaginalis is a two-layered mesothelial sac that envelops the testis almost completely, leaving the epididymal region uncovered (upper pole and posterior border).

Answer

c

3. All of the following are correct *except*:
   (a) The genital branch of the genitofemoral accompanies the spermatic vessels.
   (b) The iliohypogastric nerve supplies the lower scrotum.
   (c) The ilioinguinal nerve supplies the penile root, the upper scrotum, and the medial thigh.
   (d) The nervi erigentes (S2–S4) are responsible for erection.
   (e) The pudendal nerves provide sensory innervation to the penis and perineum.

Comments The sensory innervation of the penis, scrotum, and pubic region is provided by multiple branches of the lumbar plexus. These nerves may be subject to injury during inguinal and pelvic surgery.

The ilioinguinal nerve supplies the base of the penis, upper scrotum, and medial thigh. It is readily identified in the inguinal canal where it courses anterior to the spermatic cord, just beneath the external oblique aponeurosis. The genital branch of the genitofemoral nerve accompanies the spermatic artery and vein along the dorsal aspect of the spermatic cord. Its motor branch is responsible for the innervations of the cremaster muscle. Its sensory branch supplies the scrotum. The iliohypogastric nerve runs along the lower edge of the internal oblique muscle and supplies the skin of the pubic region [11–13].

The sensory supply of the penis is provided by the pudendal nerves which originate in the sacral plexus and course along the ischiorectal fossa. The autonomic nerves supply of the penis is provided by the nervi erigentes, which course along the pelvic sidewalls (Fig. 21.1).

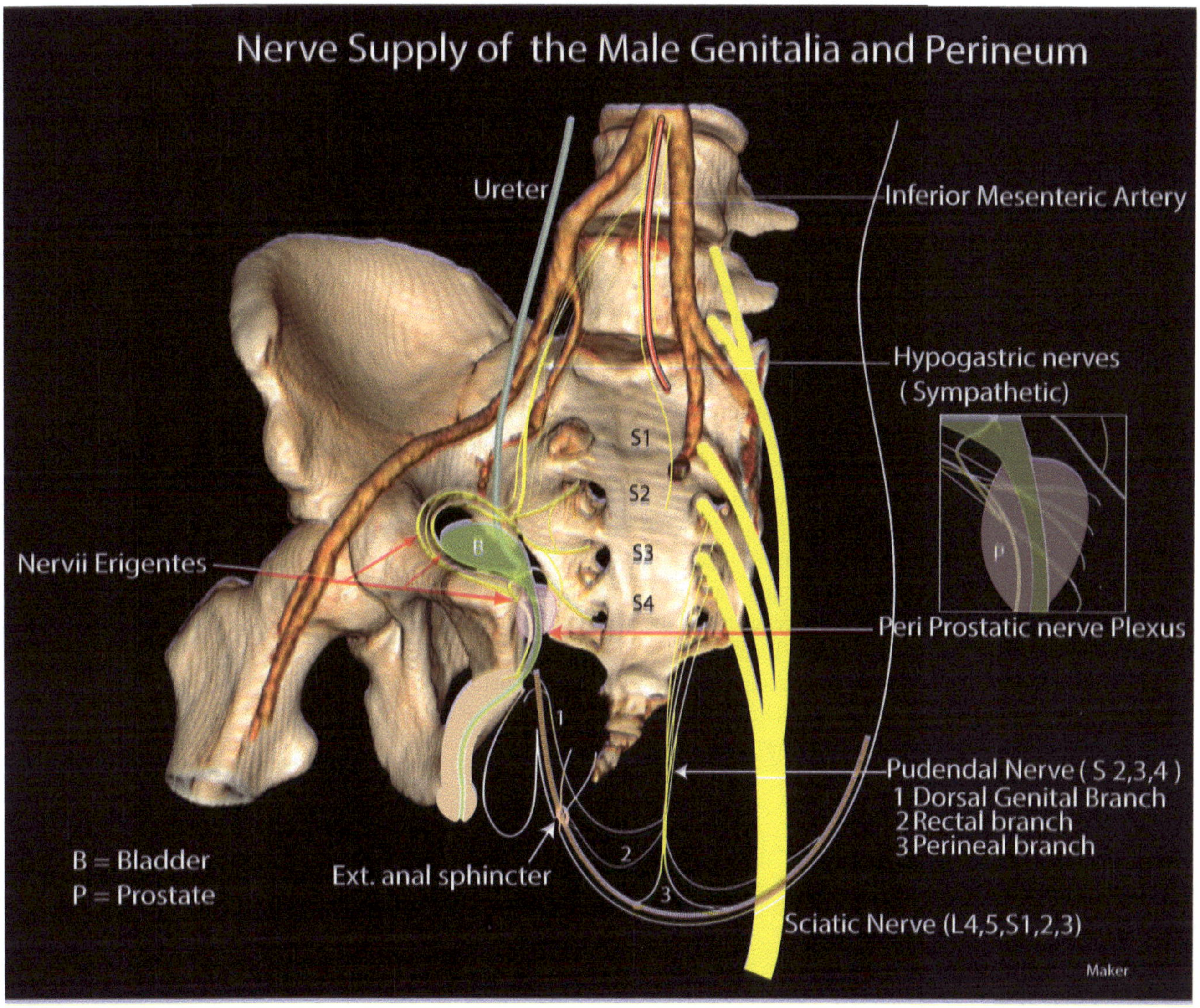

Fig. 21.1 Detailed knowledge of the nerve supply to the perineum, pelvic viscera, and genitalia is a must for the pelvic surgeon. Parasympathetic nerves come from the presacral S2, S3, and S4 foramina. Sympathetic nerves descend down from the abdomen along the gonadal vessels and the inferior mesenteric artery. The somatic innervation comes through pudendal nerves traveling from the pudendal canal on the lateral wall of the ischioanal fossa. These nerves all come together at the end organs to create a symphony of interrelated effects

Answer

b

4. All of the following are correct *except*:
   (a) Sperm granulomas result from inadequate ligation of the vas deferens during vasectomy.
   (b) The ejaculatory ducts are formed by the fusion of the vas deferens with the seminal vesicles.
   (c) The seminal vesicles store sperm cells after they exit the vas deferens.
   (d) Cowper's glands are located within the substance of the genitourinary diaphragm.
   (e) The prostatic utricle opens in the urethra and represents the male uterus.

Comments Microscopically, the testicles are divided into approximately 300 pyramidal lobules, which contain the convoluted seminiferous tubules, where spermatogenesis occurs. Posteriorly, the seminiferous tubules come together forming the rete testis that carries the sperm cells into the head of the epididymis. Testosterone is produced in the cells of Leydig, which occupy the spaces between the seminiferous tubules. Sertoli cells are modulated by testosterone and FSH, playing a key role in the maturation of sperm cells.

The epididymis is a very long and convoluted duct that lies along the posterior aspect of the testicle. Its function is to participate in the maturation and storage of sperm cells. It is divided into a head, body, and tail. The latter gives rise to the vas deferens, which forms part of the spermatic cord. Once in the pelvis, it reaches the prostate after fusing with the seminal vesicles to form the ejaculatory duct, which enters the prostate and empties into the urethra [14, 15].

Although their name may suggest otherwise, the seminal vesicles do not participate in the storage of the sperm cells. This function is carried out by the caudal aspect of the epididymis. Rather, the seminal vesicles are glands that produce a fructose- and a prostaglandin-rich fluid that makes up to 70 % of the ejaculate volume [16]. The ejaculatory ducts traverse the prostate to reach the prostatic urethra on either side of the verumontanum. The prostatic utricle is a small crypt in the central portion of the verumontanum and is thought to represent the remnants of the Müllerian system. Rarely, neoplasms similar to those found in the uterus can be found in this location. Cowper's glands are located within the genitourinary diaphragm and empty into the bulbous urethra. They produce a fluid that precedes ejaculation. Its function is thought to be the alkalinization of the urethra [17] (Fig. 21.2).

During vasectomy, the vas deferens is divided and a portion is excised. Rarely, extravasation of sperm cells may lead to the formation of an inflammatory mass known as sperm granuloma [18].

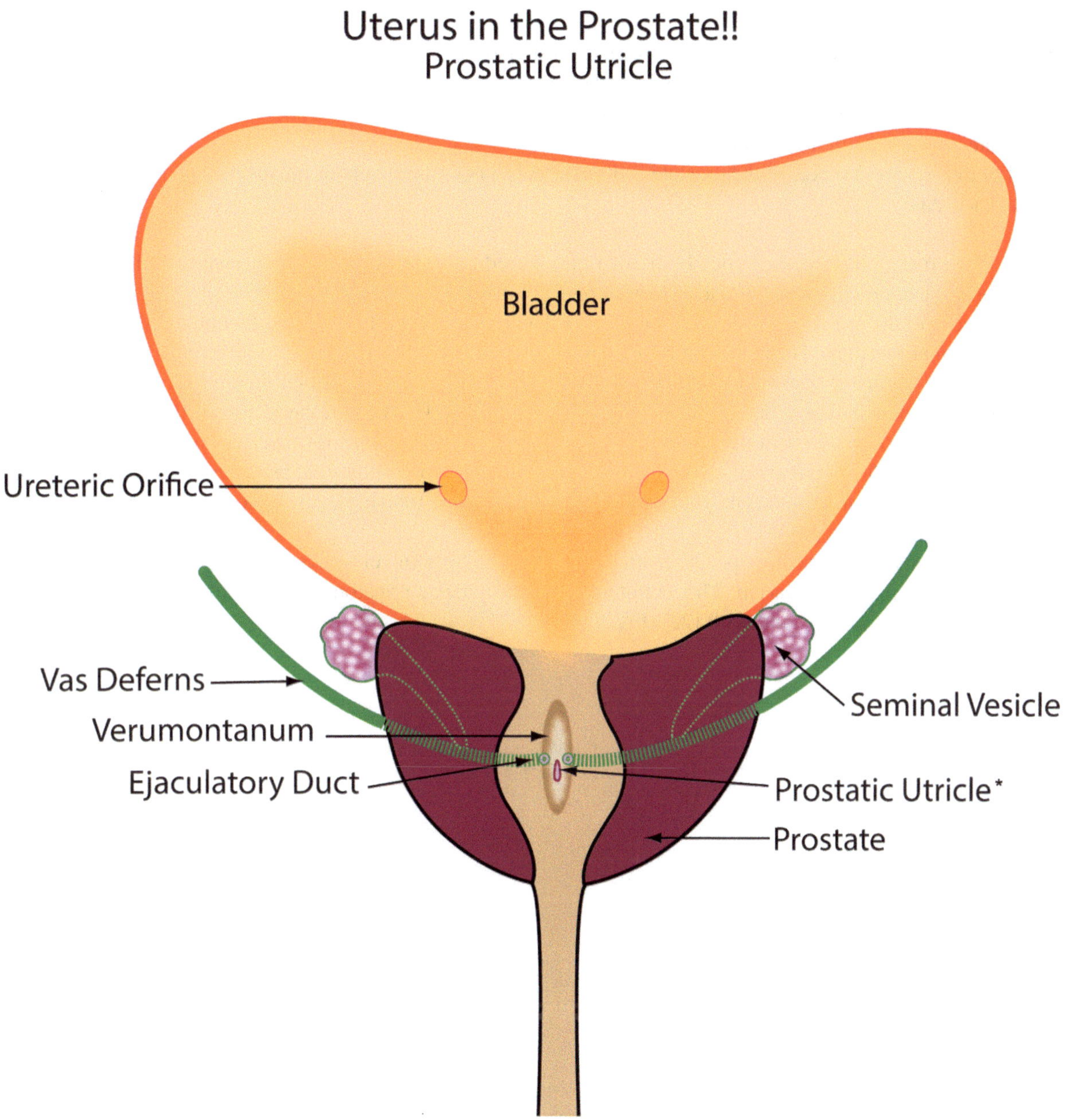

Fig. 21.2 Prostatic utricle (vagina masculina) is believed to be the Müllerian duct remnant in the prostatic urethra. Endometrial-type cancers arising in this area have been reported. *Prostatic utricle may be of urogenital sinus origin

Answer
c

5. All of the following are correct *except*:
   (a) The prostate gland has four zones: transitional, central, peripheral, and fibromuscular.
   (b) Most prostate carcinomas originate in the peripheral zone.
   (c) Benign prostatic hypertrophy arises in the transitional zone.
   (d) Prostate carcinoma often causes urethral obstruction.
   (e) Part of the venous drainage of the prostate is directed to the extradural venous plexus of Batson, explaining spine and skull metastases.

Comments The prostate had been classically divided into paired lobes. However, further anatomical studies allowed the division of the prostate into histologically and embryologically distinct zones [19].

The central zone of the prostate envelops the ejaculatory ducts and is of Wolffian origin. It comprises 25 % of the prostatic mass and is glandular in nature. The transition zone surrounds the urethra and is anterior to the central zone. It shares a common origin with the urethra. It constitutes 5 % of the prostatic mass and gives rise to benign prostatic hyperplasia (BPH). Its periurethral location explains the symptoms of urinary obstruction in BPH. The peripheral zone is the largest of the four and surrounds both the central and transitional zones posteriorly and laterally. It is also formed by glandular tissue that gives rise to prostatic carcinoma. Due to its peripheral location, masses in this zone seldom cause urinary obstruction. Finally, the anterior fibromuscular stroma contains no glands and lies anterior to the transition zone, and between the anterolateral projections of the peripheral zone [20, 21].

Prostatic venous drainage deserves special mention. It is formed by a valveless system of veins that communicates with the extradural venous plexus of Batson. This communication provides an anatomical basis for the propensity of prostate cancer to metastasize to the spine and skull [22] (Fig. 21.3).

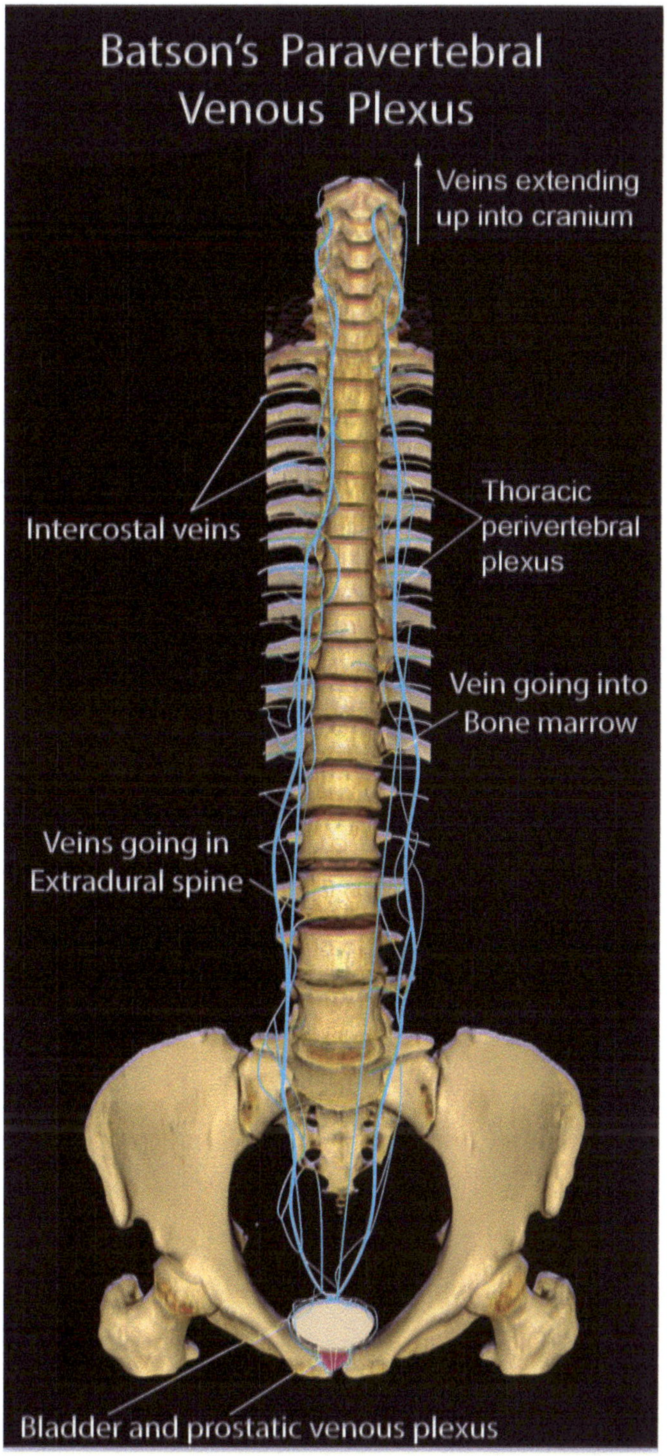

Fig. 21.3 Batson's venous plexus provides a pathway from the pelvis to the skull for the spread of metastatic and septic foci to the vertebra and cranium without systemic spread

Answer
d

6. All of the following are correct *except*:
   (a) The male urethra is divided into prostatic, membranous, and penile areas.
   (b) Urethral rupture above the urogenital diaphragm leads to urine collection in the extraperitoneal pelvis.
   (c) Urethral rupture below the urogenital diaphragm leads to subcutaneous perineal urine collection.
   (d) The urethra is preserved during TURP.
   (e) A high ridding prostate on rectal exam in perineal trauma is diagnostic of urethral rupture.

Comments The male urethra is divided into three segments: prostatic, membranous, and penile. The prostatic urethra is 1–1.5 cm in length. It receives the ejaculatory ducts and is marked by the urethral crest (a continuation of the bladder trigone), the verumontanum, and the prostatic utricle, as described previously. The membranous urethra crosses the urogenital diaphragm, which anchors it to the pelvis, making it vulnerable to shearing forces. The penile urethra starts distal to the urogenital diaphragm and ends in the urethral meatus.

Urethral injury occurs in up to 25 % of male patients with pelvic fractures. Among the fractures, the ones caused by a straddle mechanism causing sacroiliac diastasis have the highest risk. The main types of urethral injury occur above and below the urogenital diaphragm. In injuries above the urogenital diaphragm, the prostate may be displaced cephalad. Urine accumulates in the extraperitoneal pelvis, like with extraperitoneal bladder ruptures. In contrast, injury to the urethra distal to the urogenital diaphragm causes perineal infiltration with urine.

Blood at the urethral meatus, perineal ecchymoses, blood in the scrotum, inability to void, and a high riding prostate on rectal exam all suggest urethral injury. Management includes diagnosis of the injury via retrograde urethrogram. Principles of treatment include urinary diversion (usually by a suprapubic catheter) and delayed repair [22].

Answer
d

7. All of the following are correct *except*:
   (a) Testicular tumors are approached through an inguinal incision.
   (b) Needle biopsy is used to establish the diagnosis of testicular cancer.
   (c) Extratesticular germ cell tumors reside in the retroperitoneal area and may secrete large amounts of β-HCG.
   (d) Testicular tumors are more frequent in younger men.
   (e) The most common tumor of the undescended testicle is seminoma.

Comments Testicular cancer is the most common tumor in males between the ages of 15 and 34. However, its overall incidence is low, affecting only 1 % of the male population. The main risk factor is a history of cryptorchidism. Testicular cancer can arise from the germ cells (seminoma and non-seminoma tumors) as well as from the stroma (Sertoli and Leydig cell tumors).

Seminomas are the most common type of testicular cancer. They typically do not produce any markers. In contrast, non-seminomas may produce β-HCG (choriocarcinoma) and α-fetoprotein (yolk sac tumor). Teratocarcinomas are a third type of non-seminomatous tumor; it does not produce any hormones. Stromal tumors may produce androgens.

Presentation usually consists of the self-diagnosis of a testicular mass. Testicular ultrasound is the imaging modality of choice. Additional studies include tumor markers, lactate dehydrogenase, and chest X-ray. Transinguinal orchiectomy is the treatment of choice and also allows pathologic confirmation. Trans-scrotal approaches are contraindicated because they disrupt lymphatic drainage patterns and violate the multiple testicular envelopes that limit the local extension of malignant processes. Nodal staging is done through CT scanning. Seminomas are very radiosensitive, and nodal control is achieved with radiation therapy. In contrast, non-seminomas have less sensitivity and may require nodal dissection [23–25].

Answer

b

8. All of the following are correct regarding testicular torsion *except*:
   (a) A classic testicular torsion is torsion of the spermatic cord and typically exceeds 540°.
   (b) Torsion of the appendix testis produces a more focal area of pain and often a bluish discoloration over the testicular appendage.
   (c) A gangrenous testicle should be implanted in a subcutaneous pocket of the thigh to preserve testosterone production.
   (d) The bell clapper deformity predisposes to intravaginal testicular torsion.
   (e) The anatomical predisposition to torsion affects both testicles; therefore, the contralateral testicle should be similarly repaired.

Comments Classic intravaginal testicular torsion consists of 540° (1½ turns) or greater rotation of the spermatic cord including the epididymis and testicle. This is the most common type of torsion, resulting in elevation of the testicle with the epididymis in an anterior location. Presentation is that of acute onset testicular pain often accompanied by nausea and vomiting. The cremasteric reflex is abolished. The diagnosis can be confirmed by duplex ultrasound.

Less commonly testicular torsion is the result of an anatomical abnormality in which the tunica vaginalis completely surrounds the testicle and distal spermatic cord, which are freely mobile within this investment (bell clapper deformity). In this setting, the testicle and spermatic cord rotate within the tunica vaginalis.

Treatment should be prompt, with restoration of blood flow within 6 h. While medial to lateral manual detorsion might be successful, definitive treatment is surgical and consist of a trans-scrotal approach, detorsion, and orchiopexy. Contralateral orchiopexy is mandatory. If the testicle is necrotic, orchiectomy is performed.

Extravaginal torsion occurs in approximately 5 % of cases. It is often a prenatal event which occurs before testicular fixation is complete. It presents as a firm scrotal mass in the neonatal period and is not associated with the bell clapper deformity (Fig. 21.4).

Torsion of the appendix testis is an important differential diagnosis. In this scenario, there is also sudden testicular pain. However, tenderness is focal, and the infracted appendage may be seen through the scrotum (blue dot sign). The most important differential diagnosis of testicular torsion is epididymo-orchitis, which often affects the same age group. A wrong diagnosis may be devastating, as epididymo-orchitis is treated medically. The two most important diagnostic tools are ultrasonography and nuclear scan, which must be done on emergency basis because of the time limit to correct testicular torsion [26, 27] (Fig. 21.5).

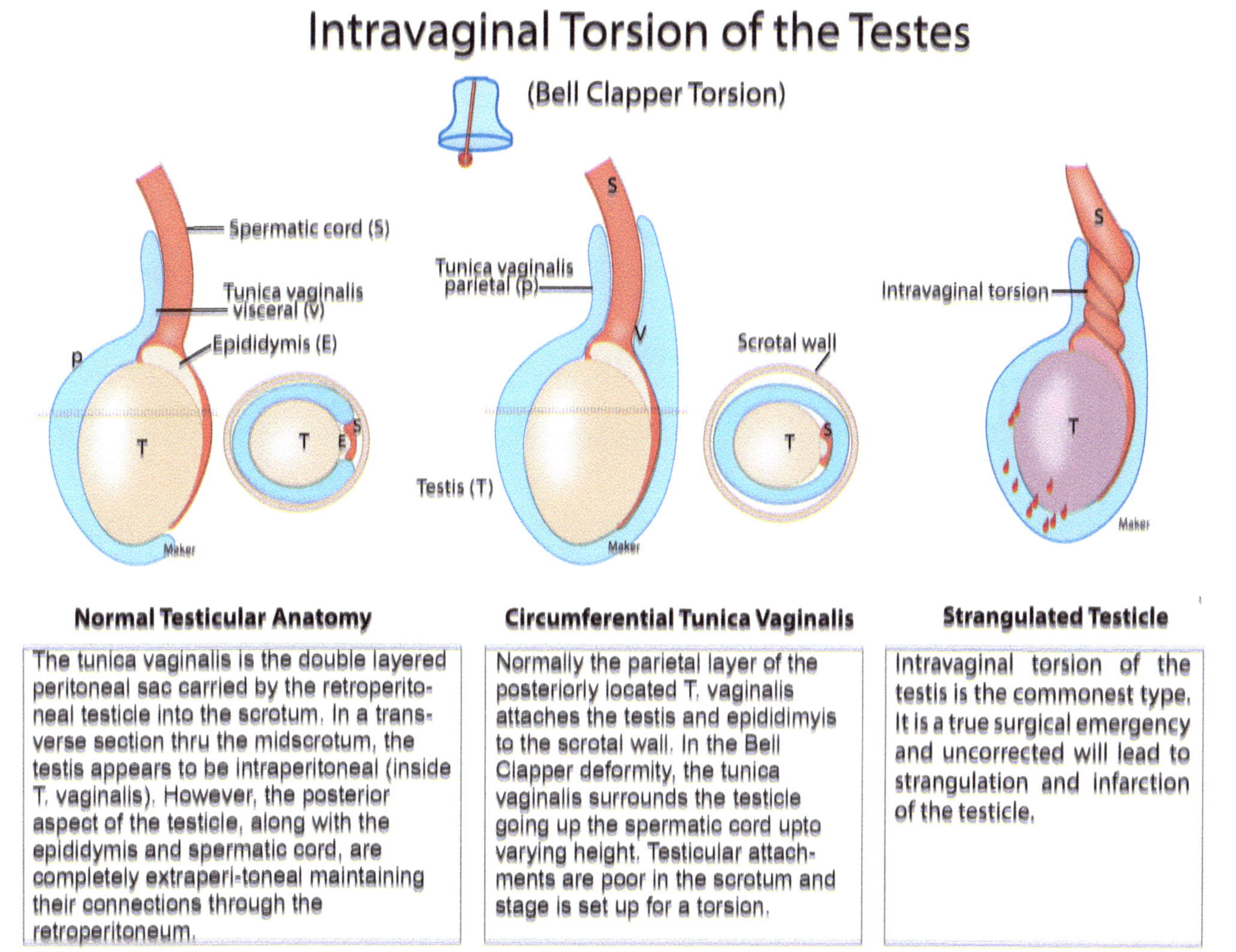

Fig. 21.4 The surgeon taking care of testicular pain must rule out the diagnosis of testicular torsion before establishing the diagnosis of epididymo-orchitis, as this may be the last chance of testicular salvage. Apart from a good history and physical exam, ancillary tests with the ultrasound and nuclear scan may be needed

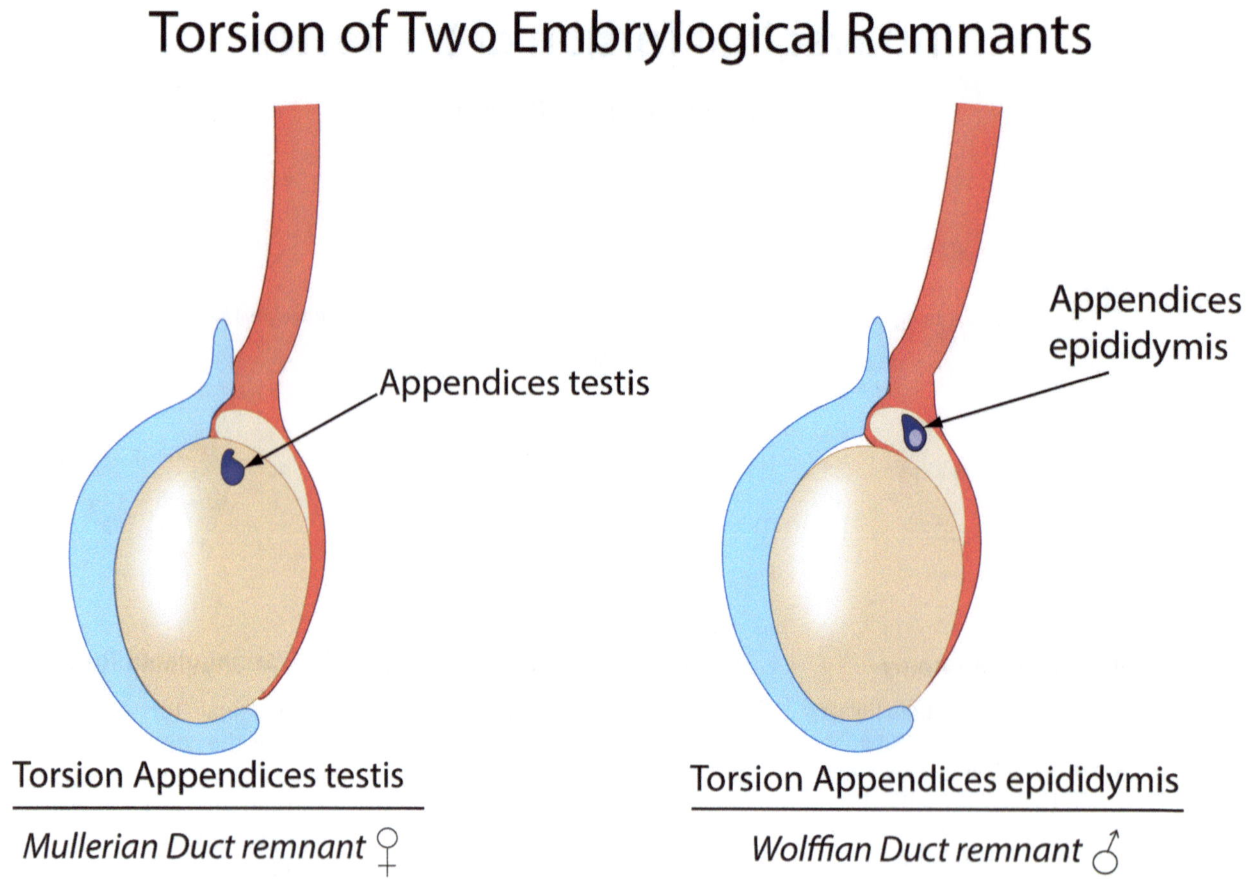

Fig. 21.5 Sudden testicular pain is a surgical emergency, and the correct diagnosis must be established. Apart from a good history and physical exam looking for a blue dot sign and localized area of tenderness; ancillary tests including an ultrasound and nuclear scan are needed

Answer

c

9. All of the following are correct regarding male sexual physiology *except*:
   (a) Penile erection is mediated by the parasympathetic system.
   (b) Ejaculation is mediated by the sympathetic nervous system.
   (c) Sensory innervation of the penis is provided by the genitofemoral nerves.
   (d) Acetylcholine is the key messenger responsible for penile erection.
   (e) Preservation of sexual function after pelvic surgery may be achieved in up to 90 % of cases.

Comments Erectile dysfunction is defined as the inability to develop and maintain an erection for satisfactory sexual intercourse. Etiology is often multifactorial, involving psychological, neurologic, hormonal, and vascular mechanisms. The key molecular signaling event in the development of penile erection is the release of nitric oxide, which induces the formation of cyclic GMP resulting in smooth muscle relaxation leading to increased arterial inflow to the penis. Sildenafil increases cyclic GMP levels by blocking phosphodiesterase type 5 [28].

From an anatomical standpoint, erection is achieved through the activity of the nervi erigentes, derived from the parasympathetic sacral plexus (S2–S4). These nerves reach the penis and form the cavernous nerves, responsible for releasing nitric oxide. Ejaculation is mediated by the sympathetic system (T11–L2). Finally, the somatic sensory innervation to the penis occurs via the paired pudendal nerves (S2–S4) [29].

Pelvic surgery and radiation therapy may injure the nerve pathways listed above. The incidence of erectile dysfunction has been estimated to be 20–46 % after rectal cancer resections, 30–80 % after radical prostatectomy, and 6–84 % after pelvic radiation therapy. Furthermore, androgen deprivation therapy in prostate cancer further compounds the problem. In addition, pelvic surgery may impair penile erection further through injury to the accessory pudendal arteries. In time, neurologic and vascular injuries lead to progressive fibrosis of the corpora cavernosa [30].

In spite of the high incidence of erectile dysfunction after rectal resections, there is evidence to suggest that denervation is never complete. Delayed recovery of sexual function may occur up to a year after surgery. Most authors recommend waiting for this period of time before embarking upon surgery for impotence. During this interval, varying degrees of success have been reported with sildenafil therapy [31].

In order to improve not only erectile function but urinary and fecal continence as well, nerve-preserving resection techniques for pelvic malignancies have been developed. The principle behind these operations is the preservation of sympathetic and parasympathetic innervations to the pelvic and genital organs, by keeping a plane of dissection close to the organs to be excised while still maintaining adequate oncologic margins. It has been shown that these techniques can preserve the capacity to sustain an erection and ejaculate in up to 90 % of cases, especially when these surgeries are done for benign disease [32].

Other instances in which the nerve pathways responsible for sexual function may be injured include surgery for anal atresia, imperforate anus, and Hirschsprung's disease [33].

Answer

c

10. All of the following are correct *except*:
    (a) The lower vagina is of ectodermal origin.
    (b) The hymen represents the primitive junction between endoderm and mesoderm.
    (c) The ectoderm-derived squamous epithelium of the lower vagina migrates cephalad to the level of the cervix.
    (d) The vagina lacks somatic innervation above the hymen.
    (e) The most common carcinoma of the vagina is adenocarcinoma.

Comments The vagina, like the anorectum, is formed by the confluence of two embryologic components, in this case, the ectoderm and mesoderm. The ectodermal urogenital sinus forms the labia and distal vagina. In turn, the mesodermal Müllerian ducts form the upper vagina, uterus, and fallopian tubes. In a manner analogous to the dentate line, the hymen marks the union of these two embryologic layers [34].

However, even though the hymen represents the fusion point between ectoderm and mesoderm, the epithelial lining is shifted in relation to this landmark. The ectoderm-derived squamous epithelium of the lower vagina migrates cephalad up to the level of the cervix, where it transitions into the glandular epithelium of the cervix. The anatomical point where this junction occurs is under hormonal influence. During high estrogen states, this transformation zone is displaced distally producing cervical ectropion. Conversely, it migrates into the cervical canal when estrogen levels are low. The importance of the cervical transformation zone is that it is in this area the squamous cervical carcinomas develop.

As would be expected by its normal epithelium, squamous cell cancer is the most common type of vaginal neoplasm, accounting for up to 90 % of cases. Vaginal adenocarcinoma is the second most common histology (2–4 %) and is notably associated with in utero diethylstilbestrol exposure. Melanomas, sarcomas, and carcinoid tumors are other rarely seen forms of vaginal cancer [35, 36].

Answer

e

11. All of the following are correct *except*:
    (a) The urethral epithelium is estrogen sensitive.
    (b) The bulk and engorgement of the female urethral epithelium contributes to urinary continence.
    (c) The internal vesical sphincter contracts in response to α-adrenergic stimulation.
    (d) The striated muscle of the pelvic floor makes little contribution to female urinary continence.
    (e) Posterior support of the bladder neck and proximal urethra is necessary for urinary continence.

Comments The female genital tract and lower urinary tract both arise from the urogenital sinus and share sensitivity the effects of estrogen. Estrogen receptors have been identified in the urethra, bladder, and pelvic floor. Estrogen deprivation has been implicated in postmenopausal urinary dysfunction. It is thought that estrogen contributes to urethral epithelial growth and increases submucosal blood flow, thus aiding in urinary continence. In addition, estrogen enhances α-1 receptor-mediated trigone contraction and β-2-mediated detrusor relaxation [37].

Anatomically, urinary continence in the female is in direct relation to the support the urethra and bladder receive from the pelvic floor. Not only does the pelvic floor act as an external voluntary urinary sphincter, but it also helps preserve urethral stability and maintain a normal urethrovesical angle. Surgical interventions for urinary incontinence attempt to restore the normal anatomic relations [38–40].

Answer
d

12. All of the following are correct *except*:
    (a) Embryologic female sexual differentiation is estrogen dependent.
    (b) The labia majora are analogous to the scrotum in the male.
    (c) The labia minora are analogous to the corpus spongiosum in the male.
    (d) The shaft of the clitoris is analogous to the corpora cavernosa.
    (e) Skene's glands are a source of prostate-specific antigen.

Comments Female sexual differentiation occurs passively in the absence of androgenic influence. In effect, it is the default pathway of differentiation. Primordial gonads have the potential to become ovaries or testes. In the male fetus, the Y chromosome carries the information to produce the H-Y antigen, which induces male gonadal differentiation. In its absence, the primordial gonads become ovaries.

Early in their development, the testes produce testosterone, which promote growth and differentiation of the Wolffian system into the vas deferens and seminal vesicles. Additionally, the testes produce Müllerian-inhibiting substance, which induces the degeneration of the Müllerian system. In the female, the absence of testosterone leads to atrophy of the Wolffian ducts, and the absence of Müllerian-inhibiting substance allows the Müllerian ducts to develop into the fallopian tubes, uterus, and vagina. Initially, external genitalia are the same. Testosterone induces masculinization of the urogenital sinus [41, 42].

In light of their common origin, there are analogies between the male and female genital organs as detailed in Table 21.1

Table 21.1 Analogies between the male and female genital organs

Male	Female
Testes	Ovaries
Gubernaculum testis	Round ligament
Prostate	Skene's glands
Prostatic utricle	Uterus
Cowper's glands	Bartholin glands
Labia majora	Scrotum
Labia minora	Penile shaft skin and corpora cavernosa
Glans penis and corpus spongiosum	Clitoris

Answer

a

13. All of the following are correct *except*:
    (a) Both ovarian arteries originate directly from the aorta.
    (b) The left ovarian vein empties into the left renal vein.
    (c) The lymphatic drainage of the ovaries is directed towards the preaortic nodes.
    (d) Ligation of the ovarian artery results in ovarian necrosis.
    (e) Ovarian pain is perceived in the epigastric region.

Comments The ovaries are paired glands that measure approximately $2 \times 3 \times 4$ cm and weigh 3–4 g each. Like the testicles, they originate in the area below the diaphragm and migrate caudally to their final location in the pelvis. This determines that they carry their blood supply from their area of origin. Bilateral ovarian arteries originate from the aorta slightly below the renal arteries. These arteries cross anterior to the ureter and iliac vessels to reach the ovaries. Unlike the testicular arteries, which are end arteries, the ovarian arteries anastomose with the uterine arteries (originating from the internal iliac on either side), creating a rich vascular arcade. The fallopian tubes share this rich arterial supply. The ovarian veins (like their male counterparts) empty into the vena cava on the right and into the renal vein on the left.

Again, like what occurs with the testis, lymphatic drainage is to the preaortic nodes. Pain from the ovaries is referred to the epigastric region, once again reflecting the site of embryologic origin [43].

Answer
d

14. All of the following are correct *except*:
    (a) The fallopian tubes are derived from the Wolffian ducts.
    (b) The fallopian tubes may be a source of elevated serum amylase.
    (c) The fallopian tubes are the most common site of ectopic pregnancy.
    (d) Ectopic pregnancy most often occurs in the ampulla of the uterine tube.
    (e) The uterine tube has dual blood supply arising from the uterine and ovarian arteries.

Comments The fallopian tubes are derived from the Müllerian duct. They are paired structures that carry the ovum from the ovary to the uterus, and they are also the site of fertilization. They are divided into four sections. The infundibulum opens into the peritoneal cavity and is responsible for capturing the ovum. Its free border gives rise to the fimbriae. The ampulla follows the infundibulum and is where fertilization occurs. The isthmus is the narrowest part of the tube. Finally, the intramural segment represents the junction of the fallopian tubes with the uterus.

While ectopic pregnancy may occur in any portion of the fallopian tube, the part most commonly affected is the ampulla. Other sites of ectopic pregnancy include the peritoneal cavity, ovaries, and cervix [44, 45].

The fallopian tube epithelium produces amylase under normal conditions. It is thought that amylase in the fallopian tube breaks down glycogen to provide glucose for the ovum and sperm cells. The tubes can become a source of elevated serum amylase in the presence of fallopian cysts and neoplasms. Ectopic pregnancy has also been quoted as a source of hyperamylasemia in the past; however, current literature does not support this view [46].

Answer

a

15. All of the following are correct *except*:
    (a) Endometriosis may present as a Blumer's shelf during a rectal exam.
    (b) Endometriosis may present as cyclic bleeding from the umbilicus.
    (c) Endometriosis may be a cause of gastrointestinal bleeding.
    (d) Gelatinous deposits on the peritoneal surface are diagnostic of endometriosis.
    (e) Endometriosis may produce massive pelvic adhesions.

Comments Endometriosis consists of the presence of endometrium-like tissue outside the uterine cavity. This tissue is responsive to the hormonal fluctuations of the menstrual cycle leading to cyclic bleeding. Endometrial implants generate a sterile inflammatory response secondary to hemosiderin deposits from old blood. Endometriosis affects up to 10 % of women of reproductive age and is an important cause of chronic pelvic pain, infertility, and dyspareunia [47].

The most common sites of endometrial implants are the rectovaginal recess (accessible via rectal exam), uterus, fallopian tubes, pelvic peritoneum, and rectosigmoid. Rarely, endometrial implants may occupy extrapelvic sites. Endometriosis has been described in nearly all body cavities. Cases of intestinal, thoracic, and umbilical (Villar's nodule) endometriosis have been reported [48–51].

Endometriosis is thought to occur due to retrograde flow of menstrual blood into the abdominal cavity. This hypothesis fails to explain while only a minority of women with retrograde menstruation develop endometriosis. Other hypotheses include celomic metaplasia and origin of endometrial implants from the circulating bone marrow-derived cells.

Endometrial implants have been shown to overproduce inflammatory mediators such as prostaglandins, cytokines, chemokines, and metalloproteinases. In addition, endometrial implant cells are resistant to the apoptotic actions of prostaglandins.

The definitive diagnosis of endometriosis is established through laparoscopy and biopsy. Laparoscopy reveals the presence of firmly adhered brownish peritoneal implants that have been likened to gunpowder burns. This must be distinguished from the gelatinous deposits (jelly belly) seen in pseudomyxoma peritonei. Medical treatment involves estrogen suppression, while surgical therapy aims to eliminate implants and restore normal anatomy by lysis of adhesions. In selected cases, oophorectomy may be required.

Answer
d

16. All of the following are correct *except*:
    (a) Meigs syndrome is caused by ovarian cancer.
    (b) Krukenberg tumor cells have a signet ring appearance.
    (c) Most ovarian cancers are of epithelial origin.
    (d) Ovarian epithelial cancer has worse prognosis than cancer derived from germinal cells.
    (e) Ovarian tumors may be a source of ectopic hormone production.

Comments Krukenberg tumors are metastatic signet ring adenocarcinomas of the ovary, comprising 1–2 % of all ovarian tumors. Approximately 76 % of them are secondary to a gastric cancer. Fourteen percent arise in the small and large intestines, 4 % in the breast (lobular carcinoma), 3 % in the biliary system, and the remainder from other sites such as the pancreas, bladder, and uterine cervix. It is thought that gastric cancer cells reach the ovaries through retrograde lymphatic flow. This hypothesis is supported by the lack of superficial involvement of the affected ovaries, lack of other peritoneal tumors, and presence of Krukenberg tumors in cases of gastric carcinomas limited to the mucosa and submucosa. In addition, the occurrence of Krukenberg tumors is associated with nodal involvement in gastric cancer. Krukenberg tumors (unlike primary ovarian neoplasms) tend to be bilateral. Their presence carries poor prognosis [52–54].

Meigs syndrome is defined as the triad of benign ovarian tumors (fibroma, thecoma, or Brenner's tumor), ascites, and hydrothorax. Rapid resolution of the effusions is observed after removal of the tumor. The same association with malignant ovarian tumors is termed pseudo-Meigs syndrome. The mechanism through which these very rare syndromes occur is thought to be the transudation of the lymph from the ovaries, which reaches the thorax via transdiaphragmatic lymphatics [55, 56].

Ovarian cancer is the most common cause of death from among the gynecologic malignancies. Due to their lack of symptoms, most tumors are diagnosed at an advanced stage and carry poor prognosis. Ovarian cancers are classified into multiple subcategories based on histological characteristics. However, based on their origin, they may be derived from either the ovarian epithelium (90 %) or the germinal and stromal cells (10 %) [57].

Ovarian epithelial tumors can spread through multiple routes: local invasion, lymph, blood, remote peritoneal implantation, and transdiaphragmatic spread. The propensity for intra-abdominal implantation is the basis for debulking surgery.

In contrast to ovarian tumors of epithelial origin, germ cell tumors have favorable prognosis and occur in younger women. Among germ cell tumors, dysgerminomas are notable for their presentation in women of reproductive age, often during pregnancy [58, 59].

Ovarian thecomas are rare tumor derived from the ovarian cells. Reflecting their origin, these tumors are hormonally active and may produce sex hormones, leading to premature puberty or masculinization depending on the hormone produced [60]. Struma ovarii is another type of stromal tumor of the ovary with endocrine activity. Struma ovarii tumors may be a source of thyroid hormones, leading to hyperthyroidism with an otherwise unremarkable thyroid [61]. There have been reports of ovarian tumors producing insulin, cortisol, and gastrin [62].

Answer

a

References

1. Hughes IA, Acerini CL. Factors controlling testis descent. Eur J Endocrinol. 2008;159 Suppl 1:S75–82.
2. Barteczko KJ, Jacob MI. The testicular descent in human. Origin, development and fate of the gubernaculum hunteri, processus vaginalis peritonei, and gonadal ligaments. Adv Anat Embryol Cell Biol. 2000;156(III–X):1–98.
3. Husmann DA. Cryptorchidism and its relationship to testicular neoplasia and microlithiasis. Urology. 2005;66:424–6.
4. Wood HM, Elder JS. Cryptorchidism and testicular cancer: separating fact from fiction. J Urol. 2009;181:452–61.
5. Ritzen EM. Undescended testes: a consensus on management. Eur J Endocrinol. 2008;159 Suppl 1:S87–90.
6. Esposito C, Caldamone AA, Settimi A, El-Ghoneimi A. Management of boys with nonpalpable undescended testis. Nat Clin Pract Urol. 2008;5:252–60.
7. Agarwal PK, Diaz M, Elder JS. Retractile testis–is it really a normal variant? J Urol. 2006;175:1496–9.
8. Brandt ML. Pediatric hernias. Surg Clin North Am. 2008;88:27–43, vii–viii.
9. De Meulder F, Wojciechowski M, Hubens G, Ramet J. Female hydrocele of the canal of Nuck: a case report. Eur J Pediatr. 2006;165:193–4.
10. Schneider CA, Festa S, Spillert CR, Bruce CJ, Lazaro EJ. Hydrocele of the canal of Nuck. N J Med. 1994;91:37–8.
11. al-dabbagh AK. Anatomical variations of the inguinal nerves and risks of injury in 110 hernia repairs. Surg Radiol Anat. 2002;24:102–7.
12. Wijsmuller AR, Lange JF, Kleinrensink GJ, et al. Nerve-identifying inguinal hernia repair: a surgical anatomical study. World J Surg. 2007;31:414–20; discussion 421–2.
13. Wijsmuller AR, van Veen RN, Bosch JL, Lange JF, Kleinrensink GJ, Jeekel J. Nerve management during open hernia repair. Br J Surg. 2007;94:17–22.
14. Cornwall GA. New insights into epididymal biology and function. Hum Reprod Update. 2009;15:213–27.
15. Nguyen HT, Etzell J, Turek PJ. Normal human ejaculatory duct anatomy: a study of cadaveric and surgical specimens. J Urol. 1996; 155:1639–42.
16. Aboul-Azm TE. Anatomy of the human seminal vesicles and ejaculatory ducts. Arch Androl. 1979;3:287–92.
17. Chughtai B, Sawas A, O'Malley RL, Naik RR, Ali Khan S, Pentyala S. A neglected gland: a review of Cowper's gland. Int J Androl. 2005; 28:74–7.
18. Deane LA, Suding PN, Lekawa ME, Narula N, McDougall EM. Sperm granuloma of the inguinal vas deferens mimicking recurrent incarcerated inguinal hernia. Urology. 2007;69:1209 e1–3.
19. Timms BG. Prostate development: a historical perspective. Differentiation. 2008;76:565–77.
20. McNeal JE. The zonal anatomy of the prostate. Prostate. 1981;2:35–49.
21. Myers RP. Practical surgical anatomy for radical prostatectomy. Urol Clin North Am. 2001;28:473–90.
22. Walz J, Graefen M, Huland H. Basic principles of anatomy for optimal surgical treatment of prostate cancer. World J Urol. 2007;25:31–8.
23. Dearnaley D, Huddart R, Horwich A. Regular review: managing testicular cancer. BMJ. 2001;322:1583–8.
24. Jones RH, Vasey PA. Part II: testicular cancer–management of advanced disease. Lancet Oncol. 2003;4:738–47.
25. Jones RH, Vasey PA. Part I: testicular cancer–management of early disease. Lancet Oncol. 2003;4:730–7.
26. Gatti JM, Patrick MJ. Current management of the acute scrotum. Semin Pediatr Surg. 2007;16:58–63.
27. Ringdahl E, Teague L. Testicular torsion. Am Fam Physician. 2006;74:1739–43.
28. Lue TF. Erectile dysfunction. N Engl J Med. 2000;342:1802–13.
29. Mauroy B, Demondion X, Drizenko A, et al. The inferior hypogastric plexus (pelvic plexus): its importance in neural preservation techniques. Surg Radiol Anat. 2003;25:6–15.
30. Nandipati KC, Raina R, Agarwal A, Zippe CD. Erectile dysfunction following radical retropubic prostatectomy: epidemiology, pathophysiology and pharmacological management. Drugs Aging. 2006;23:101–17.
31. Peltier A, van Velthoven R, Roumeguere T. Current management of erectile dysfunction after cancer treatment. Curr Opin Oncol. 2009; 21:303–9.
32. Moriya Y. Function preservation in rectal cancer surgery. Int J Clin Oncol. 2006;11:339–43.
33. Sherman JO, Snyder ME, Weitzman JJ, et al. A 40-year multinational retrospective study of 880 Swenson procedures. J Pediatr Surg. 1989;24:833–8.
34. Ulfelder H, Robboy SJ. The embryologic development of the human vagina. Am J Obstet Gynecol. 1976;126:769–76.
35. Marshall FF. Vaginal abnormalities. Urol Clin North Am. 1978;5:155–9.
36. Merino MJ. Vaginal cancer: the role of infectious and environmental factors. Am J Obstet Gynecol. 1991;165:1255–62.
37. Robinson D, Cardozo LD. The role of estrogens in female lower urinary tract dysfunction. Urology. 2003;62:45–51.
38. Di Benedetto P, Coidessa A, Floris S. Rationale of pelvic floor muscles training in women with urinary incontinence. Minerva Ginecol. 2008;60:529–41.
39. Holroyd-Leduc JM, Straus SE. Management of urinary incontinence in women: scientific review. JAMA. 2004;291:986–95.
40. McLennan MT, Melick CF, Cannon S. The position of the urethrovesical junction after incontinence surgery: early postoperative changes. Int Urogynecol J Pelvic Floor Dysfunct. 2004;15:44–8; discussion 48.
41. Rey R, Picard JY. Embryology and endocrinology of genital development. Baillieres Clin Endocrinol Metab. 1998;12:17–33.
42. Wilson JD, Griffin JE, Leshin M, George FW. Role of gonadal hormones in development of the sexual phenotypes. Hum Genet. 1981; 58:78–84.
43. Berman JR, Adhikari SP, Goldstein I. Anatomy and physiology of female sexual function and dysfunction: classification, evaluation and treatment options. Eur Urol. 2000;38:20–9.
44. Barnhart KT. Clinical practice. Ectopic pregnancy. N Engl J Med. 2009;361:379–87.
45. Pauerstein CJ, Croxatto HB, Eddy CA, Ramzy I, Walters MD. Anatomy and pathology of tubal pregnancy. Obstet Gynecol. 1986;67:301–8.
46. Bruns DE, Mills SE, Savory J. Amylase in fallopian tube and serous ovarian neoplasms: immunohistochemical localization. Arch Pathol Lab Med. 1982;106:17–20.
47. Bulun SE. Endometriosis. N Engl J Med. 2009;360:268–79.

48. Arunthari V, Sevin BU, Krishna M, Johnson MM. Catamenial pneumothorax with umbilical and diaphragmatic endometriosis: a case report and review of the literature. South Med J. 2008;101:1043–5.
49. Douglas C, Rotimi O. Extragenital endometriosis–a clinicopathological review of a Glasgow hospital experience with case illustrations. J Obstet Gynaecol. 2004;24:804–8.
50. Goldberg JM, Bedaiwy MA. Recurrent umbilical endometriosis after laparoscopic treatment of minimal pelvic endometriosis: a case report. J Reprod Med. 2007;52:551–2.
51. Victory R, Diamond MP, Johns DA. Villar's nodule: a case report and systematic literature review of endometriosis externa of the umbilicus. J Minim Invasive Gynecol. 2007;14:23–32.
52. Al-Agha OM, Nicastri AD. An in-depth look at Krukenberg tumor: an overview. Arch Pathol Lab Med. 2006;130:1725–30.
53. Young RH. From Krukenberg to today: the ever present problems posed by metastatic tumors in the ovary. Part II. Adv Anat Pathol. 2007;14:149–77.
54. Young RH. From krukenberg to today: the ever present problems posed by metastatic tumors in the ovary: part I. Historical perspective, general principles, mucinous tumors including the krukenberg tumor. Adv Anat Pathol. 2006;13:205–27.
55. Lurie S. Meigs' syndrome: the history of the eponym. Eur J Obstet Gynecol Reprod Biol. 2000;92:199–204.
56. O'Flanagan SJ, Tighe BF, Egan TJ, Delaney PV. Meigs' syndrome and pseudo-Meigs' syndrome. J R Soc Med. 1987;80:252–3.
57. Soslow RA. Histologic subtypes of ovarian carcinoma: an overview. Int J Gynecol Pathol. 2008;27:161–74.
58. Gershenson DM. Management of ovarian germ cell tumors. J Clin Oncol. 2007;25:2938–43.
59. Pectasides D, Pectasides E, Kassanos D. Germ cell tumors of the ovary. Cancer Treat Rev. 2008;34:427–41.
60. Lee MH, Moon YJ, Ha CW, Hoh JK. Ovarian thecoma with virilizing manifestations. Yonsei Med J. 2009;50:169–73.
61. Yoo SC, Chang KH, Lyu MO, Chang SJ, Ryu HS, Kim HS. Clinical characteristics of struma ovarii. J Gynecol Oncol. 2008;19:135–8.
62. Leach SD, LaMorte AI, True LD, et al. Aberrant hormone production from ovarian neoplasms: strategies for diagnosis and therapy. World J Surg. 1990;14:335–40; discussion 340–1.

22 Adrenals

1. All of the following are correct *except*:
   (a) The adrenal cortex has mesodermal origin.
   (b) The adrenal medulla has neuroectodermal origin.
   (c) Ectopic adrenal neoplasms are perivertebral in location.
   (d) Accessory cortical tissue may develop symptomatic adenomas.
   (e) The organs of Zuckerkandl represent ectopic adrenal cortical tissue.

Comments See question 2.

Answer
e

V.K. Maker, E.D. Guzman-Arrieta, *Cognitive Pearls in General Surgery*,
DOI 10.1007/978-1-4939-1850-8_22,

2. All of the following are correct *except*:
   (a) The zona glomerulosa secretes aldosterone.
   (b) The zona fasciculata produces cortisol.
   (c) The zona reticularis secretes adrenal estrogens.
   (d) The adrenal medulla secretes epinephrine.
   (e) Ectopic adrenal medullary tumors may secrete catecholamine precursors.

Comments The adrenal gland represents the union of two functionally distinct organs: the adrenal medulla and adrenal cortex. The adrenal medulla is derived from the neural crest and produces catecholamines that mediate the fight-or-flight response. The adrenal cortex is derived from the mesoderm and is responsible for producing steroid hormones that regulate electrolyte balance (aldosterone), the stress response (cortisol), and to a lesser extent sexual differentiation (adrenal androgens). Production of these three hormones is anatomically compartmentalized within the cortex into the zona glomerulosa, fasciculata, and reticularis, respectively [1].

The adrenal cortex and gonads share a common origin in the mesodermal adrenogonadal primordium. As the adrenal and gonadal primordia separate, the adrenal becomes encapsulated and differentiates into the fetal cortex which will later become the zona fasciculata and reticularis. The zona glomerulosa develops later and may be distinguished at birth.

As the adrenal cortex develops, it is invaded by neural crest-derived cells (T6–T12) during the third month of gestation. These cells will form the adrenal medulla. However, not all cells may reach the developing adrenal and may become extra-adrenal medullary tissue, found along the distal aorta in perivertebral location (organ of Zuckerkandl), kidneys, broad ligament, and spermatic cord. This ectopic tissue may give rise to symptomatic adenomas or malignant tumors [2, 3] (Figs. 22.1 and 22.2).

Interestingly, there is interdependence between the adrenal cortex and the adrenal medulla. Cortisol stimulates epinephrine synthesis by increasing the activity of phenylethanolamine N-methyltransferase, the enzyme responsible for synthesizing epinephrine, using norepinephrine as a substrate. The sympathetic system also modulates the activity of the hypothalamus–pituitary–adrenal axis. Norepinephrine produced in the locus coeruleus induces hypothalamic release of corticotrophin-releasing hormone [4].

Development of the adrenal glands is not complete at birth. In the newborn, the adrenal cortex is proportionally 20 times larger than that of the adult, and the medulla is scarcely developed, perhaps reflecting underdeveloped fight-or-flight responses. Through childhood, the cortex becomes smaller and more clearly differentiates into three distinct zones, reaching complete development around the time of puberty, in which the adrenal cortex is also thought to play an important role [5].

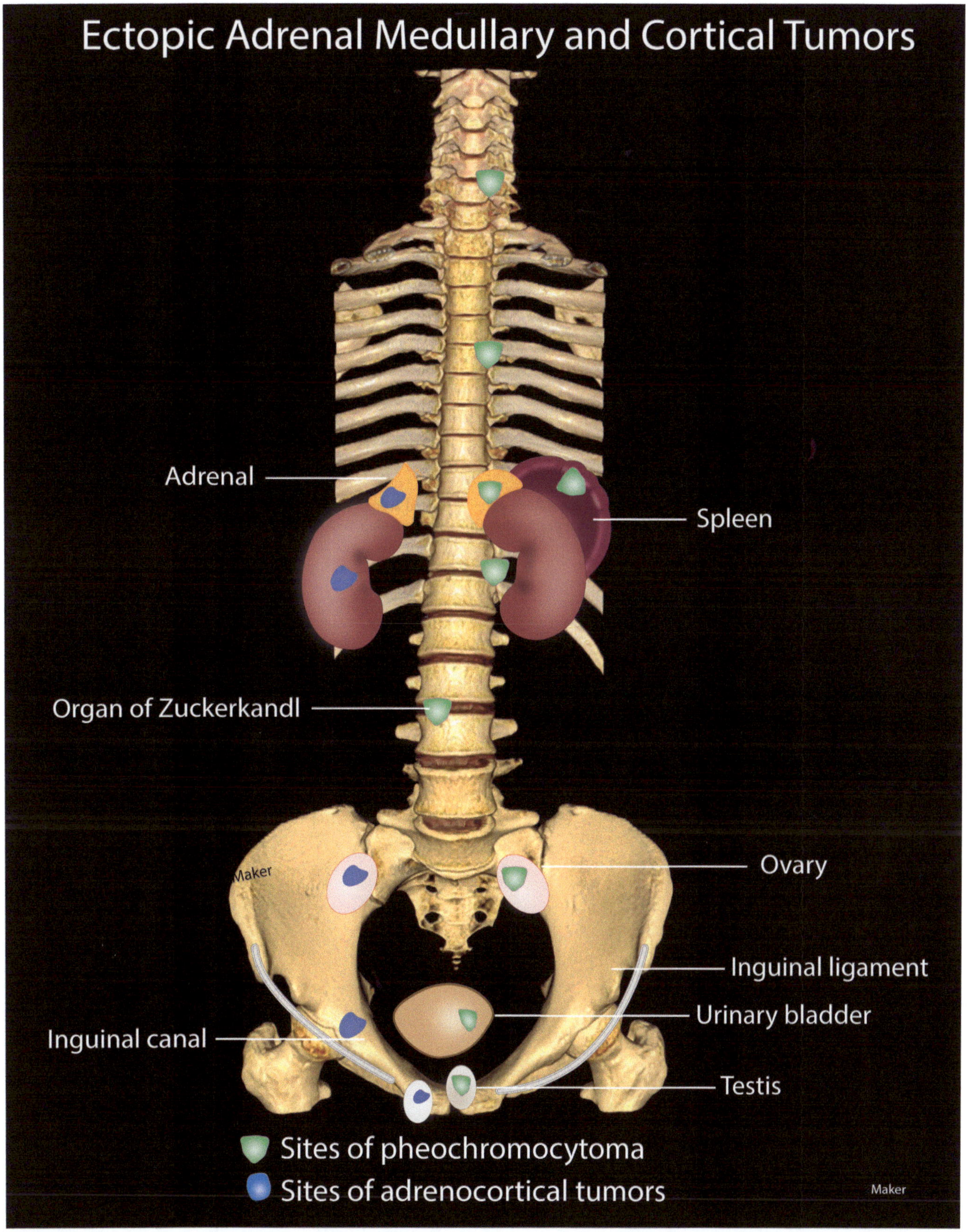

Fig. 22.1 Extra-adrenal pheochromocytomas can be found anywhere sympathetic ganglia are present. So their most common location is in the paravertebral area and rarely in the bladder and ectopic germ cell tissue of the gonads. Extra-adrenal cortical tumors have a common mesodermal origin with the gonads, and hence, the most common ectopic locations follow the gonads and their path of descent

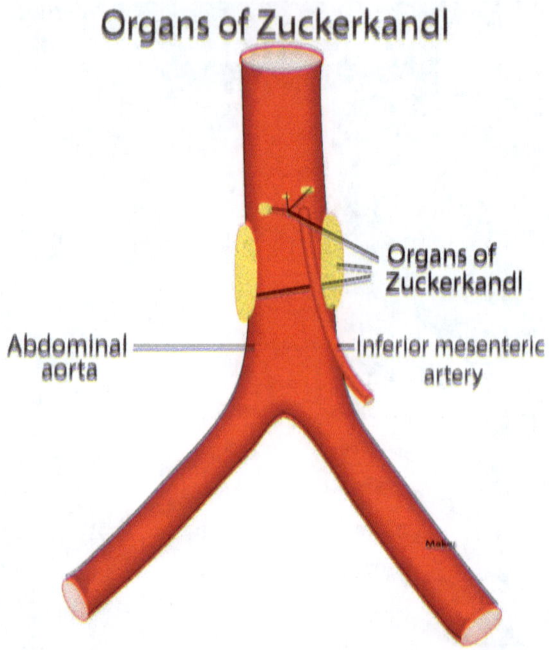

Fig. 22.2 The organs of Zuckerkandl are collections of sympathetic ganglia located around the origin of the inferior mesenteric artery. These are potential sites of an extra-adrenal pheochromocytoma (With permission from Subramanian et al. [3]. © 2006 Elsevier)

Answer

c

3. All of the following are correct *except*:
   (a) Ectopic medullary tissue tends to be distributed around the celiac and mesenteric arteries.
   (b) The majority of neuroblastomas originate in the adrenal gland.
   (c) Adrenal agenesis is commonly associated with ipsilateral renal agenesis.
   (d) The adrenal glands ascend from the pelvis together with the kidneys.
   (e) The adrenal medulla receives sympathetic preganglionic fibers.

Comments Reflecting their common origin, ectopic adrenal cortical tissue may be found in relation to the gonads or associated structures. Ectopic adrenal tissue along the spermatic cord is a fairly frequent finding during the course of pediatric groin explorations, with an incidence of 1–2 %. It is recommended that this tissue be excised [6, 7]. With less frequency, ectopic adrenal cortical tissue in the renal parenchyma has been described [8].

Extra-adrenal medullary tissue is often located along the distal aorta, particularly below the inferior mesenteric artery (organs of Zuckerkandl). They are prominent in the fetus and infant and serve as the main source of epinephrine. As the adrenal medulla develops, these aggregations of tissue involute and are usually absent by puberty. While the majority of neuroblastomas and pheochromocytomas arise from the adrenal medulla proper, extra-adrenal medullary tissue may also be affected [3, 9].

The urinary bladder is a rare site of pheochromocytoma, accounting for 0.06 % of all bladder tumors and 1 % of all pheochromocytomas. Bladder pheochromocytomas are thought to arise from chromaffin cells in the sympathetic plexus of the bladder wall. Bladder pheochromocytomas are most often located in the trigone of the bladder, which is the area with the richest sympathetic innervation. These tumors produce a unique clinical syndrome characterized by catecholamine release crisis triggered by micturition. Diagnosis is made on a biochemical basis, and localization can be made through cross-sectional imaging and cystoscopy. Similar to adrenal pheochromocytomas, bladder pheochromocytomas are hyperintense in MRI T2-weighted imaging. Like with all extra-adrenal pheochromocytomas, metaiodobenzylguanidine (MIBG) scans may be useful to localize an otherwise occult lesion. Surgical excision is the treatment of choice. It must be preceded by pharmacologic adrenergic blockade [10, 11].

Interestingly, both adrenal and extra-adrenal medullary tissues constitute functional sympathetic autonomic ganglia and synapse with afferent preganglionic fibers using acetylcholine as a neurotransmitter (nicotinic receptors).

The kidney, gonads, and adrenal cortex share a common origin in the urogenital ridge. As mentioned previously, the mesodermal urogenital ridge gives rise to the adrenogonadal primordial and the pronephros–mesonephros–metanephros sequence. Adrenal agenesis is thought to be the result of failure of the development of the urogenital ridge and, as such, is most commonly associated with renal agenesis. In contrast, renal agenesis results from failure of development of the ureteric bud, which is a later embryologic event that does not affect adrenal development [12].

Answer
d

4. All of the following are correct *except*:
   (a) The adrenal arteries arise from the inferior phrenic and renal arteries and directly from the aorta.
   (b) The adrenal gland is one of the most vascular glands in the human body.
   (c) Waterhouse–Friderichsen syndrome produces massive hemorrhage.
   (d) The superior adrenal arteries are the most constant.
   (e) The adrenal glands are a common site of hematogenous metastasis.

Comments See question 5.

Answer
c

5. All of the following are correct *except*:
   (a) Adrenal venous drainage follows the adrenal arteries.
   (b) The right adrenal vein is short and more difficult to control than the left.
   (c) The left adrenal vein drains into the left renal vein.
   (d) The right adrenal vein drains into the vena cava.
   (e) Early ligation of the adrenal vein prevents release of catecholamines from a pheochromocytoma.

Comments The adrenal gland receives its generous blood supply from multiple small branches arising from three distinct sources. The superior adrenal arteries (6–8 in number) arise from the inferior phrenic arteries; the middle adrenal artery arises from the aorta proximal to the renal arteries; lastly, the inferior adrenal arteries [1–3] arise from the renal arteries. Variations in vascular supply are common, but the superior adrenal arteries are the most constant. All the adrenal arteries branch further as they approach the gland, so that there are 50–60 small arteries piercing the adrenal capsule.

In contrast with the widely distributed arterial circulation, venous drainage of the adrenal gland is carried out by a single constant vein that emerges from the gland's hilum. Classically, the left adrenal vein is joined by the left inferior phrenic vein before emptying into the left renal vein. In contrast, the right adrenal vein follows a short course (0.5 cm) towards the vena cava, making it more difficult to control surgically than the left vein. Control of the adrenal veins is a key step in the treatment of pheochromocytomas, as it limits the release of catecholamines [13] (Fig. 22.3).

The adrenal can be very fragile, and adrenal tumors may implant if their integrity is disrupted. To this effect, the general principle of adrenal surgery is to remove the normal tissue away from the adrenal rather than the adrenal from normal tissue, considering the gland may not be grasped.

The adrenal gland is often a site of distant metastasis. Autopsy studies have shown that approximately 3 % of the general population and 25 % of cancer patients have adrenal metastasis. In fact, metastatic lesions are the second most frequent mass lesion of the adrenal after benign adenomas. The most common malignancies associated with adrenal metastasis are breast, lung, colon, and kidney cancer as well as malignant melanoma. Adrenalectomy for metastatic disease may be performed in patients with isolated metastasis [14].

Adrenal apoplexy also known as Waterhouse–Friderichsen syndrome consists of the association of adrenal hemorrhage and sepsis, most often described in the context of meningococcemia, but also reported in association to pneumococcal and staphylococcal sepsis as well as in mixed necrotizing soft tissue infections. It is thought to occur as a result of adrenal hyper-stimulation coupled with coagulation disorders induced by sepsis. While this condition is associated with high mortality, death results from overwhelming sepsis and adrenal insufficiency, rather than from the hemodynamic effects of this small volume hemorrhage [15, 16].

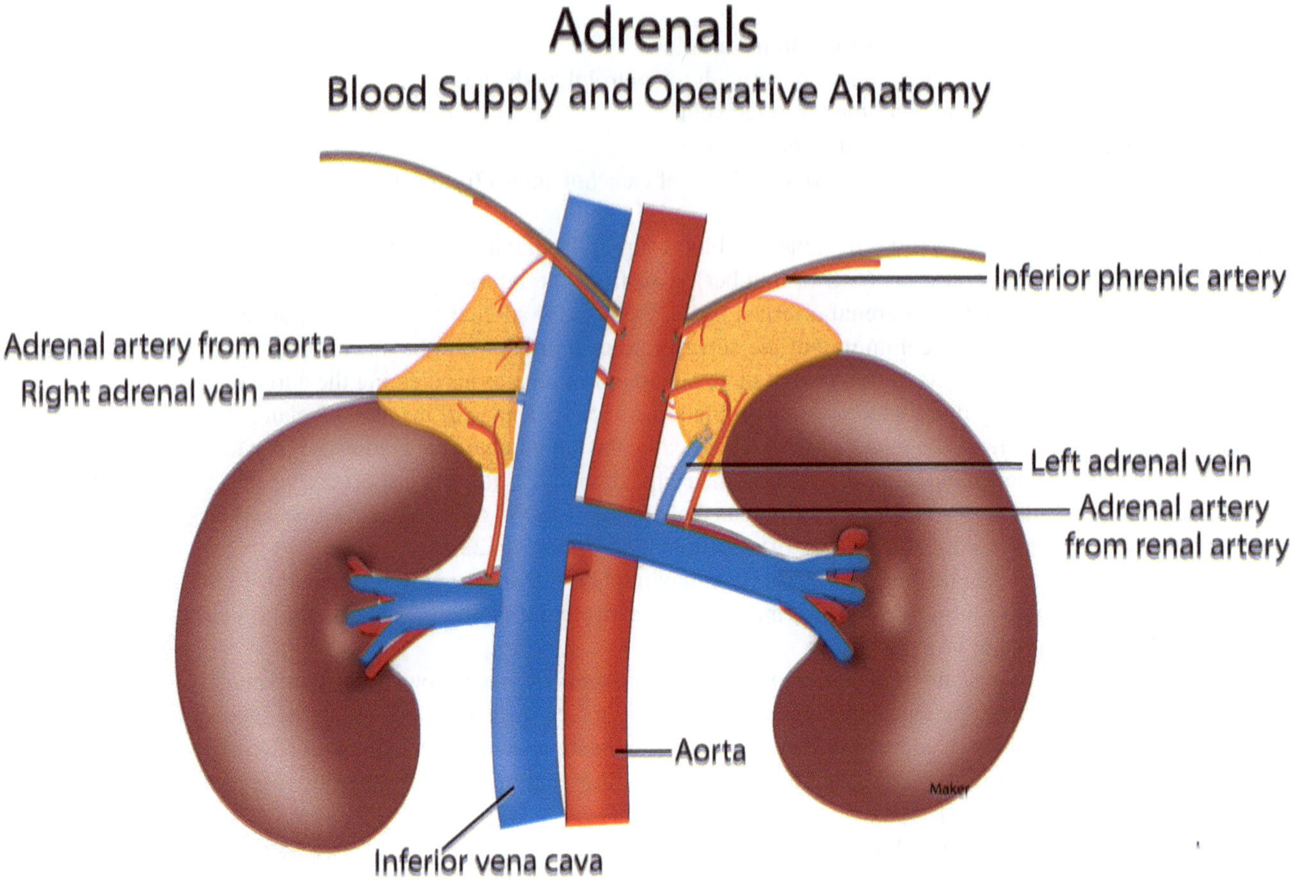

Fig. 22.3 The right adrenal vein is very short and drains directly into the inferior vena cava. Adrenal veins are almost always in the hilum of the gland, typically single, and must be controlled before any dissection of the adrenal gland. The arterial supply of the adrenal glands is comprised of multiple small vessels derived from the inferior phrenic arteries, the aorta and and the renal arteries

Answer
a

6. The most common tumor of the adrenal gland is:
   (a) Adrenal cortical adenoma producing Conn's syndrome
   (b) Adrenal cortical adenoma producing Cushing's syndrome
   (c) Pheochromocytoma
   (d) Nonfunctioning adrenal adenoma (incidentaloma)
   (e) Metastatic tumor

Comments The widespread use of computed tomography has led to the frequent identification of otherwise silent adrenal masses. The presence of such masses prompts the determination of whether these masses are malignant and/or functional. The malignant potential can be ascertained by size (greater than 6 cm), whereas functional testing is required to determine their hormone-producing capacities.

The two most important adrenocortical functional tumors are those producing aldosterone (zona glomerulosa) and cortisol (zona fasciculata). Aldosterone-producing tumors cause primary hyperaldosteronism, which is characterized by hypertension due to volume overload and hypokalemia. Additional testing reveals a high aldosterone level coupled with a low renin level. This clinical presentation is named Conn's syndrome.

Cortisol-producing tumors cause Cushing's syndrome, with all its well-known manifestations. Testing includes demonstration of elevated serum, salivary and urine cortisol, depressed ACTH levels, and positive low-dose dexamethasone suppression tests.

Pheochromocytomas are functioning tumors of the adrenal medulla. Disease manifestations are determined by excessive release of catecholamines inducing episodic hypertension, flushing, and irritability. The diagnosis can be made though demonstration of increased plasma or urine metanephrines. The diagnosis of pheochromocytoma should prompt the suspicion of multiple endocrine neoplasia (MEN) syndromes. MEN1 is characterized by pituitary, pancreatic, and parathyroid adenomas. MEN2A syndrome presents medullary carcinoma of the thyroid, pheochromocytoma, and parathyroid hyperplasia. MEN2B is characterized by medullary carcinoma of the thyroid, pheochromocytoma, neuromas, and marfanoid body habitus.

Pheochromocytomas span the spectrum of benign to malignant masses. As they dedifferentiate, their imaging characteristics change, becoming MIBG negative and PET positive. This may correlate with changes in their hormone-producing profile from epinephrine to precursors. Dopamine-producing pheochromocytomas are known to be more likely malignant, PET positive, and MIBG negative than their epinephrine- or norepinephrine-producing counterparts and overall carry a worse prognosis. The most undifferentiated form of these tumors is ganglioneuroma, which produce no hormones at all and tend to be extra-adrenal [17].

However, as important as recognizing the potential for cancer and endocrine activity in incidentally discovered adrenal masses (incidentaloma), most of these lesions are small and nonfunctional, warranting observation only [18].

Answer
d

References

1. Kim AC, Barlaskar FM, Heaton JH, et al. In search of adrenocortical stem and progenitor cells. Endocr Rev. 2009;30:241–63.
2. Adams MS, Bronner-Fraser M. Review: the role of neural crest cells in the endocrine system. Endocr Pathol. 2009;20:92–100.
3. Subramanian A, Maker VK. Organs of Zuckerkandl: their surgical significance and a review of a century of literature. Am J Surg. 2006; 192:224–34.
4. Wong DL. Epinephrine biosynthesis: hormonal and neural control during stress. Cell Mol Neurobiol. 2006;26:891–900.
5. Chrousos GP. The hypothalamic-pituitary-adrenal axis and immune-mediated inflammation. N Engl J Med. 1995;332:1351–62.
6. Mendez R, Tellado MG, Somoza I, et al. Ectopic adrenal tissue in the spermatic cord in pediatric patients: surgical implications. Int Braz J Urol. 2006;32:202–7; discussion 207.
7. Ketata S, Ketata H, Sahnoun A, FakhFakh H, Bahloul A, Mhiri MN. Ectopic adrenal cortex tissue: an incidental finding during inguinoscrotal operations in pediatric patients. Urol Int. 2008;81:316–9.
8. Ye H, Yoon GS, Epstein JI. Intrarenal ectopic adrenal tissue and renal-adrenal fusion: a report of nine cases. Mod Pathol. 2009;22:175–81.
9. Fung MM, Viveros OH, O'Connor DT. Diseases of the adrenal medulla. Acta Physiol (Oxf). 2008;192:325–35.
10. Siatelis A, Konstantinidis C, Volanis D, Leontara V, Thoma-Tsagli E, Delakas D. Pheochromocytoma of the urinary bladder: report of 2 cases and review of literature. Minerva Urol Nefrol. 2008;60:137–40.
11. Thrasher JB, Rajan RR, Perez LM, Humphrey PA, Anderson EE. Pheochromocytoma of urinary bladder: contemporary methods of diagnosis and treatment options. Urology. 1993;41:435–9.
12. Else T, Hammer GD. Genetic analysis of adrenal absence: agenesis and aplasia. Trends Endocrinol Metab. 2005;16:458–68.
13. Igwilo OC, Sulkowski RJ, Shah MR, Messink WF, Kinnas NC. Embolization of traumatic adrenal hemorrhage. J Trauma. 1999;47:1153–5.
14. Uberoi J, Munver R. Surgical management of metastases to the adrenal gland: open, laparoscopic, and ablative approaches. Curr Urol Rep. 2009;10:67–72.
15. Doherty S. Fatal pneumococcal Waterhouse-Friderichsen syndrome. Emerg Med (Fremantle). 2001;13:237–9.
16. Levin J, Cluff LE. Endotoxemia and adrenal hemorrhage. A mechanism for the Waterhouse-Friderichsen syndrome. J Exp Med. 1965; 121:247–60.
17. Dubois LA, Gray DK. Dopamine-secreting pheochromocytomas: in search of a syndrome. World J Surg. 2005;29:909–13.
18. NIH state-of-the-science statement on management of the clinically inapparent adrenal mass ("incidentaloma"). NIH Consens State Sci Statements. 2002;19:1–25.

23 Lymphatic System

1. All of the following are correct *except*:
   (a) The lymphatic system is derived from the mesoderm.
   (b) The lymphatic system originates from the venous system.
   (c) The remnant of the right thoracic duct drains the upper right hemithorax.
   (d) Congenital lymphedema (lymphedema praecox) is caused by hyperplasia of the lymphatic vessels.
   (e) Visceral lymphatics have no valves.

Comments Please see question 3.

Answer
d

V.K. Maker, E.D. Guzman-Arrieta, *Cognitive Pearls in General Surgery*,
DOI 10.1007/978-1-4939-1850-8_23, © Springer Science+Business Media New York 2015

2. All of the following are correct *except*:
   (a) Lymphatic capillaries lack a continuous basal membrane.
   (b) Extremity lymphatic vessels have valves.
   (c) The thoracic duct is interrupted by lymph nodes.
   (d) The lymph is propelled by transient increases in tissue pressure.
   (e) Reflux of blood from the jugular vein into the thoracic duct is prevented by valves.

Comments Please see question 3.

Answer
c

3. All of the following are correct *except*:
   (a) The cisterna chyli represents the confluence of the bilateral lumbar and intercostal trunks with the unpaired intestinal trunk.
   (b) The cisterna chyli gives origin to the thoracic duct and lies to the right of T12.
   (c) The thoracic duct receives multiple intercostal branches in its ascent through the thorax.
   (d) The thoracic duct traverses the diaphragm through the caval hiatus.
   (e) The rate of flow along the thoracic duct fluctuates between 60 and 190 ml/h.

Comments The lymphatic system, like the remainder of the vascular system, is thought to arise from the mesoderm. The lymphatic system arises from six primordial lymph sacs that are outgrowths of venous channels, paralleling the six aortic arches from the branchial apparatus. The first primordial lymph sacs arise at the jugular–subclavian confluences and extend into the upper extremities and head. Two unpaired sacs appear along the mesenteric and celiac trunks and form the cisterna chyli. Finally, paired femoral sacs appear and extend into the lower extremities. These six sacs become linked by a rich network of lymphatic vessels, ultimately leading from the peripheral tissues to the central veins. Lymph nodes develop at a later stage at places where lymphatic channels join.

The right and left thoracic ducts are derived from the jugular–subclavian lymph sacs. Originally, they both connect to the cisterna chyli and drain lymph towards the subclavian vessels. Later in development the distal portion of the right thoracic duct crosses over the midline behind the esophagus to join the proximal part of the left thoracic duct (T5–T7), thus forming a single duct. The caudal aspect of the left thoracic duct involutes, while the proximal part of the right thoracic duct persists and drains the lymph from the right side of the head and neck, right arm, and upper thorax into the right jugular–subclavian confluence. The thoracic duct crosses the diaphragm through the aortic hiatus. As the thoracic duct ascends though the thorax, it receives multiple intercostal branches [1].

The cisterna chyli is an elongated lymphatic sac located over T12 to L2. It receives the lymphatic drainage of the right and left lumbar trunks carrying the lymph from the lower extremities. In addition, it receives the intestinal and intercostals trunks, carrying the lymph from the GI tract and lower chest wall, respectively (Fig. 23.1).

Lymphatic flow is propelled by the cyclic compression of the peripheral lymphatics by arterial pulse waves as well as by muscular contractions and local massage. Unidirectional lymph flow is made possible by the presence of valves along the peripheral lymphatic channels. Said valves are absent in the thoracic duct and visceral lymphatics. While the thoracic duct lacks valves along its course, there exists a valve at the point where it enters the jugular vein. This valve prevents venous reflux. Even though the thoracic duct itself is not interrupted by lymph nodes, a rich network of lymphatic channels and lymph nodes surrounds it [2, 3].

The lymph flows through lymph nodes from the peripheral afferent lymphatics towards the lymph node hilum. Following this pattern, cancer cells often form subcapsular tumor deposits. From there, they may exit the node via the efferent lymphatics or the veins draining the nodes. Interestingly, sarcomas, in line with their propensity for blood-borne metastasis, may reach the lymph nodes via the artery supplying them (Figs. 23.2 and 23.3).

Lymphedema is a chronic form of protein-rich edema that results from injury to the lymphatic system. Primary lymphedema has been classified by age of presentation into congenital lymphedema (appears shortly after birth), lymphedema praecox (puberty), and lymphedema tarda (after 35 years of age). Primary lymphedema occurs due to abnormal development of the lymphatic system and tends to affect the lower extremities for unclear reasons.

Secondary lymphedema is the manifestation of the interruption of lymphatic flow due to cancer, surgery, irradiation, inflammation, or other forms of injury to the lymphatic vessels.

The treatment of lymphedema is largely supportive, involving physical therapy, elevation, massage, and external compression. Select cases may benefit from debulking and lymphovenous anastomosis [4, 5].

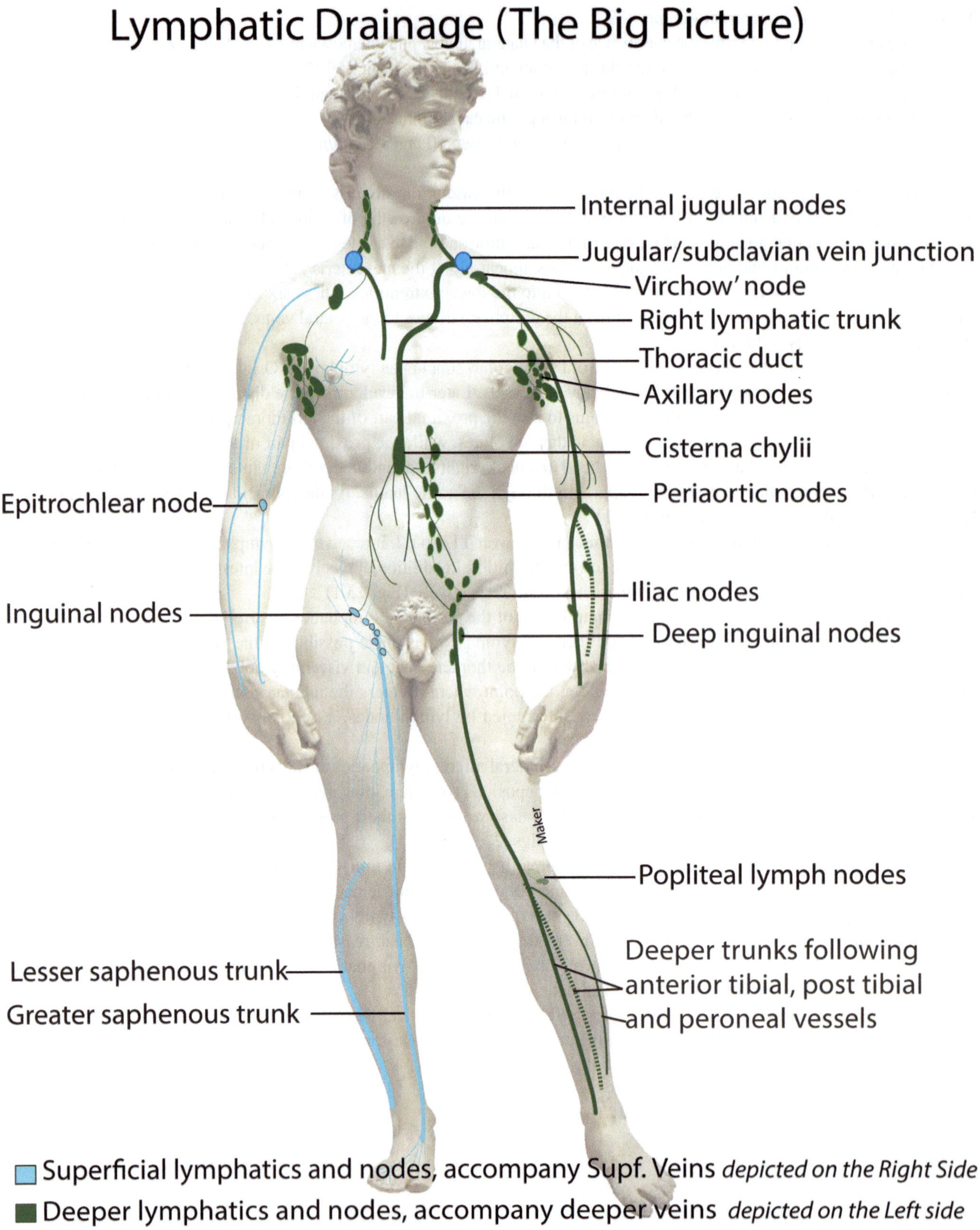

Fig. 23.1 Superficial and deep lymphatics follow their respective venous counterparts. Lymph node stations are located at the site of joints in the extremities and anatomical functional units in the head and neck. Virtually 90 % of all the lymph drains into the thoracic duct. The right lymphatic duct drains the remainder, mostly from right half of the head and neck, upper right thorax, and right upper extremity. Eventually the entire body lymph is returned to the right atrium via the superior vena cava

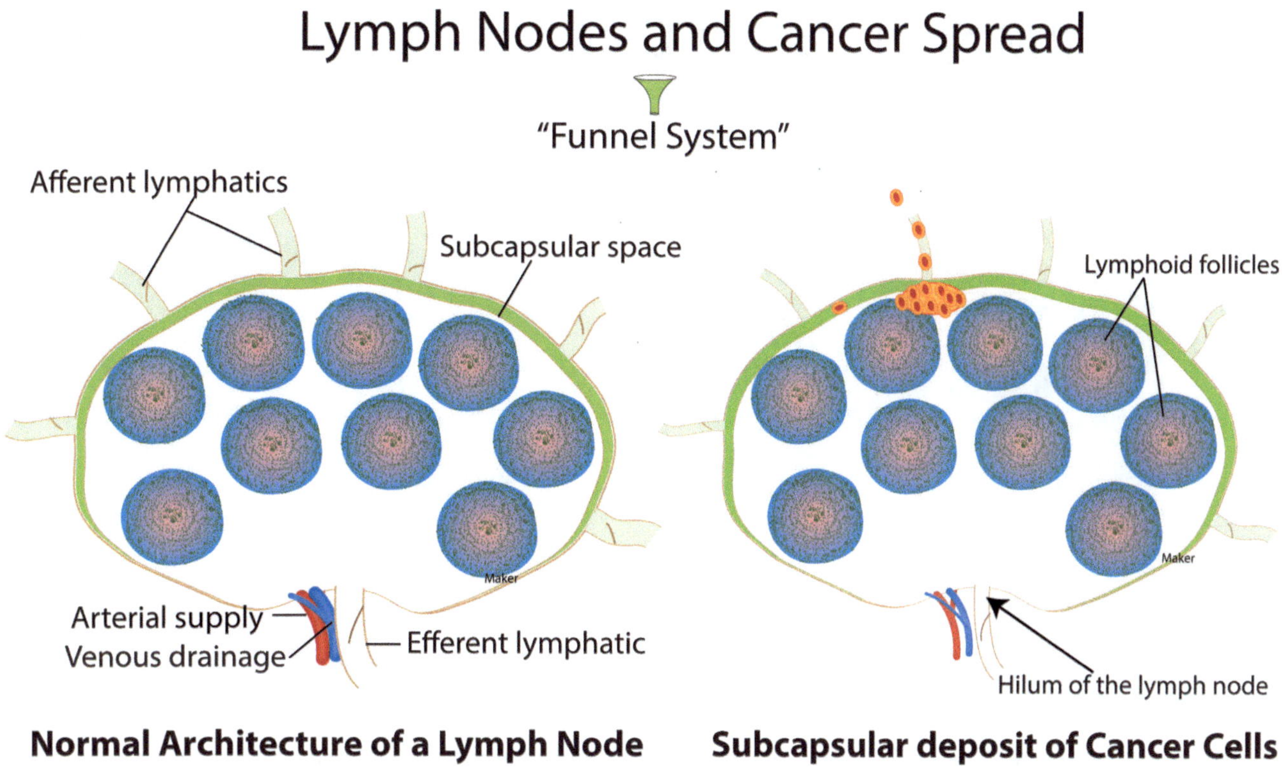

Fig. 23.2 Filtration function of a lymph node is architecturally designed on a funnel principle where a number of one-way valved afferent lymphatics drain into a subcapsular space, filter through lymphoid tissue and exit through a usually single efferent lymphatic channel. When cancer cells travel through lymphatics to a lymph node, their first site of deposit may well be subcapsular. If a metastatic lymph node deposit is large enough, gross examination at the time of surgical excision can identify a subcapsular location and give a clue that the mode of invasion was through the afferent lymphatics. Visceral lymphatics function similarly, but do not contain valves

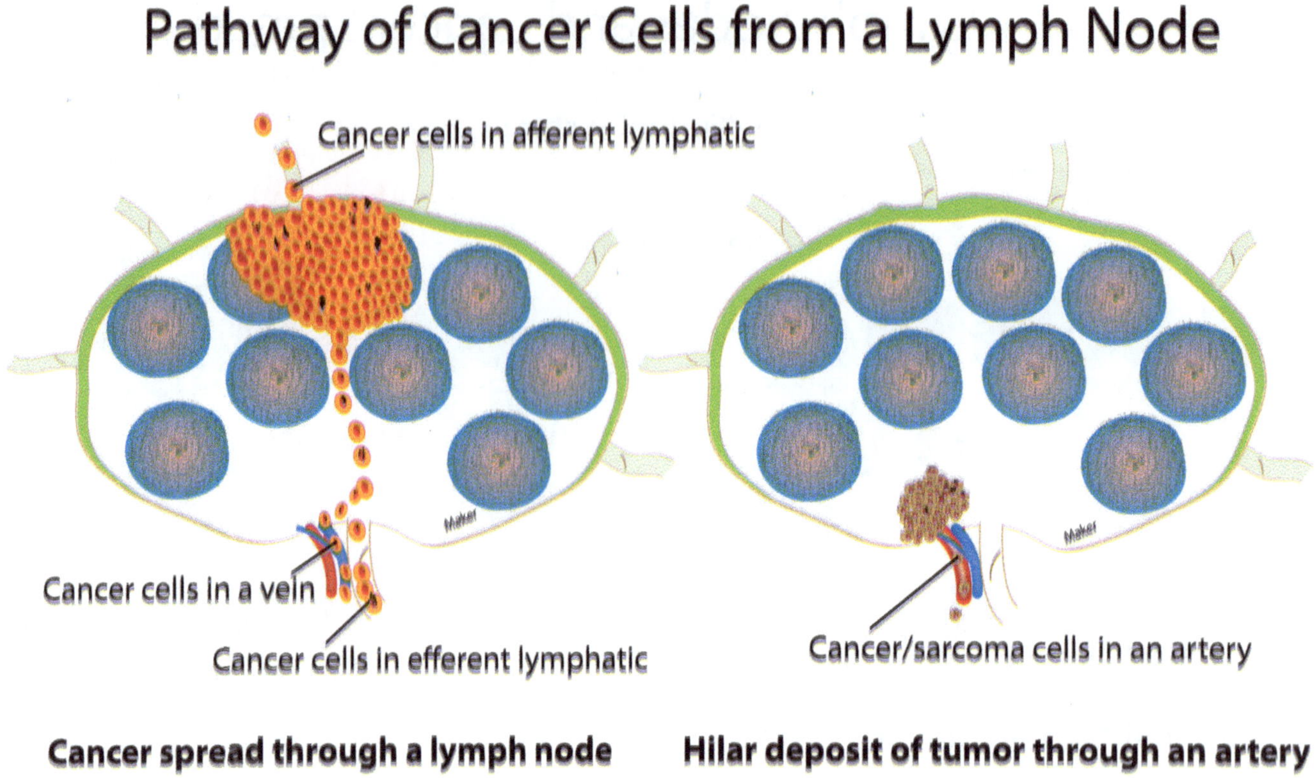

Fig. 23.3 Cancer cells that survive filtration through a lymph node exit through the efferent lymphatic at its hilum into the afferent lymphatic of the next node/nodes. Each lymph node at its hilum also has a small artery and a vein. This vein may well be a pathway for lymphovascular spread in certain cancers. The arterial blood supply at the hilum can be the source of hematogenous spread to a lymph node, in which case the initial deposits of cancer cells will be at the hilum rather than in the peripheral subcapsular space

Answer

d

4. All of the following are correct *except*:
   (a) Cystic hygromas represent a cystic dilatation of the lymphatic vessels.
   (b) Cystic hygromas fail to drain the lymph into the venous circulations.
   (c) Cystic hygromas are most common in the posterior neck region.
   (d) Cystic hygromas require radical excision with at least 1 cm margins.
   (e) Cystic hygromas may cause airway obstruction.

Comments Cystic hygromas are lymph-filled sacs that result from the failure of drainage of lymph into the venous system, resulting in stasis and dilatation of the lymphatic vessels. They most often occur in vicinity to the left internal jugular vein, consistent with the entry of the thoracic duct into the central venous system. To a lesser extent, cystic hygromas have been described affecting most anatomic regions. Cystic hygromas are benign lesions, but they may be associated with systemic lymphangiomatosis and other congenital anomalies resulting in significant morbidity.

Cystic hygromas may be congenital or appear later in life, often after viral illnesses. In the neonate, cystic hygromas may constitute a threat to the airway as they cross the midline. Although some lesions resolve spontaneously, complete surgical excision is the treatment of choice. Considering the benign nature of these lesions, broad margins or en bloc resection of affected structures is not indicated [6, 7].

Answer
d

5. All of the following are correct *except*:
   (a) Chyle is a lymph rich in chylomicrons which travels through lacteals towards the thoracic duct.
   (b) Medium-chain triglycerides are directly absorbed into the portal venous system.
   (c) The most common cause of chylous ascites is injury to the subdiaphragmatic thoracic duct during surgery.
   (d) Chylothorax is treated by urgent radiotherapy.
   (e) The most common causes of thoracic duct injury are mediastinal dissection and radical surgery of the left neck.

Comments

Chyle is a milky fluid consisting of lymph, chylomicrons, and free fatty acids, produced by intestinal fat absorption. Chyle is captured by specialized mesenteric lymphatic vessels called lacteals and carried to the cisterna chyli. From there, it reaches the venous circulation via the thoracic duct. Chyle production and flow increase dramatically with the ingestion of food, especially those rich in long-chain fatty acids. Of note, medium-chain triglycerides are absorbed directly into the portal circulation and do not contribute to chyle formation. These facts are the basis for the nutritional recommendations for the treatment of chyle leaks as well as enteral nutritional support of patients in hepatic failure, where medium-chain triglycerides are used as a major fuel for non-protein energy.

Injury to the vessels carrying chyle may result in a chyle leak. While injury to these vessels is often well tolerated thanks to the presence of collaterals, massive injury may overwhelm this compensatory mechanism, leading to chyle accumulation in the thoracic or abdominal cavities. Rarely, fistulization to the external environment may occur. The most common etiologies of chyle leaks are surgery of the mediastinum and left neck for chylothorax and retroperitoneum as well as the diaphragm for chyloperitoneum. Trauma may also be a cause of both entities.

Initial treatment of chyle leaks is nonoperative, consisting of measures aimed at reducing chyle flow while preserving nutritional health. There is no consensus on what the best treatment strategy is, but NPO status combined with total parenteral nutrition or nonfat enteral intake combined with medium-chain triglyceride supplements has been successfully implemented. Octreotide has been used as an adjunct to reduce chyle flow further. Drainage of chyle from the thorax or the abdomen is needed to maintain respiratory function. When nonoperative measures fail, surgery to control the chyle leak is indicated in both the abdomen and thorax [8–10].

Answer

d

References

1. Skandalakis JE, Skandalakis LJ, Skandalakis PN. Anatomy of the lymphatics. Surg Oncol Clin N Am. 2007;16:1–16.
2. Olszewski WL. The lymphatic system in body homeostasis: physiological conditions. Lymphat Res Biol. 2003;1:11–21; discussion 21–4.
3. Schmid-Schonbein GW. The second valve system in lymphatics. Lymphat Res Biol. 2003;1:25–9; discussion 29–31.
4. Connell F, Brice G, Mortimer P. Phenotypic characterization of primary lymphedema. Ann N Y Acad Sci. 2008;1131:140–6.
5. Harel L, Amir J, Nussinovitch M, Straussberg R, Varsano I. Lymphedema praecox seen as isolated unilateral arm involvement: case report and review of the literature. J Pediatr. 1997;130:492–4.
6. Emery PJ, Bailey CM, Evans JN. Cystic hygroma of the head and neck. A review of 37 cases. J Laryngol Otol. 1984;98:613–9.
7. Gedikbasi A, Oztarhan K, Aslan G, et al. Multidisciplinary approach in cystic hygroma: prenatal diagnosis, outcome, and postnatal follow up. Pediatr Int. 2009;51:670–7.
8. Roche-Nagle G, Walsh S, Barry MC. Chylous ascites following abdominal aortic aneurysm repair. Vascular. 2009;17:100–2.
9. Smoke A, Delegge MH. Chyle leaks: consensus on management? Nutr Clin Pract. 2008;23:529–32.
10. Nair SK, Petko M, Hayward MP. Aetiology and management of chylothorax in adults. Eur J Cardiothorac Surg. 2007;32:362–9.

Index

V.K. Maker, E.D. Guzman-Arrieta, *Cognitive Pearls in General Surgery*,
DOI 10.1007/978-1-4939-1850-8, © Springer Science+Business Media New York 2015

B

C

T